Donated to RMU

Dr K. Bhattacharjee

Therapeutic Endoscopy and Radiology of the Gut

Therapeutic Endoscopy and Radiology of the Gut

SECOND EDITION

Edited by

John R. Bennett
MD, FRCP
Consultant Physician
Hull Royal Infirmary
Kingston Upon Hull

and

Richard H. Hunt
FRCP, FRCPEd., FRCPC
Professor of Medicine and Head
Division of Gastroenterology
McMaster University Medical Centre
Canada

CHAPMAN AND HALL MEDICAL
LONDON · NEW YORK · TOKYO · MELBOURNE · MADRAS

UK	Chapman and Hall, 11 New Fetter Lane, London EC4P 4EE
JAPAN	Chapman and Hall Japan, Thomson Publishing Japan, Hirakawacho Nemoto Building, 7F, 1-7-11 Hirakawa-cho, Chiyoda-ku, Tokyo 102
AUSTRALIA	Chapman and Hall Australia, Thomas Nelson Australia, 480 La Trobe Street, PO Box 4725, Melbourne 3000
INDIA	Chapman and Hall India, R. Sheshadri, 32 Second Main Road, CIT East, Madras 600 035

First published in 1981 as Therapeutic Endoscopy
Second edition 1990

© 1990 Chapman and Hall

Typeset in 10/12 Palatino by
Rowland Phototypesetting Ltd
Bury St Edmunds, Suffolk
Printed in Great Britain at the
University Press, Cambridge

ISBN 0 412 30090 7

British Library Cataloguing in Publication Data

Therapeutic endoscopy and radiology of the gut. – 2nd. ed.
  1. Man. Gastrointestinal tract. Diagnosis. Fibre-optic
  endoscopy.
  2. Man. Gastrointestinal tract. Radiology
  I. Bennett, John R. (John Roderick) II. Hunt, Richard H.
  616.3'307545

ISBN 0–412–30090–7

Contents

Contents   vii

Contributors

D. J. Allison Professor of Radiology, Hammersmith Hospital and Royal Post-graduate Medical School, Ducane Road, London W12 0HS, UK

M. Atkinson Special Professor of Gastroenterology, Department of Surgery, University of Nottingham, University Hospital, Queen's Medical Centre, Nottingham NG7 2UH, UK

D. Auth Adjunct Professor of Bioengineering, University of Washington, c/o Heart Technology, 2515 140th NE Bellevue WA 98005, USA

A. T. R. Axon Consultant Physician and Gastroenterologist, Gastroenterology Unit, The General Infirmary, Leeds LS1 3EX, UK

J. R. Bennett Consultant Physician, Gastrointestinal Unit, Hull Royal Infirmary, Kingston upon Hull, UK

M. K. Bilbao Professor of Radiology, University of Utah School of Medicine, Chief, Radiology Service, Salt Lake City VA Medical Center, Salt Lake City, Utah, UT 84148, USA

S. G. Bown Director, National Medical Laser Centre, Department of Surgery, 5 University Street, London WC1E 6JJ, UK

H. J. Burhenne Professor and Head, Department of Radiology, University of British Columbia, Vancouver, British Columbia, Canada

D. O. Castell Professor of Medicine, Director, Division of Gastroenterology and Hepatology, Jefferson Medical College, 1025 Walnut Street, Philadelphia, Pennsylvania 19107, USA

A. H. Chapman Consultant Radiologist, St James's University Hospital, Beckett Street, Leeds LS9 7TF, UK

D. G. Colin-Jones Consultant Physician and Gastroenterologist, Department of Gastroenterology, Queen Alexandria Hospital, Portsmouth PO6 3LY, UK

J. G. C. Cox Consultant Physician, Medicine for the Elderly and General Medicine, Ashington Hospital, West View, Ashington, Northumberland NE63 0SA, UK

S. English Research Endoscopy Nurse, Temple University, Philadelphia, Pennsylvania, USA

I. C. Forgacs Consultant Physician, Departments of Gastroenterology, Dulwich and King's College Hospitals, East Dulwich Grove, London SE22 8PT, UK

A. Ghazi Clinical Associate Professor of Surgery, Mount Sinai School of Medicine, City of New York, 10 East 21st Street, New York, NY 10010

A. P. Hemingway Kodak Professor of Radiodiagnosis, Academic Dept. Radiology, Floor P, Royal Hallamshire Hospital, Glossop Road, Sheffield S10 2JF, UK

Chia-sing Ho Professor of Radiology, University of Toronto, Deputy Radiologist-in-Chief and Head, GI and Interventional Radiology, Toronto General Hospital, Toronto, Ontario, Canada

R. H. Hunt Professor of Medicine and Head, Division of Gastroenterology, McMaster University Medical Centre, Hamilton, Ontario, Canada

D. Jensen Professor of Medicine, University of California at Los Angeles, USA

G. Jiranek Clinical Assistant Professor of Medicine, ZB–30, Pacific Medical Center, 1200–12th Ave. S., Seattle, WA 98144, USA

B. H. Laurence Gastroenterology/Liver Unit, Sir Charles Gairdner Hospital, Nedlands, Western Australia

K. D. Lindor Assistant Professor of Medicine, Mayo Medical School, Rochester, Minnesota 55905, USA

M. D. McKay Section of Gastroenterology, Department of Medicine, Medical College of Georgia, Augusta, Georgia, USA

C. J. Mitchell Consultant Physician, Scarborough Hospital, Scarborough, North Yorkshire YO12 6QL, UK

H. J. O'Connor Consultant Physician, Tullamore General Hospital, Tullamore, Co. Offaly, Eire

K. M. Pagliero Consultant in Thoracic Surgery, Postgraduate Medical School, Royal Devon and Exeter Hospital, Exeter, Devon, UK

J. E. Richter MD, Professor of Medicine, Director of Clinical Research, Gastroenterology Division, University of Alabama at Birmingham, UAB Station, Birmingham, AL 35294, USA

J. D. R. Rose Consultant Physician, Ballochmyle Hospital, Mauchline, Ayrshire KA5 6LQ

C. G. Rowland Consultant and Senior Lecturer in Oncology and Radiation Therapy, Postgraduate Medical School, Royal Devon and Exeter Hospital, Exeter, Devon EX1 2ED, UK

L. Safrany Professor of Medicine, University of Muenster, Chief, Department of Gastroenterology, Reinhard-Neiter-Krankenhaus, FR Germany

K. F. R. Schiller Consultant Physician, Department of Gastroenterology, St Peter's Hospital, Chertsey, Surrey, UK

F. Silverstein Professor of Medicine, University of Washington, Seattle, Washington, USA

M. V. Sivak MD, Chairman, Department of Gastroenterology, The Cleveland Clinic Foundation, Cleveland, Ohio

P. M. Smith Consultant Physician, Llandough Hospital, Penarth, Cardiff CF6 1XX, UK

N. Soehendra MD, Professor of Surgery, Head of Department of Endoscopic Surgery, University Hospital of Hamburg – Eppendorf Martinistr. 52, 2000 Hamburg, 20, West Germany

S. Somers Associate Professor, Department of Radiology, McMaster University, Hamilton, Ontario, Canada

M. Stenzel Assistant Professor of Medicine, University of South Florida, College of Medicine, Chief, Gastroenterology Section, Bay Pines VA Medical Center, Bay Pines, Florida 33504, USA

G. Stevenson Professor and Chairman, Department of Radiology, McMaster University, Hamilton, Ontario, Canada

P. Swain Senior Lecturer and Consultant Gastroenterologist, Department of Gastroenterology, The London Hospital, Whitechapel, London E1 1BB, UK

F. J. Tedesco Section of Gastroenterology, Department of Medicine, Medical College of Georgia, Augusta, Georgia, USA

T. G. Walker Department of Radiology, St Johns Hospital, Lowell, Massachusetts, MA 01852, USA

A. C. Waltman Associate Professor of Radiology, Harvard Medical School, Department of Radiology, Massachusetts General Hospital, Boston MA 02114, USA

J. D. Waye Clinical Professor of Medicine and Chief, 650 Park Avenue, New York, NY 10021, USA

Acknowledgement

We thank KeyMed for both their interest and sponsorship of the colour plate section of this book.

Preface to the second edition

Therapeutic endoscopy and radiology has made enormous advances since the first edition of this book in 1981 and most of the procedures covered in the first volume have become standard practice in the endoscopy unit of almost every general hospital. Moreover these procedures have been further developed and refined leading to greater technical success and much safer and more cost-beneficial interventions. Critical evaluation of the indications and results have been published from an increasing number of better-controlled trials strengthening our confidence in both the practicability and the results of these procedures. Such studies have indicated that the simple approach may be just as successful and show a higher cost benefit than more expensive techniques. For example simple injection therapy for bleeding ulcers, or the use of relatively inexpensive intervention with the heater probe or bicap are as effective in controlling bleeding and reducing episodes of rebleeding as the neodynium YAG laser.

The benefits of interventional endoscopy or radiology are of special benefit in the older population who often can now avoid major surgery and maintain an excellent quality of life as the result of a relatively simple therapeutic or palliative procedure performed as an ambulatory patient.

In this volume we have sought to bring together the experience and opinions of a widely diverse group of therapeutic endoscopists and international radiologists from around the world. Their combined expertise provides us with succinct and topical advice on when and how to implement interventional endoscopic and radiological techniques. Such a volume cannot be comprehensive and in such a rapidly advancing field we have asked our contributors to concentrate on those techniques and applications which are established rather than experimental. Thus they have provided for us an overview of interventional procedures which would have been barely dreamt possible two decades ago, but have now become established practice.

John R. Bennett
Richard H. Hunt

Preface to the first edition

Operative surgery was unfairly castigated by Lord Cohen of Birkenhead as 'that accessory branch of therapeutics', and even its most ardent exponent would hardly deny that it is a means to an end; the desired end being usually the improvement or removal of a pathological condition. If that end can be achieved other than by open operation, then it is right that such means should be explored. This book records and discusses the results of two recent avenues of such exploration.

Access to the alimentary tract is now easily possible both by illuminated, flexible, fibreoptic endoscopes (inserted orally or *per anum*), and by needles and catheters under radiological control. These techniques began as purely diagnostic manoeuvres, and the therapeutic potential of fibreoptic endoscopy, in particular, was called into question (notably in a notorious letter in which a surgeon described the fibreoptic endoscope as an 'expensive piece of illuminated spaghetti'). The ingenuity and imagination of endoscopists and radiologists, supported by the constructional skills of manufacturing companies, have now made many therapeutic procedures possible without the need for surgical operation. These exploits at first seemed like legerdemain, but their practical value and feasibility are now well established.

With an ageing population we increasingly meet patients ill-fitted to withstand the stresses imposed even by modern anaesthesia and surgery; moreover, costs of medical care continue to rise. Procedures carried out by endoscopy or under radiological control have lower morbidity and mortality, and involve a shorter hospital stay, two great advantages over the operative techniques they displace. It seems certain that their application will increase.

In this book, experts in the various techniques describe them so that other endoscopists and radiologists may safely undertake them; they also record the outcome of these procedures so that they may be judged against the alternatives by referring doctors. We have thus combined an instruction manual with a scientific exposition of results, in the belief that anyone with patients' welfare at heart will more readily place at their disposal the best that can be provided in 1981. Although many of the techniques are in regular and common use they are still being developed, while others (particularly approaches to gastro-intestinal haemorrhage) are insufficiently assessed to justify wholesale adoption; these stand as pointers to the future. Many will have been refined even in the short time this book has been in preparation, and there are techniques not mentioned in the book which have been at least the subject of experimental work – endoscopic vagotomy, for example (T. V. Taylor, personal communication). Above all we show how medicine has again taken modern technology and harnessed it for patients' welfare.

John R. Bennett

CHAPTER ONE

Sterilization and preparation of endoscopes and their accessories

H. J. O'Connor
and
A. T. R. Axon

Contaminated endoscopic equipment may act as a vehicle for transmission of infection, with a number of papers reporting serious complications, occasionally with fatal consequences. The majority of endoscopy-related infections are caused by Gram-negative bacilli such as *Pseudomonas aeruginosa* (Greene *et al.*, 1974; Allen *et al.*, 1987) and salmonellae (Dean, 1977) which thrive in the moist, narrow channels and valves of the endoscope. It is inevitable that unrecognized hepatitis B-positive patients will, from time to time, undergo endoscopic procedures and at least one case of viral hepatitis B has been acquired at endoscopy (Birnie *et al.*, 1983). However, it is reassuring that none of 230 patients examined inadvertently with endoscopes used previously on HBsAg-positive patients developed hepatitis, suggesting that the risk of transmission of the virus at endoscopy is small (O'Connor and Axon, 1983).

More recently, concern about the increasing incidence and serious consequences of infection with human immunodeficiency virus (HIV) has raised the question of possible transmission of HIV by endoscopy. It must be assumed that, as with hepatitis B, unrecognized HIV carriers will undergo gastrointestinal endoscopy but endoscopy-related transmission of HIV has not yet been reported. The report of a Working Party of the British Society of Gastroenterology has recommended that all patients should be considered 'at risk' and that adequate antibacterial and antiviral disinfection is needed before and after each endoscopic procedure (Working Party Report, 1988).

Cleaning and disinfection of endoscopic equipment is a specialized procedure and properly trained staff are required to look after the equipment and ensure that each endoscopy is performed using a clean and disinfected endoscope and ancillary equipment. All endoscopic equipment should be thoroughly disinfected before the endoscopy list begins, between each patient examined and at the end of the list. During therapeutic procedures the mucosal integrity is likely to be breached, and material may be injected into normally sterile duct systems or into the circulation. The need for scrupulous disinfection in these circumstances is obvious. Adequate personnel, endoscopes and accessories should be available to allow enough time between cases for cleaning and disinfection procedures and when emergency endoscopy is performed out-of-hours fully trained assistants should be available to assist with the endoscopic examination and the disinfection of the equipment used.

1.1 PRECLEANING

Thorough manual physical cleaning is an essential prerequisite of effective instrument disinfection (Ayliffe, Babb and Bradley, 1986). After routine use endoscopes retain blood, secretions and organic material which trap contaminating microorganisms, and inactivate and resist penetration by germicidal molecules. Hence, the number of microorganisms destroyed chemically depends to a large extent on the thoroughness of the precleaning procedure before immersion in disinfectant (Spaulding, Lundy and Turner, 1977).

Most endoscopes marketed today are fully immersible, can be totally cleaned and disinfected, and have been designed so that their channels can be irrigated by positive pressure. After removal from the patient, the endoscopes should be taken straight to a sink containing fresh detergent solution. Before cleaning, the endoscope should be leak tested to avoid damage from immersion. With the light guide connector attached to the light source the flow of air and water is checked and the insertion tube, and where possible the handle of the endoscope, washed thoroughly. The biopsy valve is removed, dismantled and cleaned, and a cleaning brush repeatedly passed down the biopsy channel and out of the tip of the instrument until clean. The distal hood is removed, the tip of the instrument vigorously brushed with a soft tooth brush,

and the valve and biopsy housings cleaned with cotton buds. Detergent is injected through each channel; an all-channel irrigator is supplied with most endoscopes, but a separate syringe may be needed to clean the bridge elevator channel. The endoscope and channels are rinsed with clean water. Brushes and other cleaning equipment used must themselves be disinfected before each use.

Non-immersible and immersible endoscopes differ in design from one another and cleaning techniques may need to be modified according to the manufacturers' instructions.

1.2 DISINFECTION

A suitable disinfectant (Table 1.1) is injected into each channel and the shaft of the instrument immersed for the recommended period of time. All channels and the instrument itself are then rinsed in clean water and fresh suction and biopsy valves and distal hood fitted. Any part of the shaft of the instrument or handle which has not been totally immersed in disinfectant should be swabbed with 70% isopropyl alcohol.

1.2.1 CHOICE OF DISINFECTANT

The ideal fibrescope disinfectant is a rapid-acting, high-level liquid germicide which is

Table 1.1 Disinfectants recommended for fibrescopes and accessories

Disinfectant	Bacteria	TB	Viruses	Fungi	Disadvantages
	Activity against				
Glutaraldehyde, 2% alkaline	*†	*	*	*⎫	Staff sensitivity
Succine dialdehyde, 10%	*†	*	*	*⎬	reactions
Dettox, 8%	*†	n.k.	n.k.	*⎭	Virucidal capacity unknown
Povidone-iodine	*	*	*	*	Stains materials Inactivated by organic soil or hard water

*, active against.   †, in 2 minutes.   n.k., not known.

non-damaging to endoscope components, non-toxic for endoscopy staff, of low surface tension (to facilitate penetration and rinsing) and does not coagulate blood or protein. At present no disinfectant solution fulfils all these requirements, and aqueous 2% alkaline glutaraldehyde (Cidex, Totacide, Asep) or 10% succine dialdehyde (Gigasept) are the best available disinfectants. Studies with vegetative bacteria (O'Connor et al., 1982, 1983) have shown that 2 minutes' contact with these agents decontaminates fibrescopes adequately between procedures, although longer immersion times (at least 20 minutes) may be used both before and after lists to reduce the effect of pseudomonas overgrowth during storage. Based on expert interpretation of current data on infectivity and disinfection, a minimum immersion time of 4 minutes has recently been recommended (Working Party Report, 1988). Aldehyde solutions are non-flammable, non-corrosive and of low surface tension. Spire et al. (1984) have shown HIV to be highly sensitive to the virucidal action of glutaraldehyde in vitro, concentrations as low as 0.0125% effectively inactivating the virus in 5 minutes. Succine dialdehyde (5%) has been shown to inactivate HIV within 5 minutes (Working Party Report, 1988). Glutaraldehyde and succine dialdehyde are rapidly hepato-virucidal (Thraenhart et al., 1978; Bond et al., 1983; Kobayashi, Tsuzuki and Koshimizu, 1984).

An important disadvantage of aldehyde disinfectants is their propensity to cause sensitivity problems among endoscopy staff affecting the skin, eyes and respiratory tract (Corrado, Osman and Davies, 1986). In 1981, over one-third of endoscopy units in the UK reported that one or more members of staff were sensitive to glutaraldehyde (Axon et al., 1981). Ironically, the problem of aldehyde toxicity may have increased in the past few years as more endoscopy units have adopted recommended guidelines for disinfection procedures (Axon and Cotton, 1983). Direct and indirect exposure to aldehydes can be mini-mized by using disposable gloves and a 'closed-system' disinfecting apparatus in a well-ventilated area (O'Connor et al., 1982). Other aldehyde preparations such as Sporicidin (0.125% glutaraldehyde and 0.44% phenol when diluted for use) are promoted as being less toxic but confirmatory data are lacking. Furthermore, experiments with Sporicidin diluted to 1:16 have shown it to be less effective than 2% glutaraldehyde or succine dialdehyde in reducing bacterial counts from brush samples of the suction/biopsy channel (Ayliffe et al., 1986). Another disadvantage of aldehydes is progressive reduction of their germicidal capacity after activation due to chemical loss of active aldehyde groups. In practice, disinfectants also become diluted with water during disinfection procedures and so may need replacement sooner than the times recommended by their manufacturers.

Some endoscopy units have sought alternatives to aldehyde-based disinfectants rather than lose experienced staff. Dettox, an improved quaternary ammonium compound, is non-irritant, does not damage fibrescope components, and is effective against bacterial pathogens (O'Connor et al., 1983). However, the virucidal capacity of this compound is uncertain and preliminary reports suggest that HIV may be relatively resistant to Dettox (Working Party Report, 1988). The iodophor solution, povidine-iodine, is an effective disinfectant for endoscopic equipment but suffers the disadvantages of staining of materials (Spaulding, 1978) and rapid inactivation by organic soil and hard water. Buffered hypochlorite solutions (at concentrations of approximately 2000 p.p.m. available chlorine) are rapidly germicidal and hepatovirucidal but damage the rubber (bending section) and metal components of fibrescopes and the polyurethane coating of the insertion tube (Babb et al., 1981). Alcohol is an effective antiviral disinfectant (Bond et al., 1983; Resnick et al., 1986) but is limited in value by its flammability and capacity to damage epoxy lens cement, flexible plastic, and rubber seals on prolonged immersion. However, three major instrument manufacturers (Olympus, Fujinon and Pentax) have recently approved the use of 70% ethyl alcohol for repeated brief (4–5 minutes) soaks of the endoscope shaft and tip, if followed by thorough rinsing and drying; the control head of the endoscope may be wiped but not immersed in 70% alcohol. Chlorhexidine, chlorhexidine-cetrimide mixtures and hexachlorophene do not reliably disinfect fibrescopes but are suitable as precleaning agents.

If, as a result of staff sensitivity, aldehyde disinfectants cannot be used, total immersion in 8% Dettox for 2 minutes followed by 70% ethyl alcohol for 4 minutes as described above has been recommended as an effective second-line disinfection procedure (Working Party Report, 1988).

1.2.2 DISINFECTION MACHINES

An effective disinfection machine can add to the efficiency, safety and speed of disinfection procedures (Babb, Bradley and Ayliffe, 1984), but does not remove the need for manual cleaning of the endoscope including brushing the suction channel and instrument tip. Unfortunately, the development of suitable machines has not kept pace with that of other endoscopic equipment and commercially produced prototypes have only recently become available. Before purchase, the user should ensure that the particular model is convenient to operate, provides effective all-channel disinfection, does not damage fibrescopes, is of closed-system design and adaptable to the range of fibrescopes used within the unit. Many of the machines commercially available do not satisfy all these requirements, are relatively expensive, and some endoscopists have designed and constructed their own (O'Connor et al., 1982; Meuwissen et al., 1983). The recent report by Babb et al. (1984) provides a detailed account of the merits and defects of various disinfection systems.

1.3 RINSING, DRYING AND STORAGE

After disinfection, endoscopic equipment must be rinsed free of germicide and dried. A water rinse for 30 seconds effectively removes glutaraldehyde from disinfected equipment (Stonehill, Krop and Borick, 1963).

It is important to note that freestanding water tanks, tubes and bottles in disinfection machines are themselves readily colonized by *Pseudomonas* spp. (Axon *et al.*, 1974), leading to possible recontamination of fibrescopes during the rinse cycle. Hence, water tanks and bottles should be disinfected, stored dry and inverted overnight. Regular bacteriological monitoring is necessary, and clean water should be used each day.

After rinsing, the channels of the endoscope should be air dried, especially before storage. Endoscopes are best stored by hanging them vertically in air without valves in place as this helps to prevent contamination and proliferation of organisms in the instruments between sessions (Noy *et al.*, 1980).

1.4 CLEANING AND DISINFECTION OF ENDOSCOPIC ACCESSORIES

Accessories used during endoscopic procedures, and particularly those which are designed to breach the gastrointestinal mucosa, provide a potential source of transmission of infection.

All non-disposable accessories should be washed in detergent and rinsed prior to disinfection. Where possible, equipment should be dismantled as far as possible, and items such as biopsy forceps (which have a spiral structure and are difficult to clean) put through an ultrasonic cleaner (Sierra and Boucher, 1971). Many accessories can be autoclaved, but if this is not possible low-temperature steam and formaldehyde or ethylene oxide gas sterilization may be used, or a liquid disinfectant may be necessary. Special cleaning may be required for certain accessories and details are given below.

1.4.1 CYTOLOGY BRUSHES

After use, the spring-coiled brush should be separated from its sheath, scrubbed gently in soapy water using a toothbrush and then immersed in disinfectant. Cleaning solution followed by disinfectant is aspirated through the outer sheath. Both components are then rinsed, dried and reassembled.

1.4.2 BIOPSY AND GRASPING FORCEPS, STITCH CUTTERS

Adherent blood and mucus can be easily removed from spring-coiled forceps by short immersion in hydrogen peroxide solution. Some forceps are autoclavable (see manufacturers' instructions).

1.4.3 OESOPHAGEAL ACCESSORIES

Guide wires and introducers used for oesophageal dilatation and intubation have flexible spring-coiled ends which should be scrubbed gently in soapy water followed by brief immersion in hydrogen peroxide solution if there is still adherent blood. Cleaning solution followed by disinfectant should be aspirated through the central canal of both the introducer and dilators (Celestin, Rigiflex, etc.) and left in contact for 20 minutes.

1.4.4 PAPILLOTOMES, DORMIA BASKETS AND DILATING BALLOONS

Disinfectant solution can be injected through the length of these accessories using the contrast injection port. Drying is achieved by then blowing air down the injection port. Papillotomes, baskets and snares should be stored dry, otherwise they can rust.

1.4.5 ENDOSCOPIC INJECTION NEEDLES

Careful sterilization is essential (Elewant *et al.*, 1988). These should be carefully dismantled (taking care to avoid 'needle-stick' injury).

After washing, disinfectant is injected into the lumen of the needle and its sheath, and they are left immersed for 20 minutes. They can then be washed and dried.

ACKNOWLEDGEMENT

We are indebted to Sister Lilian Anderson, Endoscopy Unit, Selly Oak Hospital for helpful comments during the preparation of this report.

REFERENCES

Allen, J. I., O'Connor-Allen, M., Olson, M. M., Gerding, D. N. and Shanholtzer, C. J. (1987) *Pseudomonas* infection of the biliary system resulting from use of a contaminated endoscope. *Gastroenterology*, **92**, 759–63.
Axon, A. T. R., Phillips, I., Cotton, P. B. and Avery, S. A. (1974) Disinfection of gastrointestinal fibre-endoscopes. *Lancet*, **i**, 656–8.
Axon, A. T. R. and Cotton, P. B. (1983) Endoscopy and infection. *Gut*, **24**, 1064–6.
Axon, A. T. R., Banks, J., Cockel, R., Deverill, C. E. A. and Neumann, C. (1981) Disinfection in upper digestive endoscopy in Britain. *Lancet*, **i**, 1093–4.
Ayliffe, G. A. J., Babb, J. R. and Bradley, C. R. (1986) Disinfection of endoscopes. *J. Hosp. Infect.*, **7**, 295–309.
Babb, J. R., Bradley, C. R., Deverill, C. E. A., Ayliffe, G. A. J. and Melikian, V. (1981) Recent advances in the cleaning and disinfection of fibrescopes. *J. Hosp. Infect.*, **2**, 329–40.
Babb, J. R., Bradley, C. R. and Ayliffe, G. A. J. (1984) Comparison of automated systems for the cleaning and disinfection of flexible fibreoptic endoscopes. *J. Hosp. Infect.*, **5**, 213–26.
Birnie, G. G., Quigley, E. M. M., Clements, G. B., Follet, E. A. C. and Watkinson, G. (1983) Endoscopic transmission of hepatitis B virus. *Gut*, **24**, 171–4.
Bond, W. W., Favero, M. S., Petersen, N. J. and Ebert, J. W. (1983) Inactivation of hepatitis B virus by intermediate to high level disinfectant chemicals. *J. Clin. Microbiol.*, **18**, 535–8.
Corrado O. J., Osman, J. and Davies, R. J. (1986) Asthma and rhinitis after exposure to glutaraldehyde in endoscopy units. *Human. Toxicol.*, **5**, 325–7.
Dean, A. G. (1977) Transmission of *Salmonella typhi* by fibreoptic endoscopy. *Lancet*, **ii**, 134.

Elewaut, A., De Man, M., De Vos, M. and Barbier, F. (1988) Endoscopic sclerotherapy: the value of balloon tamponade and the importance of disinfection. *Endoscopy*, **20**, 48–51.

Greene, W. H., Moody, M., Hartley, R., Effman, E. and Aisner, J. (1974) Esophagoscopy as a source of *Pseudomonas aeruginosa* sepsis in patients with acute leukaemia: the need for sterilisation of endoscopes. *Gastroenterology*, **67**, 912–8.

Kobayashi, H., Tsuzuki, M. and Koshimizu, K. (1984) Susceptibility of hepatitis B virus to disinfectants or heat. *J. Clin. Microbiol.*, **20**, 214–6.

Meuwissen, S. G. M., MacLaren, D. M., Rijsberman, W. and Boshuizen, K. (1983) A simple method for cleaning flexible fibreoptic endoscopes by 'all-channel' perfusion. *J. Hosp. Infect.*, **4**, 81–6.

Noy, M. F., Harrison, L., Holmes, G. K. T. and Cockel, R. (1980) The significance of bacterial contamination of fibreoptic endoscopes. *J. Hosp. Infect.*, **1**, 53–61.

O'Connor, H. J. and Axon, A. T. R. (1983) Gastrointestinal endoscopy: infection and disinfection. *Gut*, **24**, 1067–77.

O'Connor, H. J., Rothwell, J., Maxwell, S., Lincoln, C. and Axon, A. T. R. (1982) A new disinfecting apparatus for gastrointestinal fibre-endoscopes. *Gut*, **23**, 706–9.

O'Connor, H. J., Steele, C. S., Price, J., Lincoln, C. and Axon, A. T. R. (1983) Disinfection of gastrointestinal fibrescopes – evaluation of the disinfectants Dettox and Gigasept. *Endoscopy*, **15**, 350–2.

Resnick, L., Veren, K., Salahuddin, S. Z., Tondreau, S. and Markham, P. D. (1986) Stability and inactivation of HTLVIII/LAV under clinical and laboratory environments. *J.A.M.A.*, **255**, 1887–91.

Sierra, G. and Boucher, R. M. G. (1971) Ultrasonic synergistic effects in liquid-phase chemical sterilization. *Appl. Microbiol.*, **22**, 160–4.

Spaulding, E. H. (1978) Fibreoptic endoscopes: disinfection and sterilization. Microbiological aspects of the dilemma. *Hosp. Infect. Control*, **5**, 35–9.

Spaulding, E. H., Cundy, K. R. and Turner, F. J. (1977) Chemical disinfection of medical and surgical materials. In *Disinfection, Sterilization and Preservation*, 2nd edn (ed. S. S. Block), Lea and Febiger, Philadelphia, pp. 654–84.

Spire, B., Barre-Sinoussi, F., Montagnier, L. and Chermann, J. C. (1984) Inactivation of lymphadenopathy associated virus by chemical disinfectants. *Lancet*, **ii**, 899–901.

Stonehill, A. A., Krop, S. and Borick, P. M. (1963) Buffered glutaraldehyde: a new chemical sterilizing solution. *Am. J. Hosp. Pharm.*, **20**, 458–65.

Thraenhart, O., Kuwert, E. K., Dermietzel, R., Scheiermann, N. and Wendt, F. (1978) Influence of different disinfection conditions on the structure of the hepatitis B virus (Dane particle) as evaluated in the Morphological Alteration and Disintegration Test (MADT). *Zentralbl. Bakteriol. Hyg. 1 Abt. Orig.*, **A242**, 299–314.

Working Party Report (1988) Cleaning and disinfection of equipment for gastrointestinal flexible endoscopy: interim recommendations of a Working Party of the British Society of Gastroenterology. *Gut*, **29**, 1134–51.

Hazards of endoscopy

J. R. Bennett

Diagnostic fibreoptic gastrointestinal endoscopy is a safe procedure. The addition of instrumentation in therapeutic procedures inevitably increases the risk of an accident or complication, and each type of procedure has its own hazards which are dealt with in the appropriate chapter.

Two hazards, common to all procedures, deserve particular mention. They are bacterial endocarditis and perforation.

2.1 BACTERIAL ENDOCARDITIS

Many studies have been made of bacteraemia during endoscopic procedures, and 41 such reports have been reviewed recently (Shorvon, Eykyn and Cotton, 1983; Botoman and Surawicz, 1986). Combined results of the incidence of bacteraemia are shown in Table 2.1. Despite the high incidence of bacteraemia with procedures like oesophageal dilatation, endocarditis is a rare complication, and only ten cases are found in the literature (Botoman and Surawicz, 1986). Although existing heart disease is believed to be a risk factor for developing endocarditis, half the patients who develop endocarditis have no previous cardiac lesion (Weinstein, 1972) and others have lesions which may not be detected by 'routine' clinical examination.

Table 2.1 Bacteraemia during endoscopic procedure

Procedure	Patients (no.)	Incidence of bacteraemia (%)
Diagnostic OGD	692	4.1
ERCP		
All patients	356	5.6
Pancreatic or biliary obstruction	102	11.0
Colonoscopy	528	2.2
Sigmoidoscopy	400	5.9
Rigid		
Fibreoptic		
Oesophageal dilatation	59	45
Variceal sclerotherapy	61	31
Laser disobliteration of oesophagogastric neoplasms	35	40
	(58 procedures)	(34)
Laser treatment of A-V malformations	5	0
	(8 procedures)	0

Combined results of 41 studies from Botoman and Surawicz (1986), Shorvon, Eykyn and Cotton (1983), Wolf, Fleischer and Sivak (1985) and Kohler and Riemann (1987).

With such a low incidence of endocarditis after endoscopic procedures, and given the difficulty of predicting patients at particular risk, a case can be made for making no attempt at prophylaxis. However, if prophylaxis can be achieved relatively simply it seems reasonable and prudent to use it in patients at known risk who are undergoing procedures which are particularly likely to cause bacteraemia, especially with faecal organisms. No national or international consensus exists, and individual endoscopists need to make their own decision.

2.1.1 PATIENTS AT RISK

(a) Prosthetic valves

These are susceptible to infection, and the morbidity and mortality of prosthetic valve endocarditis is high.

(b) Patients who have previously had endocarditis

(c) Known valvular heart disease

2.1.2 Procedures requiring prophylaxis

(a) Oesophageal dilatation
(b) Oesophageal variceal sclerotherapy
(c) Laser disobliteration of gastric or rectal neoplasma
(d) Insertion of prosthetic oesophagogastric tubes
(e) Colonic polypectomy
(f) ERCP with sphincterotomy
(g) Sigmoidoscopy with biopsy

2.1.3. RECOMMENDED REGIMEN (British Society for Antimicrobial Chemotherapy, 1982)

(a) If not allergic to penicillins

Amoxycillin	1 g	i.m. before the procedure
Gentamicin	120 mg	
and		
Amoxycillin	0.5 g	6 hours later

(b) If allergic to penicillins

Vancomycin	1 g	by slow i.v. infusion in 20–30 min
and		
Gentamicin	120 mg	i.v. before the procedure

2.2 PERFORATION

Endoscopic examination of the gastrointestinal tract carries a measurable risk of perforation, particularly if therapeutic procedures are performed. The incidence of such accidents is low, but it is essential that endoscopists minimize the risk and be aware of the appropriate management should perforation occur, since this will vary depending upon the anatomical location, severity, age of patient, etc.

2.2.1 OESOPHAGEAL PERFORATION

(a) Incidence

Surveys of endoscopists using fibreoptic instruments in Britain in 1972 (Schiller, Cotton and Salmon, 1972) and in the USA in 1974 (Mandelstam et al., 1974) suggested an overall incidence of 'complications' of about 3 per 1000 examinations.

Better instrumentation and training have improved performance and a 1981 survey of 38 000 examinations by members of the British Society of Gastroenterology (BSG) showed an overall perforation rate during fibreoptic oesophagogastroduodenoscopy of 0.018% (Dawson and Cockel, 1981). For dilatation of strictures the risk rose to 0.9%.

(b) Prevention

Accidents are least likely when the procedure is done by an experienced operator using an up-to-date fibreoptic endoscope in a well-equipped unit, but senior staff are not immune to accidents (Skinner, Little and De Meester, 1980).

(c) Detection

An instrumental perforation is regrettable, and prompt action is usually effective but any delay in detection increases the likelihood of a disaster (Skinner, Little and de Meester, 1980; Goldstein and Thompson, 1982; Bladergroen, Lowe and Postlethwait, 1986). No complaint of chest or abdominal discomfort, dyspnoea or pyrexia should be dismissed lightly, and after therapeutic procedures patients should be specifically questioned about such symptoms and also kept under observation without anything by mouth for several hours even if this might entail an overnight stay.

Even the remote possibility of perforation should lead the endoscopist to obtain chest radiographs (and films of the neck if indicated). However, these may be normal even if perforation has occurred (Hass et al., 1986) and continuing suspicion should lead to a water-soluble radio-opaque swallow.

In high-risk cases, particularly with the insertion of prosthetic tubes, the risks of inadvertent perforation may be minimized by prophylactic antibiotic administration (Hine and Atkinson, 1986), and routine radiological examination with radio-opaque contrast media before feeding is begun after the procedure.

(d) Treatment

Once a perforation is detected the endoscopist must choose surgical or conservative treatment. No consensus exists, and no trial has been undertaken to assist with the choice. Publications offer opinions, usually weighted towards the discipline of the authors. In young and otherwise fit patients surgical exploration may seem desirable and give good results, but this group is in best condition for conservative management too. The old and frail withstand surgery less well, but are in poor condition to undergo the rigours of prolonged conservative treatment.

There is an increasing trend among endoscopists towards conservative management (Mengoli and Klassen, 1965; Rogers, 1981; Fiasse et al., 1981; Goldstein and Thompson, 1982, Wesdorp et al., 1984; Hine and Atkinson, 1986; Mee, 1986; Van der Zee, Sloof and Kingma, 1986), and satisfactory results can be obtained by appropriate antibiotic treatment combined with nutritional support–parenteral or enteral.

As with many other difficult and dangerous gastroenterological problems, a careful assessment of each patient and an agreed management policy by experienced clinicians, both medical and surgical, is likely to give better results than rigid guidelines (Van der Zee, Sloof and Kingma, 1986). In general terms high perforations (in the neck) and perforations lower in the oesophagus which seem small by radiological examination may usually be treated conservatively. Free perforations within the chest with communication to a pleural cavity will be best treated by surgery.

If conservative management is chosen, the important measures are:

1. Nothing to be taken by mouth.
2. Parenteral antibiotics, e.g. amoxycillin and gentamicin.
3. Intravenous fluids.

Radiological studies every 3–4 days will show the progress of the leak. If there is still extravasation after a week parenteral feeding should be given. If the leak appears to have sealed the tentative introduction of liquid orally should be attempted under careful observation.

2.2.2 COLONIC PERFORATION

(a) Incidence

Perforation complicates diagnostic colonoscopy at a reported rate of 0.14–0.26%, and polypectomy in 0.29–0.42% (Rogers, 1981).

(b) Presentation

Abdominal pain, and distension occur soon after perforation; after polypectomy there may be a delay for days or weeks. Confirmation of perforation is by radiological demonstration of a pneumoperitoneum.

(c) Management

Surgical exploration, débridement, and closure of the perforation are usually advised; if there is colonic disease, such as diverticular disease or carcinoma, resection may be necessary.

Conservative non-operative management is not often recommended but has been used with success (Taylor, Weakley and Sullivan, 1978). If the patient has few symptoms or signs, and the colon has been well prepared, or if there are other medical contraindications to exploration, then conservative management with antibiotics can be considered.

REFERENCES

Bladergroen, M. R., Lowe, J. E. and Postlethwait, R. W. Diagnosis and recommended management of esophageal perforation and rupture. *Am. Thorac. Surg.*, **42**, 235–9.

Botoman, V. A. and Surawicz, C. M. (1986) Bacteraemia with gastrointestinal endoscopic procedures. *Gastrointest. Endosc.*, **32**, 342–6.

British Society for Antimicrobiol Chemotherapy (1982) The antibiotic prophylaxis of infective endocarditis. *Lancet*, **ii**, 1323–6.

Fiasse, R., Goncette, L., Pringot, J. *et al.* (1981) Traitement des perforations oesophagiennes instrumentales. *Acta Gastroenterol. Belg.*, **44**, 430–47.

Goldstein, L. A. and Thompson, W. R. (1982) Esophageal perforations: a 15 year experience. *Amer. J. Surg.*, **143**, 495–503.

Hass, S. Y., McElvein, R. B., Aldret, J. S. and Tisker, J. M. (1986) Perforation of the oesophagus: correlation of site and cause with plain film findings. *Am. J. Roentgenol.*, **145**, 537–40.

Hine, K. and Atkinson, M. The diagnosis and management of perforations of esophagus and pharynx sustained during intubation of neoplastic esophageal strictures. *Dig. Dis. Sci.*, 1986, **31**, 571–3.

Kohler, B. and Riemann, J. F. (1987) Incidence of bacteraemia after endoscopic laser treatment of stenosing processes in the upper gastrointestinal tract. *Am. J. Gastroenterol.*, **82**, 1026–8.

Mandelstam, P., Sugawa, C., Silvis, S. E. *et al.* (1976) Complications associated with esophagogastroduodenoscopy and with esophageal dilation. *Gastrointest. Endosc.*, **23**, 16–9.

Mee, A. S. (1986) Traumatic oesophageal perforation (letter). *Hosp. Update*, 601.

Mengoli, L. R. and Klassen, K. P. (1965) Conservative management of esophageal perforation. *Arch. Surg.*, **91**, 238–40.

Rogers, B. H. G. (1981) in *Colonoscopy* (eds R. H. Hunt and J. D. Waye), Chapman and Hall, London.

Schiller, K. F. R., Cotton, P. B. and Salmon, P. R. (1972) The hazards of digestive fibre-endoscopy: a survey of British experience. *Gut*, **13**, 1027.

Shorvon, P. J., Eykyn, S. J. and Cotton, P. B. (1983) Gastrointestinal instrumentation, bacteraemia and endocarditis. *Gut*, **24**, 1078–90.

Skinner, D. B., Little, A. G. and de Meester, T. R. (1980) Management of esophageal perforation. *Am. J. Surg.*, **139**, 760–5.

Taylor, R., Weakley, F. L. and Sullivan, B. H. (1978) Non-operative management of colonoscopic perforation with pneumoperitoneum. *Gastrointest. Endosc.*, **24**, 124–5.

Van der Zee, D. C., Sloof, M. J. H. and Kingma, L. M. (1986) Management of oesophageal perforations: a tailored approach. *Neth. J. Surg.*, **38**, 31–5.

Weinstein, L. (1972) Infective endocarditis: past, present and future. *J. R. Coll. Physicians Lond.* **6**, 161–74.

Wesdorp, I. C. E., Bartelsman, J. F. W. M., Huibregtse, K. *et al.* (1984) Treatment of instrumental oesophageal perforation. *Gut*, **25**, 348–404.

Wolf, D., Fleischer, D. and Sivak, M. V. (1985) Incidence of bacteraemia with elective upper gastrointestinal endoscopic laser therapy. *Gastrointest. Endosc.*, **31**, 247–50.

CHAPTER THREE

Benign oesophageal strictures

J. G. C. Cox
and
J. R. Bennett

3.1 AETIOLOGY

Although any severe oesophagitis may lead to stricturing (Table 3.1), the vast majority of oesophageal strictures in the western world are due to reflux oesophagitis. Caustic ingestion is commoner outside Britain. Iatrogenic oesophagitis may be due to drugs, nasogastric intubation, sclerotherapy and surgery. Rare causes of oesophageal stricture include Crohn's disease (Dyer, Cook and Harper, 1969; Geboes *et al.*, 1986), tuberculosis (Dow, 1981), candidiasis (Ginsburg *et al.*, 1978), rheumatoid arthritis (John, Stirling and Matthews, 1978) and ankylosing spondylitis (Hay, 1978). The causes of stricture in 254 consecutive patients treated at Hull, UK, are listed in Table 3.2.

3.2 DIAGNOSIS

3.2.1 HISTORY

Knowledge of the natural history of reflux strictures is important to differentiate them from other strictures in which management may be different.

A patient with a reflux stricture may have a long history of reflux symptoms, including posture-related chest pain, acid reflux, heartburn, intermittent vomiting, and pain on swallowing and drinking hot liquids. If oesophagitis is severe but no stricture is

Table 3.1 Aetiological classification of benign oesophageal strictures

Reflux	including Barrett's, recumbency, Nasogastric tube, vomiting (hyperemesis gravidarum), cytotoxic therapy
Drugs	Emepronium bromide
	Tetracycline
	Potassium chloride
	Quinidine
	NSAID
	Iron salts
	Steradent tabs
	Clinitest tabs
	Corrosives
Postoperative	Overtight Nissen, Angelchik
	Achlalasia dilatation or surgery
	Post-gastrectomy
	Post-oesophagectomy
	Post-sclerotherapy
Radiation	Conventional
	Endocavitary
Physical damage	Hot cheese
	Foreign body
Autoimmune disease	Scleroderma
	Rheumatoid
	Ankylosing spondylitis
Infections	Tuberculosis
	Candidiasis
Congenital	*Forme fruste* oesophageal atresia
Oesophageal dermatoses	Behçets syndrome
	Pustular pemphigoid
	Epidermolysis bullosa
Other	Crohn's disease
	Webs
	Schatski rings

Table 3.2 Frequency of types of stricture in Hull series of 254 patients

Type of stricture	Frequency (no.)
Reflux	214 (nasogastric tube implicated in 12)
Barrett's	20
Achalasia	7 (6 postsurgical, 1 postdilatation)
Scleroderma	6
Caustic	2
Oesophageal atresia	2
Web	1
Granulomatous	1
Sclerotherapy	1

Of these four developed carcinoma (risk 1.56%), one of these in a Barrett's oesophagus.

present the patient may still have painful dysphagia due to disordered oesophageal motility, and paradoxically this may be worse for liquids than solids. Dysphagia due to oesophagitis alone is characteristically variable and there may be intermittent episodes of transient total dysphagia.

However, 25% of patients develop a stricture without any preceding reflux symptoms (Patterson *et al.*, 1983). Moreover, patients with a longstanding oesophageal stricture may not complain of dysphagia, because either they have got used to it, or chew their food well or liquidize it, or because their personality affects their perception of the problem. Patients without dysphagia may then present in more subtle ways: for instance with intermittent vomiting, weight loss, hiccup, nocturnal cough (patients with obstructing oesophageal strictures may fail to clear their saliva which may be aspirated causing cough), aspiration pneumonia, or iron-deficient anaemia.

Sudden worsening of dysphagia can occur in benign as well as malignant strictures. Reasons for this include food impaction, narrowing of the stricture due to drugs (Collins *et al.,* 1979; Kikendall *et al.,* 1983; Oakes and Sherck, 1985; Agha, Wilson and Nostrand, 1986), prolonged recumbency, and use of nasogastric tubes (Banfield and Hurwitz, 1974; Zaninotto *et al.,* 1986).

A clear drug history is essential in managing stricture patients. Non-steroidal anti-inflammatory drugs (NSAID) can lead to stricture formation (Heller *et al.,* 1982; Wilkins *et al.,* 1984). Elderly patients may consider aspirin a tonic and not report its use without direct questioning. Patients may not report NSAID bought 'over the counter' rather than prescribed. Many other tablets may remain in the oesophagus causing local damage (Evans and Roberts, 1976; Channer and Virjee, 1982). The mortality of drug-induced oesophageal injury is high: 6–20% (Collins *et al.,* 1979; Oakes and Sherck, 1985).

Dysphagia after variceal sclerotherapy (Chapter 13) may be due to an oesophageal ulcer at the injection site, or a stricture; if the latter then treatment follows the usual lines (Haynes *et al.,* 1986).

Strictures in immunosuppressed patients may be induced or exacerbated by candidiasis (Ginsburg *et al.,* 1978) or viral infections. Vomiting due to cytotoxic drugs may lead to oesophagitis, which may be exacerbated by corticosteroids or NSAIDs: as vomiting is so common with cytotoxics, oesophageal disease can be easily overlooked.

Rapidly progressive dysphagia suggests a carcinoma, and a change in the character or severity of dysphagia merits further investigation. Carcinomas can arise in patients with previously benign oesophageal strictures. This is uncommon, occurring in 2.5–4% of patients (Moghissi, 1977; Ogilvie, Ferguson and Atkinson, 1980; Watson, 1984), but may be predisposed to by Barrett's oesophagus. In our series of 254 patients with benign oesophageal stricture (Table 3.2), four patients (1.56%) developed a carcinoma (one of whom had Barrett's oesophagus).

3.2.2 RADIOLOGY

A barium swallow is the first investigation in a patient with dysphagia as it allows identification of the site of any obstruction and shows the length and surface contour of a stricture. It is particularly useful for high or for gastric fundal lesions, as strictures in both of these areas can be technically difficult for the endoscopist without forewarning (Bingham *et al.*, 1986). Wide strictures may be overlooked by the endoscopist (Halpert *et al.*, 1985; Ott *et al.*, 1985), a problem increased by the tendency to use increasingly narrower endoscopes. Radiology cannot accurately distinguish a benign from a malignant stricture (Eastman, Gear and Nicol, 1978) – cytology and biopsy of the lesion is needed for this. However, it is important to take further specimens from any stricture that on radiology or endoscopy looks malignant if initial specimens are negative, as the wrong area may have been selected or the tumour may be predominantly submucosal.

The barium swallow may show a hiatus hernia and reflux, unsuspected achalasia, as well as other coincidental relevant pathology affecting management such as diverticula. In patients with high narrow strictures, a barium swallow can help in the positioning of tubes for feeding and for passage of guide-wires prior to dilatation.

The size of the stricture can be measured using a measuring stick (the black and white bands being 2 mm in width) (Figure 3.2), fully extended biopsy forceps, barium swallow, or more satisfactorily barium spheres or tablets (Figure 3.1) (Dyet *et al.*, 1983). Measurement by barium spheres is also useful in serial assessment of patients, particularly those who present unusually with weight loss or symptoms other than dysphagia. Screening the passage of a barium-coated marshmallow may give information about oesophageal motility.

A chest radiograph is necessary to assess the degree of pulmonary aspiration, to look for primary or secondary tumour related to the stricture, and is useful for comparison

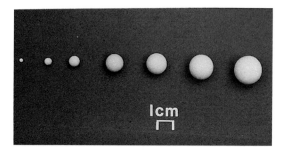

Figure 3.1   Barium impregnated wax spheres of graded sizes for measuring stricture size.

with postdilatation films if complications arise.

3.2.3 ENDOSCOPY

Particular care is needed during endoscopic examination of the patient with an oesophageal stricture. Advancement of the endoscope must be cautious and under direct vision only. The endoscopist should note features suggesting reflux, Barrett's oesophagus, achalasia or carcinoma. We record the presence of diverticula prominently on the front of the casenotes in case future attempts are made to dilate without direct vision (e.g. by Maloney bougie, balloon), a hazardous procedure if the operator directs the dilator into the diverticulum. The diameter of the stricture can be measured at endoscopy (Figure 3.2), although it is our current practice to measure using barium-coated spheres. The distance from the gums to the stricture should be recorded for use at future endoscopy or for balloon dilatation. The endoscopist must perform a full gastroduodenoscopy including a retroverted view of the fundus and hiatus hernia. If the stricture is impassable then full endoscopy should be done after dilatation. A narrow endoscope (e.g. Olympus GIFXQ10: Table 3.3) is useful for endoscopies on patients with strictures since it is more likely to pass the stricture (even though the operator may have more difficulty detecting wide strictures), making placement of the wire more

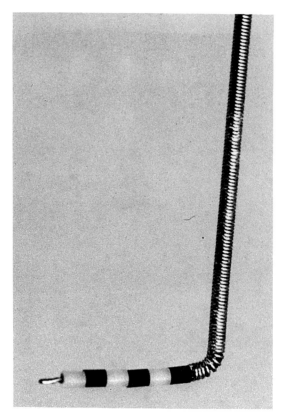

Figure 3.2   Measuring stick to be passed down the endoscope channel. Each ring is 2 mm wide.

certain. Endoscopes with a wide field of view and wide angles of movement are particularly helpful in getting easy retroverted views of the fundus. A repeat endoscopy is desirable in case other pathology emerges unnoticed: the incidence of peptic ulcer in stricture patients is 23% (Patterson *et al.*, 1983). This policy also enables the continuing benign nature of the stricture to be confirmed, although whether patients should return purely for surveillance is uncertain (Spechler *et al.*, 1983; Watson, 1987).

Brushings for cytological examination are taken by rubbing the brush up and down against the side of the stricture. This should be with firm enough pressure to disrupt the mucosa but not roughly, as if bleeding occurs and the brushings are heavily blood stained the cytologist's task is more difficult. Biopsies are best taken by toothed forceps as these provide a better grip at the angle necessary for oesophageal specimens. If biopsies are difficult to obtain from strictures that are hard or tight, biopsy after dilatation may offer a greater chance of success. The diagnostic rate is improved by taking both brushings as well as biopsies (Eastman, Gear and Nicol, 1978), but there is no good evidence that it is helpful to amputate the brush head for examination. Several biopsies are better than a single one, and we recommend taking them from all four quadrants of the stricture as well as from any suspicious area.

Table 3.3 Olympus endoscope specifications (with reference to oesophageal strictures)

Endoscope	Diameter distal end (mm)	Field of view	Angulation Up	Down	Right	Left	Max.	Channel diameter (mm)
GIFXP20	7.9	100	210	90	100	100	240	2.0
GIFP10	9	100	.210	90	100	100	240	2.5
GIFPQ20	9	100	210	90	100	100	240	2.8
GIFXQ10	9.8	100	210	90	100	100	240	2.8
GIFXQ10	11	120	210	90	100	100	240	2.8
GIFQ	11	100	180	90	100	100	200	2.8
GIFXQ20	11	120	210	90	100	100	240	2.8
GIF1T	12.8	100	180	90	100	100	180	3.7
GIF1T10	12.8	100	180	90	100	100	200	3.7

Suction biopsies taken immediately before dilatation may increase the risk of perforation (Jones and Bozymski, 1979), although conventional forceps biopsy followed by dilatation seems safe (Barkin, Taub and Rogers, 1981). Even though the case against suction biopsies is anecdotal, it is desirable to wait for results of biopsies before proceeding to dilatation, as if the stricture is malignant then dilatation is more hazardous and other treatment may be more appropriate.

3.3 MANAGEMENT

3.3.1 AIMS

The first aim of management is to improve symptoms. These are most commonly dysphagia, regurgitation and weight loss, but the patient may also have reflux symptoms and chest problems such as nocturnal coughing, wheeze and recurrent bronchitis. Many stricture patients are elderly and in these it is desirable to avoid the hazards of general anaesthesia and surgery as far as possible. Before embarking on planned treatment, it is essential that necessary steps have been taken to establish the cause, the benign nature of the condition, and the site and course of the stricture as outlined above.

There is little correlation between the degree of oesophagitis and the severity of symptoms. The success of antireflux measures should be judged on control of symptoms rather than resolution of endoscopic appearances.

Measurement of stricture size is helpful in comparing methods of treatment, but less helpful in clinical management because symptoms are poorly related to size alone.

3.3.2 CONSERVATIVE TREATMENT

If reflux symptoms are prominent, then conservative antireflux measures may improve dysphagia, even though their value in treating the stricture is unproven. These measures include the following:

(a) No smoking

Despite evidence from a large endoscopic survey in which oesophagitis was more common in non-smokers (Ainley et al., 1986), smoking is generally thought to exacerbate oesophagitis. Moreover, smoking diminishes the effectiveness of H_2 blockade in reducing acid production.

(b) Dietary measures

Avoidance of foods which tend to reduce lower oesophageal sphincter tone such as chocolate, peppermint and alcohol, those that increase gastric acid secretion such as coffee, and those which may cause pain on contact with an area of oesophagitis such as alcohol and fruit juice, may be helpful. It is sensible to avoid large meals before going to bed. Weight loss may also be helpful.

(c) Postural measures

These are elevating the head of the bed by 15 cm and avoidance of stooping. In some areas of the UK, the Social Service Departments will provide and fit blocks free and promptly, an important consideration for frail elderly patients. However, slow, immobile patients may not be safe in a tilted bed unless supervised. The importance of continuing this measure should be emphasized to those who improve, as it is commonly abandoned when the patient feels better.

(d) Avoidance of provocative drugs

NSAIDs, slow-release potassium chloride tablets (slow K) and many other drugs cause or exacerbate oesophagitis (Collins et al., 1979; Kikendall et al., 1983; Oakes and Sherck, 1985; Agha, Wilson and Nostrand, 1986). NSAIDs are misused and overprescribed (Walt et al., 1986) and should be given to such patients only when really indicated. It may not be possible for patients to stop NSAIDs, but it does not seem to help merely to avoid the oral route by taking the drugs as suppositories. NSAIDs should be continued only after explanation of the relative risks, even though these are difficult to quantify.

As the passage of many tablets through the oesophagus is delayed, especially in the elderly, they should be taken in the erect position and washed down with plenty of water (Evans and Roberts, 1976; Channer and Virjee, 1982). Edwards has shown that half of his series of 400 consecutive stricture patients had oesophageal diameters of 6 mm or less (Edwards, 1984), so drugs prescribed for stricture patients for any purpose, including healing the stricture, should be given only as small tablets or in liquid form.

(e) Measures to lower intra-abdominal pressure

Avoidance of tight clothing (belts and corsets) and weight loss reduce intra-abdominal pressure and probably diminish reflux.

(f) Drugs

There are difficulties in assessing the beneficial effects of drugs on oesophageal stricture and there is a dearth of controlled trial data. The evidence has been well reviewed by Wesdorp (1986).

(i) Antacids Antacids transiently neutralize gastric acid in the oesophagus and the stomach. Their effect on the course of the stricture is unknown.

An alginate and antacid combination seems to be better than an antacid alone (Wesdorp, 1986). Antacids with anticholinergic agents should be avoided in the elderly. Antacids with an effect against alkaline reflux may have a special role (Orlando and Bozymski, 1973).

Antacids should be given at appropriate times; e.g. regularly after meals, at night before going to bed, and as needed for heartburn.

(ii) H_2 blockade and mucosal protective agents There is no objective evidence of any beneficial effect of H_2 blockers in stricture patients. However, although treatment may not change the dilatation requirements (Ferguson, Dronfield and Atkinson, 1979; Starlinger et al., 1985), these agents are widely prescribed and it seems logical to use them for symptoms of reflux or where the stricture is accompanied by severe oesophagitis.

(iii) Sucralfate This should be useful in the elderly because of its lack of side-effects. However the size of the tablet (maximum diameter 20 mm) and its poor dispersibility limit its usefulness. The action of sucralfate is probably not pH dependent as formerly thought, so the timing of antacid therapy may no longer be important. The taste of sucralfate and the dispersible forms of cimetidine and ranitidine is disappointing.

(iv) Other drugs Bethanechol reduces reflux symptoms and improves oesophagitis (Thanik et al., 1980), but its side-effects in the elderly preclude its widespread use.

Omeprazole may have an important role in the future but no evidence is yet available of its effectiveness in stricture patients.

(g) Importance of dentition

Oesophageal strictures are more common in patients with severe tooth loss (Maxton et al., 1987). We have found that, of edentulous patients, those without false teeth tended to have the narrowest strictures. It seems best for the edentulous to use false teeth, as mastication leads to the formation of a food bolus which may dilate the oesophagus.

3.3.3 DILATATION

(a) Historical aspects

Physicians have been able to dilate oesophageal strictures for about 400 years, the first to do so being Fabricius ab Acquapendente using a wax taper (Earlam and Cunha-Melo, 1981). However, such dilatations were blind and non-guided and relied on axial pressure. The development of a bougie weighted by lead was an advance, since dilatation could be done using gravity rather than axial pressure, and this was safer for such blind dilatations. Although Kussmaul was the first to use an oesophagoscope in 1868, and Mikulicz the first to examine it with distal illumination in 1881, it was not until the end of the century that Chevalier Jackson designed his bougies for use through the oesophagoscope (Earlam and Cunha-Melo, 1981). The advent of guide-wires meant that if the guide was properly placed, the dilator would follow and the risk of perforation recede.

Eder–Puestow dilators were first used in the late 1930s although not formally described until 20 years later (Puestow, 1955). The fibreoptic bundle was developed in 1952 and incorporated into an oesophagoscope in the 1960s, and it was the use of the Eder–Puestow dilator (Lilly and McCaffery, 1971) with such an instrument that marked the beginning of modern fibreoptic endoscopic dilatation. This advance enabled elderly, frail patients with strictures to have effective treatment without self-bougineage or the greater risks of rigid oesophagoscopy (Katz, 1967; Mandelstam et al., 1976; Olsen et al., 1977; Vejlsted and Struve-Christensen, 1977; Borgeskov and Struve-Christensen, 1978; Dawson and Cockel, 1981) and general anaesthesia. The Eder–Puestow bougies have remained in the centre of the therapeutic stage ever since, joined by Savary dilators in 1980, Celestin dilators in 1981 and balloon dilators in 1981. A current innovation is the transendoscopic balloon dilator which allows dilatation under direct vision. Lastly, new materials make possible increasingly versatile dilators such as the new KeyMed advanced dilator, bringing closer the reality of an 'Ideal Dilator'.

Developments in oesophageal dilatation have changed the concepts about the need and benefit of dilatation. Bougie dilatation was once considered undesirable on the grounds that it made reflux worse (Barrett, 1960), but the overwhelming evidence is now that dilatation is the correct management, at least initially, in most patients with stricture (Price, Stanciu and Bennett, 1974; Ogilvie, Ferguson and Atkinson, 1980; Gear, 1981; Patterson et al., 1983). Not only does dilatation adequately relieve dysphagia but the need for dilatation decreases with time; indeed 50% of patients treated by one oesophageal dilatation do not require a second for 12 months (Patterson et al., 1983). Thus the majority of patients, especially those who are frail and elderly, but also those younger patients who are not keen on surgery can be managed by dilatation as a long-term option.

(b) Indications and contraindications

Dilatation may be used for all types of benign strictures listed in Table 3.1, and at any age of patient from a few months old to the nineties. Suitability for the elderly is important, as the mean age at presentation for our 254 stricture patients was 68 years, and many receive treatment when much older.

Absolute contraindications are achalasia and an uncontrolled bleeding diathesis. Dilatation techniques (using a balloon) are used for motility disorders such as achalasia, but these disorders are entirely different from benign reflux strictures.

Relative contraindications include an uncooperative patient and a recent myocardial infarction. However, a general anaesthetic and a cautious operator are the answer to the first. It is possible to dilate a patient's stricture, if necessary, a week after an uncomplicated myocardial infarction, but the additional risk should be justified by the severity of the clinical need.

Bolus food impaction, oesophageal diverticulum and ulcer, and severe (rheumatoid) disease of the cervical spine are not contraindications but all require special care by an experienced operator. Indeed, sometimes it is only by dilatation that food bolus obstruction can be safely cleared (Chapter 10) and oesophageal diverticulum and ulcer are common accompaniments of strictures that require dilatation. A guide-wire technique is needed for these particular dilatations.

(c) Personnel and site

It is vital that the operator should embark on this procedure only after adequate training – it is not for beginners. It should not be contemplated without trained nursing staff or the facilities for X-ray screening available nearby. It is clearly impossible for all dilatations to be done in centres with thoracic surgical facilities, but it is important for operators to have support from a surgeon able to tackle the oesophagus. The operator should have knowledge of how to avoid problems and be able to manage them.

(d) General principles

After initial assessment by barium swallow and diagnostic endoscopy the patient is prepared for oesophageal dilatation. Although routine clotting studies and radiographs of the neck or cervical spine are recommended by some authors, these seem irrelevant unless there is a specific indication. Similarly, while there is often blood staining of the dilator, there is no need for routine screening for HBsAg or HIV, although gloves should be worn and the instruments sterilized appropriately (Chapter 1).

The patient is fasted for 8 hours. Informed written consent is necessary. If it appears from the radiographs and the endoscopy that it is a straightforward benign stricture, dilatation may be done immediately without waiting for the biopsy results, if the patient has given consent. This saves time as well as relieving symptoms. If the two procedures are done separately, then ideally the doctor doing the endoscopy should also perform the dilatation.

Patient with valvular heart lesions, some other cardiac conditions including permanent pacemakers, as well as those with dialysis fistulas and ventriculo-atrial shunts should receive antibiotic prophylaxis (Chapter 2).

It is not necessary to wash out the oeso-phagus prior to dilatation unless there is evidence (from radiology or endoscopy) that the oesophagus is abnormally dilated and that food retention is occurring.

In the past dilatation was performed using the endoscope, but this is a dangerous practice, although occasionally it may be sufficient for webs and rings. The endoscopist should be aware of the normal appearances of the upper oesophageal sphincter at 18 cm and the gastro-oesophageal sphincter (usually at about 40 cm) and be able to negotiate the endoscope into the oesophagus under direct vision rather than by feel.

(e) Sedation

While it is possible to perform endoscopy satisfactorily without intravenous sedation, it is desirable to perform most dilatations with sedation to avoid restlessness and diminish discomfort.

Intravenous diazepam (or the oil-in-water emulsion, Diazemuls) are suitable for sedation, as in addition to their sedative properties they also induce amnesia for the event (Dundee and Pandit, 1972). Midazolam is a suitable alternative but care over the dose used is needed, especially in the elderly in whom deaths have occurred with excessive doses (Leading Article, 1988). Flumazenil, an antidote to midazolam, may be helpful but has a shorter half-life, so reversal of sedation may be only temporary (Leading Article, 1988). When used carefully, midazolam is safe (Bardhan and Hinchliffe, 1988). If benzo-diazepines do not provide satisfactory sedation, then the combination of pethidine and a smaller amount of diazepam is a useful alternative, although naloxone should be available.

The combination of topical anaesthesia to the pharynx and intravenous sedation may add to the risk of postdilatation aspiration by suppressing cough in a drowsy patient. It is wiser to use one or the other.

Special cases include self-bougienage by Maloney or Hurst bougies which can be done

Table 3.4 Technical characteristics of dilators

Dilator	Wire needed?	X-ray needed?	Min. diameter (tip) (mm)	Max. diameter (body)		Tip to max. diameter* (cm)	Angle of incidence†	Number of passages‡
				mm	Fr			
Balloon (Rigifiex)	Yes	Yes	2.8	20	60	8	—	1
Balloon (Rigiflex TTS)	Yes	No	1.8	20	60	8	—	1
Celestin	Yes	No	3.7	18	54	16	6°	2
Eder–Puestow	Yes	No	3.7	19.3	58	2.1	49°	multiple
Hurst	No	No	4.0	19.5	59	14	8°	3
KAD	Yes	No	3.0	17.3	52	8.2	12°	3 or less
Maloney	No	No	4.4	16	48	11.5	8°	multiple
Pilling	No	No	4.4	19.8	60	14	8°	multiple
Savary	Yes	No	5.0	20	60	17.7	6°	multiple
Tridil	Yes	No	3.7	18	54	2.1	46°	3 or less

*This length is from the start of the dilator proper (bougie or rod) to the maximum diameter.
†The angle of incidence is the angle at the start of the dilator subtended by the maximum diameter of the maximum bougie or rod (Figure 3.2).
‡The number of passages to achieve maximum dilatation depends on the individual circumstances.

with only topical anaesthesia. Children and alcoholics also require special consideration as both may be excitable with intravenous benzodiazepines: the former may require general anaesthesia and the latter are often more cooperative with topical anaesthesia. Facilities for cardiopulmonary resuscitation must be available. It is also essential that suction equipment is ready for oropharyngeal suction during and after the procedure.

(f) Instruments

The variety of dilators now available is still increasing, and choosing between them is made more difficult by the lack of controlled trials. An 'ideal dilator' would be capable of easy passage through the oropharynx and stricture but would allow the operator to retain tactile sensation for the stricture. Such a dilator should have as few passages through the pharynx as possible for maximum dilatation (at least 16 mm) and should produce efficient dilatation with minimum risk of perforation. It should be able to dilate narrow strictures and be radiopaque so that X-ray screening can be used as needed, without being always neces-

sary. Lastly it should be suitable for patients with small stomachs or difficult hiatus hernias.

Dilators currently available are of four main kinds: the short stubby dilator on a flexible staff (Eder–Puestow), the type where a flexible staff is itself the dilator (Maloney, Savary), the intermediate kind with long flexible dilators on flexible staffs (KeyMed Advanced Dilator) and lastly balloon dilators. Other dilators, for example Tridils or Celestins, are variations on these themes. Dilators may also be divided on whether they dilate by radial force alone (balloons) or by axial force and radial forces (all others). The characteristics of these dilators are set out in Tables 3.4 and 3.5.

(i) Weighted bougies for self bougienage: the Hurst and Maloney dilators Maloney dilators (Figure 3.3) are tapered rubber bougies filled with mercury, this giving a balance of flexibility and rigidity. They are available in sizes 7–20 mm (24–60 Fr in 2-Fr increments*).

*Fr = French gauge values. Conversion of millimetre values to the French gauge can be done by the following simple equation: XX mm × 3 = XX Fr.

Table 3.5 Longevity and cost of dilators

Dilator	Length of life in our hands or recommended	Cost per set VAT included*
Balloon (Rigiflex) 20 mm	not known >50 cases	£281 (manometer £345 extra)
Balloon (Rigiflex 20 mm TTS	not known	£370 (manometer £345 extra)
Celestin	2 years	£141 (2 dilators)
Eder–Puestow	17 years and still in use	£837 (19 olives)
Hurst	2 years recommended	Priced individually: e.g. £41 each up to 38 Fr, £59 for 40 Fr
KAD	not known	£569 (3 dilators)
Maloney	2 years recommended	Priced individually: e.g. £71 for 44 Fr, £103 for 57 or 60 Fr
Pilling	2 years recommended	Priced individually: e.g. £54 for 40 Fr
Savary	3–4 years recommended	£880 (10 dilators)
Tridil	not known (same construction as Eder–Puestow)	no longer marketed

*Guide-wire replacements cost: 250-cm steel, £21; 400-cm Teflon coated, £35.

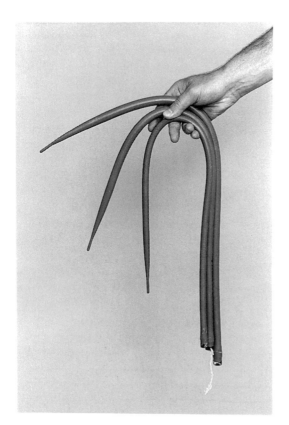

Figure 3.3 Maloney Mercury-weighted rubber dilators.

The Hurst dilator is a similar bougie except that it has a blunt round-nosed end and was more often used for patients with achalasia.

Dilatation is performed with the patient awake and seated. It is usual to spray the orpharynx with lignocaine spray but some patients manage quite well without. Lubrication using margarine or another acceptable lubricant improves tolerance of the procedure. The dilator is held between thumb and first finger – this allows the patient to get a feel of the stricture, and prevents the use of excessive force (although gravity alone is not enough). The patient swallows a 24-Fr dilator initially and then a further three dilators (or six if the stricture is particularly easy). The next dilatation would then start at 30-Fr or 36-Fr, and so on until satisfactory relief is gained. Dilatation can be done either in a supervised outpatient setting (Stoddard and Sims, 1984) or by the patient at his home once the technique had been learned (Grobe, Kozarek and Sanowski, 1984), the latter being more suitable if daily dilatation is required. The advantage of these dilators is that they are safe for simple strictures (i.e. 'wider' strictures and those not complicated by diverticula, having very tortuous paths or in patients with small stomachs). The complication rate for the correctly selected patient is low (Grobe, Kozarek and Sanowski, 1984; Stoddard and Sims, 1984). They are effective, do not require a guide-wire, radiographs, sedation or hospitalization and so are particularly suitable for those strictures which may require periods of almost daily dilatation, such as long restenosing caustic strictures. They can be used for children (Orenstein and Whitington, 1985).

Their main disadvantage is that patients' tolerance of this sort of procedure can be poor, especially in the elderly and infirm; it is preferable for these to have another method under sedation. Complicated and narrow strictures need other methods.

(ii) Eder–Puestow bougie dilators The Eder–Puestow bougie is a short olive-shaped dilator mounted on a flexible shaft and used over a guide-wire (Figure 3.4), the whole being made of steel. The bougies are available in sizes 6.66–19.33 mm (20–58 Fr) in 0.66-mm (2-Fr) increments (Table 3.4).

The biopsy channel of the endoscope and the steel guide-wire are both lubricated with silicone, and the guide-wire checked for kinks. The dilator may be lubricated also but our practice is to moisten it only with water if the patient's mouth is dry. Dilatation is performed with the patient on his left side with the neck slightly flexed. The patient should usually be flat to diminish the risk of aspiration. However, as a hiatus hernia may alter the axis of the oesophagus below the stricture, tilting the patient slightly head up (15–30 degrees) may help by straightening the path by gravity. Sedation is needed, and is best introduced through an indwelling 'butterfly' cannula to provide access later for further doses or pethidine, if required. The endoscope is inserted into the oesophagus and through the stricture. The metal guide-wire is passed through the biopsy channel of the endoscope (as this is also the suction channel, aspiration should be performed first) and through into the stomach leaving only a few centimetres protruding from the biopsy

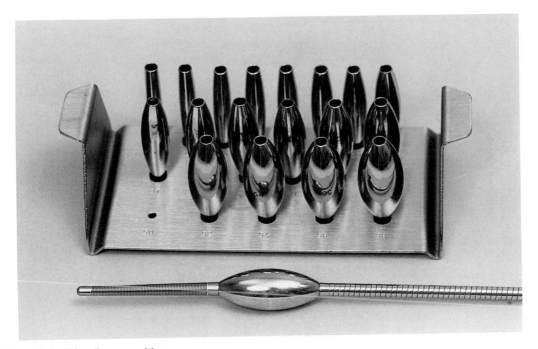

Figure 3.4   Eder–Puestow dilators.

channel. If the endoscope cannot pass through the stricture into the stomach, then the guide-wire has to be fed through the stricture blindly. Particular care is then needed to ensure that it passes smoothly and does not get looped in a hiatus hernia. The guide-wire will pass out of sight, but so long as the wire passes smoothly to an adequate length, then it can be presumed to be in a good position. If the wire meets with any resistance beyond the stricture, X-ray screening is obligatory. With the guide-wire in position (Figure 3.5), the endoscope is removed. It is the assistant's task to ensure that, when the endoscope is on the point of being removed from the mouth, the guide-wire is firmly gripped without deforming it, so that there is a substantial amount (about 80 cm) of guide-wire retained in the stomach.

The endoscope is completely removed, and then the toothguard. The prepared dilator, with an appropriately small bougie mounted, is passed smoothly over the wire which is held stationary throughout. It is simplest to hold the dilator in the left hand close to the bougie but on the right side of the doctor's body, so that it is threaded down the guide-wire which is held firmly in the right hand. The dilator is passed through the pharynx with care, as this is a sensitive area for the patient, and then slowly on a few centimetres at a time. Once the stricture is met (Figure 3.6), gentle pressure is applied at which a sensation of the stricture 'giving' is felt. The bougie is passed beyond the stricture (Figure 3.7) and then pulled back up the guide-wire, the wire itself remaining stationary. The assistant holds the guide-wire when the dilator has been re-

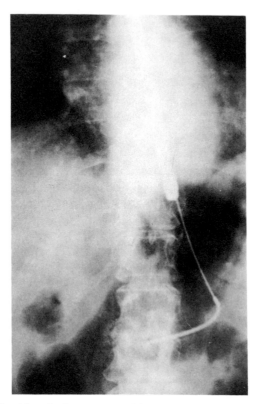

Figure 3.5   Radiograph of guide-wire in correct position.

moved so that it remains in the same position until the next dilator is passed. It is important that the patient is cooperative and lies still, as a sudden movement may make the dilator jerk through the stricture and cause damage. The process is repeated until full dilatation has been achieved, at which point the guide-wire is removed with the final dilator. It is common to find copious secretions in the mouth during and after dilatation: these should be sucked away promptly to reduce the risk of aspiration. It is not our practice to perform a further endoscopy immediately after dilatation as this is unlikely to detect all perforations and the extra instrumentation is an additional risk. The results of this method have been well described (De Carle, 1974; Price, Stanciu and Bennett, 1974; Royston, Dowling and Gear, 1976; Lee *et al.*, 1983; Patterson *et al.*, 1983; Rago, Boesby and Spencer, 1983).

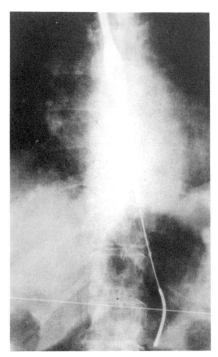

Figure 3.6 Eder–Puestow olive passing over guide-wire through stricture.

The advantages of the Eder–Puestow dilators are that they are effective and can be used over a guide-wire which gives a greater degree of safety. Although several passages of bougies through the mouth are required, the dilatation can be to a precise, predetermined diameter, and strictures can be dilated gradually through a small range of dilator sizes. They can be used for patients with tortuous strictures or small stomachs, and they are durable (Table 3.5). Disadvantages include the unpleasantness of their passage through the pharynx and over the teeth, and the multiple passages required to bring a narrow stricture up to maximum. It is difficult to dilate pinpoint strictures because of the shoulder of the bougie or high 'angle of incidence' (Table 3.4). The use of grooved olives has been described (Korompai and Hayward, 1984) but they seem to offer little real advantage.

Although a guide-wire is used to reduce complications, there are potential problems and these are common to all dilators dependent on a guide-wire. If too much wire is inserted into the stomach, or it is pushed into a blind passage, the sharp angulation of the junction of the introducer tip and the wire may result in a kink or a knot, and when the wire is removed this may perforate the oesophagus (Bancewicz, 1979; Sanderson and Trotter, 1980). The solution is to draw the wire into the dilator before removing it all together. The operator's end of the guide-wire is a potential hazard to the patient's and the operator's eyes, but if the assistant holds the tip the risk is avoided. For complete safety, the operator and assistants can wear protective spectacles or goggles.

(iii) Tridil dilators These are dilators with three olives mounted on the same staff (Figure 3.8). The range of olives on each staff is: 7.4–11 mm (22–34 Fr), 12.4–15 mm (37–45 Fr) and 16–18 mm (45–54 Fr). They were designed to reduce the number of passages through the oropharynx necessary for dilatation. They are

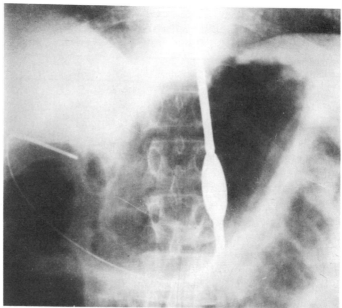

Figure 3.7 Eder–Puestow olive beyond stricture.

used in a similar manner to Eder–Puestow dilators, but with additional caution through the pharynx. Their blunt 'angle of incidence' makes them unsuitable for tough strictures. Their use has been described by Goldberg, Manten and Barkin (1986), but no comparative trials have been performed.

(iv) Celestin dilator The Celestin dilators are long tapered bougies made of the poly-

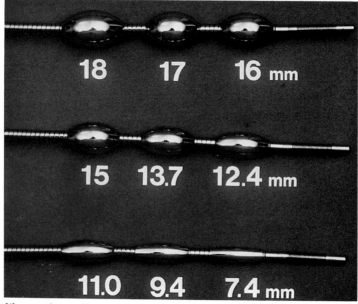

Figure 3.8 Tridil dilators: three olives on one staff.

propylene Neoplex (thermal polyvinylchloride) and may be used over the identical steel guide-wire used for Eder–Puestow dilators, or over a specially designed soft 'piano-wire' (Celestin and Campbell, 1981). They are radiopaque. There are two sizes which increase in small steps to 18 mm (54 Fr) (Figure 3.9). If full dilatation has not been performed, the diameter of the dilatation may be calculated by an equation (Table 3.6). The procedure of dilatation is the same as for the Eder–Puestow dilators, but it may help to warm the dilators to body temperature to attain optimum flexibility.

Advantages are that dilatation is smooth and can be accomplished in two passages. The texture and shape of the dilator are less unpleasant during passage through the pharynx. Celestin dilators are faster to use than Eder–Puestow bougies and the number of guide-wires damaged is significantly less (Hine *et al.*, 1984).

A disadvantage is strictures of patients who have small stomachs must be dilated with great care because of the length of dilator required to be passed to achieve dilatation. Similar difficulty can be encountered in patients with large intrathoracic hiatus hernias. Moreover the tapering shape, although

Table 3.6 Equation for calculation of the diameter (X) of dilatation using Celestin dilators: $X = 60 - (S + M)$*

X	Diameter (mm)
0–5.5	12
5.6–12	14
12.1–18	16
18.1	18

*60 = distance from tip to a 60-cm mark on dilator.
 S = distance from stricture to teeth.
 M = distance from 60-cm mark on dilator to teeth.

an advantage for smooth dilatation, leads to loss of the operator's 'feel' for the stricture or 'tactile sensation', so it may be difficult to know whether resistance is at the mouth or stricture. It is also impossible to know accurately to what diameter the stricture has been taken (despite the equation) unless the dilator is passed to the hilt. If used with the Eder–Puestow guide-wire, the dilator may impact on the flexible tip of the wire: this may damage the dilator and also requires removal of the dilator and wire together.

In a randomized study of 133 patients this dilator was shown to have similar efficacy in long-term relief of symptoms to the Eder–Puestow bougie, although no stricture measurements were made (Hine *et al.*, 1984).

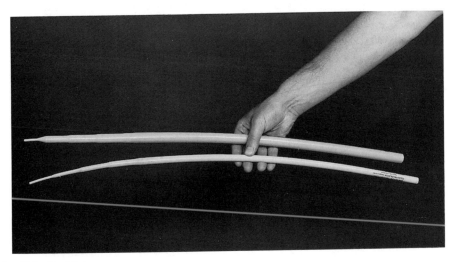

Figure 3.9   Celestin dilators.

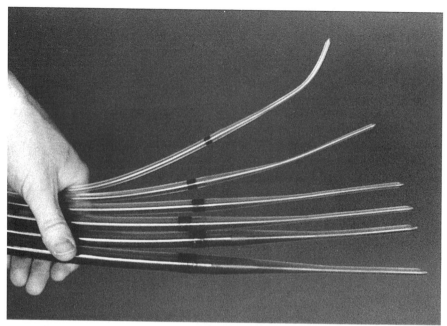

Figure 3.10   Savary dilators.

(v) Savary dilators These dilators are hollow bougies made of plastic-coated polyvinyl (Figure 3.10). They have a flexible tip which passes into a more rigid shaft and are designed to be passed over a steel guide-wire in the same way as Celestin dilators. The calibre of the dilator starts at 5 mm (15 Fr) and proceeds in 1–2 mm increments to 18 mm (54 Fr). There are two sets of differing lengths: 70 cm and 100 cm long. Each rod has a small radiopaque marker at the junction of the tip and the shaft.

The advantages and disadvantages are similar to the Celestin dilators, although a shorter length needs to be passed into the stomach; the major difference is that Savary dilators cannot achieve dilatation in two passages – multiple passages are required. Since there is no advantage over the Celestin dilators, the latter are generally to be preferred for convenience, but Savary dilators allow precise dilatation to a specific diameter. The American endoscopy dilator is a modified version of the Savary.

There have been no randomized controlled trials on their use but a retrospective survey suggested that they might be comparable to Eder–Puestow dilators (Dumon *et al.*, 1985)

(vi) The KeyMed Advanced Dilators (KAD) These are long oval-shaped dilators made of medical grade polyurethrane rubber (Fig. 3.11 a,b) in three diameters – 6.5–9 mm (20–27 Fr), 6.5–14 mm (20–42 Fr). 6.5–17 mm (20–51 Fr). The bougie screws on to a flexible shaft similar to that of the Eder–Puestow dilator. The whole apparatus is hollow and the dilator is passed over an Eder–Puestow guide-wire. X-ray screening is possible as the wire and shaft are radiopaque although the bougie is not. Advantages include the need for only three passages through the mouth for full dilatation, ease of passage through the pharynx, smooth passage over the stricture using an intermediate angle of incidence (so retaining some tactile sensation) and its suitability for use in those with small stomachs.

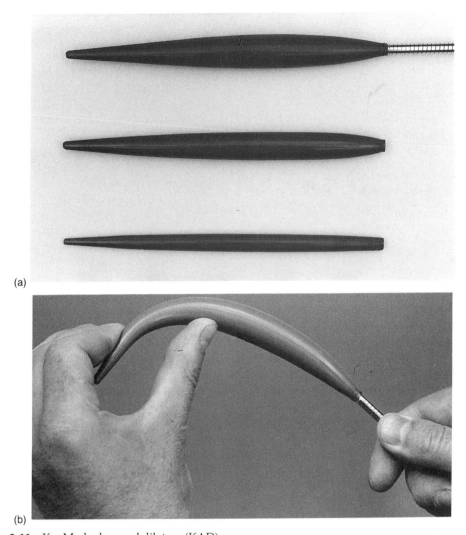

(a)

(b)

Figure 3.11 KeyMed advanced dilators (KAD).

These are significant advantages and brings it close to an 'ideal dilator' (Table 3.7).

Maximum dilatation is a little less at 17.5 mm than the maximum obtainable by Celestin (18 mm) or Eder–Puestow (19.33 mm).

There have been no controlled trials of its use, but we have reported its safe use in 79 patients (125 dilatations) without complications (Cox *et al.*, 1989).

(vii) Balloon dilators The procedure for dilatation using balloon dilators is described in Chapter 4. The results of a comparative study between balloons and Eder–Puestow bougies performed in this unit are given under section '(j) Effectiveness'.

(viii) Eska–Buess multistage bougie This is a tube-shaped dilator of medical grade plastic with an atraumatic shoulder zone which is designed to fit snuggly over a small calibre endoscope (Figure 3.12) (Buess *et al.*, 1983a). The endoscope is introduced then the stricture is dilated using the endoscope as an obturator.

Table 3.7 Characteristics desirable in an ideal dilator possessed by KAD

---

(1) Smooth, easy passage through pharynx and stricture and ability to negotiate tortuous strictures:
    Narrow tip
    Tapering contour
    Intermediate 'angle of incidence'
    Smooth passage over guide-wire
    Flexible staff or dilator
(2) Safe, effective dilatation:
    Wide effective dilating surface
    'Feel' as dilatation occurs
    Few passages needed but variable size of dilatation permitted
(3) Suitable for use in small stomachs
(4) No radiographs needed routinely, but radiopaque for screening if stricture difficult
(5) Suitable for use in a busy endoscopy list:
    Easy to use and not time consuming
    No need for special room
    Easy to clean
(6) Patient acceptability
(7) Cost equivalent to other dilators

Retroverted views of the procedure can be obtained as the operator advances the endoscope and bougie together. Narrow strictures require a separate technique and are dilated by a stenosis tip attached to the distal end of the endoscope.

The advantages of this technique are that the operator can do the dilatation under direct vision, without need for radiography or guide-wires. There is no need for an instrument change so the whole procedure takes less time than usual, unless the stenosis tip is needed.

The disadvantages are the possibility of mucosal tears despite the atraumatic shoulder zone at the distal end of the dilator, the relative difficulty in managing very narrow strictures and, although less important, the lack of range of sizes to which the stricture may be dilated. The performance of this dilator has been described by Buess *et al.* (1983b), but it has yet to see wide use, and its value is uncertain.

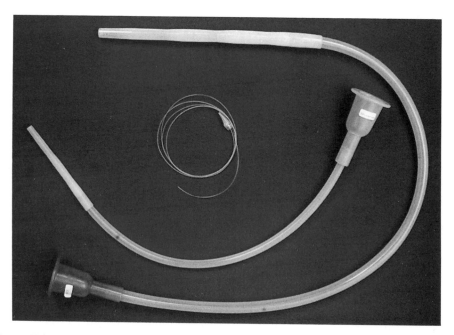

Figure 3.12   Eska-Buess dilators.

(g) Use of radiographic screening

The use of X-ray screening is not routine in the UK, but medicolegal constraints make it wise, if not obligatory, in the USA. The widespread use of balloons in the USA has led to increasing use of X-ray screening in children with strictures. Excessive X-ray screening in children should be avoided (Dawood and Hall, 1988), especially in a recurring condition. Although blind retrograde balloon dilatation may be done without radiography (Graham and Smith, 1985), we have not found this satisfactory and at present X-ray screening is desirable for balloon dilatation. In view of this, the operator caring for a child with a stricture should carefully assess whether balloon dilatation is wise and whether another method might not do as well.

The indications for X-ray screening should be as follows:

1. Where there is difficulty in positioning the guide-wire.
2. Where there is a particularly tortuous stricture or difficult hiatus hernia.
3. For all balloon dilatations.
4. For learners, when the added visibility and security improves the safety of the procedure.

(h) Aftercare and complications

It is common practice for patients to be sent home after endoscopy with instructions not to drive, go out, use machinery or drink alcohol until the next day. Those who have received dilatation are told to report back if they get any chest pain. This will probably be sufficient for the majority of patients. However, a few suffer major complications and may ignore early or mild symptoms until it is too late to salvage the situation. For this reason we have elected to admit all patients overnight for observation after dilatation. This is important not only for those patients with potential perforation but also for elderly patients who may be too drowsy after sedation to go home safely. Observations (half-hourly pulse, blood pressure and temperature) are performed for 3 hours, then if all is well they are performed hourly for a further 3 hours. The patient is allowed nothing by mouth for 6 hours and then only a drink of sterile water. A further drink is allowed 6 hours later and the next morning, breakfast.

If the patient is malnourished, it may be prudent to consider a period of several days inpatient observation to ensure that the situation is really improving, possibly with further dilatations if needed. The degree of malnutrition of such patients can be easily underestimated, so their food intake and weight should be watched carefully.

The major hazard of oesophageal dilatation is perforation (Tulman and Boyce, 1981). Recorded rates vary and the mortality is 6–25%, although this depends on the promptness of diagnosis. Such statistics include figures for dilatation of malignant strictures which are more likely to perforate as well as dilatation of achalasia as primary treatment, which should be considered separately unlike dilatation of the secondary reflux stricture in achalasia.

Even an experienced operator may cause a perforation. The possibility of perforation should be borne in mind by the whole team caring for the patient, so that any chest pain lasting longer than a few minutes (even if it subsequently goes away), pyrexia or tachycardia should be considered as potential evidence of perforation. Even if the patient later improves, he should be kept nil by mouth until investigations for perforation have proved negative. A chest radiograph may show a pneumomediastinum, a pneumothorax, air under the diaphragm or a pleural effusion, but it can be entirely normal despite perforation. A water-soluble contrast swallow (either gastrograffin or omnipaque (Seltzer, Jones and McLaughlin, 1979) is essential: barium should not be used in case a barium mediastinitis develops. Correct management at this stage will allow diagnosis within 24 hours in 94.4% of perforations (Wesdorp, 1984).

Table 3.8 Studies of dilators and their complications (since introduction of flexible oesophagoscopes)

Reference	Type of dilator	Mean age (yr)	Patients (no.)	Dilatations (no.)	Perforations (no.)*		Cancers (no.) Deaths	Cancers (no.) Included?
Adults								
Price et al. (1974)	EP	—	28	72	1	(1.4)	0	0
De Carle (1974)	EP	—	—	225	1	(0.4)	0	0
Royston et al. (1976)	EP	68	26	51	0		0	0
Huchzermeyer et al. (1977)	M/H	—	16	86	0		0	†
Croker et al. (1980)	EP	69	19	48	0		0	0
Celestin and Campbell (1981)	C	72	25	29	0		0	†
Dawson and Cockel (1981)	—	72	—	1203	13	(1.08)	6	†
Gotberg et al. (1982)	B	67	40	78	0		0	0
Wesdorp et al. (1982)	EP	62	100	665	4	(0.5)	0	0
	M				4	(0.3)	0	0
Buess et al. (1983)	MSB	—	37	113	2	(1.8)	0	†
Lee et al. (1983)	EP	—	97	309	0		0	0
	C	—		46	0		0	0
Lifton (1983)	H	—	152	279	1	(0.4)	0	†
	EP/H	—		56	0		0	†
Patterson et al. (1983)	EP/H	—	154	764	5	(0.65)	2	0
Rago et al. (1983)	EP	65	33	152	0		0	0
Grobe et al. (1984)	M	60	13	4600	0		0	0
Hine et al. (1984)	EP	—	72	69	0		0	0
	C			64	1	(1.6)	0	0
Kollath et al. (1984)	B	—	21	41	0		0	†
Stoddard and Simms (1984)	M	69	109	524	0		0	0
Watson (1984)	EP/C	70	120	309	2	(0.64)	0	0
Starck et al. (1984)	B	—	31	67	0		0	0
Webb and McDaniel (1984)	M/EP	—	289	533	1	(0.2)	1	0
Bremner (1985)	C	—	46	46	1	(2.2)	0	†
Dumon et al. (1985)	S	—	300	300	1	(0.3)	0	†
	EP	—	248	248	2	(0.8)	1	†
Goldberg et al. (1985)	T	59	35	65+	0		0	†
Graham and Smith (1985)	B	—	22	55	0		0	†
Lindor et al. (1985)	B	—	69	69+	0		0	0
Fellows et al. (1986)	C	—	100	302	0		0	0
Haynes et al. (1986)	M	57	10	28	0		0	0
Kozarek (1986)	B	—	486	—	2	(0.4)	0	0
Leahy et al. (1986)	EP	—	19	78	0		0	0
McLean et al. (1987)	B	—	48	110	0		0	†
Mandelstam et al. (1976)	M/H	—	—	13 139	12	(0.09)	0	?
	EP	—	—	9 431	33	(0.3)	0	?
Children								
Goldthorn et al. (1984)	B	2	8	46	0		0	0
Orenstein and Whitington (1985)	M/P	5	13	211	0		0	0
Johnsen et al. (1986)	B	1	10	47	0		0	0
Sato et al. (1988)	B	2.5	20	68	0		0	0

*Figures in parentheses are percentages.
† = Included.

The usual sites of perforation are the cervical oesophagus and at or just proximal to the level of the stricture (which may be either intrathoracic or intra-abdominal). Perforation in the cervical oesophagus appears to be related to faulty technique or an anatomical abnormality of the cervical oesophagus or cervical spur (Wychulis, Fontana and Payne, 1969). If perforation has occurred in the cervical oesophagus, the patient may also have pain on swallowing, a change in voice or subcutaneous emphysema. A lateral radiograph of the neck may show air in the retro-oesophageal space, but if not a contrast swallow is needed. Chest symptoms after dilatation without evidence of perforation may be due to aspiration (Royston, Dowling and Gear, 1976; Lanza and Graham, 1978). It is unwise to use both pharyngeal anaesthesia and sedation, since this may increase the risk of aspiration (Royston, Dowling and Gear, 1976).

Bacteraemia is thought to occur during most dilatations. The source may be the pharynx (Stephenson et al., 1977) and are α- or β-haemolytic streptococci or the bougie (Raines et al., 1975). Antibiotic prophylaxis is therefore needed for rheumatic and prosthetic valves and other cardiac conditions (Yin and Dellipiani, 1983; Niv, Bat and Motro, 1985), and the bougie requires careful cleaning beforehand. Metastatic abscesses are a recognized if rare complication, (Raines et al., 1975; Golladay et al., 1980; Schlitt et al., 1985), and so extra care should be taken in dilating the immunosuppressed.

Bleeding requiring transfusion is extremely rare (Mandelstam et al., 1976). Although a number of unusual complications have been reported (Palmer, 1970; Mandelstam et al., 1976; McDonald, 1978; Hasan, 1981; Lehmann et al., 1987; Sagar and Macfie, 1987), these are usually the result of bad technique or mishap. Technical failures caused by bent or broken wires and the bougie sticking on the end of the guide-wire are commoner than complications. Careless insertion or removal of a steel guide-wire may give a perforation at any level.

It is important not to allow a feeling of complacency about dilatation to blind the operation to the risks. It is not possible to predict those patients who will have complications. If, because of pressure on beds, it is necessary to discharge patients the same day as the dilatation is performed, then these patients should be young or have someone at home with them, have 'easy' strictures, and be experienced in the procedure. Those who have performed self-bougineage in the hospital setting are most suitable. It is wise for the patient to drink a glass of water before going home, and if pain results then a contrast swallow is needed.

(i) Avoidance of complications

The following are golden rules to avoid trouble:

1. Don't tackle strictures until you are an experienced endoscopist.
2. Obtain a good quality barium swallow before the first dilatation, paying special attention to the hypopharyngeal region and looking for diverticula and congenital abnormalities.
3. Ensure screening facilities are available.
4. Use good equipment, check guide-wires for kinks, and balloons for leaks beforehand.
5. Don't advance the endoscope without good vision.
6. Get a good 'feel' of the stricture; don't force the dilator.
7. Don't advance the dilator if the wire has slipped.
8. Don't try too much too soon: especially in longstanding or very tough strictures.
9. Any pain or fever after dilatation should be investigated as a possible perforation or aspiration.

The management of complications is dealt with in Chapter 2.

(j) Effectiveness

Measurement of strictures by barium balls after dilatation has showed that the diameter achieved is usually 4–8 mm less than the diameter of a 19.33 mm (58 Fr) Eder–Puestow dilator passed 1 week later (Bennett *et al.*, 1985). Despite this degree of 'rebound', the patient may still have a persisting remission from symptoms. Whether or not remission occurs depends on the persistence of the cause and its exacerbating factors, the rigidity or pliability of the stricture and the patient's perception of dysphagia and his dietary habits. Oesophagitis alone may lead to severe dysphagia without recurrence of restenosis. The best guide to progress is a combination of symptoms, the patient's weight and the serial stricture measurement.

There is good evidence that dilatation is effective: 40–60% of patients can be managed with dilatation and medical therapy (Glick, 1982; Watson, 1984). There have, however, been few controlled trials between dilators. We have examined the difference between the Eder–Puestow dilators and balloons in a prospective controlled trial (Cox *et al.*, 1988).

Table 3.9 Dysphagia score

No dysphagia	0
Dysphagia with meat	1
Dysphagia with bread	2
Dysphagia with semisolids	3
Dysphagia with liquids	4
Total dysphagia	5

Sixty-five patients with benign oesophageal stricture received dilatation to either 20 mm by the Rigiflex balloon or to 19.33 mm by Eder–Puestow bougie, the closest size bougie to the 20-mm balloon. Stricture measurements were performed before dilatation, at 1 week and thereafter at monthly intervals to 5 months by a barium sphere technique (Dyet *et al.*, 1983). Patients' dysphagia was assessed using a simple dysphagia score (Table 3.9). Antireflux measures including antacids and H_2 blockers were advised as needed for symptoms. Eder–Puestow bougies were better than balloons in maintaining stricture patency at 5 months but the difference, calculated from the mean change from the baseline measurement, was not significant ($P = 0.06$) (Figure 3.13). There was however a significantly better reduction

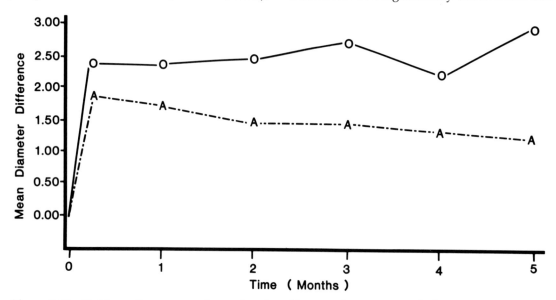

Figure 3.13 Stricture diameters at intervals after dilatation by a 20 mm balloon and a 19.3 mm Eder–Puestow olive.

of dysphagia in the bougie group, assessed from the mean change from baseline dysphagia score $(P = 0.02)$ (Figure 3.14). There were no complications in either group. The amount of sedation needed and the patient acceptability scores were similar in both groups. The mean incident skin radiation in the balloon group was 57.5 mGy: by comparison a barium meal would give an exposure of 150 mGy. Balloons might be expected to be safer than bougies as the pressures in balloon dilatation are exerted in a radial direction only, but these pressures may still be of considerable magnitude (Cox, Buckton and Bennett, 1987). As the incidence of serious complications following dilatation is small, the assessment of relative safety will depend on large surveys (Kozarek, 1986).

As balloons are less durable than bougies it seems likely that for the near future bougie dilatation will remain the preferred choice. Balloons may have a complementary role for special cases as follows:

1. Patients with particularly narrow or tortuous strictures, since the balloon may be used to open up these strictures for other techniques. The balloon must retain its suppleness to be effective in these situations, as if it is too stiff to furl it will not pass.
2. Patients who are difficult to endoscope, since the balloon can be passed without repeating the endoscopy.
3. Patients who cannot tolerate traditional dilatation with Eder–Puestow dilators.
4. Patients with small stomachs, although these may also easily be done by Eder–Puestow bougies.
5. Patients with a previous perforation in whom gentle dilatation without longitudinal force is necessary.
6. Possibly children, although there must be reservations about irradiating small children for what can be a recurring condition. A recent improvement is the transendoscopic balloon dilator (Rigiflex TTS)

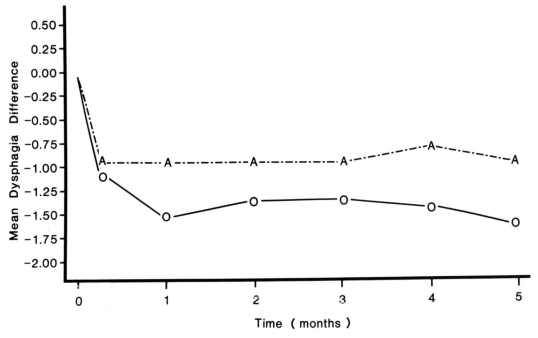

Figure 3.14 Dysphagia scores at intervals after dilatation by a 20 mm balloon and a 19.3 mm Eder-Puestow olive.

which can be passed down a 2.8-mm biopsy channel, thus excluding the need for X-ray screening and unifying the processes of endoscopy and balloon dilatation (Wilson *et al.*, 1980). The maximum size balloon is 18 mm. Unfortunately the balloon rupture rate seems to be higher than the more established balloons, and thus the cost becomes exorbitant.

(k) Frequency of dilatation

The necessary frequency of dilatation is variable and depends on severity – some strictures resolve spontaneously never requiring dilatation (Palmer, 1968), some resolve on medical treatment, and others may require frequent dilatations. Half of the patients with oesophageal strictures do not require another stretch within a year (Patterson *et al.*, 1983). Severity depends not just on diameter but on whether the stricture is primarily mucosal, or due to perioesophageal fibrosis as in caustic strictures, making them often difficult to dilate: they may require frequent dilatation and tend to recur. Strictures which have been perforated may also be tough because of perioesophageal fibrosis excited at the time of the perforation. The need for dilatation depends on the patient's symptoms – this is relatively easy if the main symptom is dysphagia, especially if the endoscopy reveals a narrow stricture. It is more difficult if the patient's symptom is not dysphagia but, for example, nocturnal cough, and measurement of stricture size may then be of help in judging when and how often to dilate. Measurement may also be helpful if the symptoms are dysphagia, vomiting or pain due to oesophagitis, as if the reduction in bore is minimal then dilatation on its own is unlikely to be enough. In general, patients with stricture measurements of 12 mm diameter are doing well and are unlikely to improve from dilatation, while those with measurements of 4 or 6 mm usually develop problems and should be watched carefully. In between these extremes lie a large number of patients in whom the management has to depend on individual assessment. It is not practical to measure all strictures, but it may be useful for patients difficult to assess or who are apprehensive about further dilatation. Measurement may also be helpful for patients with postvagotomy dysphagia, dysphagia after Nissen fundoplication or patients with systemic sclerosis and other motility disorders, as these patients are difficult to evaluate by endoscopy.

Follow-up should include regular weights at each attendance in addition to dysphagia and heartburn 'scores'. It is our practice to discharge patients who remain asymptomatic over a year or two. There is little evidence that endoscopic surveillance of patients with benign strictures is justified despite the 'malignant potential', even if they have a Barrett's oesophagus. However, this is a controversial area and some units advocate regular biopsy and cytology (Spechler *et al.*, 1983; Watson, 1987).

(l) How much?

The established principle of limiting one treatment session to a maximum of three dilators passed once the operator meets resistance is no longer strictly necessary (Lifton, 1983), and it is our practice to dilate to the maximum dilator if possible at the first attempt. However, it is important to acquire a 'feel' of what is possible – this is a different sensation with the various dilators. Attempts to dilate to the maximum by force will lead to unnecessary complications. Commonsense and caution should be the operator's guide, for each stricture is slightly different. Dilatation to 13–14 mm will relieve most patient's symptoms. Failure to dilate adequately a perforation despite careful dilatation or a speedy return to the previous bore or symptoms suggests a carcinoma (Gear, 1981).

3.3.4 OTHER TECHNIQUES

(a) Guide-wire alternatives

For difficult strictures, we use a narrow

Teflon-coated guide-wire, fed through a kifa catheter or an amputated nasogastric tube. The smallest balloon can then be passed to gain access for larger dilators. If the stricture is impassible by the steel guide-wire others have found it helpful to use narrow angiographic guide-wires, followed by an Amplatz catheter and a conventional steel guide-wire inserted by a railroading technique (Sharpe, Chalmers and Gough, 1986).

Torque controlled guide-wires may be helpful (Keshishian *et al.*, 1984) but we have never found them necessary.

Temporary stenting by an amputated nasogastric tube may buy time and allow feeding between dilatations if the stricture narrows down quickly (Barkin and Rosen, 1984), in addition to providing a route for a guide-wire if the stricture is narrow (Sawyer, 1985).

High narrow strictures can be particularly difficult and often require an ENT surgeon's expertise: urethral catheters with a screw fitting onto a variable calibre follower may be helpful here (Sawyer, 1985).

(b) Intubation

Endoscopic intubation using prosthetic tubes can be used for benign oesophageal strictures (Carenfeldt *et al.*, 1983). Although this technique undoubtedly has its place, the 'tube existence' is not a very satisfactory result for someone with benign disease. It is best reserved as an alternative to dilatation for those patients with frequently recurring strictures who wish to escape dilatation and who are unfit for surgery. There are risks attached to the process of insertion, problems inherent in the tube material (MacGown, 1980; Braniki *et al.*, 1981; Buess *et al.*, 1982), and the procedure can be complicated by stenosis proximal to the tube (Gear, 1981). For these reasons, intubation should be used only when other measures have failed.

Operative insertion of prosthetic tubes for benign disease (Wilson, 1980) should now be obsolete, although it may have a place after

oesophageal perforation (Asplund and Hill, 1985; Quayle *et al.*, 1985).

(c) Didcot dilator, laminaria tents

The Didcot dilator is a cylindrical high-strength stainless-steel wire braid placed astride a stricture to exert a slow continuous dilatation (Didcot, 1973). This offers few advantages and has been superseded by other techniques.

Laminaria tents are similar in principle to the Didcot dilator.

(d) Stenosis endoscope, tape dilator

A stenosis endoscope with a 9-mm (27-Fr) calibre tip tapering gently to a shaft of 13 mm (39 Fr) has been designed by the Fuji company (Frimberger, 1983) but seems to offer little advantage over less expensive dilators. A piece of tape wrapped round an endoscope forms the basis of the endoscopic tape dilator (Lehman and O'Connor, 1985), but this cannot be seriously recommended: all centres performing dilatation should be equipped with properly manufactured and reliable dilators.

(e) Transgastric oesophageal bougienage

Transgastric oesophageal bougienage via a feeding gastrostomy (Earlam and Cunha-Melo, 1981) has been used recently for very narrow strictures impassable by other techniques in patients unfit for more extensive surgery (Winkler *et al.*, 1985). This is worth considering under exceptional circumstances, especially as the gastrostomy helps in improving the patients' nutrition.

(f) Transendoscopic electrosurgical incision

Cautery of oesophageal strictures is another established technique but transendoscopic electrosurgical incision of webs, narrow lower oesophageal strictures or Schatzki rings via the fibreoptic gastroscope has only recently been described. At present the reports remain anecdotal (Groitl, 1982; Huchzermeyer, Freise and Becker, 1979; Luna, 1983; Raskin *et al.*,

1985), and the risks appear more striking than the advantages.

(g) Laser

While experience in laser treatment in the oesophagus is largely confined to carcinoma of the oesophagus, lasers can be used for benign strictures (Loffler, Dienst and Velasco, 1986; Sander and Poesl, 1986). Lasers may provide an effective answer for short, very tough strictures and for correctly selected patients lasers may be curative. Further comparative studies are needed.

(h) Surgery

Although conservative treatment using dilatation is effective for the majority of patients with oesophageal strictures, there are patients in whom surgery offers a more satisfactory option. Selection is all important. Even in good hands, the recurrence rate of stricture after surgery for those patients in whom initial medical treatment had failed was 25%, and the mortality 10% (Raptis and Mearns Milne, 1972).

Indications for surgery include:

1. Young patients whose stricture continues to require dilatation after 1 or 2 years.
2. Patients whose strictures require excessively frequent dilatation.
3. Patients whose oesophagus may be irretrievably damaged (for replacement).
4. Patients with oesophageal perforation with complications.
5. Patients who are temperamentally or technically unsuitable for repeated dilatation. The latter include patients with narrow, tortuous or horizontally sited strictures and some patients with systemic sclerosis (Netscher and Richardson, 1984).

The currently favoured approach is to use a standard antireflux procedure, dilating the stricture as needed (Watson, 1984; Shirazi, Schulze and Soper, 1987; Little et al., 1988, Stirling and Orringer, 1988). If an antireflux procedure is technically difficult or impossible

then a duodenal diversion using a Roux-en-Y loop may be helpful (Royston, Dowling and Spencer, 1975; Washer et al., 1984). Resection carries a high mortality. If the stricture cannot be dilated, resection and jejunal (Cranford and Cushieri, 1986) or colonic (Isolauri, 1988) replacement may need considering. Patients with anastomotic strictures after total gastrectomy may also be helped by Roux-en-Y diversion, although these patients can also be dilated.

3.3.5 SPECIAL CASES

(a) Children with strictures

A number of studies have reported the use of balloon dilators in children (Ball et al., 1984; Goldthorn et al., 1984; Stringer, Pablot and Mancer, 1985; Johnsen, Ingemann Jensen and Mauritzen, 1986; Sato et al., 1988). While this seems an attractive option, there have been no controlled trials against other methods in children and the X-ray exposure is a clear disadvantage (Dawood and Hall, 1988) if repeated dilatations are needed.

(b) Caustic burns and strictures

There are many approaches to this difficult problem and there is a lack of suitable clinical trials. Important facets of management in the acute phase are:

1. Early endoscopy to establish the extent of damage is desirable (Poelman, Hausman and Hoitsma, 1977; Oakes, Sherck and Mark, 1982).
2. There is no convincing evidence that early prophylactic dilatation is helpful, and it can be dangerous.
3. Emergency surgery seems unnecessarily dangerous except for those with gastric perforations.
4. An oesophageal stent or nasogastric tube may be helpful in the prevention of stricture (Mills, Estrera and Platt, 1979; Wijburg et al., 1985).
5. The place of penicillamine and other drugs

has yet to be proved although results of animal studies are encouraging (Gehanno and Guedon, 1981). The place of steroids is uncertain (Oakes, Sherck and Mark, 1982; Wason, 1985).

6. Careful nutrition, whether by nasogastric tube or gastroenterostomy, is important.
7. Early diagnosis and treatment of aspiration pneumonia is essential.

The risk of perforation, once a stricture has developed, seems to be higher than in reflux strictures although there is little recent work on this (Alford, Johnson and Harris, 1963; Bill, Mebust and Savage, 1963). Possible reasons are that the wall has been weakened by steroids, the strictures are tight and narrow and too much is attempted too soon, and that the fibrous reaction encasing them is hard but brittle.

(c) Food impaction

This difficult problem is often best managed by passing the guide-wire past the bolus through the stricture and performing a dilatation, the bolus then passing distally. However, if the guide-wire cannot be passed then the bolus has to be removed piecemeal and this should only be done with an overtube in place to avoid the unpleasant multiple passages of the endoscope (Chapter 10).

(d) Endoscopic surveillance

There is no evidence that continued endoscopic surveillance of uncomplicated biopsy-proven benign oesophageal strictures is necessary or desirable. The benefit of surveillance in patients with Barrett's oesophagus is also unproven, even though this is a premalignant condition.

REFERENCES

Agha, F. P., Wilson, J. A. and Nostrand, T. T. (1986) Medication-induced oesophagitis. *Gastrointest. Radiol.*, **11**, 7–11.

Ainley, C. C., Forgacs, I. C., Keeling, P. W. N. and

Thompson, R. P. H. (1986) Outpatient endoscopic survey of smoking and peptic ulcer. *Gut*, **27**, 648–51.

Alford, B. R., Johnson, J. L. and Harris, H. H. (1963) Penetrating and perforating injuries of the oesophagus. *Ann. Otol.*, **72**, 995–9.

Asplund, C. M. and Hill, L. D. (1985) Delayed lower oesophageal perforation: management with Celestin tube. *Ann. Otol. Rhinol. Laryngol.*, **94**, 114–6.

Ball, W. S., Strife, J. L., Rosenkrantz, J. *et al.* (1984) Oesophageal strictures in children: treatment by balloon dilatation. *Radiology*, **150**, 263–4.

Bancewicz, J. (1979) A hazard of the Eder–Puestow system of oesophageal dilatation. *Br. J. Surg.*, **66**, 66.

Banfield, W. J. and Hurwitz, A. L. (1974) Oesophageal stricture associated with nasogastric intubation. *Arch. Intern. Med.*, **134**, 1083–6.

Bardhan, K. P. and Hinchliffe, R. F. C. (1988) Midazolam antagonism. *Lancet*, **ii**, 388.

Barkin, J. S., Taub, S. and Rogers, A. I. (1981) The safety of combined endoscopy, biopsy and dilatation in oesophageal strictures. *Am. J. Gastroenterol.*, **76**, 23–6.

Barkin, J. S. and Rosen, H. H. (1984) Temporary stenting as an aid to oesophageal dilation. *Gastrointest. Endosc.*, **30**, 376–7.

Barrett, N. R. (1960) Hiatus hernia. *Br. Med. J.*, **2**, 247–52.

Bennett, J. R., Sutton, D. R., Price, J. D. and Dyet, J. F. (1985) Effects of bougie dilatation on oesophageal stricture size, in *Oesophageal Disorders: Pathophysiology and Therapy*, Raven, New York, pp. 221–4.

Bill, A. H., Mebust, W. K. and Savage, L. R. (1963) Evaluation of techniques of oesophageal dilatation in relation to the danger of perforation. *J. Thorac. Cardiovasc. Surg.*, **45**, 510–4.

Bingham, B. J., Drake-Lee, A., Chevretton, E. and White, A. (1986) Pitfalls in the assessment of dysphagia by fibreoptic oesophagogastroscopy. *Ann. R. Coll. Surg. Engl.*, **68**, 22–3.

Borgeskov, S. and Struve-Christensen, E. (1978) The modern treatment of oesophageal strictures using the Eder–Puestow dilators. *Acta Otolaryngol.*, **85**, 456–60.

Branicki, F. J., Ogilvie, A. L., Willis, M. R. and Atkinson, M. (1981) Structural deterioration of prosthetic oesophageal tubes: an *in vitro* comparison of latex rubber and silicone rubber tubes. *Br. J. Surg.*, **68**, 861–4.

Bremner, C. G. (1985) Combined technique of oesophageal endoscopy, dilatation, and biopsy using the celestin system of dilators, in

Oesophageal Disorders: Pathophysiology and Therapy, Raven, New York, pp. 501–3.

Buess, G., Lorenz, B., Eitenmuller, J. and Steinbrich, W. (1982) Problems of dissolution after long term placement of a Celestin oesophageal tube. *Endoscopy*, **14**, 182–4.

Buess, G., Thon, J. and Hutterer, F. (1983a) A multiple diameter bougie fitted over a small-calibre fibroscope. *Endoscopy*, **15**, 53–4.

Buess, G., Thon J., Eitenmuller, J. *et al.* (1983b) The endoscopic multiple-diameter bougie: clinical results after one year of application. *Endoscopy*, **15**, 337–41.

Carenfelt, C., Jonsell, G., Lejdeborn, L. *et al.* (1983) Permanent indwelling tubes in benign oesophageal stricture. *Acta Chir. Scand.*, **149**, 299–301.

Celestin, L. R. and Campbell W. B. (1981) A new and safe system for oesophageal dilatation. *Lancet*, **i**, 74–5.

Channer, K. S. and Virjee, J. (1982) Effect of posture and drink volume on the swallowing of capsules. *Br. Med. J.*, **285**, 1702.

Collins, F. J., Matthews, H. R., Baker, S. E. and Strakova, J. M. (1979) Drug-induced oesophageal injury. *Br. Med. J.*, **1**, 1673–6.

Cox, J. G. C., Buckton, G. K. and Bennett, J. R. (1987) Radial pressures during stricture dilatation with bougies and balloons. *Gut*, **28**, A1370–1.

Cox, J. G. C., Buckton, G. R. and Bennett, J. R. Benign oesophageal stricture – a new dilator (in press for *Gastrointestinal Endoscopy*).

Cox, J. G. C., Winter, R. K., Maslin, S. C. *et al.* (1988) Balloon or Bougie for dilatation of benign oesophageal stricture? An interim report of a randomised controlled trial. *Gut*, **29**, 1741–7.

Cranford, C. A. and Cushieri A. (1986) Benign oesophageal strictures, in *Surgery of the Oesophagus*, Baillière Tindall, London.

Croker, J. R., Vallon, A. G. and Cotton, P. B. (1980) Benign oesophageal stricture in the elderly – use of cimetidine and fibreoptic dilatation. *Age Ageing*, **9**, 53–8.

Dawood, R. M. and Hall, C. M. (1988) Too much radiation for too many children? *Br. Med. J.*, **296**, 1277–8.

Dawson, J. and Cockel, R. (1981) Oesophageal perforation at fibreoptic gastroscopy. *Br. Med. J.*, **283**, 583.

De Carle, D. J. (1974) Dilating oesophageal strictures. *Lancet*, **ii**, 224–5.

Didcot, C. C. (1973) Oesophageal strictures, treatment by slow continuous dilatation. *Ann. R. Coll. Surg. Engl.*, **53**, 112–26.

Dow, C. J. (1981) Oesophageal tuberculosis: four cases. *Gut*, **22**, 234–6.

Dumon, J., Meric, B., Sivak, M. V. and Fleisher, D. (1985) A new method of oesophageal dilatation using Savary–Gilliard bougies. *Gastrointest. Endosc.*, **31**, 379–82.

Dundee, J. W. and Pandit, S. K. (1972) Anterograde amnesic effects of pethidine, hyoscine and diazepam in adults. *Br. J. Pharmacol.*, **44**, 140–4.

Dyer, N. H., Cook, P. L. and Harper, R. A. K. (1969) Oesophageal stricture associated with Crohn's disease. *Gut*, **10**, 549–54.

Dyet, J. F., Bennett, J. R., Buckton, G. and Ashworth, D. (1983) The radiological measurement of oesophageal stricture diameter. *Clin. Radiol.*, **34**, 647–9.

Earlam, R. and Cunha-Melo, J. R. (1981) Benign oesophageal strictures: historical and technical aspects of dilatation. *Br. J. Surg.*, **68**, 829–36.

Eastman, M. C., Gear, M. W. L. and Nicol, A. (1978) An assessment of the accuracy of modern endoscopic diagnosis of oesophageal stricture. *Br. J. Surg.*, **65**, 182–5.

Edwards, D. A. W. (1984) Dysphagia. *Postgrad. Med. J.*, **60**, 737–42.

Evans, K. T. and Roberts, G. M. (1976) Where do all the tablets go? *Lancet*, **ii**, 1237–9.

Fellows, I. W., Raina, S. and Holmes, G. K. T. (1986) Celestin dilatation of benign oesophageal strictures; a review of 100 patients. *Am. J. Gastroenterol.*, **81**, 1052–4.

Ferguson, R., Dronfield, M. W. and Atkinson, M. (1979) Cimetidine in the treatment of reflux oesophagitis with peptic stricture. *Br. Med. J.*, **2**, 472–4.

Frimberger, E. (1983) Endoscopic treatment of benign oesophageal stricture. *Endoscopy*, **15**, 199–202.

Gear, M. W. L. (1981) Benign oesophageal strictures, in *Therapeutic Endoscopy and Radiology of the Gut*, Chapman and Hall, London.

Geboes, K., Janssens, J., Rutgeerts, P. and Vantrappen, G. (1986) Crohn's disease of the oesophagus. *J. Clin Gastroenterol.*, **8**, 31–7.

Gehanno, P. and Guedon, C. (1981) Inhibition of experimental oesophageal lye strictures by penicillamine. *Arch. Otolaryngol.*, **107**, 145–7.

Ginsburg, C. H., Braden, G. I., Tauber, A. I. and Trier, J. S. (1978) Oral clotrimazole in the treatment of oesophageal candidiasis. *Am. J. Med.*, **71**, 891–5.

Glick, M. E. (1982) Clinical course of oesophageal stricture managed by bougienage. *Dig. Dis. Sci.*, **27**, 884–8.

Goldberg, R. I., Manten, H. O. and Barkin, J. S. (1986) Oesophageal bougienage with triple metal olive dilators. *Gastrointest. Endosc.*, **32**, 226–8.

Goldthorn, J. F., Ball, W. S., Wilkinson, L. G. *et al.* (1984) Oesophageal strictures in children: treatment by serial balloon catheter dilatation. *Radiology*, **153**, 655–8.

Golladay, E. S., Tepas, J. J., Pickard, L. R. *et al.* (1980) Bacteraemia after oesophageal dilatation: a clinical and experimental study. *Ann. Thorac. Surg.*, **30**, 19–23.

Gotberg, S., Afzelius, L. E., Hambraeus, G. *et al.* (1982) Balloon-catheter dilatation of strictures in the upper digestive tract. *Radiology*, **22**, 479–83.

Graham, D. Y. and Smith, J. L. (1985) Balloon dilatation of benign and malignant oesophageal strictures: blind retrograde balloon dilatation. *Gastrointest. Endosc.*, **31**, 171–4.

Grobe, J. L., Kozarek, R. A. and Sanowski, R. A. (1984) Self-bougineage in the treatment of benign oesophageal stricture. *J. Clin. Gastroenterol.*, **6**, 109–12.

Groitl, H. (1982) Organische osophagusstenosen – moglichkeiten der operativen therapie, in *Endoskopische Prothetik*, Heumann, Hamburg.

Halpert, R. D., Feczko, P. J., Spickler, E. M. and Ackerman, L. V. (1985) Radiological assessment of dysphagia with endoscopic correlation. *Radiology*, **157**, 599–602.

Hasan, M. (1981) Misguided wire. *Gastrointest. Endosc.*, **27**, 109.

Hay, A. M. (1978) Stricture of the oesophagus associated with ankylosing spondylosis. *Br. Med. J.*, **1**, 1138.

Haynes, W. C., Sanowski, R. A., Foutch, P. G. and Bellapravalu, S. (1986) Oesophageal strictures following endoscopic variceal sclerotherapy: clinical course and response to dilatation therapy. *Gastrointest. Endosc.*, **32**, 202–5.

Heller, S. R., Fellows, I. W., Ogilvie, A. L. and Atkinson, M. (1982) Non-steroidal anti-inflammatory drugs and benign oesophageal stricture. *Br. Med. J.*, **285**, 167–8.

Hine, D. R., Hawkey, C. J., Atkinson, M. and Holmes, G. K. T. (1984) Comparison of the Eder–Puestow and Celestin technique for dilating benign oesophaeal strictures. *Gut*, **25**, 1100–2.

Huchzermeyer, H., Freise, J. and Becker, H. (1977) Dilatation of benign oesophageal strictures by peroral fiberendoscopic bougineage. *Endoscopy*, **9**, 207–11.

Isolauri, J. (1988) Colonic interposition for benign oesophageal disease: long-term clinical and endoscopic results. *Am. J. Surg.*, **155**, 498–502.

John, V., Stirling, A. J. and Matthews, H. R. (1978) Rheumatoid stricture of the oesophagus. *Br. Med. J.*, **1**, 479.

Johnsen, A., Ingemann Jensen, L. and Mauritzen, K. (1986) Balloon-dilatation of oesophageal strictures in children. *Pediatr. Radiol.*, **16**, 388–91.

Jones, J. D. and Bozymski, E. M. (1979) Instrumental oesophageal perforation. *Dig. Dis. Sci.*, **24**, 319–20.

Katz, D. (1967) Morbidity and mortality in standard and flexible gastrointestinal endoscopy. *Gastrointest. Endosc.*, **14**, 134–7.

Keshishian, J. M., Smyth, N. P. D., Maxwell, D. D. and Chua, L. (1984) Dilatation of difficult strictures of the oesophagus. *Surg. Gynecol. Obstet.*, **158**, 499.

Kikendall, J. W., Friedman, A. C., Oyewole, M. A. *et al.* (1983) Pill-induced oesophageal injury. *Dig. Dis. Sci.*, **28**, 174–82.

Kollath, J., Starck, E. and Vittorio, P. (1984) Dilation of oesophageal stenosis by balloon catheter. *Cardiovasc. Intervent. Radiol.* **7**, 35–9.

Korompai, F. L. and Hayward, R. H. (1984) Modification of Eder–Puestow dilators. *Ann. Thorac. Surg.*, **38**, 301.

Kozarek, R. A. (1986) Hydrostatic balloon dilatation of gastrointestinal stenoses: a national survey. *Gastrointest. Endosc.*, **32**, 15–9.

Lanza, F. L. and Graham, D. Y. (1978) Bougienage is effective therapy for most benign oesophageal strictures. *J. A. M. A.*, **240**, 844–7.

Leading Article (1988) Midazolam – is antagonism justified? *Lancet*, **ii**, 140–2.

Leahy, A. L., Gorey, T. F. and McMullin, J. P. (1986) Serial dilatation of peptic strictures of the oesophagus: a planned approached. *Ir. J. Med. Sci.*, **155**, 389–91.

Lee, M., Ravenscroft, M. M., Green, J. R. B. and Swan, C. H. J. (1983) Safe outpatient dilatation of benign oesophageal strictures. *Gut*, **24**, A1008.

Lehman, G. A. and O'Connor, K. W. (1985) Endoscopic tape dilator – a new and inexpensive method to dilate upper gastrointestinal strictures. *J. Clin. Gastroenterol.*, **7**, 208–10.

Lehmann, K. G., Blair, D. N., Siskind, B. N. and Wohlgelernter, D. (1987) Right atrial-oesophageal fistula and hydropneumopericardium after oesophageal dilatation. *J. Am. Coll. Cardiol.*, **9**, 969–72.

Lifton, L. J. (1983) Multiple oesophageal dilatations at a single session. *Gastrointest. Endosc.*, **29**, 114–5.

Lilly, J. O. and McCaffery, T. D. (1971) Oesophageal stricture dilatation: a new method adapted to the fibreoptic oesophagoscope. *Am. J. Dig. Dis.*, **16**, 1137–40.

Lindor, K. D., Ott, B. J. and Hughes, R. W. (1985) Balloon dilatation of upper digestive tract strictures. *Gastroenterology*, **89**, 545–8.

Little, A. G., Mannheim, T. S., Ferguson, M. K. and Skinner, D. B. (1988) Surgical management of oesophageal strictures. *Ann. Thorac. Surg.*, **45**, 144–7.

Loffler, A., Dienst, C. and Velasco, S. B. (1986) International survey of laser therapy in benign gastrointestinal tumours and stenoses. *Endoscopy*, **18**, 62–5 (suppl. 1).

Luna, L. L. (1983) Endoscopic therapy of benign oesophageal stricture. *Endoscopy*, **15**, 203–6.

McDonald, H. F. (1978) Right pneumothorax following fibreoptic oesophageal dilatation. *Endoscopy*, **10**, 130–2.

McLean, G. K., Cooper, G. S., Hartz, W. H., Burke, D. R. and Merantze, S. G. (1987) Radiologically guided balloon dilatation of gastrointestinal strictures, **165**, 35–40.

MacGowan, K. M. (1980) Celestin tube disruption. *Br. J. Surg.*, **67**, 421–4.

Mandelstam, P., Sugawa, C., Silvis, S. E. *et al.* (1976) Complications associated with oesophagogastroduodenoscopy and with oesophageal dilatation. *Gastrointest. Endosc.*, **23**, 16–9.

Maxton, D. G., Ainley, C. C., Grainger, S. L., Morris, R. W., and Thompson, R. P. H. (1987) Teeth and benign oesophageal stricture. Gut, **28**, 61–3.

Mills, L. J., Estrera, A. S. and Platt, M. R. (1979) Avoidance of oesophageal stricture following severe caustic burns by the use of an intraluminal stent. *Ann. Thorac. Surg.*, **28**, 60–5.

Moghissi, K. (1977) Carcinoma of the cardia and thoracic oesophagus coexisting with and following sliding hiatal hernia and peptic stricture. *Thorax*, **32**, 342–5.

Netscher, D. T. and Richardson, J. D. (1984) Complications requiring operative intervention in scleroderma. *Surg. Gynecol. Obstet.*, **158**, 507–12.

Niv, Y., Bat, L. and Motro, M. (1985) Bacterial endocarditis after Hurst bougienage in a patient with a benign oesophageal stricture and mitral valve prolapse. *Gastrointest. Endosc.*, **31**, 265–7.

Oakes, D. D. and Sherck, J. P. (1985) Drug-induced oesophagitis, in *Oesophageal Disorders: Pathophysiology and Therapy*, Raven, New York, pp. 241–6.

Oakes, D. D., Sherck, J. P. and Mark, J. B. D. (1982) Lye ingestion: clinical patterns and therapeutic implications. *J. Thorac. Cardiovasc. Surg.* **83**, 194–204.

Ogilvie, A. L., Ferguson, F. and Atkinson. M. (1980) Outlook with conservative treatment of peptic oesophageal stricture. *Gut*, **21**, 23–5.

Olsen, H. W., Lawrence, W. A., Bottarini, G. and Pises, P. (1977) The fibreoptic approach to dilatation of stenotic lesions of the oesophagus. *Gastrointest. Endosc.*, **23**, 201–2.

Orenstein, S. R. and Whitington, P. F. (1985) Oesophageal stricture dilatation in awake children. *J. Pediatr. Gastroenterol Nutr.*, **4**, 557–62.

Orlando, R. C. and Bozymski, E. M. (1973) Heartburn in pernicious anaemia – a consequence of bile reflux. *N. Engl. J. Med.*, **289**, 522–3.

Ott, D. J., Men Chen, Y., Wu, W. C. and Gelfand, D. W. (1985) Endoscopic sensitivity in the detection of oesophageal strictures. *J. Clin. Gastroenterol.*, **7**, 121–5.

Palmer, E. D., (1968) The hiatal hernia–oesophagitis stricture complex; twenty year prospective study. *Am. J. Med.*, **44**, 566–79.

Palmer, E. D. (1970) Broken nose in the endoscopy clinic. *Gastrointest. Endosc.*, **17**, 69.

Patterson, D. J., Graham, D. Y., Lacey Smith, J. *et al.* (1983) Natural history of benign oesophageal stricture treated by dilatation. *Gastroenterology*, **85**, 346–50.

Poelman, J. R., Hausman, R. H. and Hoitsma, H. F. W. (1977) Endoscopy in lye burns of oesophagus and stomach. *Endoscopy*, **9**, 172–7.

Price, J. D., Stanciu, C. and Bennett, J. R. (1974) A safer method of dilating oesophageal strictures. *Lancet*, **i**, 1141–2.

Puestow, K. L. (1955) Conservative treatment of stenosing diseases of the oesophagus. *Postgrad. Med.*, **18**, 6–14.

Quayle, A. R., Moore, P. J., Jacob, G. *et al.* (1985) Treatment of oesophageal perforation by intubation. *Ann. R. Coll. Surg. Engl.*, **57**, 101–2.

Rago, E., Boesby, S. and Spencer, J. (1983) Results of Eder–Puestow dilatation in the management of oesophageal peptic strictures. *Am. J. Gastroenterol.*, **78**, 6–8.

Raines, D. R., Branche, W. C., Anderson, D. L. and Boyce, H. W. (1975) The occurrence of bacteraemia after oesophageal dilatation. *Gastrointest. Endosc.*, **22**, 86–7.

Raptis, S. and Mearns Milne, D. (1972) A review of the management of 100 cases of benign stricture of the oesophagus. *Thorax*, **27**, 599–603.

Raskin, J. B., Manten, H., Harary, A., Redlhammer, D. E. and Rogers, A. I. (1985) Transendoscopic electrosurgical incision of lower oesophageal (Schatzki) rings: a new treatment modality. *Gastrointest. Endosc.*, **31**, 391–3.

Royston, C. M. S., Dowling, B. L. and Gear, M. W. L. (1976) Oesophageal dilatation using Eder–Puestow Dilators. *Am. J. Surg.*, **131**, 697–700.

Royston, C. M. S., Dowling, B. L. and Spencer, J. (1975) Antrectomy with Roux-en Y anastomosis in the treatment of peptic oesophagitis with stricture. *Br. J. Surg.*, **62**, 605–7.

Sagar, P. M. and Macfie, J. (1987) Iatrogenic splenic trauma – a rare complication following oesophageal dilatation. *Gastrointest. Endosc.*, **33**, 333–4.

Sander, R. and Poesl, H. (1986) Treatment of non-neoplastic stenoses with the neodymium-YAG laser – indications and limitations. *Endoscopy*, **18**, 53–6 (suppl. 1).

Sanderson, C. J. and Trotter, G. A. (1980) Eder–Puestow oesophageal dilatation: a new hazard. *Br. J. Surg.*, **67**, 300–1.

Sato, Y., Frey, E. E., Smith, W. L. *et al.* (1988) Balloon dilatation of oesophageal strictures in children. *A. J. R.*, **150**, 639–42.

Sawyer, R. (1985) Treatment of upper oesophageal strictures. *Otolaryngol. Head Neck Surg.*, **93**, 379–84.

Schlitt, M., Mitchem, L., Zorn, G. *et al.* (1985) Brain abscess after oesophageal dilatation for caustic stricture: report of three cases. *Neurosurgery*, **17**, 947–51.

Seltzer, S. E., Jones, B. and McLaughlin, G. C. (1979) Proper choice of contrast agents in emergency gastrointestinal radiology. *C.R.C. Crit. Rev. Diagn. Imaging.*, **12**, 79–99.

Sharpe, M. S., Chalmers, A. H. and Gough, K. R. (1986) Cannulation of difficult oesophageal strictures with angiographic catheters. *Br. Med. J.*, **293**, 240.

Shirazi, S. S., Schulze, K., and Soper, R. I. (1987) Long-term follow-up for treatment of complicated chronic reflux oesophagitis. *Arch. Surg.*, **122**, 548–52.

Sorensen, T. I. A., Burchath, F., Pedersen M. L. and Findall, E. (1984) Oesophageal stricture and dysphagia after endoscopic sclerotherapy for bleeding varices. *Gut.* **25**, 473–7.

Spechler, S. J., Sperber, H., Doos, W. G. and Schimmel, E. M. (1983) The prevalence of Barrett's oesophagus in patients with chronic peptic oesophageal strictures. *Dig. Dis. Sci.*, **28**, 769–74.

Starck, E., Paolucci, V., Herzer, M. and Crummy, A. B. (1984) Oesophageal stenosis: treatment with balloon catheters. *Radiology*, **153**, 637–40.

Starlinger, M., Appel, W. H., Schemper, M. and Schiessel, R. (1985) Long-term treatment of peptic oesophageal stenosis with dilatation and cimetidine: factors influencing clinical result. *Eur. Surg. Res.*, **17**, 207–14.

Stephenson, P. M., Dorrington, L., Harris, O. D. and Rao A. (1977) Bacteraemia following dilatation and oesophago-gastroscopy. *Aust. N.Z. J. Med.*, **7**, 32.

Stirling, M. C. and Orringer, M. R. (1988) The combined Collis–Nissen operation for oesophageal reflux stricture. *Ann. Thorac. Surg.*, **45**, 148–57.

Stoddard, C. J. and Simms, J. M. (1984) Dilatation of benign oesophageal strictures in the outpatient department. *Br. J. Surg.*, **71**, 752–3.

Stringer, D. A., Pablot, S. M. and Mancer, K. (1985) Gruntzig angioplasty dilatation of an oesophageal stricture in an infant. *Pediatr. Radiol.*, **15**, 424–6.

Thanik, K. D., Chey, W. Y., Ashok, N. S. and Gutierrez, J. G. (1980) Reflux oesophagitis: effect of oral bethanechol on symptoms and endoscopic findings. *Ann. Intern. Med.*, **93**, 805–8.

Tulman, A. B. and Boyce H. W. (1981) Complications of oesophageal dilatation and guidelines for their prevention. *Gastrointest. Endosc.*, **27**, 229–34.

Vejlsted, H. and Struve-Christensen, E. (1977) The effect of dilatation in the treatment of benign oesophageal strictures. *Scand. J. Thorac. Cardiovasc. Surg.*, **11**, 71–4.

Walt, R., Logan, R., Katschinski, B. *et al.* (1986) Rising frequency of ulcer perforation in elderly people in the United Kingdom. *Lancet*, **i**, 489–92.

Washer, G. F., Gear, M. W. L., Dowling, B. L. *et al.* (1984) Randomised prospective trial of Roux-en-Y duodenal diversion versus fundoplication for severe reflux oesophagitis. *Br. J. Surg.*, **71**, 181–4.

Wason, S. (1985) The emergency treatment of caustic ingestions. *J. Emerg. Med.*, **2**, 175–82.

Watson, A. (1984) The role of antireflux surgery combined with fibreoptic endoscopic dilatation in peptic oesophageal stricture. *Am. J. Surg.*, **148**, 346–9.

Watson, A. (1987) Reflux stricture of the oesophagus. *Br. J. Surg.*, **74**, 443–8.

Webb, W. A. and McDaniel, L. (1984) Endoscopic evaluation of dysphagia in two hundred and ninety-three patients with benign disease. *Surg. Gynecol. Obstet.*, **158**, 152–6.

Wesdorp, I. L. E., Bartelsman, J. F. W. M., Den Hartog Jager, F. C. A. *et al.* (1982) Results of conservative treatment of benign oesophageal strictures: a follow up study in 100 patients. *Gastroenterology*, **82**, 487–93.

Wesdorp, I. C. E. (1986) Critical evaluation of controlled trials in the treatment of reflux oesophagitis, in *Controlled Therapeutic Trials in Gastroenterology*, Raven, New York.

Wijburg, F. A., Beukers, M. M., Heymans, H. H. *et al.* (1985) Nasogastric intubation as sole treatment of caustic oesophageal lesions. *Ann. Otol. Rhinol. Laryngol.*, **94**, 337–41.

Wilkins, W. E., Ridley, M. G. and Pozniak, A. L.

(1984) Benign stricture of the oesophagus: role of non-steroidal anti-inflammatory drugs. *Gut*, **25**, 478–80.

Wilson, M. G., Bristol, J. B., Mortensen, N. J. and John, H. T. (1980) The Celestin tube in the treatment of benign oesophageal strictures. *Br. J. Surg.*, **67**, 506–8.

Winkler, W. P., Haroutiounian G., Baer, J. W. *et al.* (1985) Transgastric oesophageal bougienage via a feeding gastrostomy. *Gastrointest. Endosc.*, **31**, 277–9.

Wychulis, A. R., Fontana, R. S. and Payne, W. S. (1969) Instrumental perforation of the oesophagus. *Dis. Chest.*, **55**, 184–9.

Yin, T. P. and Dellipiani, A. W. (1983) Bacterial endocarditis after Hurst bougienage in a patient with a benign oesophageal stricture. *Endoscopy*, **15**, 27–8.

Zaninotto, G., Bonavina, L., Pianalto, S. *et al.* (1986) Oesophageal strictures following nasogastric intubation. *Int. Surg.*, **71**, 100–3.

CHAPTER FOUR

Balloon dilatation of upper digestive tract strictures

K. D. Lindor

4.1 INTRODUCTION

Dilatation with balloons offers an alternative to mechanical dilatation of oesophageal strictures and allows one to approach strictures of the pylorus or duodenum that were previously inaccessible to endoscopic dilatation. Balloon dilators are simple to use and control while dilating strictures and appear to be safe and effective.

4.2 OESOPHAGEAL STRICTURES

4.2.1 TECHNIQUES

We use Olympus GIF-XQ10 endoscopes, which have a 9.8-mm outside diameter and a 2.8-mm biopsy channel, are manoeuvrable and small enough to pass through many strictures narrow enough to cause dysphagia. Compared with smaller diameter paediatric endoscopes the XQ10 has enough rigidity to allow the operator to gain a feel for the tightness of the stricture. The 2.8-mm channel allows the use of standard biopsy forceps and 'through-the-endoscope' balloons (see below).

The patients are positioned in the left lateral decubitus position on a movable fluoroscopy table beneath a fixed fluoroscope. Patients undergoing routine diagnostic endoscopy are generally sedated with 2–5 mg midazolam given intravenously through a 21-gauge butterfly needle. Patients scheduled for dilatation are generally given 25–50 mg pethidine (meperidine) intravenously as well.

The endoscope is introduced, the stricture identified and a complete endoscopic examination of the stomach and proximal duodenum is performed, if the stricture allows passage of the endoscope. Cytological brushings and biopsies are obtained from the stricture. A guide-wire is passed into the distal stomach and the endoscope withdrawn over the wire. If the stricture is above the level of the diaphragm, the tip of the endoscope can be used to identify its position radiologically. Available guide-wires include a Teflon-coated wire 0.038 in (0.097 mm) in diameter, 300 cm long (Cook, Bloomington, Indiana, USA) and a soft-tipped steel Eder–Puestow guide-wire. Both guide-wires are radiopaque.

In patients with strictures so tight that the endoscope can not be passed, the guide-wire is positioned fluoroscopically. In these patients, we defer cytological brushing and biopsies until the stricture has been dilated because bleeding induced by brushing and biopsy may obscure the lumen and make passage of the guide-wire more difficult. Histological specimens are obtained after dilatation when the remainder of the upper gut is examined through the dilated stricture.

Balloons are available in diameters 6, 8, 10, 12, 15, 20 and 25 mm (Rigiflex balloons) which are passed over a wire (Microvasive, Milford, Massachusetts, USA) (Figure 4.1). Balloons

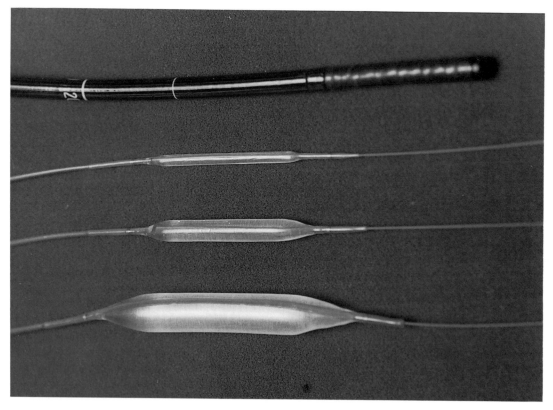

Figure 4.1 Balloon dilators for use with a guide-wire. The balloon sizes shown are 6, 10 and 20 mm. Balloons have been placed over a Cook's guide-wire. An Olympus GIF-XQ10 is shown for size comparison.

can be cold sterilized to allow repeated use. The balloon is inflated with dilute (33%) hypaque to allow easier cleansing of the balloon's interior. The use of fluid rather than air is necessary to ensure full inflation of the balloon. Air is so compressible that a rigid stricture might prevent full inflation, whereas the use of relatively incompressible liquid allows steady reproducible pressure to be applied by the balloon. The balloons are readily seen with the use of radiopaque contrast. The size of the balloon used depends on the endoscopist's judgement. Successively larger diameter balloons can be used at the same sitting or a few days later, depending on the patient's response to the initial dilatation. Especially tight or long strictures often require

multiple dilatations over the course of several days.

After a trial inflation to test for leaks and remove air bubbles, the fluid is withdrawn into a 35-cm^2 syringe. While the fluid is removed, the balloon can be folded over onto itself to decrease its width, and this position is maintained with gentle suction. This allows the balloon to be readily passed through the mouth and pharynx and reduces patient discomfort. The balloon is threaded over the guide-wire, the patient is asked to swallow, and the balloon is advanced. Radiopaque markers on the catheter distal and proximal to the balloon aid in positioning it. Once positioned in the area of the stricture, the balloon is partially inflated. The stricture indents the balloon's contour, and if necessary, minor repositioning can be done to ensure that the stricture lies at or near the middle of the balloon. The balloon is then inflated until the stricture indentation, monitored fluoroscopically, is obliterated. Once the balloon is fully inflated, full pressure is held for 30–60 seconds. We have not used manometers to measure inflation pressures but have had our endoscopic assistants apply steady pressure with a 35-cm^2 syringe. After 30–60 seconds of sustained pressure the inflated balloon can be withdrawn through the mouth to exclude the presence of other more proximal strictures. If necessary, endoscopy is repeated and biopsies taken. After the procedure the patient is moved to the recovery room and observed for an hour. If free of discomfort, they are asked to drink a small amount of water. If swallowed water or spontaneously initiated swallows elicit pain, the patients are sent for a water-soluble radiopaque radiological examination. If pain persists or extravasation is seen, the patients are admitted for observation and management of suspected or proven perforation.

4.2.2 COMPLICATIONS

Complications arising from balloon dilatation are those associated with any endoscopic or dilatation procedure: aspiration, perforation and bleeding. It has been suggested that balloons allow dilatation to be more controllable and may be associated with fewer complications, but this contention is not supported by the little comparative data available.

4.2.3 RESULTS

Our initial experience (Lindor, Ott and Hughes, 1985) was in 88 patients with oesophageal strictures; 69 were benign, and 19 were associated with malignant disease. Successful dilatation, as judged by the endoscopist at the time of the procedure, was achieved in 93% of patients. For benign stric-

tures, the success rate was 99%, while for strictures associated with malignancy (11 of 19 had previous operation for oesophageal cancer) the success rate was 89%. Follow-up was available in 95% of patients. Ninety-one per cent of patients who were alive felt that the procedure had provided symptomatic improvement lasting for a median duration of 10 months. Of patients with benign oesophageal strictures, 35% required a repeat dilatation during the period of follow-up; 73% of patients with strictures associated with malignancy required repeat dilatations, and 78% of patients with strictures associated with cancer died during the follow-up observation period.

Minor complications occurred in only three patients; pain in two patients and minor mucosal tears in one patient. None required hospitalization.

The results of our initial experience are summarized in Table 4.1 and compare favourably with other large series of patients managed with conventional dilators. Rupture or perforation are much more likely to occur with malignant than with benign structures. In a recent series of 170 dilatations in 35 patients, there were two perforations of malignant strictures (9.3%) but one in a benign stricture (0.8%) (Maynar *et al.*, 1988).

4.3 PYLORIC AND DUODENAL STRICTURES

Strictures at the pylorus or within the duodenum are difficult to dilate with conventional mechanical dilators. The length of the dilators is often insufficient to reach the stricture; and, more importantly, application of dilating pressure is often unsuccessful because of the shape of the stomach. With mechanical dilators, all force is directed in an orad-caudad direction. Redirection of this force into a transverse or caudad-orad direction relies on the dilator being turned horizontally or upward by the greater curvature of the stomach. Although occasionally successful, the guide-

Table 4.1 Results of balloon dilatation of oesophageal strictures

	Success		Complications (%)	Symptomatic improvement (%)	Further procedure done (%)
	No.	%			
Benign	69	99	1	90	35
Malignant	19	89	11	91	73

wire is usually dislodged from the pylorus, or the dilator can not be passed through the stricture. Formerly, these strictures usually required surgical correction, but the availability of balloon dilators allows endoscopic management of many of these pyloric or duodenal strictures.

4.3.1 TECHNIQUE

The patient is positioned and sedated as described previously for oesophageal strictures. The endoscope is used to examine the upper gastrointestinal tract and specifically to identify the stricture. The endoscopist has two options for balloon dilatation of these strictures, balloon dilatation over a wire or dilatation using a through-the-scope balloon.

Balloon dilatation over a wire is performed as detailed above. Briefly, a Cook's guide-wire or a stiffer Eder–Puestow guide-wire is passed via the endoscope through the stricture and positioned in the distal duodenum or proximal jejunum under fluoroscopic guidance. Next, the deflated balloon is passed over the wire and positioned within the strictured area as assessed fluoroscopically. The balloon is inflated under fluoroscopic control, held inflated for 30 seconds, deflated and withdrawn over the wire. If judged feasible, based on ease of stretching of the stricture and patient's comfort, the next larger size balloon can be introduced and the process repeated. Finally, the balloon and wire are withdrawn, and the endoscope can be re-introduced and the stricture and the area beyond inspected.

A newer approach relies on balloons (Rigiflex TTS, Microvasive, Milford, Mass-achusetts, USA) passed through the endoscope (Figure 4.2). These balloons range in size from 4 to 25 mm. They allow the endoscopist to inspect the stricture and watch through the endoscope as well as fluoroscopically as dilatation proceeds. The balloons are clear, and the stricture can be seen through the balloon with the endoscope. These balloons appear to be most useful for strictures of the pylorus, particularly in J-shaped stomachs, because the balloon catheter can be manipulated and directed through the endoscope. Disadvantages include the lack of a guide-wire passed through the stricture to provide an avenue of safe passage and the relatively stiff tip which must be passed blindly through the stricture; these features of through-the-scope balloons could potentially lead to penetration of the bowel wall distal to the stricture as the balloon is positioned. This theoretical disadvantage should not overshadow the usefulness of these balloons in dilating pyloric or duodenal strictures.

It is important that the through-the-scope balloons be lubricated with a silicone material prior to inserting them into the scope. Without lubricant it is difficult to move the balloon catheter forward or backwards. The balloon is inflated using a manometer to monitor pressure; the desired pressure varies with the size of balloon and is indicated in the manufacturer's product insert. Before removing the balloon, care must be taken to completely remove the sterile fluid used to inflate it using the size of syringe specified by the manufacturer. Failure to do so may cause the balloon to lodge in the biopsy channel of the 'scope and necessitate expensive repairs, as well as

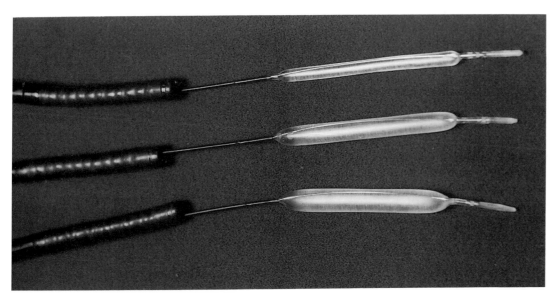

Figure 4.2   Rigiflex TTS Balloons placed through Olympus GIF-XQ10 endoscopes. The size (top to bottom), are 6, 8 and 10 mm.

damaging the balloon. Rapid decompression may be achieved by use of the endoscopic suction machine to evacuate the balloon.

4.3.2 RESULTS

We have previously reported our experience in dilating strictures of the stomach or pyloro-duodenal area in 23 patients (Lindor, Ott and Hughes, 1985). Successful dilatation with balloons passed over a guide-wire were accomplished in 87% of patients. Two-thirds of patients alive at follow-up experienced symptomatic improvement lasting a median period of 12 months. One-third of patients required further procedures such as operation or repeat dilatations. No complications were noted in this small series. Craig and Gillespie (1988) report 13 good results in 14 patients without complications.

4.4 CONCLUSIONS

Balloon dilatation of upper digestive tract strictures is both safe and effective. On theoretical grounds, the complication rate might be expected to be lower with this technique. The forces generated by balloon dilators are directed radially against the stricture and do not include longitudinal shearing forces such as those generated by conventional mechanical dilators (Abele, 1980). These longitudinal shearing forces may be responsible for some perforations, but absolute evidence of greater safety is lacking.

A major disadvantage of the balloons is their expense. The balloons that are passed over a wire cost $90 each and those that are passed through the endoscope cost $125 each. In our experience, balloons can be used an average of three times before they leak or rupture; therefore, there is considerable expense involved in keeping a wide range of balloons available. Mechanical dilators, on the other hand, can be re-used indefinitely, and the only cost associated with them is the initial purchase price.

Controlled clinical trials are needed to assess further the efficacy, indications, and any advantages in safety of these balloons before their exact role in the management of upper digestive tract strictures is known; the first such trial is reported in Chapter 3, and the results of others should be available soon.

REFERENCES

Abele, J. E. (1980) Balloon catheters and transluminal dilatation: technical considerations. *A.J.R.*, **135**, 901–6.

Craig, P. T. and Gillespie, P. E. (1988) Through the endoscope balloon dilatation of benign gastric outlet obstruction. *Br. Med. J.*, **297**, 396.

Lindor, K. D., Ott, B. J. and Hughes, R. W. (1985) Balloon dilatation of upper digestive tract strictures. *Gastroenterology*, **89**, 545–8.

Maynar, M., Guerra, C., Reyes, R. *et al.* (1988) *Radiology*, **167**, 703–6.

CHAPTER FIVE

Palliative treatment for oesophageal carcinoma

J. R. Bennett

Carcinoma of the oesophagus or cardia, if left untreated, inevitably results in relentlessly progressive dysphagia and death from nutritional impairment and fluid depletion, or from aspiration into the respiratory tract. Even with prompt diagnosis the majority have already passed the stage at which curative resection is possible, and palliation becomes the primary aim.

Palliation of incurable oesophageal carcinoma is important because radical resection carries a high mortality, and the unpleasant alternative of terminal complete oesophageal obstruction needs to be avoided. An ideal palliative technique would provide normal swallowing for the patient's remaining days by a technique which was quick, safe, painless, needing only a short inpatient stay and having a low complication rate. Attempts to secure this paradigm have resulted in many treatments, unfortunately not usually subjected to well-controlled trials.

Operation by a skilled surgeon can lead to excellent palliation because it usually relieves dysphagia completely, but the morbidity and a mortality of 7–29% is a considerable price (Belsey, 1980; Conlan et al., 1983; Cunha-Melo, 1980; McKeown, 1985; Orringer, 1984 a,b; Watson, 1982). Operations which avoid thoracotomy, intrathoracic anastomosis, multiple abdominal anastomoses and a bypassed unresected oesophagus probably give the safest surgical palliation, although Ellis, Gibb

and Watkins (1983) report 167 oesophagogastrectomies with two deaths and 22 major complications. Although age itself is not a contraindication to surgery (Mohansingh, 1976; Sugimachi et al., 1985; Williamson, 1985), some older patients will tolerate imperfect swallowing in order to avoid surgery. Nevertheless, anyone discarding surgery in favour of some other palliative manoeuvre must realize that a few patients may miss an unrecognized chance of cure, because preoperative staging is difficult even using computerized tomography and endoscopic ultrasound. Conservative management (choice of food, posture, corticosteroids) alone helps many patients (Sykes, Barnes and Carter 1988).

Simple dilatation of the malignant stricture with bougie or balloon still has a place as not all growths narrow quickly. Multiple dilatations are usually needed (Cassidy, Nord and Boyce, 1981; Moses et al., 1985) and if the need becomes frequent alternative forms of palliation should be chosen.

Tubes placed through a growth found to be inoperable at the time of surgical exploration may work well, but planned surgical intubation through a gastrotomy in patients known to have an inoperable growth has been generally abandoned because of the disproportionately high morbidity and mortality (Lishman, Dellipiani and Devlin, 1980; Watson, 1982).

Endoscopic intubation (Chapter 6) has many attractive features, especially for the frail and elderly for whom the single procedure, usually without general anaesthesia, needs only a short hospital stay and gives immediate improvement in swallowing. These are considerable therapeutic gains, but the 'tube existence' which forbids solid food, the care required to keep the tube patent and the risk of subsequent tube migration detract from it. The expertise of the operator is an essential prerequisite and frail patients may still do poorly, despite skill and experience. Reported mortality varies from 2% to 27% (Den Hartog Jager, Bartelsman and Tytgat, 1979; Diamantes and Mannell, 1983). Newly designed tubes are an improvement on earlier models, but recurrent growth sometimes blocks a previously well-placed tube.

Laser disobliteration (Chapter 7) avoids some of the shortcomings of tubes, and potentially offers better relief from dysphagia. However, the number of patients treated so far in most centres is still relatively small. Skill in its use has to be learned but practised units (Bown *et al.*, 1987; Krasner *et al.*, 1987) report the achievement of good swallowing with over a third of patients eating normally and more than a further third eating most solids; complication rates are low. Ell *et al.* (1986) reported fair results in 1359 patients with malignant upper gastrointestinal stenosis, of whom 816 had oesophageal carcinoma. They claimed success in 83% with a perforation rate for the whole series of 2.1% and a mortality of 1%. The full potential of laser treatment has probably not yet been achieved and tuneable wavelength lasers, contact laser probes, laser-resistant guide probes (Ell *et al.*, 1986), photosensitive dyes, and the additional use of local anaesthetic injections into the growth (Fleischer and Sivak, 1985) may improve results further.

The effect of palliative radiotherapy is difficult to assess (Earlam, 1984) but at least half the patients with advanced oesophageal carcinoma respond badly (Koch *et al.*, 1967; Pearson, 1981) and dysphagia is not always well relieved (Kelsen, 1982). However, the new technique of intracavitary radiation appears to offer good palliation (Chapter 12). There have not been any extensive trials of this technique but its attractive features include its ease of outpatient use and the general availability and cheapness of equipment. It may also be particularly suitable for proximal lesions.

There are other putative palliative techniques still in the research stage. Early reports on the BICAP tumour probe suggest this may be safe and cheap, although oesophageal stricture can be a complication (as it can be after laser therapy) (Johnston *et al.*, 1987; Jensen *et al.*, 1988). Combination chemotherapy has its proponents (Kelsen *et al.*, 1983; Liechman *et al.*, 1984) and phototherapy has given promising results (McCaughan, Williams and Bethell, 1985). Hypothermochemoradiotherapy is a further technique under trial (Sugimachi, Kai and Inokuchi, 1985).

There is a great need for controlled and randomized trials of palliative techniques, and assessments should include measures of the quality of life, agreed dysphagia scores and performance status and time to recurrence of symptoms, rather than simply the duration of survival. These treatments should not be considered competitive, for they can be complementary. Combined treatment schedules may allow more rapid treatment and open the possibility of outpatient management with fewer visits (Lightdale, Zimbalist and Winawer, 1987).

The management options are still increasing and if patients are to be given the best chance a strong case can be made for assessment and treatment of oesophageal carcinoma in specialized centres, as few centres can offer every treatment option and the numbers of patients are limited.

The descriptions which follow about intubation, laser treatment and intracavitary radiation give further insight into the methodology and possibilities for these therapies.

REFERENCES

Belsey, R. H. R. (1980) Palliative management of oesophageal carcinoma. *Am. J. Surg.*, **139**, 789–94.

Bown, S. G., Hawes, R., Matthewson, K. *et al.* (1987) Endoscopic laser palliation for advanced malignant dysphagia. *Gut*, **28**, 799–807.

Cassidy, D. E., Nord, H. J. and Boyce, H. W. Jr (1981) Management of malignant oesophageal strictures: role of oesophageal dilatation and peroral prosthesis. *Am. J. Gastroenterol.*, **76**, 173.

Conlan, A. A., Nicolaou, N., Hammond, C. A. *et al.* (1983) Retrosternal gastric bypass for inoperable esophageal cancer: a report of 71 patients. *Ann. Thorac. Surg.*, **36**, 396–401.

Den Hartog Jager, F. C. A., Bartelsman, J. F. W. M. and Tytgat, G. N. J. (1979) Palliative treatment of obstructing esophagogastric malignancy by endoscopic positioning of a plastic prosthesis. *Gastroenterology*, **77**, 1008–14.

Diamantes, T. and Mannell, A. (1983) Oesophageal intubation for advanced oesophageal cancer: the Baragwanath experience 1977–1981. *Br. J. Surg.*, **70**, 555–7.

Earlam, R. (1984) Oesophageal cancer treatment in North East Thames region 1981: medical audit using Hospital Activity Analysis data. *Br. Med. J.*, **288**, 1892–4.

Earlam, R. and Cunha-Melo, J. R. (1980) Oesophageal squamous cell carcinoma: a critical review of radiotherapy. *Br. J. Surg.*, **67**, 457–61.

Ell Ch. Reimann, J. F., Lux, G. and Demling, L. (1988) Palliative laser treatment of malignant stenoses in the upper gastrointestinal tract. *Endoscopy*, **18**, suppl. 1, 21–6.

Ellis, F. H., Gibb, S. P. and Watkins, E. (1983) Oesophagogastrectomy: a safe, sidely applicable and expeditious form of palliation for patients with carcinoma of the oesophagus and cardia. *Ann. Surg.*, **198**, 531–40.

Fleischer, D. and Sivak, M. V. (1985) Endoscopic Nd:YAG laser therapy as palliation for esophagogastric cancer: parameters affecting initial outcome. *Gastroenterology*, **89**, 827–31.

Jensen, D. M., Machicado, G., Bandall, G. *et al.* (1988) Comparison of low-power YAG laser and BICAP tumour probe for palliation of esophageal cancer strictures. *Gastroenterology*, **94**, 1263–70.

Johnston, J. H., Fleischer, D., Petrini, J. and Nord, H. J. (1987) Palliative bipolar electrocoagulation therapy of obstructing esophageal cancer. *Gastrointest. Endosc.* **33**, 349–53.

Kelsen, D. (1982) Treatment of advanced oesophageal cancer. *Cancer*, **50**, suppl. 2, 2576–81.

Kelsen, D., Hilaris, B., Coonley, C. *et al.* (1983) Cisplatin, Vindesine, and Bleomycin chemotherapy of local-regional and advanced esophageal carcinoma. *Am. J. Med.*, **75**, 645–52.

Koch, N. G., Lewin, E., Petterson, S. *et al.* (1967) Carcinoma of the thoracic oesophagus and cardia: a review of 146 cases. *Acta Chir. Scand.*, **133**, 375.

Krasner, N., Barr, H., Skidmore, C. and Morris, A. I. (1987) Palliative laser therapy for malignant dysphagia. *Gut*, **28**, 792–8.

Liechman, L., Steiger, Z., Seydel, H. D. and Vatkevicius, V. K. (1984) Combined pre-operative chemotherapy and radiation therapy for cancer of the oesophagus: the Wayne State University. South West Oncology Group and Radiation Therapy Oncology Group experience. *Semin. Oncol.*, **11**, 178–85.

Lightdale, C. J., Zimbalist, E. and Winawer, S. J. (1987) Outpatient management of esophageal cancer with endoscopic Nd:YAG laser. *Am. J. Gastroenterol.*, **82**, 46–50.

Lishman, A. H., Dellipiani, A. W. and Devlin, H. B. (1980) The insertion of oesophagogastric tubes in malignant oesophageal strictures: endoscopy or surgery? *Br. J. Surg.*, **67**, 257–9.

McCaughan, J. S., Williams, T. E. and Bethel, B. H. (1985) Palliation of esophageal malignancy with photodynamic therapy. *Ann. Thorac. Surg.*, **40**, 113–20.

McKeown, K. C. (1985) The surgical treatment of carcinoma of the oesophagus. *J. R. Coll. Surg. Edinb.*, **30**, 1–14.

Mohansingh, M. P. (1976) Mortality of oesophageal surgery in the elderly. *Br. J. Surg.*, **63**, 579–80.

Moses, F. M., Peura, D. A., Wong, R. K. H. and Johnson, L. F. (1985) Palliative dilation of esophageal carcinoma. *Gastrointest. Endosc.*, **31**, 61–3.

Orringer, M. B. (1984a) Transhiatal esophagectomy without thoracotomy for carcinoma of the thoracic esophagus. *Ann. Surg.*, **200**, 282–8.

Orringer, M. B. (1984b) Substernal gastric bypass of the excluded oesophagus – results of an ill-advised operation. *Surgery*, **96**, 467–70.

Pearson, J. G. (1981) Radiotherapy for oesophageal carcinoma. *World J. Surg.*, **5**, 489–97.

Sugimachi, K., Kai, H. and Inokuchi, K. (1985) Preoperative hyperthermochemoradiotherapy for esophageal carcinoma – analysis of 20 cases. *Jpn. J. Med.*, **24**, 80–3.

Sugimachi, K., Matsuzaki, K., Matsuura, H. *et al.* (1985) Evaluation of surgical treatment of carcinoma of the oesophagus in the elderly: 20 years' experience. *Br. J. Surg.*, **72**, 28–30.

Sykes, N. P., Barnes, M. and Carter, R. L. (1988)

Clinical and pathological study of dysphagia conservatively managed in patients with advanced malignant disease. *Lancet*, **ii**, 726–8.

Watson, A. (1982) A study of the quality and duration of survival following resection, endoscopic intubation and surgical intubation in oesophageal carcinoma. *Br. J. Surg.*, **69**, 585–8.

Williamson, R. C. N. (1985) Abdominocervical oesophagectomy in the elderly. *Ann. R. Coll. Surg. Engl.*, **67**, 344–8.

CHAPTER SIX

Endoscopic intubation of oesophageal malignant obstruction

M. Atkinson

Recent advances in gastrointestinal endoscopy have made accurate placement of endoprosthetic tubes both easier and safer, and a considerable range of equipment is now available for this purpose (Tytgat *et al.*, 1986). Tubes of adequate dimensions with appropriate flexibility are now obtainable, and the risk of their disintegration *in situ* has been overcome. The method used with each of the currently available systems is first to make a passage through the neoplastic stricture with the endoscope and/or a guide-wire, secondly to dilate the stricture to a luminal diameter that will accept the endoprosthesis, thirdly to assess the extent of the lesion and so select an endoprosthesis of appropriate size, and fourthly to introduce this into a satisfactory position through the stricture.

6.1 THE AIMS OF THERAPY

The placement of an endoprosthetic tube through a carcinoma of the oesophagus or cardia is done primarily to restore the ability to swallow and so allow the patient to spend his remaining life at home rather than in hospital. Nutritional status is frequently improved and the risk of aspiration into the respiratory tree is lessened. Some prolongation of life probably results from intubation, but this is to be measured in months at the most, and the principal aim is to improve the quality rather than the quantity of remaining life.

6.2 ENDOPROSTHETIC TUBES (Table 6.1)

The earliest endoprosthetic tube to be used on a widespread basis was that of Souttar which consisted of a coil of German silver wire placed using the rigid oesophagoscope (Souttar, 1927). Tubes of larger diameter and length offered obvious advantages and the advent of fibreoptic endoscopy facilitated their placement. At first latex tubes of modified Celestin type (Etienne and Celestin,

Table 6.1 Endoprosthetic tubes in common usage

Type	Manufacturer	Material	Bore	Lengths available (cm)
Atkinson	KeyMed, UK	Silicone rubber	11.7	11, 14, 19
Celestin	Medoc, UK	Activated latex	12	9, 11, 13, 15
Cook	Wilson-Cook, USA	Silicone rubber	12	11, 15, 17
Procter Livingstone	Latex Products South Africa	Latex	12	10, 15, 19
Polyvinyl (Tygon)		Polyvinylchloride		Made to measure

1979) were used, but as the latex tends to denature and disintegrate after about 7 months the trend is to use more inert tubes made of silicone rubber (Ogilvie *et al.*, 1982) or polyvinylchloride (Tytgat *et al.*, 1986). These tubes withstand exposure to acid, bile and irradiation well and rarely disintegrate even when they have been in place for 2 years or more (Branicki *et al.*, 1981).

The length of tube to be used will depend upon the extent of the growth and its relation to the cardia because it is advisable to carry the distal end below the cardia when the lower end of the neoplastic stricture lies within 3 cm of the cardia. Polyvinyl (Tygon) tubes may be manufactured at the time of insertion to appropriate length but most manufacturers provide a range of tubes of different length from which to choose. The longer the tube the more difficulty will the patient encounter in swallowing solids; hence, allowing for the length of the funnel and the distal end, the overall tube length should be about 4–5 cm greater than the length of the neoplastic stricture.

All tubes incorporate a proximal funnel which should fill the entire cross-section of the oesophageal lumen, thus catching all fluid and food coming down the oesophagus. If the funnel is constructed of material which is too hard there is a risk of its lip eroding through the oesophageal wall and causing a fatal haemorrhage from the aorta or causing an oesophagotracheal fistula. This is particularly likely when the tube is in the lower oesophagus and is subject to cardiac pulsation. On the other hand, too soft a funnel may collapse and allow distal displacement of the tube. Hence the pliability of the funnel is of crucial importance.

The design of the barrel of the tube must ensure that an adequate lumen is provided, and that the tube does not kink when bent. A lumen of 11–12 mm allows the ingestion of an adequate diet without resulting in the tube being too thick to insert comfortably. Wider tubes carry an increased risk of perforation when inserted through tight neoplastic strictures and are more difficult to remove should this become necessary at a later date. The prevention of kinking when the tube is bent in its passage through the stricture may be achieved by incorporating a nylon or metal spiral in its wall, or in the case of Polyvinyl (Tygon) tubes, moulding circular corrugations in the wall. These devices are effective in preventing kinking but the resulting elastic recoil when the tube is bent may increase pressure from the lip of the funnel against the oesophageal wall.

The distal part of the tube must incorporate a device to prevent proximal displacement since endoscopically inserted tubes, unlike those put in at operation, cannot be sutured in position. The corrugations of the barrel of the tubes used by the Amsterdam group may achieve this objective but a shoulder, either circumferential (Wilson–Cook tube) or in one dimension only (Atkinson tube), or a flange (Medoc tube) is effective and proximal tube displacement is now an unusual complication. The dimensions of the distal shoulder or flange should not be such as to prevent extraction of the tube should it be necessary to replace it with one of a larger size as the growth extends. Special tubes are used to occlude oesophagotracheal fistula (see below).

6.3 INTRODUCERS FOR ENDOPROSTHETIC OESOPHAGEAL TUBES

Endoprosthetic tubes may be introduced mounted on a tapered dilator, mounted on the endoscope itself or carried by an introducer which grips the tube from the inside. Most systems employ a pushing tube engaging in the funnel of the endoprosthetic tube which enables accurate positioning and holds the prosthesis in place while the introducing device is withdrawn. Whatever method is employed it is important that the leading end should be smoothly tapered with no sharp shouldering to cause trauma. This occasionally occurs when the tube is passed over the scope itself, since too tight a fit might cause difficulty in extricating the scope without displacing the tube during withdrawal. Any system for tube placement must permit its advancement or withdrawal until it is in a satisfactory position, and should be capable of extracting the tube from the oesophagus or stomach.

Tube placement usually takes several minutes, and longer if difficulties are encountered. Ear oximetry reveals that endoscopic equipment in the throat may cause anoxia through interference with ventilation by partial occlusion of the air passages (Bell *et al.*, 1987). To reduce this risk it is important to employ a pushing tube of minimum diameter unless the procedure is done under general anaesthesia with an endotracheal tube *in situ*. Even so, intubation equipment of too great diameter passing alongside the endotracheal tube will increase the risk of pharyngeal trauma.

6.4 EQUIPMENT CURRENTLY AVAILABLE FOR PLACEMENT OF ENDOPROSTHESIS

6.4.1 THE NOTTINGHAM ENDOPROSTHETIC TUBE INTRODUCING SYSTEM (KeyMed) (Figure 6.1)

This consists of an introducer incorporating an expanding Delrin cup which grips the tube from the inside. The stem consists of two flexible tubes, the one sliding inside the other. The Delrin cup mounted on the inner tube is expanded when a metal olive on the outer tube is slid into the cup and it can be locked in

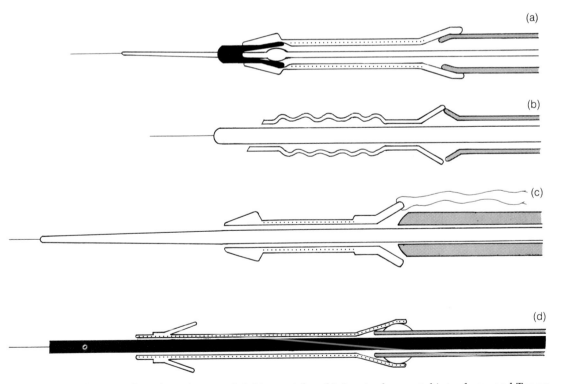

Figure 6.1   (a) Nottingham introducer and Atkinson tube. (b) Amsterdam metal introducer and Tygon tube. (c) Dumon–Gilliard introducer and Wilson–Cook tube. (d) Medoc introducer and Celestin tube.

this position by a bayonet catch on the proximal end of the introducer. A positioning tube is then passed over the introducer assembly to engage the funnel of the endoprosthesis and this is used to maintain its position whilst the introducer is removed after satisfactory positioning of the endoprosthesis through the neoplastic stricture.

The system is designed to be used with a silicone rubber (Atkinson) tube. The Nottingham system provides accurate control for tube positioning, and if extubation is required it is usually accomplished simply by reversing the procedure. It is stiffer than some other systems, and the present positioning tube is of wide diameter although the equipment can often be used without this tube when the lie of the endoprosthesis is in a straight line.

6.4.2 THE WILSON–COOK OESOPHAGEAL PROSTHESIS SET (Figure 6.1)

In this system the endoprosthesis is mounted on a polyvinylchloride Savary–Gilliard dilator with a polyvinylchloride Dumon–Gilliard positioning tube slid over the dilator behind the tube. The endoprosthesis is prevented from moving forward over the tapered tip of the dilator by a thread passed through the funnel and back alongside the positioning tube which can be released when the endoprosthesis is in position through the neoplastic stricture.

The system is more flexible than the Nottingham introducer since it is constructed of plastic materials rather than metal. It provides a less positive means of tube positioning. For extubation additional equipment is available consisting of a balloon mounted on a stem which can be inflated in the endoprosthesis to grip the endoprosthesis to enable it to be removed from the body by traction in the stem.

6.4.3 THE MEDOC INTRODUCER

This introducer, designed for use with the Medoc (Celestin) endoprosthetic tube, em-ploys a latex introducer with a balloon near its tip which can be inflated in the lumen of the tube, thus providing positive control of the assembly as it is slid into position over a mandril placed through the neoplastic stricture. Once the endoprosthesis is in a satisfactory position the balloon is deflated and the introducer is withdrawn. Medoc offer an alternative system in which the endoprosthesis is slid over the endoscope itself (Figure 6.1).

6.4.4 THE AMSTERDAM METAL INTRODUCER

This is inserted over a guide-wire and it will assume the bend of the lumen through angulated growths. It can then be gradually stiffened and straightened until a Polyvinyl (Tygon) tube can be slid into position over it, thus reducing the risk of sustaining a perforation.

6.5 TECHNIQUE FOR PLACEMENT OF OESOPHAGEAL ENDOPROSTHETIC TUBES

6.5.1 PREPARATION OF THE PATIENT

The clinician must be certain from the outset that his patient is unsuited for any attempt at curative resection of the growth and this is best decided in consultation with a surgeon. At physical examination anaemia, signs of fluid depletion, and signs of respiratory disease from aspiration of oesophageal contents should be sought and corrected if possible before intubation. Evidence of metastases such as lymphadenopathy and hepatomegaly may be present and routine laboratory investigations include a full blood count, blood urea and electrolyte levels and liver function tests, together with a chest radiography. Normally a barium swallow would already have been done. It is important to remember that once the endoprosthesis is in position the growth will not be accessible for endoscopic biopsy and a histological diagnosis should have been previously established. CT scanning and endoscopic ultrasonography are sometimes useful to determine the extent of local spread of the tumour, and to detect hepatic metastases.

6.5.2 ANALGESIA, SEDATION AND ANAESTHETIC

Intubation can usually be done under local anaesthesia using topical anaesthesia of the throat with lignocaine spray. A butterfly cannula is inserted into a vein in the arm or hand and diazepam 10–20 mg, or midazolam 5–10 mg, is administered slowly. This may be supplemented by pethidine (Demerol) 25–50 mg if the patient experiences pain or discomfort during the procedure. Should the intubation procedure be expected to be technically difficult or time consuming, as for example with tight obstructions at the cardia, general anaesthesia is preferable, and the use of an endotracheal tube ensures adequate ventilation of the lungs, obviating the possibility of mechanical obstruction of the airway by the introducer assembly.

Because of the risk of mediastinitis resulting from perforation of the oesophagus during the procedure a prophylactic injection of antibiotic (e.g. cefuroxime 1.5 g) is given immediately before the start of the procedure.

6.5.3 ENDOSCOPIC METHOD

An attempt is made to ease a thin endoscope, usually a paediatric model (e.g. Olympus XP20), through the stricture, keeping the lumen constantly in view. Once this has reached the stomach a stainless-steel guide-wire is inserted until its tip lies in the pyloric antrum and the endoscope is withdrawn. During withdrawal the distances of the diaphragmatic hiatus, the cardia and the upper and lower margins of the growth and the cricopharyngeus are recorded. If the endoscope will not pass through the stricture the guide-wire is passed under radiological control into the stomach. Should the view be

obscured by bleeding from the growth this may be controlled by washing through the 'scope or by the topical application of adrenaline solution. However, if bleeding persists it is better to postpone the intubation for 24 hours.

Once the guide-wire is in position dilatation of the neoplastic stricture is done using metal olive dilators (Eder–Puestow or Tridil) or tapered plastic (Celestin, Savary–Gilliard or KeyMed Advanced Dilators) up to a 54 French gauge (18 mm) diameter. This gives an adequate luminal diameter for insertion of the endoprosthesis.

An endoprosthetic tube of appropriate length is selected and mounted on the introducer. The distance of the upper margin of the growth to the incisor teeth is measured from the neck of the funnel and marked on the stem of the introducer by adhesive plastic. The positioning tube is slid over the introducer to engage in the tube funnel and it is marked in the same way. After lubrication the whole assembly is advanced along the guide-wire using radiological screening to check its position. Resistance is felt when the leading end of the tube reaches the upper end of the stricture and gentle pressure, rotating the assembly by a few degrees if necessary, is used to insert the tube through the stricture until the mark on the stem or positioning tube is opposite the incisor teeth. The introducer is then released and both it and the guide-wire are withdrawn through the positioning tube which is used to prevent displacement of the endoprosthesis during this manoeuvre. The positioning tube is then withdrawn watching the endoprosthesis by fluoroscopy to ensure its position is maintained.

Finally, a check is made by passing the endoscope into the oesophagus and through the tube into the stomach, noting its position in terms of distance of the lip of the funnel from the incisor teeth. A free passage into the lumen of the oesophagus or stomach should be possible and if the distal end of the tube is occluded by pressure against the gastric wall adjustment is needed or it may be preferable to use a shorter tube.

6.6 AFTERCARE

About 3 hours after completion of the intubational procedure posteroanterior and lateral chest radiographs are taken to search for air in the tissues of the mediastinum or neck which would indicate that a perforation had been sustained. Because the oesophagus is insufflated with air under pressure during endoscopy, pneumomediastinum is an almost invariable sign of perforation. If the radiographs are clear the patient is allowed fluids by mouth and next day a radiological examination is made again after swallowing of contrast material (propyliodone suspension (Dionosil, Glaxo), to assess the patency of the endoprosthetic tube.

If the tube functions adequately the patient is started on a soft diet. He should be advised:

1. To eat sitting erect.
2. To masticate carefully (and dentures should be provided if necessary).
3. To drink frequently during meals. Sometimes fizzy drinks are recommended but palatability is more important than effervescence.

It is useful for the patient and his or her spouse to meet the dietitian before discharge to be provided with written details about what to eat and what to avoid. Some patients are reluctant to take an adequate diet and unnecessarily restrict their intake of alcohol, spiced foods or fruit. The longer the endoprosthetic tube the more likely will the patient have difficulty with solid foods and he may well require dietary supplements to improve nutritional status.

Placement of an endoprosthesis usually entails 3–5 days in hospital and the majority of patients can be managed at home throughout their terminal illness. Regular monthly review in the outpatient clinic including a visit to the dietitian helps to resolve many minor prob-

lems and provides an opportunity to check nutritional indices.

The procedure-related mortality for placement of an endoprosthesis results largely from perforation of the growth. Cardio-respiratory complications, frequently present before intubation, may be aggravated but it is often difficult to be sure that death is not the result of natural progression of the disease itself which certainly accounts for the majority of deaths in hospital within 6 weeks. The outcome in a personal series of 323 intubations is shown in Figure 6.2, where it will be seen that 86% of patients left hospital swallowing satisfactorily.

6.7 COMPLICATIONS OF ENDOSCOPIC TUBE PLACEMENT

6.7.1 IMMEDIATE

Perforation of the growth represents the greatest immediate hazard of intubation. Many growths are friable and the remaining lumen through them is sometimes angulated which increases the risk. Should a perforation be recognized to have occurred during intubation the tube should still be inserted if possible since its wall will frequently help to occlude the hole and prevent spillage into the mediastinum. The incidence of perforation is of the order of 10% of intubations (Bennett, 1981) and must be accepted as an unavoidable risk even by the most skilled endoscopist unless he is unduly restrictive in his choice of

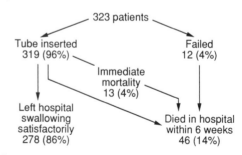

Figure 6.2 Outcome in 323 patients undergoing intubation for neoplastic strictures of the cardia.

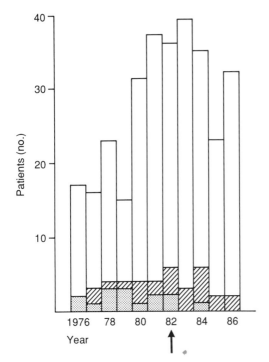

Figure 6.3   Incidence of oesophageal perforation in Nottingham over an 11-year period. Fatal perforations are shown in stipling and the non-fatal ones are hatched.

patients. The incidence of perforation has not declined over the past decade (Figure 6.3) but fortunately with active conservative management the survival rate after perforation is now in the order of 90%; the outlook is worst in those with pneumothorax and extravasation into the pleural cavity. A successful outcome depends upon the use of prophylactic antibiotics, such as i.v. cefuroxime 1.5 g q.d.s., the first dose given *before* commencement of tube insertion and administration continued until perforation has been excluded, and the prevention of extravasation of food, fluids or barium into the mediastinum. Many perforations are symptomless and can only be detected radiologically. A careful search for signs of perforation must be made along the lines already outlined in all patients before fluid or food is allowed.

If a perforation is found, no oral intake of food or fluid is allowed and feeding by a fine-bore tube inserted through the endoprosthesis with its tip in the gastric antrum is instituted (Wesdorp *et al.*, 1984; Hine and Atkinson, 1986). If the perforation is at the cardia or in the upper stomach intravenous feeding is preferable. After 5–7 days a check contrast swallow is done. This will usually show that the perforation has sealed, and oral feeding can then be commenced and the antibiotic stopped.

Other immediate complications are rare. Although some bleeding is often encountered this is seldom sufficient to necessitate blood transfusion. Aspiration of food material into the respiratory tract during the intubation procedure may occur, but this risk can be reduced by removing oesophageal food residues at the outset.

6.7.2 LONG-TERM COMPLICATIONS

(a) Blockage of the endoprosthetic tube with food

This is now an uncommon occurrence provided the patient is properly instructed about aftercare. The food is dislodged by passing a paediatric endoscope through the tube. Food blockage may be the result of overgrowth of the proximal or distal end of the endoprosthesis by the tumour and it is essential that a full endoscopic inspection be made after any food material has been removed.

(b) Overgrowth of the tube by tumour or by granulation tissue

With the passage of time, extension of the tumour may overgrow the funnel (Figure 6.4) or occasionally the distal end of the tube. Several therapeutic options should be considered in this situation. The most satisfactory, if it can be achieved, is first to dilate the ring of tumour using metal olives (Eder–Puestow) rather than tapered plastic dilators. Radiological screening is important to make sure the

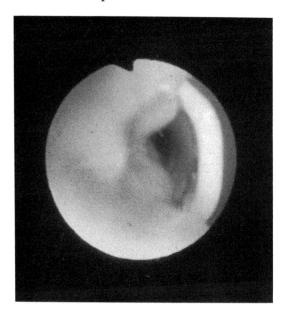

Figure 6.4 Overgrowth of an endoprosthetic growth by tumour tissue. The rim of the tube funnel is visible on the right.

dilator is not advanced too far so as to push the tube distally. Secondly, the Nottingham or Medoc introducer is passed with the tube lumen and expanded to grip the tube and allow it to be gently withdrawn through the mouth. A longer tube can then be inserted in the usual way. An alternative approach is to trim away the growth from the funnel using laser or a bipolar (bicap) probe. These procedures will probably have to be repeated at intervals of 2 or 3 weeks as the growth recurs.

Rarely the lip of the funnel excites a reaction in the healthy oesophageal wall above the tumour and a sheet of granulation tissue extends across the mouth of the funnel of the tube (Philp, Gunning and Bennett, 1983). This can usually be trimmed away with laser or the bipolar probe but care should be exercised not to ignite the tube with the laser beam.

(c) Tube displacement

If the neoplastic stricture does not grip the tube firmly, or if the patient has much vomit-ing, tube displacement may result. This is more common in a proximal than in a distal direction and the development of distal shoulders or flanges on the modern endoprosthetic tube has greatly reduced the frequency of displacement (Figure 6.5). Although it is sometimes possible to push the tube back into position by the endoscope with a pushing tube mounted over it, usually the displaced tube is removed by reversing the introducing procedure and reintubation is then under-taken.

Distal tube displacement is less common because the funnel usually prevents onward passage of the tube. Sometimes tubes can be retrieved from the stomach with the Nottingham introducer, but if not the choice lies between laparotomy or, if the patient's life expectation is limited, the tube may be left in the stomach and another inserted through the neoplastic stricture.

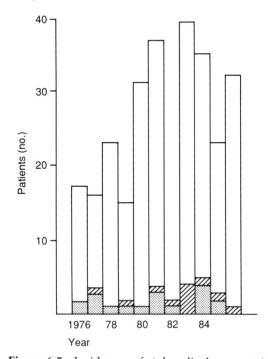

Figure 6.5 Incidence of tube displacement in Nottingham over an 11-year-period. Proximal displacements are shown in stippling and distal displacements are hatched.

(d) Erosion into other organs

The lip of the funnel may erode through the oesophageal wall, particularly if the endoprosthesis is subject to cardiac pulsation when in the lower oesophagus. Penetration of the aorta or the heart may cause fatal torrential haemorrhage. The stiffness of the tube lip is critical in this respect and the incurved tip of the Medoc (Celestin tube) is designed to reduce the likelihood of this rare occurrence which may occur through uninvolved oesophageal wall although it occurs more commonly at the site of neoplastic infiltration. Erosion into the pericardium or the pleural cavity is fortunately very rare.

6.8 TRACHEO-OESOPHAGEAL FISTULA

A tracheo-oesophageal fistula may result from breakdown of oesophageal tumour tissue or complicate bronchial neoplasms invading the oesophagus. The majority of fistulae develop spontaneously but radiotherapy, endoscopy or pressure from an endoprosthetic tube may act as precipitating factors.

Small fistulae can usually be occluded by an

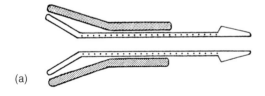

(a)

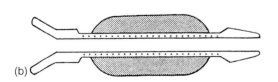

(b)

Figure 6.6 Endoprosthetic tubes used in the management of oesophagotracheal fistula. (a) An Atkinson tube wrapped with polyurethene (Ivalon) sponge. (b) A Wilson–Cook oesophageal balloon prosthesis. The balloon contains polyurethene sponge.

unmodified endoprosthetic tube which serves to prevent spillage into the respiratory tract, thus giving striking relief from a particularly unpleasant variety of dysphagia. When the opening is large the endoprosthesis has to be adapted to increase its diameter, either by wrapping it with polyurethane sponge which swells when it becomes wet, or by investing the barrel of the tube with a balloon containing polyurethane sponge (Figure 6.6) (Robertson and Atkinson, 1986; Irving and Simson, 1988). These devices are also useful if the fistula is not associated with oesophageal stricture, when an unadapted endoprosthesis would not maintain its position.

6.9 LIMITATIONS OF ENDOSCOPIC INTUBATION

6.9.1 FAILURE TO ESTABLISH A WAY THROUGH THE STRICTURE

Very tight strictures and those with angulation of the lumen are often difficult to negotiate even with the thinnest endoscope and blind passage of the guide-wire often presents problems. Fortunately with perseverance the guide-wire can be placed in more than 90% of patients and if there is bleeding obscuring the view it is advisable to wait for 24 hours before making another attempt. If this is unsuccessful laser therapy or bipolar thermocoagulation is required.

6.9.2 NEOPLASMS OF THE UPPER OESOPHAGUS

When the upper end of the growth lies within 3 cm of the cricopharyngeus the insertion of an endoprosthetic tube results in intolerable discomfort. Although tubes with a modified funnel have been used these are seldom tolerated and such growths are best treated by laser therapy or bipolar thermocoagulation.

6.9.3 UNSATISFACTORY TUBE LIE

For an endoprosthetic tube to function satisfactorily its distal end must lie in a luminal cavity large enough not to cause blockage. Recurrent growths after previous gastrectomy with oesophagojejunal anastomosis are seldom suitable for intubation and patients with a small gastric lumen or marked cup and spill configuration of the stomach may present difficulties.

Acute bending of the endoprosthetic tube when it is inserted through a neoplastic stricture in which the lumen is angulated may result in pressure on the funnel causing partial occlusion. This problem can be overcome by using a longer tube so the funnel lies further above the bend in the tube.

6.10 THE OUTLOOK AFTER ENDOPROSTHETIC INTUBATION

The endoscopist inevitably has to deal with those patients with the most advanced carcinomas and those in the worst physical condition. Placement of the endoprosthesis is possible in the great majority of such patients and the majority continue to swallow until death from the disease which occurs on average 4 months after intubation, although 10% survive a year. In the first few weeks after intubation nutrition commonly improves with an average weight gain of 3 kg in the first month (Haffjee and Angorn, 1977; Fellows, Greensmith and Atkinson, 1984). Inevitably nutritional deterioration in the later stages

results from anorexia rather than dysphagia. Nevertheless, restoration of the ability to swallow allows most patients to be managed at home in the terminal stages of their illness.

Squamous carcinoma of the oesophagus, and less frequently adenocarcinoma occurring at the cardia or in the columnar-lined oesophagus, may be treated by radiotherapy. If there is luminal narrowing it is advisable to insert an endoprosthesis before starting radiotherapy because this causes the growth to swell and become more friable which increases the risks of intubation. Although survival is longer in patients with squamous carcinoma treated by radiotherapy than in squamous or adenocarcinoma not irradiated, this is possibly the result of selection of those with least advanced carcinoma for treatment. Undoubtedly a course of radiotherapy considerably increases time spent in hospital by patients whose life expectation is limited and controlled trials are needed to establish the benefits of irradiation.

6.11 THE RELATIVE VALUE OF ENDOSCOPIC INTUBATION AND LASER THERAPY (Table 6.2)

Published reports suggest that both endoscopic intubation and recanalization by laser therapy provide effective palliation of symptoms in neoplasms of the oesophagus or

Table 6.2 Comparative value of endoprosthesis and Nd–YAG laser

	Endoprosthesis	Nd–YAG Laser
Relief of dysphagia	>90%	>90%
Ability to take virtually normal diet	23%	20%
Mean endoscopies per patient (no.)	1.2	4.7
Cumulative duration of hospitalization	Short	Longer
Upper oesophageal growths	Not applicable	Applicable
Ease of method when lumen angulated	Difficult	Easier
Occlusion of oesophagotracheal fistula	Valuable	Impossible
Perforation rate (%)	12	2
Procedure-related mortality	Comparable	
Mean survival (months)	19	18
Expense of equipment	Inexpensive	Expensive

cardia (Bown, 1986). Laser therapy requires more endoscopies since several sessions may be required to achieve adequate recanalization and tumour regrowth necessitates retreatment at intervals of usually about a month. Failure of tube function necessitates re-endoscopy in about a third of patients treated by intubation.

Perforation of the tumour is more common with intubation than with laser therapy but the resulting mortality is low and in a recent prospective comparison no procedure-related fatality was encountered with either intubation or laser therapy (Loizou et al., 1988). The improvement in swallowing is comparable between the two techniques (20–25% in each group were able to take a virtually normal diet) and there is no difference in median survival. Laser therapy offers obvious advantages with high oesophageal growths and in those patients in whom intubation has failed. Exophytic neoplasms with a polypoidal mass projecting into the oesophageal lumen are best treated by laser vapourization. Intubation may offer advantages with long strictures producing concentric narrowing and is effective in oesophagotracheal fistulae.

To summarize, at the present time both intubation and laser therapy provide good quality long-term palliation in malignant dysphagia and the two procedures should be regarded as being complementary until the results of larger long-term prospective trials are available.

6.12 BIPOLAR THERMOCOAGULATION

The high cost of a laser unit has led to thermocoagulation using bipolar electrodes to recanalize neoplastic strictures (Johnston et al., 1987). The bicap equipment consists of graded metal olives with bipolar electrodes around the circumference passed over a guide-wire inserted through the neoplastic stricture. A series of dilators of increasing diameter are used and olives with electrodes extending round only half of their circumference are

available for growths that do not involve the whole circumference of the oesophageal lumen. Care is required not to burn healthy mucosa in the oesophagus or pharynx during withdrawal. By this means a lumen can be restored but recanalization is slower than with laser and more treatment sessions are likely to be needed.

REFERENCES

Bell, G. D., Reeve, P. A., Moshiri, M. et al. (1987) Intravenous midazolam: a study of the degree of oxygen desaturation occurring during upper gastrointestinal endoscopy. Br. J. Pharmacol., 23, 703–8.

Bennett, J. R. (1981) Intubation of gastro oesophageal malignancies – a survey of current practice in Britain 1980. Gut, 22, 336–8.

Branicki, F. J., Ogilvie, A. L., Willis, M. R. and Atkinson, M. (1981) Structural deterioration of oesophageal tubes: an in vitro comparison of latex rubber and silicone rubber. Br. J. Surg., 61, 861–4.

Bown, S. G. (1986) Endoscopic laser therapy for oesophageal cancer. Endoscopy, 18, suppl. 3, 26–31.

Etienne, J. and Celestin, L. R. (1979) La prosthèse oesophagienne: passe et présent. Acta Endoscopiea, 9, 235–43.

Fellows, I. W., Greensmith, J. and Atkinson, M. (1984) The nutritional effects of endoscopic intubation for carcinoma of the oesophagus or cardia. Clin. Nutr., 2, 167–8.

Haffjee, A. A. and Angorn, I. B. (1977) Oral alimentation following intubation for oesophageal carcinoma. Ann. Surg., 186, 759–61.

Hine, K. R. and Atkinson, M. (1986) The diagnosis and management of perforation of oesophagus and pharynx sustained during intubation of neoplastic oesophageal strictures. Dig. Dis. Sci., 31, 571–3.

Irving, J. D. and Simson, J. N. L. (1988) A new cuffed oesophageal prosthesis for the management of malignant oesophago respiratory fistula. Ann. R. Coll. Surg. Engl., 70, 13–5.

Johnston, J. H., Fleischer, D., Petrini, J. and Nord, H. T. (1987) Palliative bipolar electrocoagulation therapy of obstructing esophageal cancer. Gastrointest. Endosc., 33, 349–57.

Loizou, L. A., Grigg, D., Robertson, C. S. et al. (1988) Long term palliation of malignant dysphagia. Laser v intubation. Gut, 29, A1492.

Ogilvie, A. L., Dronfield, W., Ferguson, R. and

Atkinson, M. (1982) Palliative intubation of oesophago gastric neoplasms at fibreoptic endoscopy. *Gut*, **23**, 1060–7.

Philp, T., Gunning, A. J. and Bennett, M. K. (1983) Inflammatory obstruction of oesophageal tubes. *Gut*, **24**, 960–3.

Robertson, C. S. and Atkinson, M. (1986) A modified prosthetic oesophageal tube to manage malignant oesophago respiratory fistula. *Lancet*, **ii**, 949–50.

Souttar, H. S. (1927) Treatment of carcinoma of the oesophagus based on 100 personal cases and 18 post mortem reports. *Br. J. Surg.*, **15**, 76–91.

Tytgat, G. N. J., Bartelsman, J. F. W. M., Den Hartog Jager, F. C. A. *et al.* (1986) Upper intestinal and biliary tract prostheses. *Dig. Dis. Sci.*, **31**, 575–765.

Wesdorp, I. C. E., Bartelsman, J. F. W. M., Huibregtse, K. *et al.* (1984) Treatment of oesophageal perforation. *Gut*, **25**, 398–404.

CHAPTER SEVEN

Laser disobliteration for advanced gastrointestinal malignancy

S. G. Bown

The first treatment of malignant dysphagia by insertion of a prosthetic tube was reported over 100 years ago by Symonds, in 1885. Since then, the tubes and the methods used for their placement have developed to the established techniques now available as described in the previous chapter. The first laser was developed in 1960, with a flurry of work on the medical applications, but few applications became established at that time. This was due partly to technical problems with available lasers and partly to a lack of understanding of the interactions of laser light with living tissue.

In the early 1970s it became possible to transmit high-power laser beams along fibres that were sufficiently thin and flexible to pass down the operating channel of fibreoptic endoscopes. This made endoscopic laser treatment feasible in the gastrointestinal tract. Early studies were directed at the control of haemorrhage from a range of non-neoplastic lesions, and enthusiastic reports claimed success in a high proportion of all such cases. More detailed experimental studies and clinical trials have now defined more clearly how best to use lasers in this situation as discussed elsewhere in this book (Chapter 12).

The first patients were treated for blood loss from benign lesions in 1975, but it was not until the early 1980s that reports started appearing on the use of lasers for the palliation of symptoms from advanced malignant tumours of the gastrointestinal tract (Fleischer, Kessler and Haye, 1982). Results show that endoscopic laser therapy is effective in this situation, but it should be stressed that, compared with insertion of prosthetic tubes, laser therapy is very new. The techniques are still being developed, and anyone starting work in this field should do so with a pioneering spirit and feel that they are contributing to the evolution of this new approach to therapeutic endoscopy, rather than expect to find all the answers in an article such as this.

A laser is a sophisticated light source producing light with several special properties. It is coherent, polarized and monochromatic, but most important are the ability to focus all the output of a high-power laser on to the end of a flexible fibre and the ease and precision of control. For example, the Nd–YAG (neodymium yttrium aluminium garnet) laser, which is the principal laser used in gastroenterology, has a power output up to 100 W (similar to that of a domestic light bulb), focused on to the end of a fibre less than 0.5 mm in diameter. It is necessary to look at the principles of the interaction of laser light with living tissue to understand how this is of value in tumour therapy. When light of any sort is incident on tissue, it can be reflected, transmitted, scattered or absorbed. Only absorbed light can produce a biological effect, but the extent to which the light is reflected, transmitted and scattered will determine the volume of

tissue in which the light is absorbed. The laser light is absorbed as heat, and the first effect seen is thermal contraction in the immediate vicinity of the target area. This is the mechanism employed in laser haemostasis, vessels being sealed by thermal contraction of their walls and of the surrounding tissue. As more heat is dissipated, local necrosis is produced, and if enough heat is delivered in a short time, cells are vaporized.

The ultimate fate of tissues exposed to intense laser light can be summarized as follows:

Total destruction
    Instant vaporization
    Necrosis with later sloughing
Destruction with reconstruction
    Necrosis with healing by scarring
    Necrosis with healing by regeneration
Reversible effects
    Oedema and inflammation
    Local warming only

If the laser power is high enough (e.g. over 50 W for the Nd–YAG laser) and the laser is fired for long enough at one spot, all these effects can be seen in one area. Tissue immediately under the beam is vaporized, adjacent areas below and laterally are necrosed with later sloughing or scarring and beyond this, only reversible effects are seen. Current clinical use for the palliation of symptoms from advanced gastrointestinal tumours is relatively crude, but is nevertheless effective in a high percentage of cases. New techniques are being developed which may make better use of the precision available from lasers (Matthewson et al., 1989).

7.1 UPPER GASTROINTESTINAL TRACT TUMOURS

7.1.1 INDICATIONS

Most cases of cancer of the oesophagus and gastric cardia present with dysphagia when the disease has already reached an advanced stage and there is little prospect of cure. As diagnostic techniques improve, the proportion considered unsuitable for curative surgery rises, and one has to ask which form of palliation provides the most effective symptomatic relief (both in quality and duration) with the minimum of general disturbance to the patient. The morbidity associated with palliative surgery, radiotherapy or chemotherapy is often relatively extended, which makes the endoscopic options more attractive for patients with a limited life expectancy. Endoscopic insertion of a prosthesis provides for nourishment by liquids and some solid foods in most cases. The results of endoscopic laser treatment are more variable, but many individuals may be able to return to a diet close to normal.

On technical grounds, some patients are only suitable for insertion of a prosthesis and some are only suitable for laser therapy, although in the majority of cases, both are possible. The laser works by destroying tissue under direct endoscopic vision. Thus to be effective, that part of the tumour causing the worst obstruction must be accessible. Only exophytic tumour can be treated with the laser, and not tumour that is submucosal or causing obstruction by extrinsic pressure on the oesophagus. Laser treatment cannot be definitive in patients with an oesophago-tracheal fistula, although it may help to create a lumen for the insertion of a prosthetic tube. Laser therapy is possible in areas where prostheses are poorly tolerated, as in the cervical oesophagus, or the tube cannot be inserted endoscopically, such as in the gastric outlet.

7.1.2 TECHNIQUE

Laser treatment for palliation of advanced malignant dysphagia is not as easy as might first appear. It is time consuming (individual treatment sessions can last up to 1 hour), it is hard on endoscopes and there are still many questions to be answered on which technique

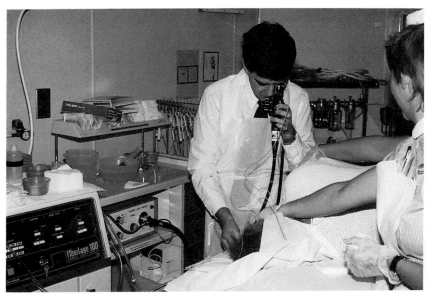

Figure 7.1   Treatment of an oesophageal carcinoma with a 100-W Nd–YAG laser. The laser fibre is seen inserted into the operating channel of the endoscope.

is best under various circumstances (Figure 7.1).

The procedure is normally carried out under sedation with intravenous diazepam 5–20 mg supplemented with 25–50 mg of pethidine (Demerol) given intravenously, the dose of each being titrated according to the individual patient's response. Pharyngeal anaesthesia is also used. Occasionally, it is necessary to use general anaesthesia.

7.1.3 INSTRUMENTATION

The currently used technique is relatively crude but the principle is simple. The high power of the laser (60–80 W) is used to burn a way through those parts of the tumour causing the worst obstruction. We use a 100-W continuous wave Nd–YAG laser, the Fiberlase 100 (Pilkington Medical Systems, Glasgow). This produces an infrared beam of wavelength 1064 nm with a visible red beam from a small helium-neon laser to use for aiming. The laser light is transmitted via a 0.6-mm diameter glass or quartz fibre. The fibre is fixed in a 2-mm diameter Teflon catheter, which can be passed through any endoscopic biopsy channel of diameter 2.8 mm or greater. The Teflon gives mechanical support to the fibre and provides a means of delivering a stream of gas (usually carbon dioxide or air) which serves to keep the tip of the fibre clean. Just before and during laser shots, a separate control on the foot switch gives a more rapid gas flow which clears the target of blood and debris, and cools the fibre tip. Great care must be taken to keep the tip clean, because firing with debris present destroys it and necessitates recleaving before that fibre can be used again.

The laser power is preset prior to use by inserting the fibre tip into a power meter built into the laser (the precise value depending on the particular lesion being treated). The exposure time for each shot can also be preset at any duration from 0.1 to 9.9 seconds, but for most tumour work the best range is 0.5–2 seconds, and the majority of shots are 1 second long. Similar lasers are manufactured by MBB (Germany), Cilas (France) and

Cooper Medical (USA), although one new feature, so far only introduced by Pilkington, is the disposable fibre. This does increase the operating costs, but is worth while for the time saved by not having to repair fibres by recleaving and fitting new metal tips.

The use of co-axial gas means that a venting system must be provided to prevent overdistension of the oesophagus and stomach. Often a separate gas escape route is required. A convenient arrangement is to pass a nasogastric tube alongside the endoscope and can be done simply if the tube is stiffened with an endoscope cleaning brush and gently slid along the side of the endoscope. Once in position the stiffening brush is removed, and the end of the tube connected to an underwater drain. Bubbles through the water give immediate confirmation that the venting system is working, and considerable smoke generated by lasering passes into the drain bottle rather than the room, which is more pleasant for both patient and staff. The only essential modification required to the endoscope is insertion of an appropriate safety filter in the eyepiece. If this is not fitted, the endoscopist must wear safety goggles. A white ceramic tip fitted to the endoscope by the manufacturer instead of the usual black plastic is another useful modification. As more difficult cases are attempted, in which the manoeuvring space for the tip of the endoscope in the tumour is smaller, it has become clear that there is a definite risk to the endoscope, which makes this worthwhile. Three golden rules before firing the laser are that the tip of the fibre should be visible through the endoscope, the aiming beam should be seen on the target area, and the fibre should not be touching the target tissue.

Endoscopic laser therapy, particularly of oesophageal tumours, presents a tough challenge to the endoscopes but one of the worst problems is channel blockage so it is important that all channels are checked frequently during the procedure. If a procedure lasts longer than 30 minutes, the instrument is removed, cleaned, and all channels thoroughly washed and cleared before continuing. Inevitably, old food debris collects above an obstructing oesophageal cancer, fragments of tumour break off during endoscopic manipulation, and laser treatment produces charred tumour tissue and debris which easily block channels. Instruments with as wide an operating channel as possible are preferable. If the operating channel is much wider than the laser fibre, the same channel can be used for the gas escape. This can be done by intermittent aspiration, or if a second port to the channel is available (as with the Fujinon UGI-CT) or a T-shaped adaptor is fixed to the top of the operating channel, this can be connected directly to the underwater drain. With the Olympus 2T-10, the second channel can be used for gas escape. The Pentax 34 JH has the advantage of a smaller outside diameter, but still with a 3.6-mm operating channel, although the air and water channels seem more vulnerable to blockage. All these endoscopes have a separate narrow channel to which a syringe can be attached to give a jet of water for washing the target. This can be used while the laser fibre is in the main channel, which is a major asset. Laser vaporization of tumour produces hot gases which may condense on the objective lens of the endoscope, particularly if the tissue is very close to the instrument. This can happen with all instruments and modification to the lens washing system may be necessary to reduce the need to remove the instrument to clean the distal lens manually during a procedure.

The final choice of endoscope is personal. Sometimes adequate venting of the co-axial gas is possible by simple aspiration, or, for high oesophageal lesions, by spontaneous escape around the instrument, although unpleasant smoke escapes into the room, which makes a separate smoke extractor desirable. Narrower endoscopes seem more vulnerable to laser damage, and the channels get blocked more easily.

7.1.4 ENDOSCOPIC TECHNIQUE

Once the endoscope has been inserted, it is important to identify the neoplastic areas causing the worst obstruction and direct treatment to these areas, although this is not always immediately possible for technical reasons. The objective is to destroy as much exophytic, intraluminal tumour as is consistent with minimal risk of perforation, and to slow down intraluminal regrowth. Several techniques can be used, depending on the nature of the tumour treated and the preference of the endoscopist. The first choice is whether to start at the top or the bottom.

The major problem in treating the tumour from above downwards is that treated areas not actually vaporized rapidly become oedematous, and impair access to more distal areas during a treatment session. This can be avoided by starting treatment distally. In some cases, despite clinically significant dysphagia, it is still possible to pass the cancer with the endoscope at the time of first examination. In these cases, to reduce immediate local oedema, it is best to start therapy at the inferior margin of the tumour and work back to the superior margin. This may also make it feasible to treat the whole tumour in one session. Even if the endoscope will not pass the obstruction initially, most lesions can be passed with a guide-wire and then dilated with bougies to create a temporary lumen wide enough for the instrument. This often assists laser treatment by making more tumour immediately accessible to the laser beam, but balloon or bougie dilatation causes considerable local tissue damage and increases the risk of perforation and the ensuing oozing of blood may make it difficult to see target areas clearly.

If the lesion cannot be passed with the endoscope or the guide-wire for dilators, treatment must start at the superior margin. The fibre tip is held 5–10 mm above the target tissue and aimed at prominent and protruding nodules of tumour, using 1-second shots at 50–80 W power. Limited access may reduce this distance, but there is a greater risk to the fibre and endoscope. Usually some vaporization of tissue is seen, with obvious necrosis of underlying layers seen as blanching or as superficial charring (any shots on to blood cause charring). This process is continued, shaving the tumour back towards the oesophageal wall, but stopping short of normal tissue. Two to three millimetres depth of necrosed tissue will slough a few days after lasering, so allowance must be made for this in deciding how much tumour can be treated safely. The amount of tumour that can be treated in one session usually depends on endoscopic access and patient tolerance. If in doubt about what is under a particular area, it is better to wait for the necrosed tissue to slough, and continue therapy at a subsequent endoscopy. When more than one endoscopy is required to complete a primary course of treatment (the average is two to three sessions per patient), the optimum time between sessions is 3–4 days. This time is required to make the necrosed areas easy to remove (and to give the patient at least 1 day's break between sessions) without inordinately prolonging treatment.

At the second procedure, previously lasered areas appear yellow-white and necrotic although if the interval from the first procedure is more than a few days, most slough separates spontaneously. As much of this necrotic material as possible should be removed before further treatment. The simplest way is to dislodge it with the endoscope itself or a stiff endoscope cleaning brush pushing debris beyond the lesion, although suction and biopsy techniques may also be effective. Once viable tumour is seen (which under these circumstances is often red, friable and haemorrhagic) this is treated as initially and this process can be repeated until the tumour is sufficiently recanalized to permit passage of the endoscope through to the stomach. Once the lumen is re-established, the whole neoplastic section of oesophagus should be carefully re-examined, and all obviously malignant areas treated. Any residual nodules may be vaporized, but at this stage, great care must be taken not to overtreat as this increases the risk of perforation. Flat malignant areas are treated with short bursts of laser energy, aiming to blanch the surface without vaporization in order to slow down intraluminal regrowth, as will be discussed later.

Two other factors can be identified which influence the technical difficulties involved.

(a) Texture

Soft, well-vascularized, pink, polypoid lesions absorb most of the laser light that falls on them, and are very easy to vaporize. In contrast, hard, white tumours reflect much of the incident light, and are much more difficult to destroy. The former respond to powers of 50–60 W while the latter require 70–80 W.

(b) Position

The easiest cancers to treat are those in the middle third of the oesophagus which is straight and there is reasonable room to manoeuvre. Cervical lesions are the most difficult as this area is uncomfortable for the patient, and access is difficult. Lesions at the gastro-oesophageal junction may cause problems if there is sharp angulation, as this may make identification of the way forward difficult.

An example of an oesophageal carcinoma before and after treatment is shown in Figure 7.2.

A further development is the introduction of artificial sapphire tips for the laser fibre known as contact laser probes (Surgical Laser Technologies, Keighley, UK). These can be attached to the end of fibre delivery systems and provide a new concept in endoscopic laser treatment. These tips are designed to be used in contact with the target, and produce their effect by a combination of the laser light transmitted through the sapphire and direct mechanical effect of the hot tip on tissue which can be rather like a hot knife on butter.

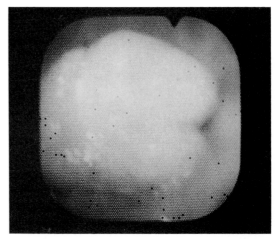

(a)

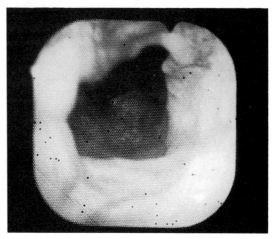

(b)

Figure 7.2 Endoscopic view of advanced, obstructing oesophageal cancer at presentation (a) and after two laser treatments (b).

The tips come in a variety of shapes (hemispherical, cylindrical, wedge shaped and spiked), and the laser power required is only 10–15 W, so a less powerful laser source can be used. This low power means that less oedema is produced in the immediate vicinity of the treated area, making it easier to work through a tight stenosis. The probes tend to stick to tissue, although this is helped by cooling them with co-axial saline rather than gas (which also eliminates the problem of venting the gas). However, there is also a greater risk of perforation with the probes, as they tend to be used to probe areas of the tumours that are not well visualized, and the endoscopist cannot always see tissue at the tip on firing. It has not yet been established whether prolonged exposure to low-power contact therapy can stimulate the fibrosis required for good long-term palliation without regrowth of intraluminal tumour as is seen after treatment with the high-power, non-contact technique. The only controlled study comparing contact with non-contact probes was performed on rectal tumours, and showed that patients found treatment more comfortable with the contact probes, but more treatment sessions were required. The early results were comparable with both types of probe, but no follow-up data was given in this report (Rutgeerts et al., 1987). In my experience, the contact probes are occasionally useful, but it is unlikely that they will replace the non-contact probes in the near future. I would advise gastroenterologists starting laser work to use a source that gives at least 80 W at the end of the fibre to have the capability of treating all types of tumour with the standard, non-contact fibres.

Laser therapy is best limited to exophytic tumours of the oesophagus, and obstruction caused by submucosal tumours or extrinsic compression should be treated by alternative methods such as a prosthetic tube. Others feel that it is occasionally reasonable to treat submucosal lesions, and this may be the case if there is supporting diagnostic information that defines the precise extent of the lesion (e.g. endoscopic ultrasound or computerized tomography). However, to treat submucosal lesions it is necessary first to burn through the overlying normal mucosa, and the risks of perforation are certainly higher than for exophytic lesions.

7.1.5 RESULTS

Since 1982, several groups from different countries have reported successful immediate relief of dysphagia in a large majority of cases with advanced malignant obstruction of the oesophagus or gastric cardia. Data is much more limited on the follow-up of these patients, although some groups have now published analyses of outcome after the initial course of laser treatment (Buset et al., 1983; Mellow and Pinkas, 1984; Riemann et al., 1985; Fleischer and Sivak, 1985; Krasner et al., 1987; Bown et al., 1987).

The early results are similar in all the major published series, with a significant relief of dysphagia achieved in 80–90% of cases. In looking at these results, the most difficult problem is quantifying the change in swallowing ability; the simplest way to do this is to grade dysphagia on a scale of 0–4.

0 = normal swallowing
1 = able to swallow most solids
2 = only able to swallow semi-solids
3 = only able to swallow liquids
4 = unable to swallow even liquids

The results from our first series of 34 patients are shown in Figure 7.3. (Bown et al., 1987); the average improvement in swallowing was 1.7 grades after the initial course of treatment. Five patients did not benefit from laser treatment. In one, the tumour was predominantly extrinsic, and therefore inaccessible to the laser, and in two others, the tumour was so advanced that it was felt unjustified to proceed with endoscopic therapy. For patients such as these last two, with severe anorexia, no form of recanalization would have helped their swallowing as the main problem was not the mechanical block. These three patients should be classified as inappropriate patient selection and the other two were laser perforations. Patients with a prosthetic tube can swallow some solids, although cannot be expected to take an entirely normal diet. Our results show that one-third of laser patients do better than the best results in those with a functioning tube, one-third have a similar result and one-third fare worse. It only takes one endoscopy to insert a

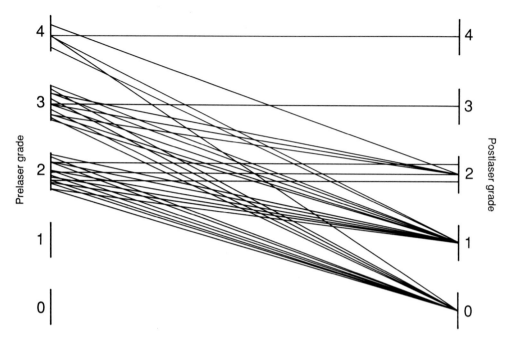

Figure 7.3 Grade of dysphagia before and after the first course of laser treatment in 34 successive patients. 0, Able to swallow all solids; 1, able to swallow most solids; 2, only able to swallow semisolids; 3, only able to swallow liquids; 4, unable to swallow even liquids. Reproduced from Bown *et al.* (1987) with permission.

prosthetic tube, and we averaged 2.7 endoscopies for an initial course of laser treatment with an average of 4400 Joules of laser energy per session. We have now treated over 100 patients and the overall pattern of results has been similar, although the average number of endoscopies for the initial course of treatment has fallen to 2.0.

Perforation is the most important acute complication, and from a review of the literature on laser complications occurs in 4.2% of cases (about half the rate for perforation following endoscopic insertion of a prosthesis) (Delvaux and Escourrou, 1985). However, the risk of perforation is higher in patients who have had previous radiotherapy (23%) compared with those who have not (3.6%). It is also higher if endoscopic dilatation is used at the time of laser treatment. A little oozing of blood is often seen during these endoscopies, but significant haemorrhage is rare, occurring in about 1%. Some degree of chest pain occurs

in about 20% after treatment, but it is rare for this to last more than a few hours. Other reasons for failure are commonly related to the position of the tumour. Some authors describe good endoscopic results for tumours in the cervical oesophagus, but the patient is still unable to swallow, presumably due to malignant involvement of muscle or nerves at that level. Problems also occur at the gastro-oesophageal junction where the angulation may frustrate all attempts at recanalization if the direction of the lumen cannot be identified.

The mean survival after laser treatment in our series was 19 weeks (range 2–44), which is similar to that in other series both after intubation and laser treatment. The most difficult factor to analyse is recurrent dysphagia after laser therapy. There appear to be two forms of this, as summarized in Table 7.1.

Recurrence due to regrowth of exophytic tumour can be retreated with the laser, with

Table 7.1 Follow-up after successful laser treatment of malignant dysphagia (28 patients)

	Patients	
	No.	%
No recurrent dysphagia	10	36
Recurrence treatable by laser	13	46*
Recurrence not treatable by laser	5	18†

* After mean of 5 weeks.
† After mean of 10 weeks.

good results, but our recent analysis suggests that this form of recurrence may be at least partly preventable. Post-mortem examination of oesophageal tumours treated successfully with the laser showed considerable fibrosis in the laser-treated areas, even in patients who had not received radiotherapy or any other treatment (Figure 7.4). Such fibrosis may be slowing down local tumour regrowth, so if *all* areas of neoplastic mucosa are coagulated, even areas that do not require debulking to relieve obstruction, local regrowth may be reduced. However, fibrosis in treated areas can also have disadvantages. In a small number of patients, recurrent dysphagia has been due to a benign-looking stricture in the previously treated area, presumably due to contraction in fibrous tissue. As shown in Table 7.1, these strictures occur later than exophytic recurrences, and are usually tough strictures which are difficult to treat by dilatation with or without insertion of a prosthetic tube. Some of the other late recurrences are due to pressure from extrinsic tumours, and, like fibrous strictures, can only be treated by mechanical dilatation and intubation (Bown *et al.*, 1987).

In an attempt to anticipate some of the problems of recurrent dysphagia, we carry out follow-up endoscopy about 4 weeks after initial laser treatment, at which time any recurrent exophytic tumour can be treated with the laser, or a developing fibrous stricture can be dilated. If left until symptoms develop,

fibrous strictures can be extremely tough and may perforate on dilatation. Fibrous, post-laser strictures occur most often in tumours at the gastric cardia, and may in part be due to reflux oesophagitis which can occur after laser recanalization as the anti-reflux mechanism has been destroyed by the tumour. Anti-reflux measures may reduce the incidence of these strictures.

The best results after laser recanalization are better than after other endoscopic techniques, but the results are very variable. Better ways of using lasers endoscopically may develop, but to extend the duration of good palliation,

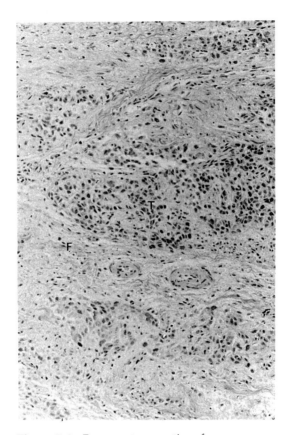

Figure 7.4 Post-mortem section from an oesophageal carcinoma treated 8 months previously and not requiring any subsequent treatment for dysphagia. Areas of tumour (T) are apparent, surrounded by extensive fibrous tissue (F) in laser-treated areas.

it may be appropriate to develop complementary techniques to treat tumour outside the lumen of the oesophagus which is not accessible to the laser. The most promising of these is intracavitary radiotherapy, as discussed in Chapter 8, as this does not have the prolonged morbidity often associated with external beam radiotherapy. Rapid relief of dysphagia with the laser followed by intracavitary irradiation to give an extended period of local palliation could be the best option for the future (Bader *et al.*, 1986).

Dysphagia is by far the commonest local symptom of advanced tumours of the oesophagus and gastric cardia. However, chest pain and bleeding may also be troublesome and neither responds to laser treatment as well as dysphagia does, but both may be alleviated in at least some patients. Several of our patients with a vague continuous retrosternal pain commented that this was relieved following successful recanalization, and others with pain on swallowing were also helped. Significant haemorrhage from oesophageal tumours is unusual although it occurs more frequently from lesions in the gastric cardia.

7.2 LOWER GASTROINTESTINAL TRACT TUMOURS

The vast majority of colorectal cancers are best treated by surgery. However, there are some cases, particularly of rectal cancer, who are unsuitable for surgery either due to the extent of local disease or metastases or poor general condition (Goligher, 1984). These patients have distressing local symptoms, and a range of techniques has been attempted to relieve them without resorting to major surgical intervention. Radiotherapy, cryotherapy, electrocoagulation and, more recently, lasers have proved effective under appropriate circumstances, but the precise treatment under direct vision, which is possible with the laser, gives this approach several advantages. It can be applied safely to lesions that extend above

the peritoneal reflection, using a flexible sigmoidoscope with little or no sedation and day-case therapy is often possible.

The principles of treatment are exactly the same as for the upper gastrointestinal tumours. The tumour bulk is usually greater in the rectum than in the oesophagus, but there is also more room to manoeuvre the endoscope. The objective of therapy is to debulk as much exophytic tumour as possible, with care not to coagulate too deeply, and avoid perforation. This relieves symptoms of rectal bleeding, tenesmus, diarrhoea and incontinence as well as obstruction. Abdominal radiographs of a patient with an obstructing rectal cancer before and after laser treatment are shown in Figure 7.5. In three recent series (Vliegen and Tytgat, 1986; Bown *et al.*, 1986; Brunetaud, Mosquet and Houcke, 1987) significant symptomatic improvement was achieved in 80–90% of patients with advanced tumours. In the largest series (Brunetaud *et al.*, 1987), better results were achieved for relieving rectal bleeding and diarrhoea than for obstructive symptoms, and circumferential tumours were less satisfactory to treat than those that did not completely encircle the bowel. Complications were rare but perforations were reported in the two large series (two of 95 by Brunetaud *et al.* (1987) and six of 84 by Vliegen and Tytgat (1986)). These were fatal in four cases, in two of whom the perforations occurred above the peritoneal reflection. It is not clear why control of blood loss seems more effective in lower than upper gastrointestinal tract tumours, but perhaps the better access in the rectum makes it easier to coagulate larger volumes of tumour effectively. This may also explain the lower proportion of patients who need subsequent intervention for recurrent local symptoms compared with those requiring repeated treatment for dysphagia (23% versus 64% in our experience), although the average survival after treatment in each group was similar (15 versus 19 weeks).

Laser therapy may be useful as a prelude to

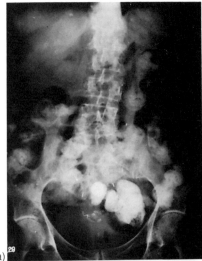

(a)

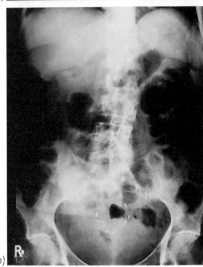

(b)

Figure 7.5 Rectal carcinoma. Anastomotic recurrence after anterior resection 1 year earlier. (a) Plain abdominal X-ray 1 week after a barium enema, showing gross faecal impaction and prolonged retention of the barium. (b) Plain abdominal X-ray after three laser treatments. The colon has cleared and now contains air.

surgery in high-risk patients who present with large bowel obstruction due to carcinoma. Endoscopic laser recanalization can overcome the obstruction temporarily so the patient can be in optimum condition for a one-stage definitive surgical procedure. A recent survey has shown that in-hospital

mortality for resection of colorectal cancers rises from 9% for unobstructed lesions to 22% for obstructed cases (Phillips *et al.*, 1985).

Laser treatment may be definitive treatment for villous adenoma (Brunetaud, Mosquet and Houcke, 1985) or small carcinoma of the large bowel in patients who are unfit for surgery due to advanced age or other serious disease, and disease-free survival for up to 3 years has been reported (Brunetaud *et al.*, 1987). However, until laser effects can be more precisely controlled so that the extent of laser necrosis closely matches the extent of the neoplasm being treated, surgery must remain the best option for cure if the patient is otherwise fit.

7.3 PHOTODYNAMIC THERAPY

Photodynamic therapy (PDT) has attracted considerable interest as a non-thermal approach to the local treatment of malignant tumours with lasers that has the potential for tumour selectivity (Doiron and Gomer, 1984). It is based on the systemic administration of sensitizing drugs – the best known of which is HpD (haematoporphyrin derivative) – which are retained with some degree of selectivity in areas of severe dysplasia or frank malignancy. These drugs fluoresce under ultraviolet light, which may be of value in localizing early lesions and can be activated by visible light of a wavelength matched to an absorption peak to produce singlet oxygen, which has a local cytotoxic effect. Local tumour destruction is possible but it is in an early stage of development, and many of the factors involved are poorly understood. It is far from clear what role it may have to play in the treatment of human disease.

The mechanism of PDT necrosis appears to involve shutdown of tumour vasculature rather than any effect on individual malignant cells. Also, healing seems to be different; in contrast to thermal necrosis, as seen after Nd –YAG laser treatment, which heals with at least some fibrosis, animal tumours treated by

PDT disappear completely although normal colon heals by regeneration after PDT necrosis (Barr *et al.*, 1987). This has considerable implications when choosing lesions to treat clinically, as necrosed tumour may slough without a surrounding area of scarring, leaving a defect which is only functionally and mechanically acceptable if there is enough supporting tissue present. Extensive necrosis from PDT of tumours involving the full thickness of the oesophageal wall could thus cause a perforation or lead to major haemorrhage, and it is likely that PDT will be of more value in treating small, early lesions than advanced obstructing tumours. It has already been used in Japan to treat early gastric carcinoma in patients unfit for surgery, with encouraging results (Kato *et al.*, 1986). There have been anecdotal reports of PDT for advanced oesophageal cancers but the results described mix PDT and Nd–YAG laser hyperthermia, and use laser powers for PDT that could produce thermal effects, and the results are difficult to interpret (McCaughan *et al.*, 1984).

REFERENCES

Bader, M., Dittler, H. J., Ultsch, B. *et al.* (1986) Palliative treatment of malignant stenoses of the upper gastrointestinal tract using a combination of laser and afterloading therapy. *Endoscopy*, **18**, supp. 1, 27–36.

Barr, H., Tralau, C. J., Krasner, N. *et al.* (1987) Photodynamic therapy of the normal rat colon with phthalocyanine sensitisation. *Br. J. Cancer*, **56**, 111–8.

Bown, S. G., Barr, H., Matthewson, K. *et al.* (1986) Endoscopic treatment of inoperable colorectal cancers with the Nd–YAG laser. *Br. J. Surg.*, **73**, 949–52.

Bown, S. G., Hawes, R., Matthewson, K. *et al.* (1987) Endoscopic laser palliation for advanced malignant dysphagia. *Gut*, **28**, 799–807.

Brunetaud, J. M., Maunoury, V., Ducrotte, P. *et al.* (1987) Palliative treatment of rectosigmoid carcinoma by laser endoscopic photoablation. *Gastroenterology*, **92**, 663–68.

Brunetaud, J.M., Mosquet, L. and Houcke, M. (1985) Villous adenoma of the rectum. Results of endoscopic treatment with argon and Nd–YAG lasers. *Gastroenterology*, **89**, 832–7.

Buset, M., Dunham, F., Baize, M. *et al.* (1983) Nd–YAG laser – a new palliative alternative in the management of oesophageal cancer. *Endoscopy*, **15**, 353–6.

Delvaux, M. and Escourrou, J. (1985) Complications observed during laser treatment of tumours of the upper digestive tract. *Acta Endoscopica*, **15**, 13–8.

Doiron, D. R. and Gomer, G. J. (1984) *Porphyrin Localisation and Treatment of Tumours*, Alan R. Liss, New York.

Fleischer, D., Kessler, F. and Haye, O. (1982) Endoscopic Nd–YAG laser therapy for carcinoma of the oesophagus: a new palliative approach. *Am. J. Surg.*, **143**, 280–3.

Fleischer, D. and Sivak, M. V. (1985) Endoscopic Nd–YAG laser therapy as a palliation for oesophagogastric cancer. *Gastroenterology*, **89**, 827–30.

Goligher, J. (1984) *Surgery of the Anus. Rectum and Colon*, 5th edn, Baillière Tindall, London, pp. 741–3.

Kato, H., Kawaguchi, M., Konaka, C. *et al.* (1986) Evaluation of photodynamic therapy in gastric cancer. *Lasers Med. Sci.*, **1**, 67–74.

Krasner, N., Barr, H., Skidmore, C. and Morris, A. I. (1987) Laser therapy for malignant dysphagia. *Gut*, **28**, 792–8.

Matthewson, K., Barton, T., Lewin, M. R. *et al.* (1988) Low power interstitial Nd–YAG laser photocoagulation in normal and neoplastic rat colon. *Gut*, **29**, 27–34.

McCaughan, J. S., Hicks, W., Laufman, L. *et al.* (1984) Palliation of oesophageal malignancy with photoradiation therapy. *Cancer*, **54**, 2905–8.

Mellow, M. H. and Pinkas, H. (1984) Endoscopic therapy for oesophageal carcinoma with Nd–YAG laser: prospective evaluation of efficacy, complications and survival. *Gastrointest. Endosc.*, **30**, 334–9.

Phillips, R. K. S., Hittinger, R., Fry, J. S. and Fielding, L. P. (1985) Malignant large bowel obstruction. *Br. J. Surg.*, **72**, 296–302.

Riemann, J. F., Ell, C., Lux, G. and Demling, L. (1985) Combined therapy of malignant stenoses of the upper gastrointestinal tract by means of laser beam and bougienage. *Endoscopy*, **17**, 43–8.

Rutgeerts, P., Van Trappen, G., D'Heygere, F. and Geboes, K. (1987) Endoscopic contact Nd–YAG laser therapy for colorectal cancer – a randomised comparison with non-contact therapy. *Lasers Med. Sci.*, **2**, 69–72.

Vliegen, E. M. H. and Tytgat, G. N. T. (1986) Nd–YAG laser photocoagulation in gastroenterology – its role in palliation of colorectal cancer. *Lasers Med. Sci.*, **1**, 75–80.

CHAPTER EIGHT

Intracavitary irradiation for oesophageal malignancy

C. G. Rowland
and
K. M. Pagliero

In the early part of this century radioactive sources were placed into many tumours including those of the oesophagus (Guisez, 1925). These 'brachytherapy' techniques have a number of attractions for radiation delivery and are enjoying a world-wide renaissance. Apart from gynaecological practice widespread use has been discouraged mainly by safety factors. Developments were few until the advent of afterloading treatment systems such as the Selectron which allows safe, precise (anatomical and physical) placement of radioactive sources loaded by a microprocessor-controlled machine after placement of unloaded applicators. This equipment is now widely available in, or accessible to most hospitals (Nucletron Trading Ltd, Rijksstraatveg 269, PO Box 110, 3956 C P Leersum, The Netherlands). In cancer of the oesophagus little impact has yet been made on overall survival despite encouraging reports from small selected series. For many patients the most realistic treatment goal is effectively to relieve dysphagia, one of the most unpleasant symptoms of any cancer. Any improvement in palliation of dysphagia would be welcome.

Some 3 years ago we set out to develop a treatment technique which would provide simple, safe palliation of dysphagia for a large number of patients (Rowland and Pagliero, 1985).

8.1 TECHNIQUE

1. A standard fibreoptic endoscope is used to visualize the upper and lower tumour limits and to biopsy the tumour. Skip lesions are carefully noted. In about 30% minimal bougie dilatation is used to facilitate visualization of the lower tumour.

2. The oesophageal applicator is a flexible outer tube 8 mm in diameter. At its tip is an angled guide channel allowing passage of a flexible guide-wire. The inner tube which transmits the caesium-137 sources is locked into the outer applicator. It allows treatment of the lower 13 cm of oesophagus. If a decision is made to treat virtually the whole oesophagus a shorter insert tube can be used to treat the proximal 13 cm of oesophagus sequentially. The total length that can be treated is 26 cm. The applicator is inserted under local or general anaesthetic. The endoscope is passed and the tumour limits defined under screening control. The flexible guide-wire is then passed via the endoscope side channel through the tumour into the stomach. The endoscope is removed and the oesophageal applicator passed down the guide-wire and using radiological screening is positioned to straddle the tumour. Finally, the guide is removed and the

applicator fixed to a facemask containing an insert to protect the tube should the patient have teeth. The mask is held in place with Velcro straps around the head (Figures 8.1–8.3).

3. The patient is returned to the Selectron suite (radiation protected room) and connected to the machine which is then programmed to give the required dose and time. The radioactive sources consist of 48 pellets of caesium-137 which are transferred pneumatically into the applicator.

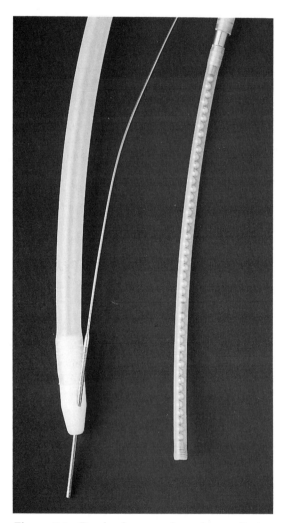

Figure 8.1 Rowland oesophageal applicator, guide-wire and insert tube.

Throughout treatment the patient is observed on closed circuit television. If staff need to enter the room the treatment can be stopped by command or a failsafe interlock on the door, the sources being automatically returned to the machine. The Selectron will reprogramme itself regarding treatment time (Figure 8.4).

4. In our study we have aimed for rapid treatment and have used a single dose of 15 Gy (1500 rads) at a reference point 1 cm off the central axis of the applicator. The surface dose in contact with the tumour is much higher than this. The target volume is thus represented by a cylinder 2 cm in diameter and 13 cm in length. Using all 48 sources gives a treatment time of about 1.14 hours (this adjusted for source decay) or 2.28 hours if the whole oesophagus is treated.

8.2 PATIENTS AND ASSESSMENT

One hundred and twenty patients (median age 76 years, oldest patient 93 years) have been treated; four have been unable to tolerate the tube for the requisite time. Only occasionally has further sedation been required. All cases have been unsuitable for radical surgery or radiation therapy because of metastases, size of primary tumour (over 5 cm in length) or performance status. The response of the patients' dysphagia at 6 weeks has been defined as a movement of 0–2 or 1–3 on the following scale:

0 = complete obstruction
1 = fluids only
2 = puree, mince or mash
3 = normal swallowing

8.3 RESULTS

Squamous carcinoma had a 70% response at 6 weeks (range 6–80 weeks); adenocarcinoma (cardia) had a 60% response at 6 weeks (range 6–110 weeks). In a limited number of patients (due to the logistics of recall) barium studies

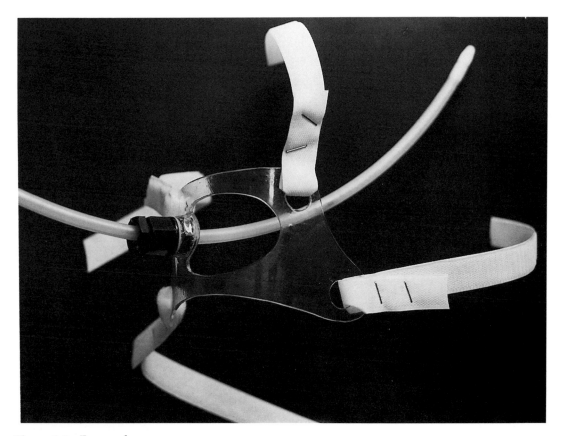

Figure 8.2 Facemask.

confirmed these responses. About 10% of patients survive beyond 1 year with disease, but are symptom free. This is clearly related to their tumour biology but is an example of how this group might bias curative trials.

8.4 TOXICITY

This has been minimal, allowing most patients to return home the day after treatment. Five patients have had sore throat, four transient oesophagitis, five epigastric pain/discomfort, two nausea and two diarrhoea. One patient developed a fistula – a contributing factor here may have been previous radiation therapy for carcinoma of the breast. In one case the oesophagus was perforated but this responded to conservative treatment,

intubation being performed at a later date. The two cases of radiation stricture have been successfully dilated.

8.5 DISCUSSION

Previous experience in our centre with pulsion intubation gave a mortality of 14.3% with a hospital stay of 8.3 days (Unruh and Pagliero, 1985). Recurrent tube blockage was common. Our results with intracavitary irradiation appear significantly better; this is now used as our first-line palliation – later intubation for failures is not precluded. In the entire group there has been no need to readmit acutely for dysphagia.

Over the past 3 years, inclusion of

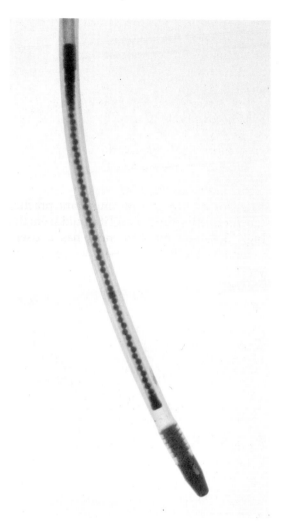

Figure 8.3 Dummy sources in applicator.

are few, oesophagitis being far less than with external beam. We have experienced only two cases of fistula (one still alive at 3 years). Other workers (Hishikawa *et al.*, 1987) have given higher figures but this is in combination with high-dose external beam radiation – in other series multimodality treatment has been used and it seems difficult to sort out the contributory factors. We feel strongly that in the majority of patients that we see, cure is only a false hope and aggressive treatment not justified; here, the risk of fistula is low from intracavitary treatment alone. Again it emphasizes

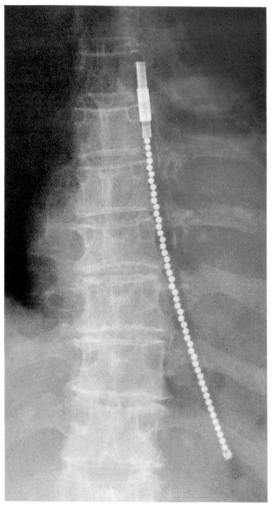

Figure 8.4 Dummy sources in position.

brachytherapy for palliation has resulted in a reduction of in-hospital mortality and longer survival than with intubation. Its efficacy in palliation has further improved results by discouraging palliative resection. The overall result of the entire series is double the number of survivors at 2 years compared with previously reported results and allows us to review the disease as a whole with a little less pessimism (Kaul, Rowland and Pagliero, 1988).

The side-effects of intracavitary treatment

the importance of knowing the effects of intracavitary irradiation when used alone at this and other sites before its integration into other schedules.

Detailed costing has shown that in our centre palliative intubation costs around £1500, intracavitary irradiation £250. These factors clearly cannot be ignored by any health care providers. Intracavitary irradiation is effective in relieving dysphagia and is a simple, safe and economical treatment. As we have aimed at palliation we have used a single 'shot', although other fractionation schedules can be used especially when combining this with external beam radiation, surgery and chemotherapy attempting cure. In Vancouver (Flores et al., 1985, 1986) a further large series of patients has been safely treated with a combination of intracavitary and external beam radiation and the authors conclude this treatment should be explored as a palliative treatment in all cases; as a potentially curative treatment in the upper oesophagus; and as a preoperative adjuvant in lower oesophagus and cardia. More recently this group has shown a significant increase in therapeutic ratio for the use of intracavitary irradiation (Flores, 1988). Allowing for different philosophies (attempted cure as against palliation) between North America and Europe, it seems that intracavitary irradiation has a significant role.

High dose-rate machines which allow an intense iridium source to be transmitted through 2-mm diameter catheters with treatment times of around 10 minutes may improve results further, and are currently under assessment.

The advantages of this technique compared with other methods of palliation are:

1. Outpatient treatment.
2. Short treatment times.
3. Minimal nursing care.
4. No major positional changes during treatment.
5. Accurate, failsafe treatment control.
6. The tumour is actually treated (not cut or bypassed).
7. Staff are protected from radiation hazards.
8. Significant saving in health-care costs may result.
9. A simple, safe technique not restricted to high-technology centres.

Radiation has been and seems likely to remain for a long time an important practical tool for treating cancer, and it would seem that high dose-rate brachytherapy has a useful potential contribution to make in the next few years.

REFERENCES

Flores, A. D. (1988) Cancer of the Oesophagus and Cardia: An Overview of Radiotherapy. Brachytherapy 2 (Proceedings Brachytherapy Working Conference, *5th International Selectron User's Meeting* (1988) (ed. R. F. Mould) pp. 427–38.

Flores, A. D., Stoller, J. L., Nelems, B. and Hay, J. (1985, 1986) Intracavitary irradiation for esophageal cancer. *Lancet*, **ii**, 1365; Selectron Users Meeting, Vancouver, 4 September 1986.

Guisez, J. (1925) Malignant tumors of the esophagus. *J. Laryngol. Otol.*, **40**, 213–32.

Hishikawa, Y., Kamikonya, N., Tanaka, S. and Miura, T. (1987) Radiotherapy of esophageal carcinoma: role of high dose rate intracavitary irradiation. *Radiother. Oncol.*, **9**, 13–20.

Kaul, T. K., Rowland, C. G. and Pagliero, K. M. (1988) Carcinoma of the oesophagus: treatment with radical surgery or brachytherapy. Brachytherapy 2 (Proceedings Brachytherapy Working Conference, *5th International Selectron Users Meeting*, 1–3 September (1988) (ed. R. F. Mould), pp. 449–58.

Rowland, C. G. and Pagliero, K. M. (1985) Intracavitary irradiation in the palliation of carcinoma of the esophagus and cardia. *Lancet*, **ii**, 981–3.

Unruh, H. and Pagliero, K. M. (1985) Pulsion versus traction intubation for obstructing carcinoma of the esophagus. *Ann. Thor. Surg.*, **40**, 337–42.

CHAPTER NINE

Balloon dilatation for the treatment of achalasia

J. E. Richter
and
D. O. Castell

Achalasia is a motility disorder of the oesophagus characterized by loss of peristalsis and failure of relaxation of the gastro-oesophageal sphincter on swallowing (Castell, 1976). Although the age of onset is usually between 20 and 40 years, cases have been recorded in infants and the elderly. The classic symptom is progressive dysphagia, gradual in onset and usually painless, which may be precipitated by solids or liquids. Frequent regurgitation of undigested food is common, particularly at night. As the underlying pathophysiological defect cannot be reversed, treatment is directed towards symptomatic relief of the disorder, by disrupting the circular muscle fibres of the gastro-oesophageal sphincter. Thomas Willis performed the first oesophageal dilatation with a whale bone in the seventeenth century. Today the two-currently accepted forms of therapy for achalasia are pneumatic dilatation of the gastro-oesophageal sphincter and a distal oesophagomyotomy; the modified Heller procedure. Our discussion will review the various instruments and techniques for pneumatic dilatation, the results, complications, and comparison with surgical therapy.

9.1 PRELIMINARY EVALUATION AND INDICATIONS

Patients with suspected achalasia should have a thorough evaluation prior to definitive therapy in order to confirm the diagnosis and exclude an occult carcinoma. Achalasia is usually suggested by the clinical history and barium swallow. Upper gastrointestinal endoscopy, oesophageal manometry and nuclear scintigraphic studies subsequently may be needed to confirm the diagnosis.

Classically, the barium swallow shows widening of the oesophageal lumen often associated with tortuosity. The distal oesophagus shows a smooth, symmetrical, tapered narrowing. An air-fluid level may be seen on a chest radiograph or barium swallow in addition to retained particulate matter in the oesophagus. Tertiary contractions of the barium column in the oesophageal body are common.

The endoscopic appearances depend upon the stage of the disease. Many patients have normal mucosa, but as the oesophagus dilates from retention of ingested material mild diffuse erythema may be noted distally. Later still, white thickening of the mucosa results from stagnation oesophagitis. As the endoscope approaches the gastro-oesophageal junction resistance may be noted, but with gentle forward pressure the instrument should 'pop' into the stomach. Inability to pass the endoscope easily into the stomach raises a suspicion of malignancy or a benign stricture. Once in the stomach, careful inspection of the gastro-oesophageal junction should be noted on retroflexed view to exclude an infiltrating carcinoma of the cardia.

It is desirable to confirm the diagnosis manometrically. The characteristic manometric features include:

1. Absence of peristalsis in the oesophageal body.
2. Incomplete or absent relaxation of the gastro-oesophageal sphincter with swallowing (Cohen and Lipshutz, 1971).
3. Elevation of resting gastro-oesophageal sphincter pressure.
4. Resting intra-oesophageal pressures greater than or equal to intragastric pressures.

The traditional manometric diagnosis of achalasia has rested on the demonstration of at least the first two abnormalities. However, we have recently observed a subset of individuals with symptoms suggestive of achalasia in whom oesophageal manometry demonstrated aperistalsis but complete, albeit short duration, relaxation of the gastro-oesophageal sphincter (Katz et al., 1986). These patients appear to have 'early achalasia' since they report a shorter duration of symptoms and less weight loss than a comparable group with classic achalasia.

In atypical cases of achalasia, nuclear scintigraphic studies may help in defining and quantitating the functional defect in oesophageal emptying (Gross, Johnson and Kaminski, 1979; Holloway et al., 1983). In the normal subject, a labelled test meal should empty rapidly (less than 5 minutes) from the oesophagus into the stomach with the patient in the upright position. We have found that patients with classic achalasia retain approximately 75% of the solid test meal at 5 minutes while patients with early achalasia retain 25–

50% and more rapidly empty their oesophagi over the next 15 minutes than their classic counterparts (Katz et al., 1986).

After the diagnosis is confirmed, we believe pneumatic dilatation should be the initial form of therapy for most patients with achalasia. When properly performed, the success rate of pneumatic dilatation approaches that of surgery, and the likelihood of subsequent gastro-oesophageal reflux is less, the duration of hospitalization required for the procedure is shorter, and overall morbidity is considerably less than that of surgical cardiomyotomy. Indications for surgical treatment include:

1. Several unsuccessful attempts at pneumatic dilatation.
2. Inability to exclude oesophageal carcinoma.
3. Children and psychotic patients who are unable to cooperate (Castell, 1976; Vantrappen and Hellemans, 1980).

The last indication is relative since pneumatic dilatation can be safely performed under general anaesthesia (Fellows, Ogilvie and Atkinson, 1983). With the development of guide-wires and balloons which can be positioned endoscopically, the extremely tortuous 'sigmoid' oesophagus is no longer a contraindication to pneumatic dilatation. Diverticula of the lower segment of the oesophagus, however, increase the risk of perforation during dilatation, and a myotomy may be safer in these patients (Vantrappen and Hellemans, 1980).

9.2 MECHANICAL AND PNEUMATIC DILATORS

The specifications of currently available dilators are listed in Table 9.1. Four types of dilators are available:

(a) Mechanical

The Starck dilator (Starck, 1924) is a device with expanding metal arms where the dilating

Table 9.1 Specifications of the most popular pneumatic dilators

Dilator	Type	Company	Diameter (cm)
1. Mosher	Pneumatic	Pilling, USA	3.0, 3.6
2. Hurst–Tucker	Pneumatic	Pilling	3.0
3. Browne–McHardy	Pneumatic	Pilling	3.0, 3.6
4. Sippy	Pneumatic		3.0, 3.5, 3.8, 4.0, 4.2, 4.5, 5.0
5. Rider–Moeller	Pneumatic	Eder Instruments, USA	2.9, 3.8, 4.8
6. Rigiflex	Pneumatic	Microinvasive, USA	3.0, 3.5, 4.0
7. Witzel	Endoscopic	Wimmed Med Technik, FR Germany	4.0

diameter is determined by manual force. It was the first commercially available dilator but generally has been replaced by pneumatic balloon dilators. The rigidity of the instrument precludes its use in a tortuous oesophagus.

(b) Hydrostatic

Single bags of fixed diameter which are distended with water under various pressures. They too have generally been replaced by pneumatic dilators.

(i) Negus (Thomas, Negus and Bateman, 1955) Positioned through a large endoscope under visual direction. Usually requires general anaesthesia.

(ii) Plummer (1908) Usually passed over a previously swallowed string and positioned by measurement of distance from the incisors.

(c) Pneumatic

Bag dilators distended with air under various pressures. The maximum diameter of these bags is fixed by a silk, nylon, or plastic cover.

(i) Mosher (1923) Cylindrical bag with six stripes of radiopaque material set into the wall.

(ii) Sippy (Kurlander et al., 1963; Van Goidsenhaven, Vantrappen and Verbeke, 1983) A series of bags from 3 to 5 cm in diameter which can be placed sequentially on a metal bougie. The bags are hourglass shaped. The bougie can be passed over a guide-wire.

(iii) Hurst–Tucker (Tucker, 1939) and Browne–McHardy (Browne and McHardy, 1939) These are virtually identical dilators with cylindrical radiopaque balloons. The mercury-filled rubber tube is heavy yet pliable. A guide-wire cannot be used, so they may be difficult to pass in a sigmoid oesophagus.

(iv) Rider–Moeller (Rider et al., 1969) Hourglass-shaped bag of variable size. The bag is not radiopaque. Dilator is passed over a guide-wire.

(v) Rigiflex (Cox, Buckton and Bennett, 1986) Similar in design to the Grunkzig angioplasty catheter. The cylindrical balloon is made of non-radiopaque polyethylene and mounted on a flexible bougie. The dilator can be passed over a guide-wire.

(d) Endoscopic

A new method of oesophageal dilatation has been described (Tytgat and Derltartogjager, 1977; Witzel, 1981) that is similar to conventional pneumatic dilatation, except that the dilator is mounted on a forward-viewing endoscope making it possible to position the dilator under directed vision. The Witzel dilator is made of non-radiopaque polyethylene.

The selection of a pneumatic dilator rests on personal preference since comparative studies are not available. Over the past 15 years, we have performed pneumatic dilatations with the Browne–McHardy, Rider–Moeller and, most recently, the Rigiflex dilators. For patients who have had previous unsuccessful pneumatic dilatations, or have a sigmoid oesophagus, it may be helpful to use variable-sized dilators directed into the stomach over a guide-wire. The Rider–Moeller, Rigiflex or Sippy dilators fulfil this purpose.

9.3 TECHNIQUE OF DILATATION

The oesophageal dilatation technique described below is the one performed by the authors at both the National Naval Medical Center, Bethesda, Maryland and Bowman-Gray School of Medicine, using primarily the Browne–McHardy and Rider–Moeller dilators.

Prior to pneumatic dilatation the inflatable bag is inspected by: (1) checking for leaks, (2) closely observing the symmetry of the bag during inflation and (3) measuring the maximum inflated circumference of the centre and outer aspects of the bag. The diameter of the bag at maximum distensions may vary from dilator to dilator. Wong and Johnson (1983) have noted a variation of 1.1 cm in dilators from the same manufacturer. A variation of 0.3 cm in diameter may be noted between the centre and outer aspects even of a 'symmetrical' bag. A small air leak from the bag may be acceptable, but large leaks signal the need for a replacement.

The patient is fasted overnight and taken to the radiology suite where the entire procedure is performed. A wide-bore (e.g. Ewald) tube is used to empty and irrigate the oesophagus. Premedication with local anaesthetic spray to mouth and throat, pethidine (meperidine) 50–75 mg i.v., and diazepam 2–10 mg i.v., is given as necessary to produce mild sedation and subsequent anaesthesia. With the patient sitting, the dilator is passed through the mouth until it is about 40–50 cm from the incisors. The patient then lies in the right anterior oblique position on the X-ray table. Under fluoroscopic guidance, the bag is positioned until it straddles the diaphragm. The bag is then inflated to 155 mmHg (3 p.s.i.) while noting the waist deformity of the bag. The waist must be maintained in the centre of the bag. As the diameter of the bag increases, the waist may tend to ride up the bag. If this happens, the bag should be deflated and then slowly reinflated with firm, upward traction on the dilator to maintain the waist in the centre of the bag. After the bag is confirmed to be in a proper position, inflation pressure is increased until the waist is entirely obliterated. The pressure usually required to dilate the adult oesophagus is between 9 and 15 psi 464 and 774 mmHg (9 and 15 p.s.i.). At this point patients usually experience moderate to severe discomfort across the lower chest. The high pressure is maintained for 60 seconds and then released. Several minutes later, the bag is reinflated for 60 seconds. During the repeat dilatation, loss of the waist at less than 309 mmHg (6 p.s.i.) is evidence of successful dilatation. No more than two dilatations are performed at a single session. A few streaks of blood are frequently seen on the balloon when it is withdrawn, but absence of blood does not necessarily indicate an unsuccessful dilatation.

After removal of the dilator, the oesophagus is examined radiographically. A nasoesophageal tube is inserted, the patient placed in a semi-erect position, and the oesophagus screened initially with water-soluble contrast material. If no obvious perforation is seen, this material is aspirated and the examination repeated with barium sulphate suspension. Films of the oesophago-gastric region are obtained and compared with the predilatation oesophagram. This examination is to identify complications and not to assess the adequacy of dilatation or predict the clinical response of the patient (Ott *et al.*, 1989). If a small 'confined' perforation or intramural haematoma is noted, the patient is not allowed to eat or drink, and is observed closely for 24 hours. These minor complications are frequently asymptomatic or can be treated conservatively with antibiotics and intravenous feedings. If barium is observed to flow freely into the mediastinum and left chest, immediate surgery is indicated.

If recovery proceeds normally, the patient is allowed to drink 4–6 hours after the procedure. The patient remains in hospital overnight and receives a normal breakfast in the morning. If the dysphagia is improved, we discharge the patient without repeating another barium swallow (Bennett and Hendrix, 1970) or performing a nuclear emptying study (Holloway et al., 1983), because subsequent relief of dysphagia and weight gain are the best indicators of a successful outcome. Occasional patients complain of intermittent pain for several days. Radiology does not show a perforation, and the pain may be due to mucosal trauma, mild acid reflux, or reactive 'spasm'.

Table 9.2 lists dilatation techniques reported in several series. It is difficult to evalu-ate the merits and drawbacks of the different techniques for pneumatic dilatation as prospective controlled comparisons have never been done. Furthermore, it is not known which is the most important variable: the diameter of the bag, the filling pressure of the bag, the duration of maximum bag inflation, or the number of dilatations.

9.4 OVERALL OUTCOME OF PNEUMATIC DILATATION

9.4.1 COMPLICATIONS

The reported incidence of immediate complications of pneumatic dilatation range from 1% to 20% (Table 9.3), mostly chest pain, fever, or gastrointestinal haemorrhage. The incidence of oesophageal perforation ranges from 1% to 16%, the majority being small, localized leaks. These small perforations can be managed conservatively with antibiotics and intravenous nutrition (Vantrappen and Hellemans, 1980). Only 20 of the 53 perforations reported (Table 9.3) required surgery.

Table 9.2 Techniques of pneumatic dilatation for achalasia

Authors	Dilator	Premedication	Dilator diameter (cm)	Pressure	Duration
Olsen et al. (1951)	Plummer	–	3.6	492–534 mm Hg	Several seconds
Schindler (1956)	Stark	–	Size determined by manual force		Continued squeeze until waist disappears
Nanson (1962)	Mosher	+	3.6	778 mm Hg	15 s – repeated 3 times
Vantrappen et al. (1963)	Sippy	–	3.0–5.0	200 mmHg and 300 mmHg	1 min at each pressure
Bennett and Hendrix (1970)	Hurst–Tucker	+	3.0	467–778 mmHg	30–60 s
Fellow et al. (1983)	Rider–Moeller	General anaesthesia	2.9 for most	280–300 mmHg	3 min
Dellipiani and Hewetson (1986)	Browne–McHardy	+	3.0	778 mmHg	15 s – repeat times one
Agha and Lee (1986)	Witzel	+	4.0	300 mmHg	2 min

Table 9.3 Results and complications of pneumatic dilatation in series with over 40 achalasia patients

Authors	Dilator	Patients (no.)	Response (%)			Complications (%)			
			Good	Fair	Poor	Perforation	Others	GER*	Death
Vantrappen and Hellemans (1980)	Sippy	537	77	9	14	2.6	1.7	1	0.2
Sanderson et al. (1970)	Plummer	456	65	16	19	3.5	1.1	—	0
Olsen et al. (1951)	Plummer	452	60		40	2.2	7.5	—	0.4
Lawrance and Shoesmith (1959)	Negus	100	59		41	1.0	—	2	0
Schindler (1956)	Stark	84	95		5	2.0	4	—	0
Kurlander et al. (1963)	Sippy	62	32	56	8	13.0	3	—	0
Fellow et al. (1983)	Rider–Moeller	50	76	10	2	2.0	2	34	0
Bennett and Hendrix (1970)	Hurst–Tucker	48	70	11	19	6.0	0	17	0
Yon and Christensen (1975)	Mosher	48	46	—	—	0	4	7	0
Dellipiani and Hewetson (1988)	Browne–McHardy	45	86		14	8.8	11		0
Ott et al. (1989)	Browne–McHardy	42	85		15	9.5	3	—	2.3

—, Not discussed or applicable.
*GER: gastro-oesophageal reflux.

No deaths were reported from the series in which small perforations were treated by medical therapy alone. Recent surgical literature also supports conservative treatment of localized oesophageal perforations (Cameron et al., 1978; Michel, Grillo and Malt, 1981). This is an important concept because routine use of postdilatation barium studies is likely to reveal small mucosal tears simply as a consequence of dilatation. Gastro-oesophageal reflux is not a significant postdilatation problem. Vantrappen and Hellemans (1980) found less than 1% evidence of reflux utilizing a modified reflux test and Csendes et al. (1981) reported a positive reflux test in 7% of patients. Fellows, Ogilvie and Atkinson (1983) noted that 34% of patients had symptoms of heartburn after pneumatic dilatation but none had evidence of peptic stricture.

9.4.2 A SUGGESTED PHILOSOPHY REGARDING THE RISK OF OESOPHAGEAL PERFORATION

A small, but definite, risk of perforation accompanies the use of pneumatic dilatation. We approach this directly and positively from the beginning. The patient is advised about the two accepted methods of treatment for their achalasia (pneumatic dilatation or myotomy). They are also informed of the small possibility of perforation during dilatation and that, if it occurs, surgery similar to the other alternative (myotomy) may have to be performed. It is also made clear that, in most cases, the dilatation will eliminate the need for surgery. Possible perforation resulting from appropriate pneumatic dilatation should offer no major deterrent to this procedure if it is recognized early and treated as indicated.

9.4.3 RELIEF OF SYMPTOMS

The best indicator of the therapeutic efficacy of pneumatic dilatation seems to be the degree of oesophageal stasis several years after treatment. However, this is not simple to determine. The height of the barium column remaining in the oesophagus after a barium meal depends not only on the volume and density of the barium suspension, but also on the degree of dilatation and tortuosity of the oesophagus as well as the gastro-oesophageal sphincter tone (Vantrappen and Hellemans, 1980). Scintigraphy may be a simpler and more reliable method for assessing oesophageal emptying (Holloway et al., 1983), but has not so far been used to evaluate the long-term efficacy of pneumatic dilatation. Clinical indices, such as the degree of dysphagia, are difficult to quantify, and are not comparable from one study to another because of variable definition of dysphagia. Few studies indicate how often the patients experience dysphagia, how long it lasts, and whether the patient is forced to stop eating or to regurgitate.

Realizing these limitations in the evaluation of long-term efficacy, Table 9.3 summarizes the results and complications of pneumatic dilatation in series with greater than 40 achalasic patients. These reports indicate that 32–95% of patients have a good clinical result (usually defined as no further dysphagia) after pneumatic dilatation. In one study of patients who failed to improve after the first dilatation, 38% and 19% improved after the second and third dilatations respectively (Olsen et al., 1951). The efficacy of pneumatic dilatation was not related to the size of the dilator or duration of dilatation. Patients undergoing progressive pneumatic dilatations have lower success rates with the smaller size dilators, but overall less complications (Vantrappen and Hellemans, 1980). In the extensive experience of the Louvain (Belgium) group, Vantrappen and Hellemans (1980) obtained their best results in patients over the age of 45 years, in patients with a history of dysphagia for more than 5 years' duration, and in patients with only moderately dilated oesophagi.

9.4.4 RADIOGRAPHIC AND MANOMETRIC IMPROVEMENT

Pneumatic dilatation may result in an immediate and sustained reduction in the diameter of the oesophagus (Vantrappen and Hellemans, 1980), but a return to normal diameter is usually only observed if the oesophageal diameter before treatment was not larger than 70 mm. Unfortunately, the elongation and tortuosity of the oesophagus is not modified by pneumatic dilatation. We have observed an increase in the mean diameter at the oesophagogastric junction from 4.2 mm before dilatation to 7.5 mm immediately following dilatation (Ott et al., 1989). Vantrappen and Hellemans (1980) have reported similar results with the mean diameter increased from 2 mm (before) to 9 mm many months after pneumatic dilatation. These authors also noted that before treatment the gastric bubble was absent in 85% of the patients, and in only 10% many months later.

Manometric studies report significant decreases in gastro-oesophageal sphincter pressure and intra-oesophageal pressure immediately after dilatation but sphincter pressure tends subsequently to increase (Mellow, 1976; Holloway et al., 1983). Relaxation of the sphincter with swallowing does not return after dilatation but the 'residual pressure' is lower. The traditional impression has been that oesophageal peristalsis does not return after pneumatic dilatation (Mellow, 1976), but this has recently been questioned by several case reports (Mellow, 1976; Vantrappen et al., 1979) and the experience of the Cleveland Clinic (Lamet, Fleshler and Achkar, 1989). The latter group demonstrated a return of distally progressive peristaltic contractions in seven of 34 (20%) patients with achalasia successfully treated by pneumatic dilatation. There was no correlation between the appearance of such waves and the clinical status, the decrease in sphincter pressure, or in the radiographically measured diameter of the oesophagus.

9.5 COMPARISON OF PNEUMATIC DILATATION AND SURGERY

There is only one prospective randomized study comparing medical versus surgical treatment for achalasia. Csendes *et al.* (1989) compared pneumatic dilatation in 39 patients with a modified Heller's myotomy in 42 patients. After a 24–156 mo. follow-up, 95% of the operated patients were asymptomatic, while 65% of the dilated patients were asymptomatic after one or more dilatations. Positive acid reflux tests were noted in 28% of the postoperative versus 8% of the postdilatation group. In both groups, pretreatment gastro-oesophageal sphincter pressures were similar and decreased significantly after treatment, the surgical group having a consistently lower mean sphincter pressure (10.13 mmHg) than the postdilatation group (15.6 mmHg). These results suggest that surgery may be more efficacious than pneumatic dilatation in treating achalasia, but this conclusion is valid only for the pneumatic and surgical techniques used by the authors. Partial or absent improvement in their dilatation group may have been related to technical deficiencies. In this study, maximal dilatations with the Mosher bag lasted 2–5 seconds, this being considerably shorter than most reports of 15 seconds to 3 minutes (Table 9.2). Atropine was also used as premedication which might relax the sphincter and render the stretching less effective (Vantrappen and Janssens, 1983).

A choice between pneumatic dilatation and surgery must still primarily be based on personal experience and retrospective studies. The two large studies that are reasonably comparable as to the number of patients, the duration of follow-up period, morbidity and mortality, and late complications are the surgical report from the Mayo Clinic (Ohike *et al.*,

1979) and the Belgium progressive dilatation study (Vantrappen and Hellemans, 1980; Vantrappen and Janssens, 1983). The number of excellent or good results is higher in the myotomy series (85% versus 77%), while early morbidity (1% versus 2.6%) and mortality (0.2% versus 0.2%) are similar. Late strictures occurred in only 0.7% of the Belgium patients compared with 3% in the Mayo Clinic series. In most series, patients who have failed to benefit from pneumatic dilatation seem to respond to myotomy as well as if they had not had previous treatment. Therefore, we would agree with the early observations of the Mayo Clinic group (Olsen *et al.*, 1951) that a reasonable approach is to perform pneumatic dilatation as the initial therapy and reserve a Heller myotomy for those few individuals who fail to benefit from two to three pneumatic dilatations.

REFERENCES

Agha, F. P. and Lee, H. H. (1986) The esophagus after endoscopic pneumatic balloon dilatation for achalasia. *A.J.R.*, **146**, 25–9.

Bennett, J. R. and Hendrix, T. R. (1970) Treatment of achalasia with pneumatic dilatation. *Med. Treat.*, **7**, 1217–28.

Browne, D. C. and McHardy, G. (1939) A new instrument for use in esophagospasm. *JAMA*, **113**, 1963–4.

Cameron, J. L., Kieffer, R. F., Hendrix, T. R. *et al.* (1978) Selective non-operative management of contained intrathoracic disruptions. *Ann. Thorac. Surg.*, **27**, 404–8.

Castell, D. O. (1976) Achalasia and diffuse esophageal spasm. *Arch. Intern. Med.*, **136**, 571–9.

Cohen, S. and Lipshutz, W. (1971) Lower esophageal sphincter dysfunction in achalasia. *Gastroenterology*, **61**, 814–20.

Cox, J., Buckton, G. K. and Bennett, J. R. (1986) Balloon dilatation in achalasia: a new dilator. *Gut*, **27**, 986–9.

Csendes, A., Braghetto, I., Henriquez, A. and Cortés, C. (1989) Late results of a prospective randomized study comparing forceful dilatation and esophagomyotomy in patients with achalasia. *Gut*, **30**, 299–304.

Dellipiani, A. W. and Hewetson, K. A. (1986)

Pneumatic dilatation in the management of achalasia: experience of 45 cases. *Q. J. Med.*, **58**, 253–8.

Fellows, I. W., Ogilvie, A. L. and Atkinson, M. (1983) Pneumatic dilatation in achalasia. *Gut*, **24**, 1020–3.

Gross, R., Johnson, L. F. and Kaminski, R. J. (1979) Esophageal emptying in achalasia quantitated by a radioisotope technique. *Dig. Dis. Sci.*, **24**, 945–9.

Holloway, R. H., Krosin, G., Lange, R. C. *et al.* (1983) Radionuclide esophageal emptying of a solid meal to quantitate results of therapy. *Gastroenterology*, **84**, 771–6.

Katz, P. O., Richter, J. E., Cowan, R. and Castell, D. O. (1986) Apparent complete lower esophageal sphincter relaxation in achalasia. *Gastroenterology*, **90**, 978–83.

Kurlander, D. J., Raskin, H. F., Kirsner, J. B. and Palmer, W. L. (1963) Therapeutic value of the pneumatic dilator in achalasia of the esophagus: long-term results in sixty-two living patients. *Gastroenterology*, **45**, 604–13.

Lamet, M., Fleshler, B. and Achkar, E. (1985) Return of peristalsis in achalasia after pneumatic dilatation. *Am. J. Gastroenterol.*, **80**, 602–4.

Lawrance, K. and Shoesmith, J. H. (1959) A review of the treatment of cardiospasm. *Thorax*, **14**, 211–5.

Mellow, M. H. (1976) Return of esophageal peristalsis in idiopathic achalasia. *Gastroenterology*, **70**, 1148–51.

Michel, L., Grillo, H. C. and Malt, R. A. (1981) Operative and non-operative management of esophageal perforation. *Ann. Surg.*, **194**, 57–63.

Mosher, H. P. (1923) Cardiospasm. *Post. Med. J.*, **26**, 240–6.

Nanson, E. M. (1962) Treatment of cardiospasm by the expanding bag technique. *Canad. Med. Assoc. J.*, **86**, 1107–11.

Ohike, N., Payne, W. S., Neufeld, D. M. *et al.* (1979) Esophagomyotomy versus forceful dilation for achalasia of the esophagus: results in 899 patients. *Ann. Thorac. Surg.*, **28**, 119–25.

Olsen, A. M., Harrington, S. W., Moersch, H. J. and Anderson, H. A. (1951) The treatment of cardiospasm: analysis of a twelve-year experience. *J. Thorac. Cardiovasc. Surg.*, **22**, 164–87.

Ott, D. J., Richter, J. E., Wu, W. C. *et al.* (1989) Radiographic evaluation of the esophagus immediately after pneumatic dilatation for achalasia. *Dig. Dis. Sci.*, **32**, 962–7.

Plummer, H. S. (1908) Cardiospasm with a report of forty cases. *J.A.M.A.*, **51**, 549–54.

Rider, J. A., Moeller, H. C., Puletti, E. J. and Desai, D. C. (1969) Diagnosis and treatment of diffuse oesophageal spasm. *Arch. Surg.*, **99**, 435–40.

Sanderson, D. R., Ellis, F. H. and Olsen, A. M. (1970) Achalasia of the esophagus: results of therapy by dilation, 1950–1967. *Chest*, **58**, 116–21.

Schindler, R. (1956) Observations on cardiospasm and its treatment by brusque dilatation. *Ann. Intern. Med.*, **45**, 207–15.

Starck, H. (1924) Die Behandlung der spasmogenen Speiserohrenerweiterung. *Munch. Med. Wochenschr.*, **71**, 334–6.

Thomas, S., Negus, V. E. and Bateman, G. H. (1955) Disease of the nose and throat, in *A Textbook for Students and Practitioners*, 6th edn, Cassel, London, p. 776.

Tucker, G. (1939) Cardiospasm: a pneumatic-mercury dilator. *Ann. Otol.*, **48**, 808–16.

Tytgat, G. N. and Derltartogjager, F. L. (1977) Non-surgical treatment of cardio-esophageal obstruction – role of endoscopy. *Endoscopy*, **9**, 211–5.

Van Goidsenhaven, G. E., Vantrappen, G. and Verbeke, S. (1983) Treatment of achalasia of the cardia with pneumatic dilatations. *Gastroenterology*, **45**, 326–34.

Vantrappen, G., Goidsenhaven, G. E., Verbeke, S. *et al.* (1963) Manometric studies in achalasia of the cardia, before and after pneumatic dilations. *Gastroenterology*, **45**, 317–25.

Vantrappen, G. and Hellemans, J. (1980) Treatment of achalasia and related motor disorders. *Gastroenterology*, **79**, 144–54.

Vantrappen, G. and Janssens, J. (1983) To dilate or to operate? That is the question. *Gut*, **24**, 1013–9.

Vantrappen, G., Janssens, J., Hellemano, J. and Coremans, G. (1979) Achalasia, diffuse esophageal spasm, and related motility disorders. *Gastroenterology*, **76**, 450–1.

Witzel, L. (1981) Treatment of achalasia with a pneumatic dilator attached to a gastroscope. *Endoscopy*, **13**, 176–7.

Wong, R. K. H. and Johnson, L. F. (1983) Achalasia, in *Esophageal Function in Health and Disease* (eds D. O. Castell and L. F. Johnson), Elsevier Biomedical, New York, p. 109.

Yon, J. and Christensen, J. (1975) An uncontrolled comparison of treatments for achalasia. *Ann. Surg.*, **82**, 672–6.

CHAPTER TEN

Foreign bodies in the upper gastrointestinal tract

K. F. R. Schiller
and
I. C. Forgacs

10.1 INTRODUCTION

The variety of foreign bodies ingested by their fellow men whether by accident or design may surprise and, occasionally, amaze clinicians. Endoscopists have met the challenge of removing such objects with an ingenuity and enthusiasm that does full justice to their art. Fortunately for the patient (and perhaps also for the endoscopist) the majority of ingested foreign bodies traverse the gastrointestinal tract without harm. This chapter will concentrate on the 20% or less of swallowed foreign bodies that have the potential to cause harm, and the various methods that have been proposed and employed for their endoscopic removal.

The flood of reports of endoscopic management of ingested foreign bodies in the gastroenterological literature of the 1970s has diminished to a trickle in the 1980s. This may reflect the lack of novelty of what has become an almost commonplace event. It is also possible that the profusion of ever more resourceful techniques for removal of foreign bodies had so stretched the limits of credulity that the whole subject now lacks gravitas.

10.2 FOREIGN BODIES FOUND IN THE UPPER GASTROINTESTINAL TRACT

It is convenient to classify ingested foreign bodies arbitrarily into four groups: swallowed foreign bodies; bezoars; iatrogenic items, such as drugs or retained surgical suture material; and a miscellaneous group.

10.2.1 SWALLOWED FOREIGN BODIES

(a) Types of swallowed foreign bodies

An extraordinary variety of swallowed objects has been reported. The list in Table 10.1 is selective but suggests that the only limiting factor in what can and has been swallowed is the size of the oropharynx. The type of foreign body swallowed is less important than the possible consequences of so doing.

(b) Who swallows foreign bodies?

Because children, especially infants, are fond of putting objects to, or into, their mouth they form the largest group of patients seen with ingested foreign bodies. Mentally disturbed patients, on the other hand, present with the largest number of foreign bodies per patient (Eldridge, 1961; Bitar and Holmes, 1976). Chalk and Foucar (1927) surgically removed 2533 objects from the stomach of a female patient with manic depressive psychosis. Foreign body ingestion was once common in prisoners (Manegold, 1973) but, perhaps because extraction became progressively easier,

Table 10.1 Types of swallowed foreign bodies

Personal effects	Coins, keys, razor blades, dentures, hairgrips
Writing utensils	Pencils, ball-point pens
Sewing equipment	Buttons, needles, safety pins
Cutlery	Knives, forks, spoons
Miscellaneous household effects	Paperclips, drawing pins, batteries, assorted tools, wire, ball-bearings, nails, glass fragments
Articles of food	Chicken and fish bones, fruit stones, fruit pulp, meat bolus
Medication	Methycellulose and antacid tablets
Medical equipment	Pieces of tubing, hypodermic needles, dental reamer, thermometer
Worms and insects	Anasakis larvae, yellow jacket

the incidence in this group is waning. A new occupational disease has been recognized in smugglers who deliberately ingest foreign bodies. It is unlikely that this method of concealing contraband is novel, but several instances of smuggling, particularly of dangerous drugs, have been reported in recent years. Although the contraband usually appears in the stool in whatever package it had been ingested (often a condom), the packaging has occasionally ruptured with results for the smuggler that are potentially more unpleasant than merely attracting the attentions of customs officials (McCarron and Wood, 1983; Caruana et al., 1984). Apart from these rather special cases, ingestion of foreign bodies in adults is unusual, but it is the elderly, the edentulous, the inebriated and the careless who are most at risk. These high-risk groups were of course defined long before the advent of fibreoptic endoscopy and there are valuable reviews in the older literature (Carp, 1927).

(c) The fate of swallowed foreign bodies

Eldridge (1961) reported, from his experience

with the mentally handicapped, that almost all foreign bodies were eventually passed. About four-fifths of all foreign bodies traverse the gastrointestinal tract spontaneously without doing harm (Carp, 1927; McCafferey and Lilley, 1975; Selivanov et al., 1984). In the normal upper gastrointestinal tract foreign bodies may be held up at the level of the cricopharyngeus, the oesophagogastric junction, the pylorus and the duodenojejunal flexure. The anatomically abnormal gut may delay transit of foreign bodies, for example, where a paraoesophageal hernia presses on the oesophagus (Pillari et al., 1979), in diverticula (Munsell and Walker, 1972; Armengol-Miro et al., 1977), above strictures, rings and webs, at a narrowed pylorus, or by stenosing tumours (Kassner et al., 1975). In children, congenital abnormalities or previous surgery, such as repair of a tracheo-oesophageal fistula, seem to increase the risk of complications from foreign body ingestion (Spitz, 1971). Oesophageal impaction may be particularly important. Spitz reported that in two-thirds of oesophageal foreign bodies the site of impaction was the upper third of the oesophagus; 20% had impaction in the middle third and only 14% in the lower third.

(d) Complications of foreign body ingestion (Table 10.2)

Oedema or occlusion of the upper airways may be caused by damage during ingestion, and a foreign body may abrade the upper gastrointestinal tract. We have performed an oesophagoscopy on a patient who had experienced severe pain after swallowing a piece of apple. A 10-cm incomplete tear of the oesophageal wall was seen but the patient made a good recovery. A recent important

Table 10.2 Hazards of foreign body ingestion

Respiratory problems	Perforation
Abrasion	Abscess formation
Retention	Haemorrhage
Penetration	Migration

addition to the long list of ingested foreign bodies has been the button battery. Impaction of button batteries in the oesophagus have caused mucosal burns and, in one instance, a tracheo-oesophageal fistula (Litovitz, 1985). A sharp foreign body may penetrate the wall of the oesophagus or stomach causing it to be retained and subsequently to require removal; for example, a dental reamer penetrating the wall of the gastric antrum as described below. A foreign body may perforate the wall of a viscus without clinical evidence of peritonitis (Sartory and Trabant, 1978). After symptomless perforation a foreign body may appear elsewhere in the body. For example, a swallowed hairgrip in a child eventually caused haematuria after its migration to the right kidney. Abscess formation is a well-known complication, and mediastinal abscesses have involved the aorta, with fatal results.

Perforation is a serious complication of foreign body ingestion. In two recent publications, the rates of perforation from foreign bodies were 1% (Vizcarrondo, Brady and Nord, 1983) and 7% (Selivanov, Sheldon and Cello, 1984) of patients who had reported to hospital following foreign body ingestion. Unsurprisingly, sharp objects are particularly likely to result in this complication. Mac-Manus' series in 1941 showed that almost half of foreign body-induced perforations of the intestine were caused by animal bones, especially the bones of fish and chicken. A similar proportion were caused by metallic objects. Ashby and Hunter-Craig (1967) thought that chicken and fish bones were more likely to cause gastrointestinal perforation than sharp, metallic objects. In 313 cases seen by Savary and Miller (1978) there were 17 perforations, all in adults, fifteen due to ingested bone fragments. In Miller's series (1975) the frequency of perforation was distributed equally between stomach and duodenum, small bowel, appendix and caecum, and colon and rectum, but MacManus (1941) reported that almost three-quarters of foreign body-associated perforations occurred in the ileocaecal region. In one patient a button battery caused perforation of a Meckel's diverticulum (Temple and McNeese, 1983). Norburg and Reyes (1975) described the sad case of a child who developed serious colonic complications after swallowing a glass Christmas tree light. Perforation may also be due to local pressure necrosis which is revealed only when the foreign body is extracted (Classen et al., 1976). In one of our patients, when removing an impacted meat bolus piecemeal and subsequently studying the fragments microscopically, it was apparent that some of the necrotic muscle fibres were of human and not bovine origin, suggesting that there had been undiagnosed mural pressure necrosis which had not yet progressed to perforation.

Obstruction of a viscus from an impacted foreign body is most likely to occur in the oesophagus, particularly in its upper third, or when associated with an oesophageal stricture. Prompt removal of foreign bodies lodged in the oesophagus is important, not least to protect the airway. Less commonly, obstruction may occur at the gastric outlet or in the intestine.

An impacted foreign body may cause bleeding. We have experience of a patient who swallowed a chicken bone. After 1 week he presented with severe haematemesis. The offending wishbone was easily removed endoscopically using a snare; it had caused a deep oesophageal ulcer which had bled. There was no rebleeding and the ulcer healed under medical treatment.

While radiographic assessment may help in the detection of metallic objects, it should be noted that some non-ferrous metals, such as aluminium (in ring pulls from canned drinks), may be difficult to demonstrate radiologically (Burnington, 1976). Contrast radiology of the gastrointestinal tract may reveal a foreign body as a filling defect. This technique can be particularly helpful in the oesophagus, although sometimes, in difficult cases, soft-tissue techniques may be necessary. Furthermore, radiological interpretation can be complicated by the foreign body having both radiolucent and radiopaque components. Endoscopy may, of course, be useful in diagnosis as well as therapy.

10.2.2 BEZOARS

Bezoar is derived from the Arabic *badzehr*, the Persian *padzahr* and the Turkish *panzehir*, each of which means antipoison or antidote (DeBakey and Ochsner, 1938). Thus bezoars derived from the entrails of animals were believed to have useful properties in, for example, the treatment of weakness of the heart and loss of sexual powers (Elgood, 1935). Murdock (1934) expands on the magical property of bezoars and comments on their use by Elizabeth I.

(a) Trichobezoars

Trichobezoars (hairballs) are uncommon and may be asymptomatic for years. They are found mainly in young women who ingest their own hair. There is no medical or endoscopic treatment and, if removal is indicated, this must be surgical.

(b) Phytobezoars

Plant bezoars are composed of leaves, roots, skins, pulp and other plant residue. They occur most commonly in patients with disturbed gastric motility or after partial gastrectomy. Of special interest is the phytobezoar caused by ingestion of persimmons: these bezoars occur in subjects with normal stomachs; 14% of the pulp of this fruit is made up of pectin and gum (Murdock, 1934); gastric acidity causes a coagulum to form. In the series of phytobezoars reported by DeBakey and Ochsner (1938, 1939) those derived from persimmons accounted for 73%. Symptoms may include dyspepsia, nausea, vomiting, ulceration and obstruction. The diagnosis may be confirmed radiologically or by endoscopy. Enzymic dissolution has been described (Dann *et al.*, 1959; Pollard and Block, 1968), but surgery may be indicated. Endoscopic methods of treatment include the instillation of cellu-

lase into the bezoar (Gold *et al.*, 1976), fragmentation of the bezoar using biopsy forceps (Lukash, Fornes and Johnson, 1970; McKechnie, 1972; Brady, 1978) and removal of the bezoar (Munsell and Walker, 1972; McLoughlin *et al.*, 1979). Armengol-Miro *et al.*, 1977) describe removal of a prepapillary, intra-diverticular bezoar which had caused obstructive jaundice. Yeast bezoars occur not uncommonly in Scandinavia (Bong *et al.*, 1966; Perttala *et al.*, 1975).

10.2.3 IATROGENIC FOREIGN BODIES

Retained non-absorbable sutures usually do not give rise to symptoms, but they are occasionally thought to cause ulceration at the suture line. Hoare and Alexander-Williams (1977) doubt that sutures are the cause of ulcers and do not advocate their removal, but occasional case reports suggest that sutures can give rise to problems. Belber (1978) describes a patient in whom a single suture had 'transfixed an artery and for many months had acted as a wick which led to severe chronic blood loss'. Occasionally long sutures have traversed the lumen of the oesophagus or stomach causing episodic obstruction. Retained sutures can be detected and removed endoscopically – usually with ease – so that surgical intervention should not be necessary.

Enteric-coated preparations of potassium chloride have long been recognized as causes of inflammation, ulceration and, on occasions, stricture formation within the gut. Various methods of drug delivery have been devised to circumvent this problem, but even the slow-release polymer-coated preparation of potassium chloride, which had hitherto been thought not to be associated with mucosal damage, may become adherent to the gastric mucosa resulting in local inflammation (Graham *et al.*, 1987). More strangely, concretions of medication may obstruct the intestine and such polypharmaceutical conglomerations may weigh up to 2 kg (DeBakey and Ochsner, 1938; Townsend *et al.*, 1973).

Weese *et al.* (1987) report the endoscopic removal of an indwelling hepatic artery catheter which had eroded through the duodenal wall.

Prostheses placed across benign or malignant oesophageal lesions may migrate upwards, downwards into the stomach or may disintegrate (Schiller, Cockel and Hunt, 1986). They can be removed by reversing the method used for their introduction, by snaring or by other means as appropriate.

10.2.4 MISCELLANEOUS FOREIGN BODIES

Gallstones may migrate into the lumen of the gastrointestinal tract to cause intestinal obstruction (Torgerson *et al.*, 1979). Worms and insects could be categorized as foreign bodies. The vagaries of *Ascaris lumbricoides* are well known, although obstruction of a gastrojejunostomy (Lefton, 1976) is uncommon. Less is known of the genus *Anisakis*, larvae of which may be ingested in areas where there is a predilection for raw fish. Anisakiasis may now be managed endoscopically (Akasaka *et al.*, 1979). The consequences of the inadvertent ingestion of a yellow-jacket have also been described (Houston, 1975). In Bangladesh fishermen may inadvertently swallow whole live fish held between their jaws, causing asphyxia or death (Ahmed, 1988).

Even more unusual is the appearance of a foreign body in the gastrointestinal tract years after a war injury. Weithofer *et al.* (1977) described the emergence of a rifle bullet in the duodenum 32 years after wounding in the back. The bullet was seen endoscopically to be entering the duodenal wall but was passed spontaneously before arrangements could be made for endoscopic removal. The record interval between ingestion of a foreign body and the appearance of symptoms is held by a Japanese man who underwent removal of a

chopstick some 60 years after ingesting it (Yamamoto, Mizuno and Sugarawa, 1985).

10.3 INDICATIONS FOR REMOVAL OF A FOREIGN BODY

The decision to remove a foreign body from the gut should be made in the light of several considerations, not least the fact that at least 80% of them will pass spontaneously and harmlessly. Before coming to a decision about management, two questions should be asked:

1. Is the foreign body causing, or likely to cause, any harm?
2. Is the risk of removing it greater than the risk of allowing it to remain in situ?

In some instances, the decision to intervene is not difficult. Where obstruction, perforation, serious inflammation or haemorrhage have resulted, there can be little doubt about removing the foreign body. Equally, as in the situation of a button battery lodged in the oesophagus, the risk of serious damage to the mucosa is so great that its removal is essential (Blatnik, Toohill and Lehman, 1977; Shabino and Feinberg, 1979; Litovitz, 1983; Temple and McNeese, 1983; Votteler, Nash and Rutledge, 1983). Impaction of a foreign body within the oesophagus is generally an indication for its removal or, under certain circumstances, dislodgement forward into the stomach.

When the risk of the foreign body causing harm is less clear cut, it may be prudent to observe the patient's progress. This applies to ingested foreign bodies that have reached the stomach even if they are sharp pointed. It is not easy to provide guidelines for making a decision on the management of individual patients, such is the variety of foreign body (and indeed of patient) that may be involved. Selivanov, Shelden and Cello (1984) have proposed guidelines on general management which have been adapted into the algorithm (Figure 10.1) of Henderson, Engel and Schlesinger (1987).

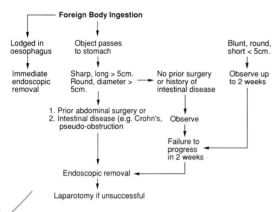

Figure 10.1 Algorithm to guide management of ingested foreign bodies. After Henderson, Engel and Schlesinger (1987).

10.4 ENDOSCOPIC TREATMENT OF FOREIGN BODIES

In this section, instrumentation, patient preparation, general and specific points of technique and the complications of foreign body extraction will be discussed using selected examples to illustrate the endoscopic management. For some years, it has been clear that laparotomy is hardly ever indicated for removal of a foreign body which lies proximal to the duodenojejunal flexure (Manegold, 1977). Even when partial perforation has occurred, endoscopic removal may be possible (Schiller and Salmon, 1973; Honaas and Shaffer 1977; Sartory and Trabant, 1978).

10.4.1 INSTRUMENTATION

The traditional rigid oesophagoscope has, in the main, been replaced by the fibreoptic instrument, but no special modification of the fibreoptic endoscope itself has been necessary for efficient extraction of foreign bodies. Standard biopsy forceps are usually unsuitable, as

it is difficult to obtain a grip on the foreign body with them, especially if they have a central spike or thorn. Several specially designed devices are now commercially available (Figure 10.2). There are various types of toothed forceps, graspers, suture-cutting devices, snares of different shapes and sizes, Dormia baskets and Fogarty catheters. Many such devices are described in detail by Chung (1987) in an excellent review. An ingeniously devised retractable snare has recently been

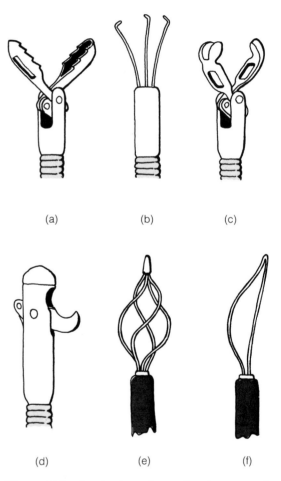

Figure 10.2 A selection of grasping forceps and other extraction devices. (a) Alligator-jawed forceps. (b) Three-nail grasping forceps. (c) Rat-tooth forceps. (d) Suture cutting forceps. (e) Dormia basket. (f) Wire snare.

reported by Hennig and Seuberth (1988). The ingenuity of endoscopists has added other items not primarily designed for the extraction of foreign bodies; for example, the condom was rescued from its pre-AIDS obscurity by Wren and Cockel (1978) to assist in the removal of a ball-bearing from the stomach. It is advised that any hospital offering a gastro-intestinal endoscopy service should equip itself with a range of extraction devices so as to be prepared to intervene quickly if the situation so requires.

Nevertheless, there is still a place for rigid oesophagoscopy in the removal of certain foreign bodies such as dentures.

10.4.2 PREPARATION OF THE PATIENT

In general, there is no need to employ general anaesthesia for extraction of foreign bodies. The decision may be more difficult in children, in patients already on psychotropic drugs and where the procedure may be prolonged or difficult. In other respects, patient preparation is as for routine endoscopy.

10.4.3 GENERAL POINTS OF TECHNIQUE

Whenever relevant, there should be radiographic confirmation of the size, shape, nature and position of the foreign body. It is prudent to perform a 'dummy run' with the extraction device on the bench, using an object as similar as possible to that which it is proposed to remove. After introduction of the most suitable available endoscope to identify the foreign body, attempts at its manipulation and extraction may well require the assistance of a second endoscopist as well as the usual support of an endoscopy nurse assistant. Ideally these supporting personnel should be able to see what the endoscopist sees, e.g. by the use of a teaching side-arm, closed circuit colour television or a video–endoscopy system.

Unless the foreign body is fixed by wedg-ing, impaction or penetration, or lies conveniently in a diverticulum, it is often necessary to prevent its moving every time it is touched with the extraction device. Coins in the stomach are particularly difficult to secure. If possible, it is advisable to move the foreign body into the most advantageous position and even to wedge it. In order to accomplish this, it may be necessary to alter the patient's position on the endoscopy table, or to compress the abdominal wall. We have occasionally resorted to passing a smaller diameter endoscope in parallel with the first, using it to hold the foreign body in position for mechanical extraction by a device passed through the primary endoscope.

A larger foreign body should be grasped or otherwise secured so that during extraction its long axis lies in the line of extraction, otherwise it will be impossible to pull it through the oesophagus. Similarly, it is essential that sharp foreign bodies should be extracted with their sharp points caudad rather than cephalad for fear of impaction or perforation during extraction. For long and sharp foreign bodies, the sheathing tube methods described by Witzel et al. (1974) and later by Rogers (1979), Martin et al. (1979) and Spurling, Zaloga and Richter (1983) are particularly recommended. Chung (1987) advances some particularly ingenious ideas in this respect, for example a right-angled snare for removing a swallowed pencil.

The extraction of foreign bodies is usually simple, safe and quick, but even experienced endoscopists will occasionally run into difficulties. The endoscopic management of ingested foreign bodies in the upper gastro-intestinal tract is not for the novice.

10.4.4 TECHNIQUES FOR ENDOSCOPIC REMOVAL OF FOREIGN BODIES

This section describes some of the more important methods that have been described for the retrieval of foreign bodies from the upper gastrointestinal tract.

(a) Simple grasping forceps

One of the commonest foreign bodies to be ingested is a coin. It is not possible to grasp a foreign body firmly using normal biopsy forceps, especially if the forceps have a central spike. Miederer (1977) has devised a special snare for smooth-rimmed coins, but it is likely that toothed forceps (Figure 10.2(a)) would suffice in most circumstances. The coin is manoeuvred into the best position, firmly gripped between the jaws of the grasping forceps and removed (Figure 10.3). Grasping forceps are invaluable for the removal of a variety of foreign bodies including, from our own experience, a golden half-sovereign, a bunch of keys, a dental reamer and surgical sutures. More unusual objects removed with forceps have included *Anisakis* larva, from the stomach wall (Aksaka *et al.*, 1979), and a species of *Ascaris lumbricoides* from a gastro-jejunostomy (Lefton, 1976).

(b) Forceps as an expanding extraction device

Certain ingested foreign bodies have an orifice through which biopsy forceps can be passed

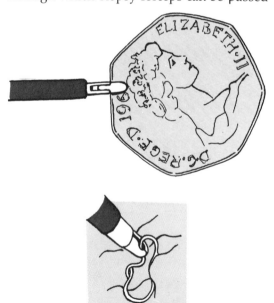

Figure 10.3   Toothed forceps grasping a coin.

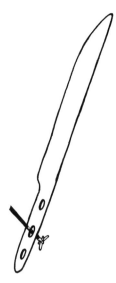

Figure 10.4   Extraction of knife blade using biopsy forceps. After Manegold (1973).

and then opened, the diameter of the opened forceps being greater than that of the orifice 'cannulated', enabling the foreign body to be extracted. Manegold (1973) successfully removed a knife blade by this method (Figure 10.4). An ingested piece of plastic tubing was removed by Gupta, Ricca and Ingegno (1977), biopsy forceps having been passed through the lumen of the tubing (Figure 10.5).

(c) Mobilization and removal

Certain foreign bodies may have to be mobilized before attempted removal, for example because of impaction or penetration of the organ wall. In our hands a dental reamer was disembedded from the gastric antral wall and removed endoscopically with no prior or subsequent evidence of perforation.

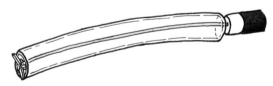

Figure 10.5   Extraction of plastic tubing using biopsy forceps. After Gupta, Ricca and Ingegno (1977).

A step forward

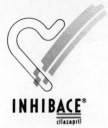

INHIBACE®
cilazapril

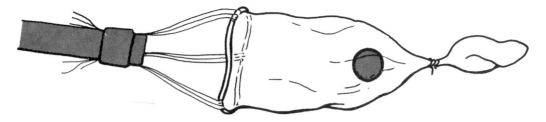

Figure 10.6   Extraction of ball-bearing using a modified condom. After Wren and Cockel (1978).

(d) Simple snaring

A polypectomy snare is so designed that, by pulling the wires back into the covering insulating sheath, the loop is reduced. This means that snares of the various sizes and shapes designed for endoscopic resection of colonic polyps are well suited for the extraction of ingested foreign bodies. Altman and Gottfried (1978) describe the use of a snare to close an opened safety pin before its endoscopic removal from the stomach.

(e) Foley catheters and Dormia baskets

Foley catheters have been passed beyond impacted foreign bodies which have then been mobilized and removed (Bigler, 1966). Similarly, small foreign bodies may be trapped in an endoscopically passed Dormia basket.

(f) Cutting and removing retained suture material

Gear and Dowling (1970) and Roesch (1970) reported simple endoscopic removal of retained sutures. Sutures may prove difficult to remove by attempting simply to pull with forceps. Seifert (1973) designed an endoscopic cutting device (Figure 10.2(d)) for such problems, while others have suggested cutting the sutures with a diathermy snare (Classen and Roesch, 1974).

(g) Trawling

The method described by Wren and Cockel (1978) is ingenious. A 4-year-old swallowed a 17-mm diameter steel ball-bearing that was retained in the stomach for 6 weeks. A contraceptive sheath was attached by three cotton ties to the tip of the endoscope, the detachable hood being used to anchor the threads (Figure 10.6). The ball-bearing was made to roll into the self-opening trawling net and was safely removed. Garrido and Barkin (1985) describe a similar device fashioned from a urinary condom catheter, while P. Mainguet (personal communication, 1978) has constructed an endoscopic trawling net from a more readily available source – a nylon stocking.

(h) Loop technique

Middleton and Nava (1978) describe an ingenious technique for the removal of a large rubber tube. A silk suture was tied to the tip of a nasogastric tube which was passed into the stomach. The suture was grasped tightly by endoscopic forceps, trapping the rubber tube (which had been retained in the stomach postoperatively) and thus removing it successfully (Figure 10.7). Dunkerley et al. (1975) used a loop of umbilical tape passed by the endoscopist to retrieve a swallowed ring.

(i) Large diameter sheathing tubes

Witzel et al. (1974) modified an earlier overtube technique that had found favour with rigid oesophagoscopists, and applied the method to removing ingested razor-blade segments. A plastic tube (80-cm long, 15-mm inner diameter) was slipped over the distal tip of the endoscope, the assembly passed into the stomach and the overtube advanced beyond the

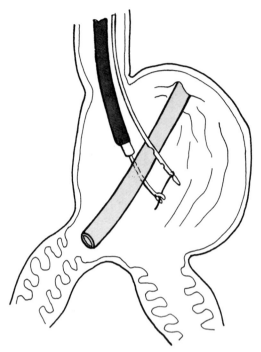

Figure 10.7 Extraction of tubing by the loop technique. After Middleton and Nava (1978).

10.4.5 PROBLEMS WITH SPECIFIC FOREIGN BODIES

(a) Food bolus impaction

In a variation of the steak house syndrome a large piece of meat may be held up in the oesophagus. A number of non-endoscopic as well as endoscopic methods have been suggested for disimpaction of a meat bolus. Ferrucci and Long (1977) and Glauser *et al.* (1979) successfully disimpacted meat boluses from the oesophagus using an intravenous injection of glucagon. Rice, Spiegel and Dombrowski (1983) had a 100% success rate in eight patients by treatment with the gas-forming combination of tartaric acid and sodium bicarbonate. An enzymic papain-containing compound was first used by Richardson (1945) and was successful in treating 16 out of 17 patients with meat bolus obstruction. A revealing insight into how this supposed enzymic treatment might actually work came from Goldner and Danley (1985). They studied the papain preparation

tip of the endoscope. Six razor blade fragments were in turn seized through the tube by wire snare and withdrawn together with the endoscope while the overtube was left *in situ* (Figure 10.8). Martin *et al.* (1979) slid a colonoscopy stiffening tube over an upper gastrointestinal endoscope into the oesophagus. Two long foreign bodies (a pencil and a ballpoint pen) were then pulled one at a time into the stiffening tube and safely extracted (Figure 10.9). We have treated a patient who swallowed several whole razor blades, albeit covered by adhesive tape: usually patients only swallow half-blades. The tape floated off in the stomach, leaving the blades free. They were grasped in turn by a snare, broken against the distal end of an overtube and the pieces extracted individually. The overtube was damaged but open operation rendered unnecessary.

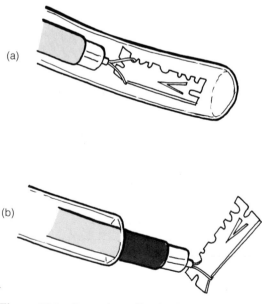

Figure 10.8 Extraction of broken razor blade with snare using overtube method. After Witzel *et al.* (1974).

Provided there is nothing to suggest an obstructive lesion below the bolus, the tip of the fibre-endoscope may be used to push the bolus into the stomach (Roesch *et al.*, 1974). Endoscopy has even been helpful where there is narrowing of the oesophageal lumen: Graham *et al.* (1978) described an instance where 'the endoscope was used as a bougie to guide a hot-dog through an oesophageal stricture'. Alternatively, under radiological control, a guide-wire can be passed through impacted foodstuff and the stenosing stricture, followed by dilating bougies to push the food and dilate the stricture simultaneously.

(b) Button batteries

The hazards of button battery ingestion have been discussed above. The United States National Button Battery Ingestion Study was established in March 1982 to encourage centralization of case reports of button battery ingestion so that guidelines for treatment could be established. Litovitz (1985) reported on 119 episodes of button battery ingestion. Ninety per cent of batteries passed spontaneously, over four-fifths of them within 72 hours. Symptoms were present in 11 patients but were minor in all but one. In an 11-month-old infant, oesophageal burns and a tracheo-oesophageal fistula resulted from a mercuric oxide battery that lodged in the oesophagus. Lodgement in the oesophagus is clearly an indication for an attempt at endoscopic removal. It may be possible to extract the battery using a balloon or some form of trawling system, in which case consideration must be given to protection of the airway, if necessary with general anaesthesia. Alternatively, the button can be pushed through the cardia into the stomach and either left to pass or possibly retrieved with a snare, Dormia basket or magnet. Volle *et al.* (1986) have removed metallic foreign bodies, including button batteries, from eight patients (seven children) using an orogastric tube magnet and fluoroscopy. In our limited experience of this technique fluoroscopy has not been necessary. The

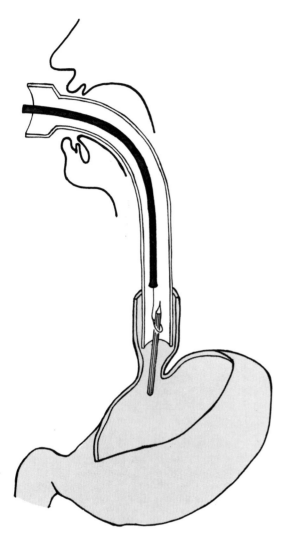

Figure 10.9 Extraction of pencil with snare using colonic stiffening tube method. Martin *et al.* (1979).

Adolph's Meat Tenderizer (AMT), and found that it had no proteolytic activity on a meat bolus *in vitro*. If given with acid and pepsin *in vivo*, severe oesophageal damage resulted. Davis, Thomas and Guice (1987) noted marked oesophagitis after AMT therapy of meat bolus impaction. It has been suggested that the success of papain treatment may relate more to the inflammatory response it produces in the oesophagus than to digestion of the impacted meat.

orogastric magnet and a slim endoscope are passed in parallel. The magnet is manoeuvred under endoscopic visual control until the button battery becomes firmly attracted. The endoscope is then withdrawn together with the magnet holding the battery, the extraction being visually controlled. X-irradiation is therefore avoided.

10.4.6   COMPLICATIONS

Any of the recognized complications of gastrointestinal endoscopy may occur during endoscopic removal of foreign bodies (Table 10.2), including trauma to the gastrointestinal tract, resulting in inflammation, haemorrhage or perforation (Classen *et al.*, 1978). Recovery may be incomplete and the foreign body may be left impacted in the oesophagus or in the bronchial tree. Oesophageal perforation following attempted removal of an impacted object may sometimes be due to pressure necrosis from the foreign body rather than the attempt to remove it (Classen *et al.*, 1976).

The relative lack of reports of the complications of extraction of foreign bodies possibly reflects the safety of such procedures. While we do not advocate an ultraconservative approach, the wise endoscopist would do well to curb the understandable enthusiasm to 'do something' when asked to assist in the management of patients with foreign bodies in the upper gastrointestinal tract, and should first give serious consideration as to whether an attempt at removal is justified. Usually it is not; *ergo primum non nocere.*

REFERENCES

Ahmed, A. H. H. (1988) Swallowed foreign bodies. *Saudi Med. J.*, 343–4.

Akasaka, Y. *et al.* (1979) Endoscopic management of acute gastric anisakiasis. *Endoscopy*, **2**, 158–162.

Altman, A. R. and Gottfried, E. B. (1978) Intragastric closure of an ingested safety pin. *Gastrointest. Endosc.*, **24**, 294.

Armengol-Miro, J. R. *et al.* (1977) Prepapillary intra-

diverticular bezoar as cause of obstructive jaundice. *Endoscopy*, **9**, 247–9.

Ashby, B. S. and Hunter-Craig, I. D. (1967) Foreign body perforation of the gut. *Br. Med. J.*, **54**, 382–4.

Banks, W. and Potsic, W. P. (1978) Unsuspected foreign bodies of the aerodigestive tract. *Ann. Otol. Rhinol. Laryngol.*, **87**, 515–8.

Belber, J. P. (1978) Gastroscopy and duodenoscopy, in *Gastrointestinal Disease* (eds M. H. Sleisenger and J. S. Fordtran), Saunders, Philadelphia.

Bigler, F. E. (1966) The use of a Foley catheter for removal of blunt foreign bodies from the oesophagus. *Thorac. Cardiovasc. Surg.*, **51**, 759.

Bitar, D. E. and Holmes, T. W. (1975) Polybezoar and gastrointestinal foreign bodies in the mentally retarded. *Am. Surg.*, **41**, 497–504.

Blatnik, B. S., Toohill, R. J. and Lehman, R. H. (1977) Fatal complications from an alkaline battery foreign body in the oesophagus. *Ann. Otol. Rhinol. Laryngol.*, **86**, 611–5.

Bong, I. *et al.* (1966) Massive growth of yeasts in resected stomach. *Gut*, **7**, 244–9.

Brady, P. G. (1978) Gastric phytobezoars consequent to delayed gastric emptying. *Gastrointest. Endosc.*, **24**, 159–61.

Burnington, J. D. (1976) Aluminium 'pop-tops' – a hazard to a child health. *JAMA*, **235**, 2614–7.

Carp, L. (1927) Foreign bodies in the intestine. *Arch. Surg.*, **15**, 575–91.

Caruana, D. S., Weinbach, B., Goerg, D. *et al.* (1984) Cocaine packet ingestion: diagnosis, management and natural history. *Ann. Intern. Med.*, **100**, 73–4.

Chalk, S. G. and Foucar, H. D. (1928) Foreign bodies in the stomach: Report of a case in which more than 2500 foreign bodies were found. *Arch. Surg.*, **16**, 494–500.

Chung, R. S. (1988) *Therapeutic Endoscopy in Gastrointestinal Surgery*, Churchill Livingstone, New York.

Classen, M. and Roesch, W. (1974) Endoscopic cutting of persisting suture material. *Gastrointest. Endosc.*, **20**, 130.

Classen, M. *et al.* (1976) Endoskopische Fremdkoerperentfernung aus den oberen Verdauungstrakt. *Dt. Aert.*, **73**, 1969–71.

Classen, M. *et al.* (1978) Operative and therapeutic techniques, in *Clinics in Gastroenterology: Endoscopy*, vol. 7, (ed. K. F. R. Schiller), Saunders, London.

Dann, S. *et al.* (1959) The successful medical management of a phytobezoar. *Arch. Intern. Med.*, **103**, 598–601.

Davis, M., Thomas, L. C. and Guice, K. S. (1987)

Esophagitis after papain. *J. Clin. Gastroenterol.*, **9**, 127–30.

DeBakey, M. and Ochsner, A. (1938) Bezoars and concretions. *Surgery*, **4**, 934–63.

DeBakey, M. and Ochsner, A. (1939) Bezoars and concretions. *Surgery*, **5**, 132–60.

Dunkerley, R. E. *et al.* (1975) Fiberendoscopic removal of large foreign bodies from the stomach. *Gastrointest. Endosc.*, **21**, 196.

Eldridge, W. W. (1961) Foreign bodies in the gastrointestinal tract. *J.A.M.A.*, **178**, 665–7.

Elgood, C. (1935) A treatise on the bezoar stone. *Ann. Med. Hist.*, **7**, 73–80.

Ferrucci, J. T. Jr and Long, J. A. Jr (1977) Radiologic treatment of esophageal food impaction using intravenous glucagon. *Radiology*, **125**, 25–8.

Garrido, J. and Barkin, J. S. (1985) Endoscopic modification for safe foreign body removal. *Am. J. Gastroenterol.*, **80**; **21**, 957–8.

Gear, M. W. L. and Dowling, B. L. (1970) Suture-line ulcer after gastric surgery caused by non-absorbable suture materials. *Br. J. Surg.*, **57**, 356–8.

Glauser, J., Lilja, G. P., Greenfield, B. and Ruiz, E. (1979) Intravenous glucagon in the management of esophageal food obstruction. *JACEP*, **8**, 228–31.

Gold, M. H., Patteson, T. E. and Green, G. I. (1976) Cellulase bezoar ingestion. A new endoscopic technique. *Gastrointest. Endosc.*, **22**, 200–2.

Goldner, F. and Danley, D. (1985) Enzymatic digestion of esophageal meat impaction – a study of Adolph's Meat Tenderizer. *Dig. Dis. Sci.*, **30**, 456–9.

Graham, D. Y. *et al.* (1978) Value of fibreoptic gastrointestinal endoscopy in infants and children. *South. Med. J.*, **71**, 558–60.

Graham, D. Y., Smith, J. L., Jones, R. D. *et al.* (1987) Gastroscopic localization of a micro-encapsulated KCl preparation in the human stomach. *Gastrointest. Endosc.*, **33**, 220–3.

Gupta, J. K., Ricca, J. J. and Ingegno, A. P. (1977) Removal of inadvertently swallowed endotracheal tube from the stomach through an oesophagostomy stoma with the fiberoptic endoscope. *Gastrointest. Endosc.*, **23**, 31–2.

Henderson, C. T., Engel, J. and Schlesinger, P. (1987) Foreign body ingestion: review and suggested guidelines for management. *Endoscopy*, **19**, 68–71.

Hennig, A. E. and Seuberth, K. (1988) Endoscopic removal of foreign bodies using a newly developed extractor. *Endoscopy*, **20**, 72.

Hoare, A. M. and Alexander-Williams, J. (1977) Thread ulcers seen on gastroscopy: do they cause ulcers or indigestion? *Br. Med. J.*, **2**, 996–7.

Honaas, T. O. and Shaffer, E. A. (1977) Endoscopic removal of a foreign body perforating the duodenum. *Can. Med. Assoc. J.*, **116**, 164–9.

Houston, H. E. (1975) Unusual esophageal foreign body: dead or alive. *Arch. Surg.*, **110**, 1516 (letter).

Kassner, E. G., Rose, J. S., Kottmeier, P. K. *et al.* (1975) Retention of small foreign objects in the stomach and duodenum. *Radiology*, **114**, 683–6.

Lefton, H. B. (1976) Endoscopic discovery and removal of *Ascaris lumbricoides*. *Gastrointest. Endosc.*, **22**, 87–8.

Litovitz, T. L. (1983) Button battery ingestions: a review of 56 cases. *JAMA*, **249**, 2495–2500.

Litovitz, T. L. (1985) Battery ingestions: product accessibility and clinical course. *Pediatrics*, **75**, 469–73.

Lukash, W. M., Fornes, M. F. and Johnson, R. B. (1970) Gastric bezoars. *Gastroenterology*, **58**, 1070 (abstract).

McCafferey, T. D. and Lilley, J. O. (1975) The management of foreign affairs of the gastrointestinal tract. *Am. J. Dig. Dis.*, **20**, 121–6.

MacManus, J. E. (1941) Perforations of the intestine by ingested foreign bodies. *Am. J. Surg.*, **53**, 393–402.

McCarron, M. M. and Wood, J. D. (1983) The cocaine 'body packer' syndrome. *JAMA*, **250**, 1417–20.

McKechnie, J. C. (1972) Gastroscopic removal of a phytobezoar. *Gastroenterology*, **62**, 1047–51.

McLoughlin, J. C., Love, A. H., Adgey, A. A. *et al.* (1979) Intact removal of a phytobezoar using fibreoptic endoscope in patient with gastric atony. *Br. Med. J.*, **1**, 1466.

Manegold, B. C. (1973) Fiberendoskopische fremdoerperextraktion aus magen und duodenum. *Chirurg*, **44**, 523–6.

Manegold, B. C. (1977) Endoskopische Fremdkoerperextraktion und intraoperatiuve Endoskopie. *Lang. Arch. Surg.*, **345**, 299–302.

Martin, W. C., Jones, S. A., Nagai, N. and Texter, E. C. Jr (1979) Fiberendoscopic removal of long foreign bodies from the stomach using a colon stiffening tube as a protection sheath. *Am. J. Gastroenterol.*, **71**, 505–7.

Middleton, P. E. and Nava, H. (1978) Retrieval of a large rubber tube from the stomach by a loop technique. *Gastrointest. Endosc.*, **24**, 295–6.

Miederer, S. E. (1977) A snare for the endoscopic extraction of coins. *Endoscopy*, **9**, 99–100.

Miller, S. F. (1975) Foreign body ingestion. *Am. Fam. Physician*, **11**, 123–6.

Munsell, J. and Walker, P. (1972) Persimmon bezoars, in an epiphrenic esophageal diverticulum with endoscopic removal. *Gastrointest. Endosc.*, **18**, 163–4.

Murdock, H. (1934) Persimmon bezoars occurring around Tulsa, Oklahoma. *J. Okla. State Med. Assoc.*, **27**, 442–7.

Norberg, H. P. and Reyes, H. M. (1975) Complications of ornamental christmas bulb ingestion. *Arch. Surg.*, **110**, 1494–7.

Perttalla, Y. *et al.* (1975) Yeast bezoar formation following gastric surgery. *Am. J. Roentgenol*, **125**, 365–73.

Pillari, G. *et al.* (1979) Meat bolus impaction of the lower esophagus associated with a para-oesophageal hernia. *Am. J. Gastroenterol.*, **71**, 287–9.

Pollard, H. B. and Block, G. E. (1968) Rapid dissolution of phytobezoar by cellulase enzyme. *Am. J. Surg.*, **116**, 933–6.

Rice, B. T., Spiegel, P. K. and Dombrowski, P. J. (1983) Acute esophageal food impaction treated with gas-forming agents. *Radiology*, **146**, 299–301.

Richardson, J. R. (1945) A new treatment for esophageal obstruction due to meat impaction. *Ann. Otol. Rhinol. Laryngol.*, **54**, 328–48.

Roesch, W. (1970) Suture material and suture-line ulcer following gastric surgery. *Endoscopy*, **2**, 237–8.

Roesch, W. *et al.* (1974) Operative endoscopy of the upper gastrointestinal tract. *Gastrointest. Endosc.*, **20**, 108–9.

Rogers, B. H. R. (1979) A new method for extraction of impacted meat from the esophagus using a flexible fiberoptic endoscope and an overtube. *Gastrointest. Endosc.*, **25**, 47.

Sartory, A. and Trabant, G. (1978) Endoscopic extraction of a perforating paperclip from the stomach. *Endoscopy*, **10**, 217–8.

Savary, M. and Miller, G. (1978) *The Esophagus: Handbook and Atlas of Endoscopy*, Gassmann, Solothurn.

Schiller, K. F. R., Cockel, R. and Hunt, R. H. (1986) in, *A Colour Atlas of Gastrointestinal Endoscopy*, Chapman & Hall, London.

Schiller, K. F. R. and Salmon, P. R. (1973) Extraction of foreign bodies utilizing fibre-endoscopy. *Gut*, **14**, 920–1 (abstract).

Seifert, E. (1973) Appliances for surgical endoscopy. *Endoscopy*, **5**, 96–00.

Selivanov, V., Sheldon, G. F. and Cello, J. P. (1984) Management of foreign body ingestion. *Ann. Surg.*, **199**, 187–91.

Shabino, C. L. and Feinberg, A. N. (1979) Oesophageal perforation secondary to alkaline battery ingestion. *JACEP*, **8**, 360–2.

Spitz, L. (1971) Management of ingested foreign bodies in childhood. *Br. Med. J.*, 469–72.

Spurling, T. J., Zaloga, G. P. and Richter, J. E. (1983) Fiberendoscopic removal of a gastric foreign body with overtube technique. *Gastrointest. Endosc.*, **29**, 226–7.

Temple, D. M. and McNeese, M. C. (1983) Hazards of battery ingestion. *Pediatrics*, **71**, 100–3.

Townsend, C. M. Jr, Remmers, A. R. Jr, Sarles, H. E. and Fish, J. C. (1973) Intestinal obstruction from medication bezoar in patients with renal failure. *N. Engl. J. Med.*, **288**, 1058–9.

Torgerson, S. A., Greening, G. K., Juniper, J. K. and Farrell, R. L. (1979) Gallstone obstruction of duodenal cap (Bouveret's syndrome) diagnosed by endoscopy. *Am. J. Gastroenterol.*, **72**, 165–7.

Vizcarrondo, F. J., Brady, P. G. and Nord, H. F. (1983) Foreign bodies of the upper gastrointestinal tract. *Gastrointest. Endosc.*, **29**, 208–10.

Volle, E., Hanel, D., Beyer, P. and Kaufmann, H. J. (1986) Ingested foreign bodies: removal by magnet. *Radiology*, **160**, 407–9.

Votteler, T. P., Nash, J. C. and Rutledge, J. C. (1983) The hazard of ingested alkaline disc batteries. *J.A.M.A.*, **249**, 2504–6.

Weese, J. L., Wissler, D. W., Magary, J. A. and Ramirez, G. (1987) Endoscopic transduodenal removal of an hepatic artery catheter. *Gastrointest. Endosc.*, **33**, 246–7.

Weithofer, G. *et al.* (1977) Spontaneous expulsion of a migrating infantry missile impacted in the duodenum and common bile duct 32 years after wounding. *Endoscopy*, **9**, 106–9.

Witzel, L., Scheurer, J., Muhlemann, A. and Halter, F. (1974) Removal of razor blades from the stomach with fibreoptic endoscope. *Br. Med. J.*, **2**, 539.

Wren, C. and Cockel, R. (1978) Endoscopic removal of a swallowed ballbearing from stomach of a four year old child. *Br. Med. J.*, **2**, 252–3.

Yamamoto, M., Mizuno, H. and Sugarawa, V. (1985) A chopstick is removed after 60 years in the duodenum. *Gastrointest. Endosc.*, **31**, 51–2.

CHAPTER ELEVEN

Gastrointestinal haemorrhage

R. H. Hunt

Acute haemorrhage can occur from anywhere in the gastrointestinal tract, often presenting as an acute event necessitating emergency hospital admission, rapid evaluation, and therapeutic intervention. There has been little change in mortality over the past 40 years, due largely to the increasing mean age of patients over the age of 60 years from about 20% in 1940 to over 60% by 1980. An additional important factor is the increasing number of patients with portal hypertension and variceal haemorrhage. In addition to these acute presentations, extensive investigation may be required for patients suspected of chronic intestinal blood loss.

Patients with gastrointestinal bleeding are best managed in a joint medical–surgical–gastroenterology environment with specialized support provided in diagnostic and therapeutic endoscopy, interventional radiology, and radionuclide scanning techniques. This combined approach employing an aggressive diagnostic policy leaves only a small residue of patients in whom the site of bleeding is not detected. Such a policy, which is advocated by many experienced units, does not accept a negative diagnosis, but aims to repeat endoscopy, especially if the initial examination under emergency conditions was carried out under less than optimal circumstances or by less experienced staff.

The chapters dealing with gastrointestinal bleeding emphasize the spectrum of local endoscopic and radiological diagnostic and therapeutic approaches which are now available, and particularly emphasize sclerotherapy, electrocoagulation, laser, and embolic therapeutic techniques. Laser therapy is now an established technique in many units but one which has been controversial due to difficulties in applying laser therapy effectively at all anatomical sites, particularly the duodenal cap. Furthermore, the bipolar probe or the heater probe require considerably less initial investment in equipment, while electrocoagulation needs only a conventional diathermy unit. There has been increasing interest in injection techniques which require no significant additional equipment, and may be undertaken almost anywhere that endoscopy is performed.

Sophisticated angiographic techniques and the widespread use of colonoscopy have changed our perspective of lower gastrointestinal bleeding, especially in the elderly. In addition to colonic polyps and carcinoma, angiodysplasia, and diverticular disease are increasingly found to be the cause of bleeding.

Location of a colonic bleeding site may be attempted endoscopically some 2 hours after balanced electrolyte bowel preparations such as Golytely are taken orally or administered via nasogastric tube, and local endoscopic therapy is often possible. If bleeding is severe, isotope scanning may locate a lesion, or angiographic studies with guided intra-arterial infusion of drugs may arrest haemorrhage. In those few patients in whom bleeding persists, the ability more precisely to locate the site of bleeding has given the surgeon the opportunity to direct his intervention more accurately to the bleeding lesion, with a subsequent reduction in morbidity and mortality.

11.1 INJECTION TECHNIQUES

The use of injection techniques for sclerosis of varices is now well accepted and widely practised, but the choice of sclerosants has remained controversial. The wide variety of agents available is confusing, and few controlled trials in patients have been published. An ideal agent for intravariceal sclerosis should produce immediate clotting with progressive sclerosis, and should have no adverse effect in the extra-oesophageal circulation. The agent should be safe and efficacious, easily injected through the small-gauge injection needle, not be associated with any allergic reaction, and produce few side-effects such as chest pain, fever or pleural effusion.

The sclerosant solutions most widely advocated include ethanol, sodium tetradecyl sulphate, ethanolamine oleate, and sodium morrhuate. The Capetown group believe that sodium tetradecyl sulphate is too damaging (Terblanche *et al.*, 1982).

Paravariceal injection has been more popular in Europe than in Britain and North America, but agents favoured for paravariceal injection, such as polidocanol, have not been widely available in the USA. The use of methylene blue or fluorescein helps to detect extravasation from intravariceal injection, helping to avoid ulceration. If the paravariceal route is intended, dilute sclerosant should be used to avoid ulceration. In practice, however, those performing endoscopic sclerosis employ both of these techniques, and the endoscopist should beware of large volumes of sclerosant being injected alongside a varix. In clinical studies, Rose and Smith have shown that intravariceal injection is more effective, and this was confirmed by Sarin *et al.* (1987) from India, who showed that intravariceal sclerosis was more effective at controlling

bleeding, and was faster at obliterating varices with fewer injection sessions required.

11.1.1 PROPHYLACTIC SCLEROTHERAPY OF VARICES

Prophylactic sclerotherapy for patients with large varices that have never bled has been advocated by some (Paquet, 1982; Witzel, Wolbergs and Merki, 1985). This strategy is questioned by Rose and Smith who are supported by a recent large comparative study from the USA performed in the VA (Gregory *et al.*, 1987), which showed that patients with alcoholic liver disease who had prophylactic sclerotherapy did worse than controls. A recent review of 9 trials confirms that prophylactic sclerotherapy cannot be justified outside of trials and that those subgroups who might benefit still need to be defined (Salena and Sivanek, 1990).

11.1.2 INJECTION FOR NON-VARICEAL LESIONS

The injection techniques for upper gastrointestinal lesions advocated by Soehendra are simple and cheap. The use of polidocanol 1%, either alone or preceded by 1 : 10 000 adrenaline, has been most frequently used, although 100% ethanol or hypertonic saline may be substituted for polidocanol. The techniques described are clearly effective in arresting acute haemorrhage in several randomized controlled trials (Salena and Sivak, 1990).

11.1.3 BICAP AND HEATER PROBES

In contrast, extensive animal work and controlled trials have been undertaken with the BICAP, which has been shown to be safe, and has improved the outcome in patients with active bleeding. The heater probe appears promising in uncontrolled studies and in two recent controlled trials from CURE and Glasgow was superior to the BICAP (Jensen *et al.*, 1986; Fullarton *et al.*, 1989).

11.2 LASER TREATMENT

Four controlled trials of laser therapy for upper gastrointestinal bleeding have been reviewed by Salmon and Jong (1986). Two trials showed a reduction in rebleeding, and need for surgery, a single study showed a reduction in mortality for laser-treated patients, while two studies showed no significant differences between laser and control patients. A further negative study was reported from the USA (Kreys et al., 1987). Problems with the negative results include small numbers entering the study, low bleeding rates, more severe bleeders with potentially most to gain, not giving consent to randomization, and laser power settings too low.

However, it is reasonable to conclude that for those patients who were eligible for, and consented to enter, laser trials haemostasis can be achieved and rebleeding, operation and mortality reduced.

A comparative study of the BICAP with Nd–YAG laser therapy in bleeding peptic ulcer was undertaken, with all patients pre-treated with local adrenaline injection (Rutgeerts, 1986), and suggested that initial haemostasis is as good with a similar surgical and mortality rate. A subsequent randomized controlled study (Matthewson et al., 1987) showed a reduction in rebleeding and mortality with the laser when compared to controls in contrast to a non-significant beneficial trend with the heater probe.

For most centres the more economical approach with a BICAP or heater probe may be just as effective.

11.3 VASCULAR ABNORMALITIES

Vascular abnormalities are increasingly recognized throughout the gastrointestinal tract. Lesions are commonly found to be the source of blood loss in the stomach and colon, although a recent report by Danesh et al. (1987) has suggested that angiodysplasia of the colon is still an uncommon condition

occurring in only 3% of patients investigated for rectal bleeding or anaemia.

Nevertheless, diagnosis can usually be made endoscopically, and angiography should be reserved for those patients in whom colonoscopy has failed to make a diagnosis but angiodysplasia is still suspected. True comparative studies between colonoscopy and angiography have been few. In a study from the Massachusetts General Hospital (Richter et al., 1984) colonoscopy had a sensitivity of 81%, but the authors assumed that angiography had a sensitivity of 100%. In a study from the Hammersmith Hospital, London, a sensitivity of 68% was found for colonoscopy, but examination to the caecum was complete in only 75% of cases (Salem et al., 1985).

Treatment of angiodysplasia has been reported using electrocoagulation with the hot biopsy technique, BICAP or the heater probe with comparable efficacy and safety, but no comparative trials have yet been undertaken. The place of laser therapy for vascular lesions, especially angiodysplasia, is promising, with rebleeding occurring in 18% of patients in one study (Rutgeerts et al., 1985). However, all patients with Osler–Rendu–Weber syndrome, or with angiomas associated with coagulation disorders due to von Willebrand's disease, had a recurrence of bleeding after laser therapy. Analysis of long-term follow-up data in 57 patients with vascular abnormalities showed a statistically significant reduction of rebleeding and transfusion requirements after laser therapy as compared with a similar pre-treatment control period.

11.4 ANGIOGRAPHY

The development of steerable catheters has transformed diagnostic selective visceral angiography into an important potential therapeutic technique in patients with severe haemorrhage from the gastrointestinal tract. Diagnosis may be achieved, with control of haemorrhage by vasopressin infusion, in up to 75% or 80% of patients with bleeding in the territory of the left gastric or coeliac arteries. In the pyloroduodenal region, the success rate falls to between 55% and 65%, while at other sites in the gastrointestinal tract experience is somewhat less and figures therefore less reliable. In addition to vasopressin infusion, embolization is also possible using gelfoam, ivalon particles, liquid adhesives or detachable balloons. Experience with these techniques is still limited and success is largely dependent upon selective catheterization of the bleeding vessel since there is a real risk of infarction of the bowel wall, gallbladder, liver or spleen.

Despite the significant advances in both diagnostic and therapeutic angiography, these procedures should only be undertaken if endoscopy is unavailable or has failed to make a diagnosis. Furthermore, therapeutic angiography is of most benefit in arresting initial haemorrhage at the time of diagnosis or may be attempted in patients who are considered poor surgical candidates or those who develop bleeding as a postsurgical complication.

The following chapters on the diagnostic and therapeutic implications of interventional endoscopy and radiology for gastrointestinal haemorrhage clearly demonstrate the dramatic advances which have been made in recent years. They also emphasize the importance of the team approach to gastrointestinal haemorrhage and the complementary nature of radiological and endoscopic techniques.

REFERENCES

Danesh, B. J. Z., Spitradis, C., Williams, C. B. *et al.* (1987) Angiodysplasia – an uncommon cause of colonic bleeding: colonoscopic evaluation of 1050 patients with rectal bleeding and anemia. *Int. J. Colorect. Dis.*, **2**, 218–22.

Fullarton, G. M., Birnie, G. G., Macdonald, A. *et al.* (1989) Controlled trial of heater probe treatment in bleeding peptic ulcers. *Br. J. Surg.*, **76**, 541–4.

Gregory, P., Hartigan, P., Amodeo, D. *et al.* (1987) Prophylactic sclerotherapy for esophageal varices in alcoholic liver disease: results of a VA cooperative randomized trial. *Gastroenterology*, **92**, 1414.

Jensen, D. *et al.* (1986) BICAP v heater probe for venostasis of severe ulcer bleeding. *Gastrointest. Endosc.*, **32**, 143A.

Krejs, G. J., Little, K. H., Westergaard, H. *et al.* (1987) Laser photocoagulation for the treatment of acute peptic-ulcer bleeding – a randomized controlled clinical trial. *NEJM*, **316**, 1618–21.

Matthewson, K., Swain, C. P., Bland, M. *et al.* (1987) Randomized comparison of Nd–YAG laser, heater probe and no endoscopic therapy for bleeding peptic ulcer. *Gastroenterology*, **92**, 1522.

Paquet, K. J. (1982) Prophylactic endoscopic treatment of the esophageal wall in varices – a prospective controlled randomized trial. *Endoscopy*, **14**, 4–5.

Richter, J. M., Hedberg, S. E., Athanasontis, C. A. *et al.* (1984) Angiodysplasia: clinical presentation and colonoscopic diagnosis. *Dig. Dis. Sci.*, **29**, 481–5.

Rutgeerts, P., VanGrompel, F., Beboes, K. *et al.* (1985) Longterm results of treatment of vascular malformations of the gastrointestinal tract by neodynism YAG laser photocoagulation. *Gut*, **26**, 586–93.

Rutgeerts, P. (1986) Randomized trial of BICAP electrocoagulation and Nd–YAG photocoagulation for hemostasis of severely bleeding ulcers. *Gastrointest. Endosc.*, **32**, 150A.

Salem, R., Wood, C. B., Rees, H. C. *et al.* (1985) A comparison of colonoscopy and selective visceral angiography in the diagnosis of angiodysplasia. *Ann. R. Coll. Surg. Engl.*, **67**, 225–6.

Salena, B. J. and Sivak, M. V. Jr (1990) Injection therapy in the treatment of upper gastrointestinal hemorrhage. *Eur. J. Gastroenterol. and Hepatol.* (in press).

Salmon, P. R. and Jong, M. (1986) Endoscopic hemostasis of the upper GI tract. *Clin. Gastroenterol.*, **15**, 321–33.

Sarin, S. K., Nanda, R., Sochdor, G. *et al.* (1987) Intravariceal v paravariceal sclerotherapy. A prospective controlled randomized trial. *Gut*, **28**, 657–62.

Terblanche, J., Jonker, M. A. T., Bornman, P. C. *et al.* (1982) A five year prospective randomized controlled clinical trial of sclerotherapy after esophageal variceal bleeding. *S. Afr. J. Surg.*, **20**, 176–7.

Witzel, L., Wolbergs, E. and Merki, H. (1985) Prophylactic endoscopic sclerotherapy of oesophageal varices. A prospective controlled trial. *Lancet*, **i**, 733–5.

CHAPTER TWELVE

Gastrointestinal haemorrhage: laser control

P. Swain

12.1 INTRODUCTION

Gastrointestinal haemorrhage is a common cause for emergency admission to hospital. Most patients do well with conservative treatment but about a quarter of them have recurrent bleeding and it is this group, particularly if elderly, that pose difficult management problems and retain a stubbornly high mortality rate.

Epidemiological studies in the UK suggest that there are about 100 admissions per 100 000 population per year (Morgan *et al.*, 1977), so 30 000 patients are admitted each year with upper gastrointestinal bleeding and 3000 die as a consequence (Allan and Dykes, 1976); Schiller, Truelove and Williams, 1976).

Although there has been a striking increase in accurate diagnosis of cause and site of gastrointestinal bleeding with the advent of urgent endoscopy, as well as apparent improvements in medical and surgical therapy, these advances have not been shown to improve the mortality from this condition (Conn, 1981; Peterson *et al.*, 1981; Collins and Langman, 1985) which has remained at about 10% over the last 30 years (Allan and Dykes, 1976; Silverstein, 1981). Although the failure to improve the mortality might in part be explained by a rise in the number of elderly patients (Allan and Dykes, 1976), another explanation is that current conventional treatment is inadequate.

Rebleeding after hospital admission remains the single most important adverse prognostic factor (Avery-Jones, 1956) and is associated with a ten-fold increase in mortality; if this could be reduced by non-operative means, the high mortality from complications of emergency surgery would diminish.

Laser photocoagulation is one of several potential endoscopic methods to prevent rebleeding, and is certainly the best studied.

12.2 HISTORY OF THE LASER

Einstein predicted that the decay of an excited atom or molecule to release a photon of light could happen not only spontaneously but also by interaction with another photon of the same energy (Einstein, 1917). The incident photon remains unchanged, while the newly emitted photon is identical to the incident photon with respect to direction of propagation, wavelength, phase and polarity. This process is called 'stimulated emission' and is the principle upon which the laser is based.

Scientists working with very high frequency microwaves in the 1950s developed methods to amplify these signals which were not amenable to conventional electronic means of amplification. It was found that a photon emitted by an excited atom or molecule could, by initiating a chain of repeated interactions with other excited atoms or molecules of the same species, stimulate the emission of numerous other identical photons. In this way, the intensity of the electromagnetic wave associated with the original photon could be amplified. A difficult prerequisite for the achievement and maintenance of this state of stimulated emission is that a 'population inversion' must be created in which more atoms or molecules exist in the excited state than in the ground state, otherwise photons would tend to be absorbed by atoms in the ground state rather than stimulate emission of further photons from atoms in excited states.

Gordon, Ziegler and Townes in America and Basov and Prokhorov in Russia simultaneously in 1955 reported the first successful solution to the problem of obtaining such a population inversion and constructed the first masar (an acronym for Microwave Amplification by Stimulated Emission of Radiation), and in 1958, Townes and Schawalow described the conditions necessary for Light Amplification by Stimulated Emission of Radiation, the laser (Schawalow and Townes, 1958).

The first practical laser emitting pulses of light was reported in 1960 by Maiman, working in the Research Laboratories of the Howard Hughes Aircraft Corporation and was a pulsed ruby laser (Maiman, 1960).

12.3 BACKGROUND TO THE PHYSICS OF LASER PHOTOCOAGULATION

An atom may be regarded in terms of electrons circling about a dense nucleus of protons and neutrons. As the orbiting electrons gain speed, and hence energy, they increase the size of their orbit, and if they gain sufficient speed they may leave the nucleus core which becomes ionized. A fundamental concept of quantum atomic theory is that electrons cannot increase their orbital energies in a continuous fashion, but do so in jumps or 'quanta'. The relationship between the wavelength of light and its energy per photon Ep is given by the equation $Ep = hc/\lambda$ where h is Planck's constant, c is the speed of light, and λ is the wavelength. Light of a particular wavelength may therefore be considered a collection of photons of equal energy.

The emission of light by an atom can occur at any time provided that its electrons can drop to a particular energy state which nature allows for it. This kind of emission is referred to as 'spontaneous emission' and is familiar as the emission of a conventional light source. Photons released by these 'spontaneous' radiative transitions (unlike stimulated emissions) are random in phase, polarity and direction of propagation. The decay of an excited atom or molecule to release a photon (Figure 12.1) can happen not only spontaneously, but also (as predicted by Einstein) by interaction with another photon of the same energy. This photon remains unchanged and the newly emitted photon is identical, being 'coherent' with it in terms of wavelength and direction of propagation.

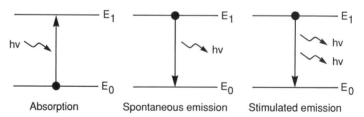

Figure 12.1   Emission and absorption processes in a two-level atomic system. **Absorption:** The atom is originally in a ground state E_0. An incident photon of energy hv $= E_1 - E_0$ strikes the atom. The photon energy is absorbed causing the atom to change to an excited state E_1. **Spontaneous emission:** The atom is in an excited state E_1. Due to the normal short lifetime of the excited state, the energy of the atom falls to the ground state E_0 spontaneously. Energy is released in the form of a photon of the magnitude hv $= E_1 - E_0$. **Stimulated emission:** The atom is in the excited state E_1. An incident photon of energy hv $= E_1 - E_0$ strikes the atom, 'stimulating' the atom to fall to the ground state E_0. As a consequence, two photons of identical wavelength, polarity and direction of propagation are emitted. These photons add together in such a way as to amplify the incident photon.

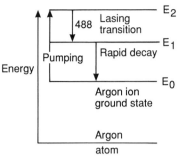

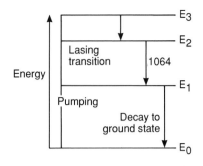

(a) Three-level laser system   (b) Four-level laser system

Figure 12.2   The atomic systems of lasers are multilevel. (a) The argon ion laser uses a three-level atomic system. Collisions between argon atoms ionized by electrical energy pump the ions to E_2, a high-level absorption state. The fall to E_1 is the transition which can emit laser radiation. The fall from E_1 to the ground state of the argon ion is a rapid decay, non-radiative transition. (b) The Nd–YAG laser uses a four-level atomic system. Atoms in the ground state E_0 are excited to the highest metastable level E_3 and descend non-radiatively to metastable intermediate E_2. E_1 is high enough above ground state E_0 to be almost empty and so a comparatively small population in E_2 is needed to achieve a population inversion between E_2 and E_1. Laser emission can take place between these levels with comparative efficiency.

If a photon strikes an atom with either its ground state or excited state occupied, the probabilities of absorption or stimulated emission are equal. Normally, due to thermal equilibrium, the higher energy states are much less populated and consequently stimulated emission is unlikely to occur. In order for the stimulated emission process to become dominant, the population of energy levels must become inverted. Only when the higher state energy levels are more populated than the lower states can the transition probability for stimulated emission overcome the probability for spontaneous emission.

A two-level atomic system has been discussed so far, projecting the idea of a ground state and an excited state with a lifetime long enough to allow a sufficient population inversion to be sustained. In practice most laser systems, including those in common use in gastroenterology, use three- or four-level atomic systems which allow a population inversion to be achieved and sustained more efficiently (Figure 12.2). In the three-level case (exemplified by the argon ion laser) the population inversion occurs between the intermediate state and the ground state. In the four-level case (of which the neodymium-YAG laser and helium neon laser are examples) population inversion occurs between two intermediate states. Since the lowest level of the lasing transition is not the ground state of the system, it will normally have a smaller population. In consequence, a substantial population inversion can be achieved more easily between this intermediate state and the excited state with the result of greater efficiency in producing stimulated emission.

12.4 THE NATURE OF A LASER SYSTEM (Figure 12.3)

The list of substances which can produce laser emission has grown to an impressive number of different solids, liquids, gases and junction diodes. There are three features which are common to the configuration of all laser systems:

(a) The laser medium

This can be a solid, liquid, gas or junction between two dissimilar metals, which is capable (because of its atomic or molecular makeup) of sustaining stimulated emission.

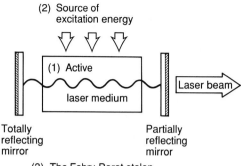

Figure 12.3   Three features ((1)–(3)) common to the configuration of all laser systems. The Fabry–Perot etalon is a pair of mirrors aligned facing one another, between which light can oscillate forming a standing wave.

(b) The source of excitation energy

A redistribution of the number of atoms in excited energy states is required in order to generate a laser beam. This process requires an external source of excitation energy often called the 'pump' energy.

(c) A Fabry–Perot etalon or interferometer

This device is a pair of mirrors aligned facing each other. Light oscillates between the two end mirrors, forming a standing wave. In the case of the laser, one mirror is placed at each end of the laser medium. Usually one mirror is a total reflector, the other a partial reflector (i.e. it allows part of the laser beam which is generated within the active medium to pass outside the interferometer). A photon released by one excited atom will stimulate another excited atom in its path also to release a photon of excess energy. This interaction results in the combination of two photons with identical coherence properties or phase relationships so that they add together to produce a beam of twice the intensity. As the beam passes through the excited laser medium, its amplitude will be rapidly increased while the coherence properties remain unchanged. When these coherent photons reach the total internal reflection mirror, the beam direction is completely reversed, thus allowing another pass through the excited laser medium so that the beam can be amplified further. When the beam reaches the partially reflecting mirror, a proportion of the beam escapes, forming the active emission of the laser. This process can continue for as long as sufficient pump energy is supplied to the laser medium.

There are several ways of pumping energy into laser media to achieve population inversion:

(i) Optical pumping This method uses a high-intensity light source, such as a xenon or krypton flash lamp, to supply sufficient photon flux in a given spectral range. Population inversion has been achieved in solids and liquids using this method, which is the basis for exciting the Nd–YAG laser. Since only a small fraction of the lamp emission is used to excite the medium the process is inefficient. Maiman made the first laser by wrapping the flash lamp in a helix around a ruby crystal. The Nd–YAG crystal and flash lamp form the two foci of an ellipsoidal reflector to improve efficiency of optical coupling in the Nd–YAG laser.

(ii) Ionization This method uses an electrical current discharge in an inert gas to produce inversion by ionizing the gas. Collisions between the ions in the discharge tube provide the source of inversion energy. Ionization is the basis of excitation for the argon laser.

(iii) Neutral atom discharge This method involves the use of low current electrical discharges in gases; an energy exchange between two gases forms the process by which inversion is achieved. This method is the basis of helium-neon laser emission, commonly used as the aiming beam for Nd–YAG laser systems.

12.5 THE PROPERTIES OF LASER LIGHT (Figure 12.4)

There are certain properties common to the light beam emitted from all lasers which distinguish their outputs from other sources of radiation. Some of these properties make lasers especially useful in therapeutic endoscopy. The properties are:

1. Emission of a collimated slowly spreading beam with well-defined wavefronts.
2. A beam of enormous intensity.
3. A nearly single frequency emission of low bandwidth; an almost pure monochromatic light beam.
4. A beam that maintains a high degree of temporal and spatial coherence.
5. A beam that is highly plane polarized.
6. A beam with enormous electromagnetic field strengths.

It is the first three properties which make laser light useful for endoscopic photocoagulation. Because of the low beam divergence of laser light, the full power of the laser beam may be focused to a small spot. This enables almost all the power of the laser to be coupled and transmitted to tissue by a small diameter fibreoptic waveguide which can be passed down the operating channel of a flexible fibreoptic endoscope.

An important consequence of the high collimation of a laser beam is that its irradiance (power per unit area) is high and can remain

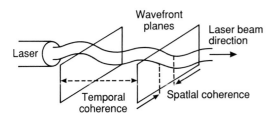

Figure 12.4 Properties of laser light: the coherence factors of a laser beam. A constant time relationship between two wavefronts defines the temporal coherence and a constant relationship across any wavefront defines the spatial coherence of a laser beam.

so up to great distances, even though the total power output may be less than that of a fluorescent lamp or light bulb. A light bulb emits light in all directions as an incoherent spherical wave, so its irradiance falls off in proportion to the inverse square of the distance. It is virtually impossible to arrange a conventional light source to produce a coherent beam of light with an irradiance comparable to that of the laser.

Another important property of laser light is that it is almost purely monochromatic. Lasers emit one or a very few narrow bands of specific wavelength and are consequently a source of pure colour of light. Light from a conventional light source is spread over a much broader band of wavelengths. This monochromaticity of laser light is a consequence of its high temporal coherence (Figure 12.4).

The practical clinical importance of the monochromaticity of laser light is that tissue components tend to absorb or scatter light of one wavelength more strongly than another. Thus, the blue-green light of the argon laser is strongly absorbed by blood (oxyhaemoglobin) and therefore tends to heat blood-containing vessels selectively, coagulating them with proportionately less heat damage to tissue structures of other colours. It is scattered superficially, penetrating to a depth of about 1 mm which makes argon laser light safe for coagulation in the gastrointestinal tract. The near infrared light emitted by the Nd–YAG laser is about five times as deeply penetrating. This enables it to pass through a film of blood to coagulate the bleeding vessel underneath, but its deeper penetration carries a greater risk of perforating a viscus.

12.6 THE COMBINATION OF LASER LIGHT WITH FIBREOPTIC TRANSMISSION

The development of low-loss optical fibre waveguides has allowed beams of laser light to be transmitted through a single fibre bundle which can be passed through the biopsy channel of a conventional endoscope. Without low-loss characteristics, an optical fibre would overheat and destroy itself if high-power laser light were confined. Indeed, when impurities of carbonized material or blood come in contact with the optical fibre, usually at its distal tip, the temperature can rise until the fibre melts and is destroyed.

The optical fibres used in endoscopes are about 10 μm diameter, but those used for laser waveguides are made of a glass or quartz cylinder of 200–600 μm. These fibres combine enough flexibility for endoscopic use with a sufficiently large diameter to allow easy focusing of the beam from the output coupling mirror of the laser on to the proximal end of the laser waveguide. To minimize power loss, the two ends of the fibre must be cleaved into a flat surface perpendicular to the fibre's longitudinal axis. The surfaces have to be kept clean as any dirt will absorb energy, get hot, and melt the fibre tip. The risk of tip contamination may be reduced by using a coaxial jet of CO_2.

The coherent beam of laser light that enters the waveguide emerges from the distal end of the fibre as a spatially incoherent, divergent cone of light, the angle of which is related to the acceptance angle of the fibre, but is typically about 10°. The irradiance at the tissue surface is dependent upon the cone angle and the distance between the tip and the tissue.

12.7 THE NATURE OF THE ARGON ION LASER

The argon ion laser, an example of the 'ion gas' laser, was invented by William Bridges in 1964. The laser medium is ionized argon gas held in a water-cooled tube of beryllium oxide sealed at each end by glass windows. A high current, constrained by a magnetic field and flowing between electrodes positioned within each end of the tube, ionizes the gas and excites the ions to high-energy states. Transitions between the high-energy states and a lower energy level atomic system releases photons in the blue-green part of the spectrum. The output of this laser is a beam of light made up of a number of different spectral lines or wavelengths lying between 347 nm and 529 nm. Eighty per cent of the power is equally divided between two spectral bands, one at 488 nm and the other at 514.5 nm. The argon laser is a three energy-level atomic system (Figure 12.2). It is inefficient in terms of power consumption for power output: an 8-W output (as generally used for photocoagulation) requires an electrical input of 20 kW.

12.8 THE NATURE OF THE NEODYMIUM YTTRIUM ALUMINIUM GARNET LASER

The rare earth neodymium was shown to have lasing properties by Snitzer in 1961 when this metal was 'doped' in glass. The success of neodymium as a medium for laser emission stems from the four levels of energy transitions available, with its lower lasing level some 2000 cm^{-1} above ground level. Because this lower level is virtually empty at room temperature, it is easier to achieve a population inversion than with three-level atomic systems.

Laser pumping threshold and efficiency are greatly dependent on the optical properties of the host material into which the neodymium atoms are doped. The laser material of the Nd–YAG laser is a synthetic crystal rod of yttrium aluminium garnet (YAG) in which is held ('doped') a small concentration of neodymium atoms. Blue-green light, emitted by a krypton lamp and focused into the rod by an elliptical reflector, excites or pumps the neodymium atoms in the form of trivalent ions into a broad band of high-energy states which then decay via non-radiative transitions to relatively long-lived metastable states. Lasing, predominantly at the near infrared 1064-nm wavelength, results from transitions of these metastable states to lower energy states, which then decay rapidly via non-radiative transitions to the ground state. The laser cavity is completed by mirrors positioned at each end of the crystal rod. The output mirror is only partially silvered, while the other mirror is usually multicoated to allow only the desired wavelength to lase.

The physical characteristics of YAG, a man-made crystal which can be worked with great optical precision, explains its superior performance during continuous wave laser operation. It has little thermal birefringence and distorts very little at the high temperature of laser emission as its high thermal conductivity makes its cooling efficient. YAG was first used in conjunction with neodymium as a laser medium by Geusic, Marcos and Van Uitert in 1964.

The overall efficiency achievable by a Nd–YAG laser is 1–2%, 10 kW of electrical energy are required to generate 100 W of laser radiation energy for the Nd–YAG laser as currently used in gastroenterology. This is an order of magnitude more efficient than the argon laser, but the high input power requires a three-phase electrical supply and high-flow water cooling of the laser head which tends to limit the portability of this laser system.

Because the Nd–YAG laser emits in the near infrared part of the spectrum which is not visible, a low-power (5 mW) beam of red light at 630 nm from a helium–neon laser is coupled into the beam path of the Nd–YAG laser output to assist visual targeting.

12.9 INTERACTIONS OF LASER LIGHT WITH TISSUE DURING PHOTOCOAGULATION

Photons of laser light striking a tissue surface have four possible fates; they may be reflected, absorbed, scattered and then absorbed, or may pass right through the tissue, being transmitted (Figure 12.5). The most important interaction of laser light is absorption and scattering within the tissue, with subsequent conversion of laser light energy to heat in the area where the laser beam is scat-

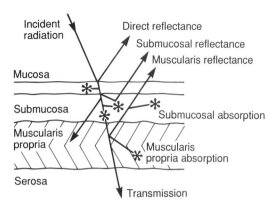

Figure 12.5   The possible fates of a photon of light striking the gut wall.

tered within the tissue. The effect of the heat developed within the tissue varies with the temperature achieved. Between 37°C and 60°C heating accelerates temperature-dependent enzyme reactions and alters membrane permeability characteristics. Between 60°C and 80°C protein denaturation occurs, with loss of cell metabolic and membrane function and degeneration of structural proteins. Haemoglobin pigment oxidizes and turns black at 80°C. At 100°C boiling of water causes cells to explode producing superficial tissue erosion. At higher temperatures charring with carbonization and smoke production occur as tissue is vaporized.

The effects are much the same as those observed when grilling steak: initially slight local swelling as membrane integrity is lost; then the appearance of opalescence as proteins lose their tertiary structure; tissue contraction occurs, mainly due to alterations of fibrous tissue proteins; crackling and spitting can be heard as cells swell and explode; dehydration and further loss of volume takes place as the temperature exceeds 100°C and there is evaporation of tissue water; at higher temperatures charring, carbonization and smoking occur with loss of mechanical strength; the meat may catch fire if temperatures are maintained at 600–1000°C.

Because of varied absorption of light by

tissue components at different wavelengths, lasers will produce a variety of tissue effects depending on their wavelength. The different effects of the argon, Nd–YAG and CO_2 lasers in tissue can be explained by considering their differing absorption in blood and water (Figure 12.6). The blue-green light of the argon laser is hardly absorbed at all by water but is almost 100% absorbed in 1 mm of red blood. In consequence this laser tends to coagulate to a depth of 2 or 3 mm at optimal settings if there is no intervening pool of blood to absorb its energy. The Nd–YAG laser light in the near infrared region penetrates water less well than the argon laser but penetrates blood better; less than a quarter of its energy will be absorbed by 1 mm of blood. This laser can produce a coagulative effect to a depth of 5 mm at optimal haemostatic settings. The CO_2 laser light is emitted in the far infrared part of the electromagnetic spectrum and is intensely absorbed by water. In consequence light at this wavelength is superficially absorbed by tissue water and this laser tends to coagulate to a depth of less than a millimetre.

Because of wide scattering of photons within the tissue, all these lasers produce tissue damage lateral to the small area where the beam strikes the tissue. This effect is more obvious histologically 1 week after treatment than immediately. The Nd–YAG laser not only penetrates more deeply than other lasers but produces a wider tissue effect because lateral scattering is greater. Because the Nd–YAG laser heats a larger volume of tissue, almost ten times more energy is required to achieve an optimal haemostatic effect when compared with the argon laser which produces more tissue damage.

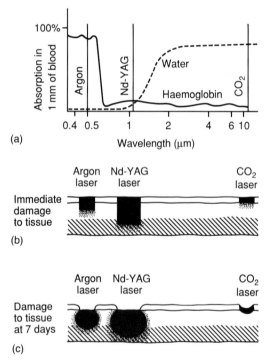

Figure 12.6 (a) Absorption characteristics in water and haemoglobin of argon, Nd–YAG and CO_2 lasers. (b), (c) Comparison of the immediate and delayed tissue effects of the argon, Nd–YAG and CO_2 lasers at optimal haemostatic settings.

12.10 STUDIES OF LASER PHOTOCOAGULATION IN EXPERIMENTAL ANIMAL STUDIES

The clinical practice of laser photocoagulation is based on considerable experimental work on animals to establish optimum power, energy and duration of laser pulse for safety and efficacy of haemostasis.

12.10.1 ANIMAL MODELS OF ULCER BLEEDING

The earliest studies of experimental laser photocoagulation (Fruhmorgen et al., 1974; Dwyer et al., 1975; Waitman et al., 1975; Silverstein et al., 1976) used mechanically or chemically induced bleeding erosions but these were unsatisfactory since they did not bleed reproducibly and were easy to stop.

The most important model has been the 'standard' bleeding canine gastric ulcer (Protell et al., 1976). Acute ulcers 1 cm in diameter were made in canine gastric mucosa using a suction biopsy capsule called the Quinton

Ulcer Maker which cut into the vascular sub-mucosa without damaging the muscularis propria. They cut through an average of five bleeding points which oozed briskly, and did not stop bleeding spontaneously because the animals were heavily heparinized. The advantages of this model were that multiple ulcers could be produced quickly, so that different settings or methods of haemostasis could be rapidly compared, and it allowed different workers to compare results. This model can be criticized because the bleeding is still fairly easy to stop, the bleeding vessels are smaller (Dennis *et al.*, 1981) than those encountered in human ulcer bleeding (Swain *et al.*, 1986a) and are not pathologically degenerate, while the absence of scar tissue and a large single bleeding vessel make this model a relatively poor analogy for bleeding peptic ulcer in man.

Other models used in animal studies of laser photocoagulation include single vessel models of ulcer bleeding (Dennis *et al.*, 1981; MacLeod, Bow and Joffe, 1982) and larger vessel bleeding using serosal, mesenteric or other arteries, either in isolation or laid over gastric or duodenal mucosa (Mills *et al.*, 1983; Swain *et al.*, 1984b; Johnston, Jensen and Auth, 1987).

12.10.2 ARGON LASER PHOTOCOAGULATION IN ANIMALS

The first report of argon laser photocoagulation via a flexible endoscope was from Munich by Nath *et al.* in 1973. Subsequent experimental studies of photocoagulation with this laser in animal studies (Fruhmorgen *et al.*, 1974; Dwyer *et al.*, 1975; Waitman *et al.*, 1975) used low powers of 1 W or less. Silverstein *et al.* (1976), using the newly introduced standard ulcer model, showed that low power (1 W) was ineffective while higher power (5–7 W) was highly effective in stopping bleeding from these ulcers. The argon laser's ability to stop bleeding was impaired in rapidly bleeding ulcers (because the energy was absorbed

superficially by the blood), and two groups (Fruhmorgen *et al.*, 1977; Silverstein, Protell and Piercey, 1977) independently developed the technique of coaxial flow of CO_2 gas passing down the laser waveguide to clear blood from the ulcer surface. Coaxial gas flow significantly decreased the number of pulses required to stop bleeding and increased the number of ulcers effectively coagulated (Silverstein, Protell and Piercey, 1977; Johnston *et al.*, 1981). Tissue injury could be minimized if the total energy delivered was limited to 50 J (Bown *et al.*, 1979), by holding the laser tip 1–2 cm from the ulcer (as closer proximity caused tissue erosion and sometimes made the bleeding worse), and avoiding gaseous overdistension of the stomach (which thinned the area to be treated and increased tissue damage (Johnston *et al.*, 1981)). When experiments were carried out at endoscopy rather than at laparotomy about twice as many pulses were required to achieve haemostasis because of the increased technical difficulty (Johnston *et al.*, 1981). In the dog duodenum and oesophagus argon laser photocoagulation caused more full-thickness tissue injury than had been reported in the thicker stomach (Machiacado *et al.*, 1979).

12.10.3 EXPERIMENTAL ANIMAL STUDIES WITH Nd–YAG LASER PHOTOCOAGULATION

Nath and Fidler (1972) described the passage of Nd–YAG laser radiation through a flexible delivery system for surgical use, and in the following year Nath, Gorish and Kiefhaber (1973) described transmission of both argon and Nd–YAG laser radiation through a flexible fibreoptic transmission system within an endoscope. Investigators were initially concerned about the greater depth of penetration and wide scattering in tissue of this near infrared laser beam which requires more power and energy than the argon laser for optimal haemostatic effect. Animal studies were to show that Nd–YAG laser caused a higher incidence of full-thickness tissue damage than the argon laser but was more effective at coagulating bleeding vessels. The fact that Nd–YAG laser photocoagulation was to prove safe in clinical use was not immediately apparent to early investigators (Protell *et al.*, 1978). Animal experiments established optimal settings for efficacy and safety and have contributed to the safety of laser photocoagulation.

12.11 STUDIES OF POWER AND EFFICACY

Silverstein *et al.* (1979) and Silverstein *et al.* (1977 and 1978) showed that the Nd–YAG laser was relatively ineffective at 15 W but became effective at higher powers, but high-power settings caused full-thickness damage in two-thirds or more of these ulcers.

The Nd–YAG laser can deliver its energy to the vessel even in the presence of active bleeding and, unlike the argon laser, coaxial gas does not enhance haemostatic efficacy or diminish injury.

In clinical practice, the depth of tissue damage is only important if perforation is produced. Dixon, Berenson and McCloskey (1979) used a 55-W Nd–YAG laser in standard experimental ulcers to study perforation risk, and showed that full-thickness tissue damage common with Nd–YAG laser photocoagulation was not synonymous with perforation.

12.11.1 RELATIONSHIP OF POWER AND PULSE DURATION TO DEPTH OF TISSUE DAMAGE

Effective coagulation of experimental ulcers requires a pulse energy greater than 20 J; 30 J is optimal except in the presence of spurting arterial haemorrhage which requires 40 J. Optimal pulse duration is between 300 and 500 ms; shorter (50–100 ms) or longer durations are less effective (Bown *et al.*, 1980). Johnston *et al.* (1980) found optimal settings to be 70 W at 0.5 s although full-thickness damage occurred in over half the ulcers treated.

Coaxial gas did not enhance efficacy or safety and modification of the Nd–YAG laser wavelength from 1.06 to 1.34 nm did not reduce tissue injury.

Short pulses of Nd–YAG laser radiation of 60 W at 1 s or 70 W at 0.5 s caused less deep injury than continuous 60-W irradiation (Rutgeerts *et al.*, 1981). There was no difference in terms of efficacy.

12.11.2 LIMITS OF LASER PHOTOCOAGULATION

There is a limit to the size of vessel that can be occluded by a beam of laser light with the Nd–YAG laser. Small vessels of up to 0.5 mm can be esily sealed (Dennis *et al.*, 1981; Johnston, Jensen and Auth, 1987) but vessels greater than 1 mm in diameter are sealed with increasing difficulty (Mills *et al.*, 1983; Swain *et al.*, 1984b; Johnston, Jensen and Auth, 1987). However, it is possible to stop bleeding from small holes in much larger vessels without occluding that vessel (MacLeod, Bow and Joffe, 1982; Jensen *et al.*, 1983; Mills *et al.*, 1983). Arteries in gastric ulcers in patients that rebleed requiring operation are 0.1–1.8 mm with a mean of 0.7 mm diameter (Swain *et al.*, 1986a). Some arteries that bleed in human ulcers are too large for effective coagulation by a Nd–YAG laser beam – five out of 27 arteries in this last series were greater than 1 mm.

12.11.3 MECHANISMS OF LASER HAEMOSTASIS

Vessel shrinkage is the single most important mechanism involved in the initial instantaneous haemostatic effect of the laser (Gorisch and Boergen, 1982). The instantaneous contraction is mainly due to alterations in structural protein, especially collagen in the vessel wall. Histological examination of sections from ulcers treated with argon or Nd–YAG lasers does not suggest that intravascular thrombosis is important (Kelly *et al.*, 1980, 1983). Oedema around the bleeding point (Dwyer, 1981; Buchi and Brunetaud, 1987) is probably not important as injection of water around vessels in experimental ulcers has no haemostatic effect (Swain *et al.*, 1984a) and lasers can effectively coagulate isolated vessels (Dennis *et al.*, 1981; Mills *et al.*, 1983; Johnston, Jensen and Auth, 1987). Some postulated mechanisms of laser haemostasis are shown in Figure 12.7.

12.11.4 COAPTIVE ENHANCEMENT OF LASER PHOTOCOAGULATION

Sigel and Dunn (1965) and Sigel and Hatke (1967) contrasted obliterative coagulation (heating the vessel by light touch with a monopolar electrode to cause vessel shrinkage for haemostasis) with 'coaptive' coagulation (where a metal clamp was used to occlude blood flow followed by the application of monopolar electrical current to the clamp to weld the flattened endothelial surfaces of the vessel together), and showed that light touch was only effective for small arteries (less than 1 mm diameter), whereas coaptive coagulation was effective with arteries of 2–4 mm diameter. Mills et al. (1983) similarly found that endoscopic bipolar forceps designed to exert considerable coaptive pressure was effective in sealing arteries of 2–4 mm. In practice a vessel in the floor of an ulcer is often not in a suitable configuration to be squeezed flat by a forceps method at endoscopy, but it is possible to use this principle of coaptation to enhance the coagulative capacity of a laser. A fibreoptic waveguide which could exert compressive force on a vessel during laser photocoagulation was capable of occluding large arteries (1–2 mm diameter) achieving high weld strengths. These arteries could not be occluded by non-contact Nd–YAG or argon laser with a contact endcap of high-grade polytetrafluoroethylene (PTFE) which transmits and scatters laser light but absorbs little laser energy. There is little back scattering of laser light, and because there is no blood flow through the vessel carrying away the heat

(an effect sometimes called the heat sink) lower total energies are required to achieve coagulation.

A ceramic material of artificial sapphire, an oxide of aluminium which has a higher melting temperature than PTFE, has also been used for the manufacture of experimental contact laser tips (Daikuzono and Joffe, 1985). These sapphire tips have been used mainly for tumour work, and their use in the treatment of bleeding peptic ulcer (Joffe, 1986) has not yet been reported in controlled studies.

12.12 UNCONTROLLED CLINICAL EXPERIENCE WITH THE ARGON LASER

After first description by Fruhmorgen of the use of the argon laser in treating bleeding angiomata in the human colon (Fruhmorgen, Bodem and Kaduk, 1975; Fruhmorgen *et al.*, 1976), he described treating 300 variously bleeding lesions in 100 patients with successful termination of bleeding in 95%; 10% had rebleeding which was subsequently recoagulated with the laser (Fruhmorgen, Bodem and Reidenbach, 1978). Three uncontrolled studies of argon laser photocoagulation reported stopping active bleeding in 86% of 33 patients (Brunetaud *et al.*, 1975) 80% of 60 patients (Laurence *et al.*, 1980) and 76% of 67 patients (Bown *et al.*, 1981). Argon laser photocoagulation appears to be very safe in that perforations have not yet been reported in clinical studies of the treatment of human gastrointestinal bleeding.

12.13 UNCONTROLLED CLINICAL STUDIES WITH THE Nd–YAG LASER

The Nd–YAG laser was first used by Kiefhaber in 1975 to treat active bleeding in the gastrointestinal tract (Kiefhaber, Nath and Moritz, 1977) and this laser has been widely used in uncontrolled studies.

A survey of Nd–YAG laser users organized

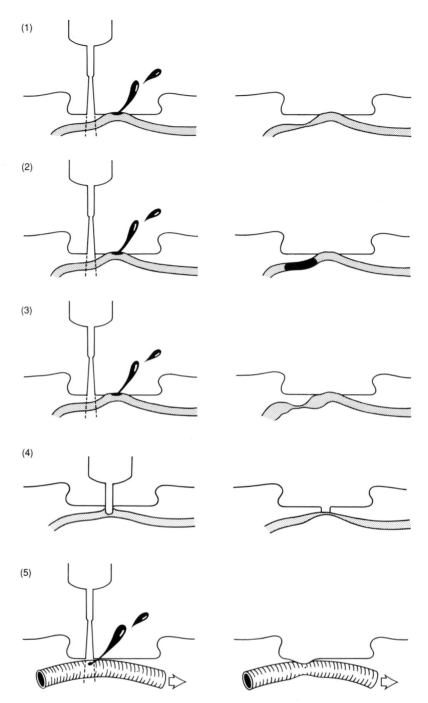

Figure 12.7 Some proposed mechanisms of laser haemostasis. (1) Obliterative coagulation; probably the most important mechanism of laser haemostasis. (2) Intravascular thrombosis; can occur as a selective mechanism of laser haemostasis, importance in ulcer bleeding uncertain. (3) Oedema exerting hydraulic compression on a bleeding vessel. Probably a canard. (4) Coaptive compression with a laser endcap. Experimentally, this method can occlude larger vessels than a laser beam used without coaptive contact. (5) Sealing a small puncture in a large vessel. The laser energy causes local contraction at the puncture site but does not occlude blood flow through the large vessel.

by Kiefhaber (1979) reported that 1776 actively bleeding lesions had been treated in 1533 patients with 'success', i.e. initial haemostasis in 87%. Kiefhaber *et al.* have recently (1983) reported the huge experience of this group: 837/888 (94%) of active bleeding episodes were successfully treated, i.e. primary haemostasis secured.

Perforations were under 2%, occurring more commonly in 'acute', i.e. thin-walled ulcers, and in lesions requiring repeated treatment. These figures are similar to those of Johnston (1982) who reported a 1% perforation rate and a 4% incidence of increased bleeding.

Unfortunately uncontrolled studies of therapy in gastrointestinal bleeding are of limited value. They may give indications of safety and technical practicality but they cannot test clinical efficacy. The 80% spontaneous remission rate (Allan and Dykes, 1976) and its varied clinical pattern demand careful trial design and choice of null hypothesis, large numbers of patients, and effective prospective stratification to concentrate high-risk groups.

12.14 CONTROLLED CLINICAL TRIALS WITH THE ARGON LASER

Vallon *et al.* (1981) reported the first controlled trial of argon laser photocoagulation from Barcelona. Of 322 patients admitted with gastrointestinal bleeding, 136 had peptic ulcers. Of 28 with active bleeding at endoscopy, 10/15 (67%) laser-treated patients had their bleeding permanently stopped, while only 4/13 (31%) of control patients stopped bleeding spontaneously. Five laser-treated patients died compared with 10 controls, but these results did not reach statistical significance. Analysis of the results overall and of other subgroups retrospectively did not show statistical benefit for this laser. There was little evidence that the argon laser prevented rebleeding in patients with a non-bleeding peptic ulcer with a red spot or visible vessel in its

crater, although there was a non-significant trend favouring laser treatment.

Another controlled trial of argon laser photocoagulation was reported from London (Swain *et al.*, 1981). Of 330 consecutive admissions for upper gastrointestinal bleeding, all 76 patients having stigmata of recent haemorrhage in a peptic ulcer were randomized if accessible to laser therapy. Of the 52 patients with a visible vessel, 8/20 patients treated by laser and 17/28 control patients had further bleeding ($P<0.05$). No laser-treated, but seven control patients died ($P<0.02$). The conclusion of this trial was that when endoscopy revealed an ulcer with a visible vessel in its floor accessible to laser therapy, argon laser photocoagulation reduced the incidence of rebleeding and mortality.

In Los Angeles 16 hospitalized patients with spurting or non-bleeding visible vessels were randomized to argon laser photocoagulation or to control treatment (Jensen *et al.*, 1984). Using an overall patient score the mean overall outcome for argon laser-treated patients (1.43) was significantly ($P<0.005$) lower than the score of the laser treated patients (2.44). The mean cost for care was less for argon laser-treated patients than for controls. The method of analysis used here is unusual and interesting, claiming to show a statistical benefit when assessed on a ranked outcome analysis; larger numbers are probably required for convincing demonstration of benefit.

Despite evidence of its effectiveness the argon laser is no longer widely used for treating bleeding ulcers because the Nd–YAG laser is more effective and has been found to be safe in clinical practice despite initial anxieties concerning its deep penetration. Gastroenterologists are also more likely to choose a Nd–YAG laser because of its superior performance in the treatment of obstructing gastrointestinal cancers. A few units with both the argon and Nd–YAG laser prefer to use the argon laser to treat vascular malformations, especially in the thin-walled colon, and to treat multiple colon polyps because of the argon laser's greater margin of safety (Buchi and Brunetaud, 1987).

12.15 CONTROLLED TRIALS OF ND–YAG LASER PHOTOCOAGULATION IN BLEEDING PEPTIC ULCERS

A controlled trial of Nd–YAG laser photocoagulation in bleeding peptic ulcers was reported from London (Swain *et al.*, 1986b) using a protocol identical to the same group's argon laser study (Swain *et al.*, 1981). Five hundred and twenty-seven consecutive patients admitted with haematemesis and/or melaena were considered for entry into this trial. Entry depended on the patients having stigmata of recent haemorrhage (SRH) (Foster, Miloszewski and Losowsky, 1978) at endoscopy, and for the bleeding lesion to be accessible to laser therapy. One hundred and thirty-eight patients with SRH found to be accessible to laser therapy were included in this trial (26 (10%) were inaccessible, 96 had no SRH).

The overall results are given in Table 12.1. These results demonstrate a significant reduction in rebleeding rate, need for emergency surgery and a reduction in mortality at convincing levels of statistical significance. Pros-

pectively randomized subgroups such as those with spurting bleeding (2/10 versus 8/10), non-bleeding visible vessels (4/29 versus 15/31) and active bleeding (2/21 versus 10/20) also all showed significant reductions in the incidence of rebleeding when laser-treated were compared with control-treated patients.

None of the 96 patients without SRH had further bleeding or died. They would not have benefited from laser treatment and their inclusion would have diluted the results demanding a much larger study population to demonstrate benefit. No patients were excluded because they were too ill for this treatment – the least fit patients have most to gain by avoiding operation. Only 10% had to be excluded, mainly because of endoscopic inaccessibility due to a stenosed or deformed duodenum. The mean age of the patients was high (69 years); old age correlates with high mortality.

One hundred and fifty-two patients with upper gastrointestinal bleeding were studied in a controlled trial of different design from Belgium (Rutgeerts *et al.*, 1982). The rebleeding rate in those with non-spurting active bleeding was significantly reduced by laser treatment (2/38 [5%] laser-treated patients rebled versus 12/36 [36%] control-treated patients). The need for urgent surgery was also reduced.

Of 45 patients in another controlled trial of Nd–YAG laser photocoagulation (MacLeod *et al.*, 1983) 25 had minor SRH or 'spots' and all settled without evidence of rebleeding. Twenty patients had bled from visible vessels and all eight who were randomized to the control group rebled, underwent emergency surgery and two died. Although 12 patients bleeding from visible vessels were allocated to laser therapy four did not receive it for technical reasons; all rebled, and had emergency surgery with one death. Of the eight who received laser therapy, two rebled and one required emergency surgery. The occurrence of further bleeding and the need for emergency surgery was reduced (*P*<0.01 and

Table 12.1 Results of a radiological trial of Nd–YAG Laser for bleeding peptic ulcer

	Patients (no.)	Results (no.)		
		Rebleed	*Surgery*	*Died*
Laser	70	7	7	1
Control	68	27	24	8
		P<0.001	*P*<0.001	*P*<0.05

Swain *et al.*, 1986.

$P<0.001$ respectively) when laser treatment (as given) was compared with control treatment. The occurrence of further bleeding in the whole group randomized to laser treatment on an 'intention to treat' basis was also reduced ($P<0.05$) as was the need for emergency surgery ($P<0.02$).

The trials described above have all reported clear benefit from Nd–YAG laser photocoagulation with statistically significant reduction in rebleeding rate and requirement for urgent surgery, without which no improvement in mortality can be expected. Krejs *et al.* (1987) has reported a negative result for Nd–YAG laser treatment of bleeding peptic ulcers from Dallas, Texas. Over 43 months, 491/1062 consecutive patients admitted with upper gastrointestinal bleeding gave consent to enter the trial, and patients with active bleeding or stigmata of recent haemorrhage were randomized to standard treatment with or without laser photocoagulation. One hundred and seventy-four patients were randomized; active bleeding was seen in 32. No benefit was observed when the laser-treated group was compared with the control group. Nor was benefit observed when subgroups were analysed. In the visible vessel subgroup rebleeding occurred in 5/14 (36%) receiving laser treatment but only 2/15 (13%) receiving control treatment, with laser treatment precipitating bleeding in four patients, two of whom required emergency surgery. There are certain flaws in the construction and execution of this trial but despite these criticisms it is a negative result and its existence must be welcomed if only to underline the difficulties in delivering an unequivocal answer (Collins and Langman, 1985).

In addition, a meta-analysis of trials of laser photocoagulation for bleeding peptic ulcer has been published recently (Henry and Whyte, 1988). Eight trials of laser photocoagulation randomized 448 laser treated and 458 control patients. The overall trends strongly favoured laser photocoagulation over control for all endpoints (rebleeding $P<0.025$, operation $P<0.005$, death $P<0.005$).

12.16 COMPARISONS OF LASERS WITH ALTERNATIVE THERMAL DEVICES IN THE TREATMENT OF PATIENTS WITH GASTROINTESTINAL BLEEDING

Lasers appear to be superior to other thermal methods of endoscopic haemostasis in experimental animal studies using bleeding ulcers; the Nd–YAG laser comes first or first equal in most studies in terms of efficacy, the argon laser comes first in terms of safety (Escourrou *et al.*, 1979; Silverstein *et al.*, 1979; Johnston, Jensen and Mautner, 1982). Lasers do not touch or mechanically disturb the bleeding point. Optical energy is easier to control than radiofrequency current, whether monopolar or bipolar, and is quicker and more precise than the thermal diffusion of the heat probe. However, the advantages in animal studies are not great when lasers are compared with bipolar, monopolar or heat probe methods and in some models of experimental bleeding, especially those using large isolated vessels, devices that can exert coaptive pressure on the vessel may work better than the laser used as a non-contact device (Mills *et al.*, 1983; Johnston, Jensen and Auth, 1987).

Lasers are expensive when compared with probes – £35 000–£50 000 – while monopolar, bipolar or heat probe devices cost £3000–£7000. Are lasers the best available means for controlling gastrointestinal bleeding when compared with these cheaper more portable devices? A few comparative clinical studies have been reported.

Rutgeerts *et al.* (1987) reported a randomized comparison of Nd–YAG laser and 3.2 mm (10 Fr) 'Bicap' bipolar probe in 100 patients presenting at endoscopy with a peptic ulcer and a spurting or oozing vessel or a non-bleeding visible vessel. All were pre-treated with an injection of 4–8 ml of 1:10 000 adrenaline (Rutgeerts *et al.*, 1984). Twenty patients had a second treatment because of recurrent bleeding. There was little to choose between these devices in clinical performance.

Johnston *et al.* (1985) reported a non-randomized study which contrasted his initial (somewhat unfavourable) experience with the Nd–YAG laser with his subsequent experience with the heat probe for which he has become an enthusiastic proponent. He reported that he used much more energy (mean 4798J versus 347J) with the laser than with the heat probe, the treatment took much longer (mean 70 min versus 25 min) and required general anaesthesia or endotracheal intubation more frequently. Neither method caused perforation but the laser caused bleeding in ten of 35 patients, which did not occur with the heat probe.

However, Matthewson *et al.* (1987) carried out a randomized and controlled comparison. One hundred and forty-three consecutive patients with SRH accessible to laser therapy were included in their trial (Table 12.2). Rebleeding was significantly reduced when laser was compared with control groups. There is a non-significant trend suggesting that the heat probe had a lower incidence of rebleeding than the control group.

It can be seen that a final answer to the question of comparability of lasers and probes has not yet emerged.

12.17 Nd–YAG LASER TREATMENT OF BLEEDING OESOPHAGEAL VARICES

Elegant experimental studies using a bleeding oesophageal variceal model in dogs demon-

Table 12.2 Results of a randomized trial, comparing Nd–YAG Laser, heat probes and control treatment for bleeding peptic ulcer

	Patients (no.)	Rebleeding rate		Death	
		No.	%	No.	%
Nd–YAG laser	44	9/44	20	1/44	2
Heat probe	57	16/57	28	6/57	10
Control	42	18/42	42	4/42	9

Matthewson *et al.*, 1987.

Table 12.3 Results of a randomized trial of Nd–YAG laser for treatment of bleeding

	Patients (no.)	Results (no.)		
		Initial haemostasis	Rebleeding	Death
Laser	10	7	7	4
Control	10	0	7	7
P value		<0.01	NS	NS

Fleischer, 1985.

strated that the Nd–YAG laser was highly effective in arresting bleeding from needle puncture holes in these varices. It proved slightly more effective than sclerotherapy in terminating acute bleeding but did not cause subsequent thrombosis of the varix as did sclerotherapy (Jensen *et al.*, 1983). Although there have been enthusiastic clinical reports (Dwyer, 1981) on the efficacy of Nd–YAG laser treatment of oesophageal variceal bleeding in man, the most experienced operator, Kiefhaber (1983), reported that the Nd–YAG laser was effective in terminating 160/174 acute bleeding episodes, but because of a high incidence of rebleeding (30%) he recommended that sclerotherapy be performed early for more definitive treatment. Ihre *et al.* (1981) in an early controlled trial of Nd–YAG laser treatment included patients with oesophageal varices and showed no benefit in this group. Fleischer (1985) has conducted the only randomized trial of Nd–YAG laser treatment of varices in patients with active bleeding at urgent endoscopy. In this study initial haemostasis was significantly greater in the laser-treated group than the control group but the incidence of rebleeding was equal in both groups (Table 12.3). He concluded that laser therapy may be useful for controlling acute bleeding and be of some interim benefit but does not represent definitive treatment.

Hashimoto, Miyohara and Yoshimura (1986) reported the use of the Nd–YAG laser in prophylactic treatment of varices and for inaccessible gastric varices. They used an innovative lateral radiation fibre (Hashimoto, 1987) with a prism mounted on the waveguide tip allowing the laser beam to exit at 90° or 45° with respect to the axis of the fibre.

12.18 LASER TREATMENT OF VASCULAR MALFORMATIONS

The intermittent chronic blood loss associated with vascular malformations in the bowel remains difficult to treat. Some patients require repeated hospital admission and transfusion for bleeding. These vascular malformations are particularly amenable to laser therapy since their bright red colour selectively absorbs laser light, and as they are small and round it is easy to coagulate many of them in a single treatment session.

In a recent large series (Rutgeerts *et al.*, 1985) 482 lesions in 59 patients were treated. Twenty-five patients had upper gastrointestinal lesions, 31 had colonic lesions and three had both. Only 17 of 59 had rebleeding requiring hospitalization during a mean follow-up period of 11.5 months. The apparent reduction of rebleeding and transfusion requirement were statistically significant at 1, 6 and 12 months when periods before and after treatment were compared. Two patients developed caecal perforation following laser treatment which required right hemicolectomy, while a third patient developed peritonism which responded to conservative therapy. No deaths appeared to be laser related. Kiefhaber *et al.* (1983) reported treating 30 patients with vascular malformations, eight having multiple haemangiomas due to Osler–Weber–Rendu syndrome in stomach and duodenum and 22 having colonic angiodysplasias. In only one of 30 patients was operative resection required because of recurrent bleeding. There was a single perforation. Other groups have reported smaller series (Etienne, Raimbert and Dorme, 1981 (3 patients); Fleischer, 1981 (5 patients); Bown *et al.*, 1985 (29 patients)), claiming efficacy and

sometimes striking reductions in transfusion requirements without perforations.

The safety of the argon laser may make it superior to the Nd–YAG laser, especially for colonic work since the thinner-walled colon is more susceptible to laser perforation than the stomach (Buchi and Brunetaud, 1987). Several centres have reported clinical use of the argon laser to treat vascular malformations since 1975 (Fruhmorgen, Bodem and Kaduk, 1975). Waitman, Grant and Chateau (1982) reported 50 patients with telangiectasia; bleeding was stopped in 33 and transfusion requirements markedly reduced in the other 17. Jensen and Machicado (1985) reported similarly impressive results in 25 patients with apparently significant reductions in transfusion requirements when a period of several months' follow-up was compared with the same time period prior to laser treatment. Bowers and Dixon (1982) reported results in the treatment of 40 patients with vascular malformations in colon and stomach: 36/40 had bleeding abolished or markedly reduced with a follow-up period of 1–40 months.

Buchi and Brunetaud (1987) pooled the results from Utah and Lille to report the treatment of 126 patients; 80 patients with upper gastrointestinal lesions, 26 with colonic lesions and nine with both. Twenty had Osler–Weber–Rendu syndrome. They reported 95% success in controlling blood loss in patients with 'sporadic' vascular malformations, and reduction of bleeding in patients with Osler–Weber–Rendu syndrome. No perforations occurred in this series of patients, the majority of whom were treated with the argon laser.

Some less common causes of gastrointestinal vascular malformation appear to do well when treated with laser. Alexander and Dwyer (1985) reported the use of Nd–YAG laser to treat bleeding from malformations associated with chronic radiation proctocolitis in nine patients, while Buchi and Dixon (1987) reported treating three patients with the same condition with the argon laser. Bleeding was controlled in all patients. Buchi and Brunetaud (1987) also reported effective control of bleeding in 3/4 patients with the blue rubber bleb naevus syndrome.

There are some difficulties in assessing the value of laser treatment of vascular malformations because the natural history is variable and some patients will go years between manifest bleeds. Controlled trials have not been performed, and the number of patients required would make such a study difficult. Comparison of transfusion requirements before and after treatment is poor evidence of efficacy since bleeding may stop spontaneously. Vascular malformations may be found without clinical evidence of bleeding (Boley et al., 1979) and these should probably be left alone by the therapeutic endoscopist. New lesions may appear, especially with Osler–Weber–Rendu syndrome, so these patients require careful follow-up. Bleeding is commonly caused by laser treatment (50% in our series) (Bown et al., 1985), but this will usually stop spontaneously. The aim of treatment is not to stop observed bleeding but rather to damage the abnormal vasculature so that subsequent scarring and healing prevent the reformation of these vessels. Some vascular lesions are too large for successful or safe endoscopic laser therapy and these are better dealt with surgically.

12.19 THE PREDICTIVE VALUE OF STIGMATA OF RECENT HAEMORRHAGE

One result of the controlled trials of laser therapy has been a critical and prospective examination of the predictive value of the presence or absence of stigmata of recent haemorrhage (SRH) in the floor of ulcers of patients who have recently bled. The presence of blood either as clot adherent to the ulcer floor or as free blood, whether or not associated with active bleeding in the ulcer crater, was reported to be of prognostic value by Foster, Miloszewski and Losowsky (1978).

Griffiths, Neumann and Welsh (1979) stressed the importance of the predictive value for further bleeding of the endoscopic finding of the 'visible vessel', which in their retrospective series was reported as being associated with a 100% incidence of further bleeding and a high mortality. A prospective study (Storey et al., 1981) suggested that the incidence of rebleeding with visible vessels was lower (56%) but that if this finding was carefully sought with gentle endoscopic washing, the incidence of further bleeding and death was almost entirely confined to patients with a visible vessel in an ulcer and that patients without stigmata did not have further bleeding. A visible vessel was defined as a raised spot or mound in the floor of an ulcer of a patient with recent bleeding, darker in colour than other structures in the ulcer floor, being dark red, blue or black, often associated with the freshest clot in the ulcer, and resistant to endoscopic washing. The predictive value of finding a visible vessel has been confirmed in other series, e.g. Vallon et al. (1981), 50%; Swain et al. (1986b), 60%; Papp (1981), 80% and MacLeod et al. (1983), 100%. One series (Wara, 1985) has questioned the value of this observation; his non-bleeding visible vessels only rebled at a rate of 32%. However, his series endorses the low incidence of rebleeding associated with the absence of SRH and usefully indicates a high rebleeding rate for visible vessels observed in the duodenum (46%) and stomach (41%) if prepyloric ulcers with visible vessels are excluded. The differences between these series are probably due to differences of definition (some groups include spurting arterial bleeding as an indication of a visible vessel) and difficulty in distinguishing adventitious clot adherent to a non-bleeding part of the ulcer crater from the vessel wall proper or clot adherent to the eroded vessel at the true bleeding point.

Our prospective study of visible vessels and SRH included 826 consecutive patients admitted because of gastrointestinal bleeding over a 4-year period (Swain et al., 1986b).

Table 12.4 Clinical courses in patients with peptic ulcer, according to features of ulcer at endoscopy*

Ulcer feature	Total	Further bleeding		Urgent surgery		Death	
		No.	%	No.	%	No.	%
Visible vessel	93	54	58	48	52	16	17
Stigmata of recent haemorrhage other than a visible vessel	36	2	6	2	6	1	3
No stigmata of recent haemorrhage	107	0		0		0	

*Ulcers inadequately visualized at endoscopy or treated with argon or Nd–YAG laser are not considered in this table.

Peptic ulcers (gastric, duodenal or stomal) were identified in 402 of 826 patients (49% at urgent endoscopy within 12 hours of admission) and full examination of the ulcer crater was possible in 329 patients (82%). A visible vessel was identified in 156 patients (39%), other SRH (i.e. flat small red or black macules in the crater floor) were observed in 66 (20%) and no such stigmata in 103 (33%). In the other 73 (18%) full examination was not possible because of problems of access in a scarred duodenal bulb or difficulty in removing overlying clot by endoscopic washing. Since argon or Nd–YAG laser treatment may have influenced the natural history, prospective predictive analysis of the subsequent clinical course is restricted to ulcers not treated with the laser (Table 12.4). These results show that patients with visible vessels rebled, required urgent surgery and died more frequently than those with other SRH. No patient without SRH rebled, required emergency surgery or died. Fifty-four of 93 patients (58%) with visible vessels rebled compared with two of 36 (6%) of patients with other SRH ($P<0.001$). Sixteen of 93 patients with visible vessels died compared with one of 36 with other SRH ($P<0.02$) and none of 107 with no SRH ($P<0.001$). Forty-three of 56 (77%) of patients with further bleeding did not have active bleeding at their initial diagnostic endoscopy.

Pathological studies have gone some way towards validating the endoscopic identification of the visible vessel and explaining why ulcers bleed (Swain *et al.*, 1986b, Swain, 1986b). In our series 27 of 54 patients with visible vessels that had recurrent bleeding bled from gastric ulcers that were subsequently removed at urgent gastrectomy and these specimens were examined with postoperative angiography and histology to establish the presence and nature of the visible vessel. The endoscopically identified visible vessel could be identified as the bleeding point at pathological examination in 26 (96%). Histology showed that the vessel wall protruded above the surface of the ulcer crater as commonly (37%) as clot (37%) which sometimes formed a pseudoaneurysmal roof in continuity with the vessel wall, covering the breach. Occasionally, a plug of thrombus occluding the breach extended downwards into the intact vessel. Johnston (1984) has suggested that the visible vessel is something of a misnomer, that the protruding nipple-like appearance recognized at endoscopy should be regarded as a 'sentinel clot' with the vessel invisible well below the ulcer floor. Sometimes neither vessel nor clot protruded above the surface at histology although the vessel had presented an appearance which was correctly recognized as the bleeding point ('visible vessel') at endoscopy. Although it may be difficult and not particularly useful at endoscopy to distinguish necrotic wall from pseudoaneurysm or plug of clot, the appearance that is recognized as a visible vessel by most endoscopists seems useful for the prediction of recurrent haemorrhage and is the essential target within the ulcer crater for endoscopic therapy. These observations support the contention that the source of bleeding or the bleeding point in an ulcer crater can almost always be found at endoscopy and at histology and that this appearance might as well be called a visible vessel, a phrase with a catchy, alliterative ring.

12.20 WHICH PATIENTS SHOULD BE TREATED?

It is essential to predict which patients are at risk from further bleeding and death, since endoscopic therapy directed at ulcers in patients without risk of further bleeding will not help and might harm patients; also such inappropriate therapy might dilute the results and render ineffective controlled clinical assessment of such therapy.

Therapeutic endoscopy also demands that the endoscopist should identify the source of bleeding within the floor of the ulcer since it is neither safe, effective or practical to burn the whole of the floor of an ulcer in the hope of coagulating a bleeding artery.

There seems no question that it is reasonable to attempt to terminate spurting arterial bleeding when seen. Although this is an uncommon finding at urgent endoscopy (seen in 5–10% of these series), it is the finding associated with the highest risk of further bleeding (Forrest et al., 1974). Only 13% of such patients had no evidence of further bleeding in our series (Swain, 1986a). Early studies of therapeutic endoscopy showed that active bleeding was a poor marker because it excluded many patients at risk of further bleeding and death, and did not force the endoscopist to find the bleeding point or vessel within the actively bleeding ulcer. Three-quarters of patients at risk of further bleeding and death were not bleeding at initial endoscopy in these series.

The problem of treating non-bleeding lesions in ulcers is that a large number of such ulcers will stop bleeding spontaneously and require no treatment; indeed treating such patients may harm them by causing perforation or precipitating further bleeding. Results of trials suggest that it is beneficial to treat patients with non-bleeding visible vessels, but not patients with minor SRH since few rebleed, or patients with overlying clot, since the energy is not likely to reach the bleeding vessel and terminate the bleeding.

The results in Table 12.5 suggest that endoscopic therapy is effective in preventing recurrent bleeding only in patients in whom a visible vessel can be identified.

It seems sensible not to treat patients with bleeding Mallory–Weiss tears or bleeding erosions, except under special circumstances, since these will almost all settle spontaneously. The treatment of variceal bleeding with the laser is probably ineffective but might be considered as a means of temporary termination of acute bleeding. The treatment of vascular malformations is probably valuable, but

Table 12.5 Incidence of rebleeding in non-bleeding visible vessel subgroups (randomized prospectively) in two trials of laser photocoagulation

	Laser treated		Control		Significance	
	No.	%	No.	%		
Argon laser trial non-bleeding visible vessel*	4/17	23.5	13/24	54	$P<0.05$	(Swain et al. 1981)
Nd–YAG laser trial non-bleeding visible vessel†	4/28	14.3	15/31	48	$P<0.005$	(Swain et al. 1986b)

*Swain et al. (1981).
†Swain et al. (1986b).

should be avoided in patients without evidence of bleeding. If they are treated it is best to treat large ones, those that are seen to bleed spontaneously or can be easily caused to bleed with gently washing, and to be scrupulous in the exclusion of other potential sources of gastrointestinal blood loss. There is some evidence that laser treatment can reduce bleeding from tumours, especially in the colon (Mathus-Vliegen and Tytgat, 1986).

12.21 TECHNIQUE OF LASER ENDOSCOPY IN GASTROINTESTINAL HAEMORRHAGE

Laser therapy can be done during the initial diagnostic endoscopy; it is best if both diagnosis and treatment can be carried out soon after admission to diminish the chance of further bleeding in hospital. The laser should be left running during the procedure, having been tuned to give appropriate power and pulse duration before the patient is intubated. During the endoscopy, particular attention is given to identification and preparation of the bleeding site for treatment. If there is loose clot, or blood in the floor of the ulcer, this can usually be removed by gentle endoscopic washing using a syringe full of water (either attached to the biopsy channel, or to a washing catheter, or 'pipe' inserted through the biopsy channel) and aimed at loose clot, blood or debris on the ulcer floor. This technique is safe; we have never observed washing to precipitate bleeding. It is gentle, exerting about ten times less force than the lightest touch with endoscopic biopsy or brush. The aim is not to disturb the vessel with its pseudoaneurysm or plug of clot but to clear the rest of the floor so that it can be fully examined. The use of washing enhances the diagnostic yield of urgent endoscopy since it facilitates the recognition of the precise source of bleeding within an ulcer and deciding if active bleeding is present – often a difficult decision when there is oozing or intermittent

bleeding. Overlying clot can absorb laser energy preventing penetration to the underlying artery.

Once the bleeding point has been identified, the laser waveguide is passed through the biopsy channel. The aiming beam is identified and is moved over the target to check accessibility. Ideally the laser tip is held 1 cm from the bleeding point, but estimating distance at endoscopy is not easy. One technique which can help is to advance the tip of the waveguide until it almost touches the target, and then withdraw the fibre by a centimetre at the biopsy port holding the endoscope steady.

The use of an initial 'sighter' pulse of laser energy delivered to mucosa on the thick edge of the ulcer may be helpful, allowing a biological test of the laser's function. At effective coagulative powers, a single pulse should produce a ring of blanched mucosa but should not cause erosion of the surface of the mucosa.

Using the Nd–YAG laser most laser endoscopists try to deliver a tight ring of pulses around the vessel (Figure 12.8). There are two reasons for this strategy. A pulse aimed at the centre of an exposed vessel may cause bleeding, since the visible protrusion is either a degenerate aneurysmally dilated part of the bleeding vessel or a plug of clot protruding from the eroded side of the bleeding artery. The other reason is that it is necessary to cause heat damage to the intact artery up- and down-stream of the bleeding point, and since it is not usually possible to guess the line of the artery at endoscopy, it is necessary to treat in a circle in order to ensure that the artery is effectively treated. The target may be missed frequently, but provided the misses are scattered this does not matter. Once the artery has been treated with a ring of pulses, the protruding centre of the visible vessel is treated to check that the artery does not bleed. Occasionally this will cause spurting bleeding but this can usually be stopped with further laser pulses or it may stop spontaneously. If spurting is not stopped with the first few laser pulses, it is often helpful to wait, since the

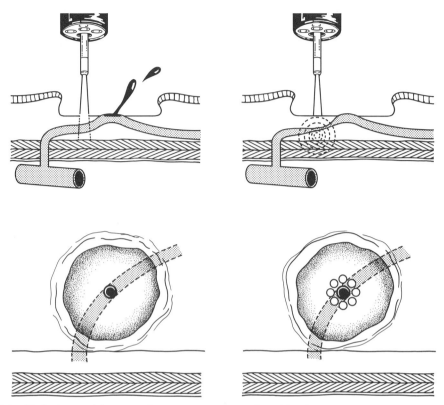

Figure 12.8 Technique of laser endoscopy in peptic ulcer bleeding. Most endoscopists treating a bleeding or non-bleeding vessel visible in the floor of an ulcer recommend placing about 8 pulses of energy which will produce visibly blanched spots in a tight ring around the vessel to coagulate both the efferent and afferent limb of the feeding vessel. Only then should the central protrusion be treated to check efficacy of coagulation (Papp, 1982, Swain, 1983).

situation usually improves with time. It may be helpful to alter the line of fire to other points near the apparent bleeding point, since a jet of blood can richochet off a bump in the ulcer crater misleading the endoscopist into treating that bump rather than the vessel. It is important not to keep firing at the same spot since this will increase the risk of perforation.

Major upper gastrointestinal bleeding from ulcers is common in two sites; the postero-inferior aspect of the duodenal bulb and the high posterior aspect of the lesser curve. Both these sites are sometimes difficult to treat and are usually approached at acute angles of between 0° and 45° using forward-viewing endoscopes. Duodenal deformity or stenosis is the commonest cause of endoscopic inaccessibil-

ity, but occasionally a blood-filled duodenum is difficult to clear for treatment. Usually adequate inflation will lift high lesser curve ulcers out of a pool of blood to allow treatment. Access is frequently improved by curving the endoscope with a J manoeuvre, and rotation of the endoscope with its eccentrically placed biopsy channel sometimes gives a more useful angle of approach.

Treating vascular malformations may be helped by modifying the technique. It seems best to find the largest lesion, which is the most likely to be the source of significant bleeding, and to aim for the central arteriole with the first pulse. Big vascular malformations usually bleed during treatment and once they start to bleed it may be difficult to identify the central arteriole. It is less important to stop any acute bleeding than to heat damage the centre of the vascular malformation, causing fibrosis and regeneration without recurrence of the anomalous vasculature.

12.22 LASER SAFETY

The main risk to the endoscopist or to others in the endoscopy room while the laser is being used is of inadvertent eye damage. The Nd–YAG, argon and dye lasers currently used in gastroenterology are all graded 'Class 4' lasers, which is the most dangerous class, denoting a laser system that can produce an optical hazard from direct or specular reflections but also from diffuse reflections. In addition, these lasers may produce electrical, fire and flood hazards and can burn the skin. Since the light of the Nd–YAG laser is in the invisible part of the spectrum, this laser may be more dangerous, since the eye will not blink automatically when light from this laser strikes the retina.

Up to 40% of Nd–YAG laser emission is scattered backwards when fired at gastric mucosa. Although this is likely to be widely scattered, it is possible for the light to strike a mirror-like pool of liquid which could reflect a large proportion of the light back up the endoscope. Measurements have shown that sufficient light could be scattered back up an endoscope to cause retinal damage. The endoscope should be fitted with a filter or the endoscopist must wear filtered goggles. It is possible to fit a filter inside the eyepiece of some endoscopes (which should then have 'filter fitted' engraved on the eyepiece). Unfortunately the geometry of some endoscopes, including the OES Olympus endoscopes, does not allow enough space for a filter to be placed and for these an external filter can be easily constructed (although this may interfere with the attachment of side viewers or television cameras). Very high quality filters exist which can filter the near infrared emission of the Nd–YAG laser without perceptible loss in the visible spectrum. Most Nd–YAG laser goggles seem to be made of cheaper filtered material with a variable green tinge which does diminish the endoscopist's ability to see red colours. Since the aiming beam is red, the displays of laser output power may be red, blood is red and it may be important to see that the patient's colour is red, this loss of colour perception can be important. Different filters and different sets of goggles will be needed if lasers with other wavelengths, such as argon or dye lasers, are used.

It is essential that all the staff and the patient have protective goggles and wear them, especially in a situation where direct or specular reflections are a potential hazard.

It seems sensible when commissioning a laser system to seek the advice of the local laser safety officer who may be a hospital physicist. Most laser endoscopy units incorporate the following safety features: a red warning light outside the room indicating that the laser is switched on, yellow laser hazard signs on all entrances, mirrors should be removed, reflective surfaces dulled or removed, windows covered. Many units incorporate safety interlock systems which will stop the laser from working automatically if the endoscopy room door is opened. 'Panic buttons' within the room are often provided to allow the laser to be turned off quickly if necessary. An on–off key is an obligatory requirement for medical laser systems; this should be removed when the laser is not in use.

A limited number of designated trained users should be allowed access to use the laser and the user endoscopist should consider himself responsible for the safety of those with him in the endoscopy room. The endoscopist needs a system of clearly understood instructions when the laser is running so that the laser is only switched to operational firing mode when needed. I tend to say 'enable laser please' or 'disable laser please'.

The key to laser safety is responsible use by experienced personnel.

12.23 WAVE-GUIDE CARE

The tip of the wave-guide has a relatively short lifespan and often burns out after a few thousand joules of Nd–YAG laser energy have been delivered. It is essential to have access to more than one wave-guide during treatment sessions so that another can be plugged in if one burns out during treatment. Care in their preparation, use and maintenance will prolong the working life of the waveguide tip.

It is well worth the laser endoscopist or technician learning how to replace tips. Most manufacturers supply kits for tip replacement, although it requires a little patience, skill and practice to cut an optically perfect cleave through the glass fibre, remove the cladding the required distance, glue on the metal tip and then insert the tip into the Teflon outer tubing.

The quality of cleave (which can be improved by careful polishing) will influence the life-expectancy. The quality of the cleave is best assessed by passing the helium neon aiming beam through the fibre after a cleave and assessing the shape of the beam on a flat surface. A good cleave produces a perfect circle of light with a clear circular paler penumbra and a moving speckled pattern due to coherent interference patterns. A less good cleave will show lateral flares. With some makes of laser it is possible to compare the power level emitted at the laser head with the power emitted at the tip of the laser. Losses in fibreoptic transmission should be at most only a few per cent.

There are two common causes of the wave-guide tip burning out. Failure to use the co-axial gas is one such cause. It is wise to check the flow rate of gas by putting the tip under water before use and to remember that gas cylinders can run out during use. Mucus, blood, or laser 'plume' which land on the wave-guide tip during use will deform the beam and tend to produce burn-out. Because light energy is scattered onto the metal tip by

this extraneous material, the temperature of the tip rises above the melting temperature of the Teflon tubing (250°C), which first swells then buckles, causing more laser light to strike the metal tip, and the temperature rises until the Teflon tubing, the cladding and the glass fibre ignite and a yellow flash is seen. If firing ceases this localized fire is rapidly extinguished by the CO_2.

If the tip inadvertently touches tissue (tissue sometimes seems to rush at the endoscope with alarming speed with sudden changes in intra-abdominal pressure) it is best to withdraw the wave-guide, temporarily disabling the laser, to clean the tip or at least check that the clear circle of the aiming beam is unimpaired. An eyeglass makes it easier to see if the tip is contaminated. Cotton wool on a stick is helpful for cleaning, as are impregnated tissues for lens cleaning. We leave the wave-guide in hydrogen peroxide for 20 minutes with the gas flow on after use.

12.24 CONCLUSION

Several conclusions have emerged from studies of laser control of gastrointestinal haemorrhage. Endoscopic intervention with laser therapy is capable of altering the outcome of bleeding from peptic ulcers, reducing rebleeding, the requirement for urgent surgery and mortality. The recognition of active bleeding is not enough; the therapeutic endoscopist has been forced to identify more precisely the bleeding point within the ulcer so that the treatment can be delivered precisely. Observations from these studies have helped to define the predictive value of the visible vessel and other stigmata of recent haemorrhage, and have aided selection of patients for treatment. Treatment of spurting or oozing from visible vessels will include virtually all ulcer patients at risk from further bleeding or death. Not all bleeding lesions are accessible to laser treatment, some arteries are too large for endoscopic occlusion with laser while treatment of bleeding varices with laser seems at best of temporary value. Larger controlled studies, with prospective randomization of high-risk groups, are required if benefit or its absence is to be demonstrated. Lasers may eventually be replaced by a superior technique for the control of gastrointestinal haemorrhage, but the study of their use in gastrointestinal bleeding has generated a new sense of optimism that it is now possible to improve the morbidity and mortality of this condition.

REFERENCES

Alexander, T. J. and Dwyer, R. M. (1985) Endoscopic Nd–YAG laser treatment of severe radiation injury of the gastrointestinal tract. *Gastrointest. Endosc.*, **31**, 152.

Allan, R. and Dykes, P. (1976) A study of the factors influencing mortality rates from gastrointestinal haemorrhage. *Q. J. Med.*, **45**, 533–50.

Avery-Jones, F. (1956) Haematemesis and melaena with special reference to causation and to the factors influencing the mortality from bleeding peptic ulcers. *Gastroenterology*, **30**, 166–9.

Basov, N. G. and Prokhorov, A. M. (1955) Possible methods of obtaining active molecules for a molecular oscillator. (In Russian.) *Zh. Ebsperim. Theor. Fiz.*, **28**, 249. Translation in *Soviet Phys. J.E.T.P.*, **1**, 184.

Boley, S. J., Sammartano, R., Brandt, L. J. and Sprayregen S. (1979) Vascular ectasias of the colon. *Surg. Gynecol. Obstet.*, **149**, 353–9.

Bowers, J. H. and Dixon, J. A. (1982) Argon laser photocoagulation of vascular malformations in the GI tract: short term results. *Gastrointest. Endosc.*, **28**, 126.

Bown, S. G., Salmon, P. R., Kelly, D. F. *et al.* (1979) Argon laser photocoagulation in the dog stomach. *Gut*, **20**, 680–7.

Bown, S. G., Salmon, P. R., Storey, D. W. *et al.* (1980) Nd–YAG laser photocoagulation in the dog stomach. *Gut*, **21**, 818–25.

Bown, S. G., Storey, D. W., Swain, C. P. *et al.* (1981) Argon laser photocoagulation for upper gastrointestinal haemorrhage: is technique the key to success? *Digestion*, **11**, 918–20.

Bown, S. G., Swain, C. P., Storey, D. W. *et al.* (1985) Endoscopic laser treatment of vascular anomalies of the upper gastrointestinal tract. *Gut*, **26**, 1338–48.

Bridges, W. B. (1964) Laser oscillations in singly ionized argon in the visible spectrum. *Appl. Phys. Lett.* **4**, 128–30.

Brunetaud, J. M., Enger, A., Herjot, A. *et al.* (1975) La photocoagulation per endoscopique des lésions digestives hemorrhagiques (nos premiers results chez l'homme a l'aide d'un laser à argon de moyenne puissance). *Gastroenterol. Clin. Biol.*, **2**, 557–8.

Buchi, K. N. and Brunetaud, J. M. (1987) Endoscopic laser therapy, in, *Surgical Application of Lasers* (ed. J. A. Dixon), Year Book Medical, Chicago, pp. 95–118.

Buchi, K. N. and Dixon, J. A. (1987) Argon laser treatment of hemorrhagic radiation proctitis. *Gastrointest. Endosc.*, **33**, 27–30.

Collins, R. and Langman, M. (1985) Treatment with histamine H_2 antagonists in upper gastrointestinal hemorrhage. Implications of randomized trials. *N. Engl. J. Med.*, **313**, 660–3.

Conn, H. O. (1981) To scope or not to scope? *N. Engl. J. Med.*, **304**, 967–9.

Daikuzono, N. and Joffe, S. N. (1985) Artificial sapphire probe for contact photocoagulation and tissue vaporization with the Nd:Yag laser. *Med. Instrum.*, 173–8.

Dennis, M. B., Silverstein, F. E., Gilbert, D. A. and Peoples, J. E. (1981) Evaluation of Nd–YAG photocoagulation using a new experimental ulcer model with a single bleeding artery. *Gastroenterology*, **80**, 1522–7.

Dixon, J. A., Berenson, M. M. and McCloskey, D. W. (1979) Neodymium-YAG laser treatment of experimental canine gastric photocoagulation. Acute and chronic studies of photocoagulation, penetration and perforation. *Gastroenterology*, **77**, 647–51.

Dwyer, R. M. (1981) The technique of gastrointestinal laser endoscopy, in *The Biomedical Laser* (ed. L. Goldman), Springer, New York, pp. 20–8.

Dwyer, R. M., Haverback, B. J., Bass, M. and Cherlow J. (1975) Laser-induced hemostasis in the canine stomach. Use of a flexible fibreoptic delivery system. *JAMA*, **231**, 486–9.

Einstein, A. (1917) Zur Quanten Theorie der Strahlung. *Phys. Zeit.*, **18**, 121–8.

Escourrou, J., Frexinos, J., Balas, D. *et al.* (1979) Comparison of a new method of electrocoagulation and YAG laser photocoagulation in the treatment of bleeding canine gastric ulcers. *Gastroenterology*, **76**, 112A.

Etienne, J., Raimbert, P. and Dorme, N. (1981) Successful Nd–YAG laser photocoagulation in Rendu Osler's and Willebrand's diseases, in *Laser Tokyo '81* (eds K. Atsumi and N. Nimsakul), Inter Group Corp, Tokyo, pp. 5-26–5-27.

Fleischer, D. (1981) ND–YAG laser photocoagulation for upper gastrointestinal angiodysplasia. *Gastrointest. Endosc.*, **27**, 122.

Fleischer, D. (1985) Endoscopic Nd:YAG laser therapy for active esophageal variceal bleeding. *Gastrointest. Endosc.*, **31**, 4–9.

Forrest, J. A. H., Findlayson, N. D. C. and Shearman, D. J. C. (1974) Endoscopy in gastrointestinal bleeding. *Lancet*, **ii**, 394–6.

Foster, D. N., Miloszewski, K. J. A. and Losowsky, M. S. (1978) Stigmata of recent haemorrhage in diagnosis and prognosis of upper gastrointestinal bleeding. *Br. Med. J.*, **1**, 1173–7.

Fruhmorgen, P., Bodem, F. and Kaduk, B. (1975) First endoscopic coagulation in the human gastrointestinal tract. *Dtsch. Med. Wochenschr.*, **100**, 167.

Fruhmorgen, P., Bodem, F. and Reidenbach H. D. (1978) Endoscopic photocoagulation by laser irradiation in the gastrointestinal tract of man. *Acta Hepatogastroenterol.*, **25**, 1–5.

Fruhmorgen, P., Bodem, K., Reidenbach, H. D. *et al.* (1976) Endoscopic laser coagulation of bleeding gastrointestinal lesions with the report of the first therapeutic application in man. *Gastrointest. Endosc.*, **23**, 73–5.

Fruhmorgen, P., Reidenbach, H. D., Bodem, F. *et al.* (1974) Reports on new instruments and new methods. Experimental examinations of laser endoscopy. *Endoscopy*, **6**, 116–22.

Fruhmorgen, P., Reidenbach, H. D., Bodem, F. *et al.* (1977) Report on preliminary experimental and clinical experiences with a new type of endoscopic argon laser photocoagulator. *Endoscopy*, **9**, 191.

Geusic, J. E., Marcos, H. M. and Van Uitert, L. C. (1964) Laser oscillations in Nd-doped Yttrium Aluminium, Yttrium Gallium and Gadolinium Garnets. *Appl. Phys. Lett.*, **4**, 182–4.

Gordon, J. P., Ziegler, H. J. and Townes, C. H. (1955) Molecular microwave oscillator and new hyperfine structure in the microwave amplifier, frequency standard and spectrometer. *Phys. Rev.*, **99**, 1266–74.

Gorisch, W. and Boergen, K-P. (1982) Heat induced contraction of blood vessels. *Lasers Surg. Med.*, **2**, 1–13.

Griffiths, W. J., Neumann, D. A. and Welsh, J. D. (1979) The visible vessel as indicator of uncontrolled or recurrent gastrointestinal hemorrhage. *N. Engl. J. Med.*, **300**, 1173–7.

Hashimoto, D. (1987) The development of lateral radiation probes. *Gastrointest. Endosc.*, **33**, 240–3.

Hashimoto, D., Miyohara, T. and Yoshimura K. (1986) A lateral radiation probe in Nd–YAG laser therapy. *Gastrointest. Endosc.*, **32**, 124–5.

Henry, D. A. and Whyte, I. (1988) Endoscopic coagulation for gastrointestinal bleeding. *N. Engl. J. Med.* **318**, 186–7.

Ihre, T., Johansson, C., Seligman, V. and Torregren, S. (1981) Endoscopic YAG laser treatment in massive upper gastrointestinal bleeding. Report of a controlled randomised study. *Scand. J. Gastroenterol.*, **16**, 633–40.

Jensen, D. M. and Machicado, G. A. (1985) Bleeding colonic angioma: endoscopic coagulation and follow-up. *Gastroenterology*, **88**, 1433.

Jensen, D. M., Machicado, G. A., Tapia, J. I. and Elashoff, J. (1984) Controlled trial of endoscopic argon laser for severe ulcer haemorrhage. *Gastroenterology*, **86**, 1125A.

Jensen, D. M., Silpa, M. L., Tapia, J. I. *et al.* (1983) Comparison of different methods of endoscopic hemostasis of bleeding canine esophageal varices. *Gastroenterology*, **84**, 1455–61.

Joffe, S. N. (1986) Contact neodymium : YAG laser surgery in gastroenterology: a preliminary report. *Lasers Surg. Med.*, **6**, 155–7.

Johnston, J. H. (1982) Complications following endoscopic laser therapy. *Gastointest. Endosc.*, **28**, 135.

Johnston, J. H. (1984) The sentinel clot and invisible vessel: Pathologic anatomy of bleeding peptic ulcer. *Gastrointest. Endosc.*, **30**, 313–5.

Johnston, J. H., Jensen, D. M. and Auth, D. (1987) Experimental comparison of endoscopic Yttrium-Aluminium-Garnet laser, electrosurgery and heater probe for canine gut arterial coagulation. *Gastroenterology*, **92**, 1101–8.

Johnston, J. H., Jensen, D. M., Mautner, W. and Elashoff, J. (1981) Argon laser treatment of bleeding canine lesions: limitations and guidelines for endoscopic use. *Gastroenterology*, **80**, 708–16.

Johnston, J. H., Jensen, D. M. and Mautner, W. (1982) Comparison of endoscopic electrocoagulation and laser photocoagulation of bleeding canine gastric ulcers. *Gastroenterology*, **82**, 904–10.

Johnston, J. H., Jensen, D. M., Mautner, W. and Elashoff, J. (1980) YAG laser treatment of experimental bleeding canine gastric ulcers. *Gastroenterology*, **79**, 1256–61.

Johnston, J. H., Sones, J. Q., Long, B. W. and Posey, E. L. (1985) Comparison of the heater probe and YAG laser in endoscopic treatment of major bleeding from peptic ulcers. *Gastrointest. Endosc.*, **31**, 175–81.

Kelly, D. F., Bown, S. G., Calder, B. M. *et al.* (1983) Histological changes following Nd–YAG laser photocoagulation of canine gastric mucosa. *Gut*, **24**, 914–20.

Kelly, D. F., Bown, S. G., Salmon, P. R. *et al.* (1980) Nature and extent of histological changes induced by argon laser photocoagulation in canine gastric mucosa. *Gut*, **21**, 1041–7.

Kiefhaber, P. (1979) Results of a Coagulation Enquiry. Reported by Fruhmorgen, P. (1981) in *Colonoscopy* (eds R. H. Hunt and J. D. Waye), Chapman and Hall, London, p. 229.

Kiefhaber, P., Nath, G. and Moritz, K. (1977) Endoscopical control of massive gastrointestinal haemorrhage by irradiation with a high-power Neodymium-YAG laser. *Prog. Surg.*, **15**, 140–55.

Kiefhaber, P., Kiefhaber, K., Huber, F. and Nath, G. (1983) Endoscopic applications of Neodymium-YAG laser radiation in the gastrointestinal tract, in *Neodymium-YAG Laser in Medicine and Surgery* (ed. S. N. Joffe), Elsevier, New York, pp. 6–14.

Krejs, G. J., Little, K. H., Westergaard, H. *et al.* (1987) Laser photocoagulation for the treatment of acute peptic-ulcer bleeding. A randomized controlled clinical trial. *N. Engl. J. Med.*, **316**, 1618–21.

Laurence, B. H., Vallon, A. G., Cotton, P. B. *et al.* (1980) Endoscopic laser photocoagulation for bleeding peptic ulcers. *Lancet*, **i**, 124–7.

Machiacado, G. A., Jensen, D. M., Tapia, J. I. and Mautner, W. (1979) Argon laser photocoagulation and bipolar electrocoagulation in the treatment of bleeding duodenal and esophageal ulcers. *Gastroenterology*, **76**, 119A.

MacLeod, I. A., Bow, C. R. and Joffe, S. N. (1982) A quantifiable bleeding gastric ulcer model in dogs for assessing the neodymium Yag laser. *Endoscopy*, **14**, 9–10.

MacLeod, I. A., Mills, P. R., MacKenzie, J. F. *et al.* (1983) Neodymium yttrium aluminium garnet laser photocoagulation for major haemorrhage from peptic ulcers and single vessels: a single blind controlled study. *Nucl. Med. J.*, **286**, 345–8.

Maiman, T. (1960) Stimulated optical radiation in ruby. *Nature*, **187**, 493–4.

Mathus-Vliegen, E. M. H. and Tytgat, G. N. (1986) Laser photocoagulation of colorectal malignancies. *Cancer*, **57**, 396–9.

Matthewson, K., Swain, C. P., Bland, M. *et al.* (1987) Randomised comparison of Nd–YAG laser heater probe (HP) and no endoscopic therapy for bleeding peptic ulcer. *Gastroenterology*, **92**, 1522.

Mills, T. N., Swain, C. P., Dark, J. M. *et al.* (1983) The 'hot squeeze' bipolar forceps. A more effective endoscopic method for stopping bleeding from large vessels in the gastrointestinal tract. *Gastrointest. Endosc.*, **29**, 184–5.

Morgan, A. G., McAdam, W. A. F., Walmsley, G. L. *et al.* (1977) Clinical findings, early endoscopy and multivariate analysis in patients bleeding from the upper gastrointestinal tract. *Br. Med. J.*, **2**, 237–40.

Nath, G. and Fidler, J. (1972) High power Nd–YAG laser surgery with a flexible delivery system, in *Conference Proceedings of 1st European Electro-Optics Market and Technology Conference, Geneva.*

Nath, G., Gorisch, W. and Kiefhaber, P. (1973) First laser endoscopy via a fiberoptic transmission system. *Endoscopy*, **5**, 208–13.

Nath, G., Gorisch, W., Kreitmair, A. and Kiefhaber, P. (1973) Transmission of a powerful argon beam through a fiberoptic flexible gastroscope for operative gastroscopy. *Endoscopy*, **5**, 213–5.

Papp, J. P. (1981) Electrocoagulation in upper gastrointestinal bleeding. *Dig. Dis. Sci.*, **26**, 41–3.

Papp, J. P. (1982) Endoscopic electrocoagulation in the management of upper gastrointestinal tract bleeding. *Surg. Clin. North. Am.*, **62**, 797–806.

Peterson, W. L., Barnett, C. C., Smith, H. J. *et al.* (1981) Routine early endoscopy in upper gastrointestinal bleeding: a randomized controlled trial. *N. Engl. J. Med.*, **304**, 925–9.

Protell, R. L., Silverstein, F. E., Auth, D. C. *et al.* (1978) The neodymium-Yag laser is dangerous for photocoagulation of experimental gastric ulcers when compared with the argon laser. *Gastroenterology*, **74**, 1082.

Protell, R. L., Silverstein, F. E., Piercey, J. *et al.* (1976) A reproducible animal model of acute bleeding ulcer – the 'ulcer maker'. *Gastroenterology*, **71**, 961–4.

Rutgeerts, P., Van Gompel, F., Geboes, K. *et al.* (1985) Long term results of treatment of vascular malformations of the gastrointestinal tract by neodymium YAG laser photocoagulation. *Gut*, **26**, 586–93.

Rutgeerts, P., Vantrappen, G., Broeckaert, L. *et al.* (1984) A new and effective technique of YAG laser photocoagulation for severe upper gastrointestinal bleeding. *Endoscopy*, **16**, 115–7.

Rutgeerts, P., Vantrappen, G., Broeckaert, L. *et al.* (1982) Controlled trial of YAG laser treatment of upper digestive hemorrhage. *Gastroenterology*, **83**, 410–6.

Rutgeerts, P., Vantrappen, G., Geboes, K. and Broeckaert, L. (1981) Safety and efficacy of Neodymium-Yag laser photocoagulation: an experimental study in dogs. *Gut*, **22**, 38–44.

Rutgeerts, P., Vantrappen, G., Van Hootegem, Ph. *et al.* (1987) Neodymium-YAG laser photocoagulation versus multipolar electrocoagulation for the treatment of severely bleeding ulcers: a randomized comparison. *Gastrointest. Endosc.*, **33**, 199–201.

Schawalow, A. L. and Townes, C. H. (1958) Infrared and optical lasers. *Phys. Rev.*, 1444–9.

Schiller, K. R. F., Truelove, S. C. and Gwyn Williams, D. (1970) Haematemesis and melaena with special reference to factors influencing the outcome. *Br. Med. J.*, **2**, 7–14.

Sigel, B. and Dunn, M. R. (1965) The mechanisms of blood vessel closure by high frequency electrocoagulation. *Surg. Gynecol. Obstet.*, **121**, 823–31.

Sigel, B. and Hatke, F. L. (1967) Physical factors in electrocoaptation of blood vessels. *Arch. Surg.*, **95**, 54–8.

Silverstein, F. E., Auth, D. C., Rubin, C. E. and Protell, R. L. (1976) High power argon laser treatment via standard endoscopes. 1. A preliminary study of efficacy in control of experimental erosive bleeding. *Gastroenterology*, **71**, 558–63.

Silverstein, F. E., Gilbert, D. A., Tedesco, F. J. *et al.* (1981) The national ASGE survey on upper gastrointestinal bleeding. *Gastrointest. Endosc.*, **27**, 73–102.

Silverstein, F. E., Protell, R. L., Gilbert, D. A. *et al.* (1979) Argon vs neodymium-YAG laser photocoagulation of experimental canine ulcers. *Gastroenterology*, **77**, 491–6.

Silverstein, F. E., Protell, R. L., Gulcsik, C. and Auth, D. C. *et al.* (1978) Endoscopic laser treatment. III. Development and testing of a gas assisted argon laser waveguide in control of bleeding experimental ulcers. *Gastroenterology*, **74**, 232–9.

Silverstein, F. E., Protell, R. L. and Piercey, J. (1977) Endoscopic laser treatment. II. Comparison of the efficacy of high and low power photocoagulation in control of severely bleeding experimental ulcers in dogs. *Gastroenterology*, **73**, 481–6.

Snitzer, E. (1961) Optical laser action of Nd^{3+} in a barium crown glass. *Phys. Rev. Lett.*, **7**, 444–6.

Storey, D. W., Bown, S. G., Swain, C. P. *et al.* (1981) Endoscopic prediction of recurrent bleeding in peptic ulcers. *N. Engl. J. Med.*, **305**, 1411–3.

Swain, C. P. (1983) Endoscopic Nd YAG laser control of gastrointestinal bleeding, in *Neodymium-YAG Laser in Medicine and Surgery* (ed. S. N. Joffe), Elsevier, New York, pp. 16–28.

Swain, C. P. (1986a) Forrest 11 bleeding: indications for treatment and results of laser therapy. *Endoscopy*, **18**, Suppl. 1, 14–6.

Swain, C. P. (1987) When and why do ulcers bleed and what can be done about it? *Aliment. Pharmacol. Therap.*, **1**, 455S–76S.

Swain, C. P., Bown, S. G., Salmon, P. R. *et al.* (1986b) Controlled trial of Nd–YAG laser photocoagulation for bleeding peptic ulcer. *Lancet*, **i**, 1113–6.

Swain, C. P., Bown, S. G., Storey, D. W. *et al.* (1981) Controlled trial of argon laser photocoagulation in bleeding peptic ulcers. *Lancet*, **ii**, 1313–6.

Swain, C. P., Mills, T. N., Dark, J. M. *et al.* (1984a) A comparative study of the safety and efficacy of liquid and dry monopolar electrodes in experimental bleeding ulcers using computerized energy monitoring. *Gastroenterology*, **86**, 93–103.

Swain, C. P., Mills, T. N., Matthewson, K. *et al.* (1984b) Development and testing of contact endoscopic thermal methods which are more effective than conventional lasers and diathermy electrodes in controlling bleeding from the gastrointestinal tract. *Gut*, **25**, A1186.

Swain, C. P., Storey, D. W., Bown, S. G. *et al.* (1986a) Nature of the bleeding vessel in recurrently bleeding gastric ulcers. *Gastroenterology*, **90**, 595–608.

Waitman, A. M., Spira, I. A., Chryssanthou, C. P. and Stenger, R. J. (1975) Fiberoptic-coupled argon laser in the control of experimentally produced gastric bleeding. *Gastrointest. Endosc.*, **21**, 78–81.

Waitman, A. M., Grant, D. Z. and Chateau, F. (1982) Argon laser photocoagulation treatment of patients with acute and chronic bleeding secondary to telangiectasia. *Gastrointest. Endosc.*, **28**, 153.

Wara, P. (1985) Endoscopic prediction of major rebleeding – a prospective study of stigmata of haemorrhage in bleeding ulcer. *Gastroenterology*, **88**, 1209–14.

Vallon, A. G., Cotton, P. B., Laurence, B. H. *et al.* (1981) Randomised trial of endoscopic argon laser photocoagulation in bleeding peptic ulcers. *Gut*, **22**, 228–33.

CHAPTER THIRTEEN

Endoscopic oesophageal variceal obliteration

J. D. R. Rose
and
P. M. Smith

13.1 INTRODUCTION

Bleeding from oesophageal varices is a medical emergency with a high mortality rate. The risk of bleeding depends principally on variceal size, rather than intravariceal pressure (Lebrec *et al.*, 1980). The bigger the varix, the thinner its wall and the greater the wall stress.

Resuscitation is the first priority in management. Blood transfusion is life saving, but attempts to correct clotting factors and platelet counts are of little value in an emergency, since their half-life is short and they are unlikely to affect variceal bleeding. Under no circumstances should intravenous saline be used, since it may induce oedema and ascites.

13.2 DIAGNOSIS

The presence of liver palms, spider naevi, loss of body hair, Dupuytren's contracture, ascites, jaundice, hepatosplenomegaly and hepatic fetor or drowsiness may indicate that an upper gastrointestinal bleed has an oesophageal variceal origin. However, peptic ulcers are common in cirrhotics and haemorrhagic gastritis can occur in alcoholics. In addition, a congestive gastropathy has been described in portal hypertension (McCormack *et al.*, 1985). Upper gastrointestinal endoscopy should therefore be performed as soon as possible, even if varices have previously been demonstrated by radiology.

Endoscopy, if done within 24 hours of the upper gastrointestinal bleed, should identify the source of the haemorrhage with over 90% accuracy. The presence of large varices in the lower 5 cm of the oesophagus should be sought. Occasionally a varix is actively bleeding. At other times a tiny break in the mucosa over a varix, sometimes with an attached clot, may be seen. Indicators of a high risk of bleeding include large varices, a bluish colouration of the variceal wall, small vessels over the varix or the presence of round red blisters (haematocystic spots) (The Italian Liver Cirrhosis Project, 1987).

Gastric varices in the fundus may be the source of bleeding in portal hypertension in 5–10% of patients, and are easy to overlook. They have a high risk of rebleeding, and the survival rate is lower than for oesophageal bleeders (Trudeau and Prindiville, 1986).

13.3 HISTORY OF SCLEROTHERAPY

Although oesophageal variceal injection was first described in 1939 (Crafoord and Frenckner, 1939), the technique was not adopted widely, and portacaval shunts became an accepted treatment for bleeding varices. In 1974, however, controlled trials of portacaval shunts were published demonstrating no advantage over simple medical treatment, the frequency of liver failure and encephalopathy outweighing the advantages of reduced haemorrhage. Sclerotherapy was therefore taken up again, the advent of the fibrescope simplifying the procedure, and over 500 papers have been published in the past 5 years.

Whereas the original papers described the direct injection of sclerosant into the lumen of the oesophageal varix, a newer technique was introduced by Wodak (1960). He injected sclerosant alongside the varix, the aim being to create a submucosal layer of fibrosis over the varix (wall sclerosis) to prevent it from bleeding but leaving it as a functional collateral to decompress the portal system. This method was widely adopted in Europe thereafter, while the intravariceal route was preferred in the UK and the USA.

13.4 AIMS OF SCLEROTHERAPY

The aim of sclerotherapy is to:

1. Stop variceal haemorrhage.
2. Prevent recurrent haemorrhage by obliteration of the varices.

13.5 TECHNIQUE

13.5.1 PREPARATION

The patient should be fasted and given the usual premedication as for a routine upper gastrointestinal endoscopy. Since visualization of the oesophagus is the main concern, special efforts to empty the stomach of blood are not essential.

A minimum of two assistants in addition to the endoscopist is required. One must be a fully trained nurse but experience and commonsense under these circumstances count for more than qualifications. One assistant is designated to look after the patient and in particular the airway while at the same time keeping an eye on the safety of the endoscope in the mouth. Toothguards frequently become dislodged unnoticed. The second assistant helps the endoscopist with the injection. It is advisable for all personnel to be immunized against hepatitis B virus.

The patient lies in the left lateral position with the head on a firm pillow and disposable absorbent towelling around the mouth. Intravenous sedation is preferred to general anaesthesia which, while having the advantage of a cuffed endotracheal tube in the airways, requires a skilled anaesthetist in addition to the other personnel. Between 5 and 20 mg of emulsified diazepam (Diazemuls, Kabivitrum Ltd, UK) are given intravenously depending on age and agitation. Emulsified diazepam produces less thrombophlebitis than the unemulsified form, but shorter acting benzodiazepines such as midazolam, 2.5–7.5 mg (Hypnoval, Roche Products Ltd, UK), are gaining favour. It is common experience that heavy drinkers react paradoxically to benzodiazepines and become uncooperative and often aggressive. Intravenous pethidine 50–100 mg is effective for these patients.

Varices are best seen in a paralysed oesophagus. Hyoscine n-butyl bromide (Buscopan, Boehringer Ingelheim Ltd, UK), 20–40 mg intravenously, at the time of sedation greatly assists proper assessment of variceal size and subsequent injection. Glucagon (Novo Laboratory Ltd, UK; Eli Lilly & Co. Ltd, UK), 0.5–1 mg, is an alternative.

13.6 EQUIPMENT

As for routine endoscopy all equipment must be carefully cleaned and then sterilized. However, because of the chance of bleeding during variceal sclerotherapy the risks of contamination are greater and the cleaning process must be all the more rigorous.

13.6.1 ENDOSCOPES

Sclerotherapy can be performed with almost any end- or oblique-viewing fibrescope, but some make the procedure easier. Injections are aimed diagonally into the varices, so a medium-sized endoscope which can be angled within the oesophageal lumen is ideal.

Table 13.1 Endoscopes particularly suitable for sclerotherapy

Make	Type	Vision	Bridge	Fully immersible	External diameter (mm)	Internal diameter (mm)
Olympus	GIFK 10	Fore/oblique	Yes	Yes	11.4	3
Olympus	GIF1T 10	Fore	No	Yes	12.6	4
Fujinon	UGI-G2	Fore/oblique	Yes	Yes	11.3	2.8
Fujinon	UGI-CT2	Fore	No*	Yes	12.1	3.7
Pentax	FG34 JH	Fore	No	Yes	11.5	3.5
Wolf	EF760 1†	Fore	No	Yes	13	3.7
Wolf	EGDTF 7649	Fore	No	Yes	13	3.7

*10° angle on a channel.
†Has built in distal slot to fix varices and a proximal balloon to compress them.

Paediatric endoscopes are too flexible and insubstantial to provide a firm base for injection. Large-diameter or twin channel endoscopes have the advantage of good suction but are difficult to angle within the lumen. This problem is overcome by the use of a bridge to angle the injector needle. Table 13.1 provides a list of endoscopes considered suitable for sclerotherapy. Rigid endoscopes are difficult to use, require a general anaesthetic, are employed only by a few surgeons particularly experienced in their use (Johnston and Rogers, 1973; Terblanche et al., 1979) and are associated with more complications (Kahn et al., 1985).

13.6.2 INJECTOR NEEDLES

All injection devices consist of a fine needle at the tip of a long thin flexible plastic tube, whose proximal end is a luer connection, within an outer protective sheath through which the needle can be protruded and retracted. There are two basic types. In the first, the outer sheath is also a plastic tube. It is cheap, relatively stiff and easy to clean, but the open distal end of the outer sheath permits contamination between the sheath and the tube. In the second, the outer sheath is a coiled spring similar to that used for endoscopy biopsy forceps and its distal tip is well engineered to reduce contamination between the tube and the sheath. It is more expensive, more flexible but more difficult to clean. Once

taken apart re-assembly is often tedious, and can be impossible. Concern to avoid infection favours equipment which is easy to clean. Most manufacturers supply injectors compatible with their own instruments (Figure 13.1). In addition, some independent suppliers are listed in Table 13.2.

13.6.3 SCLEROSANTS

A wide variety of chemicals has been used to produce vascular thrombosis. Most modern sclerosants are detergents which damage the endothelium of varices in the same way as Teepol lyses red cells. Thrombosis results from the exposure of the vessel wall beneath the damaged endothelium. Sclerosants are

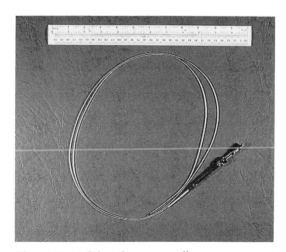

Figure 13.1   Sclerotherapy needle.

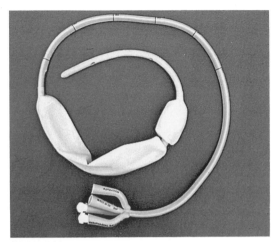

Figure 13.2   4 lumen Sengstaken tube.

not in themselves thrombotic, in fact they inhibit the action of clotting factors. At present the commonest sclerosants used in the UK are:

(a) Ethanolamine oleate (B.P.)

This is a viscous yellow alkaline liquid which is used as a 5% solution. Its viscosity makes it difficult to inject unless the ampoules are placed in hot water before use. Two-millilitre syringes also make the task easier, or a syringe 'gun' may be used with a larger syringe.

(b) Sodium tetradecyl sulphate (STD Pharmaceuticals Ltd, UK)

This is a clear neutral 3% solution of low viscosity which can be injected with 5-ml syringes.

In Europe hydroxypolyethoxydodecane (proprietary name polidocanol, commercial name Aethoxysklerol) is used extensively for

Table 13.2 Independent suppliers of sclerotherapy needles

Company	Item
Diagmed, UK	TW 1V/6
	TW 1V/6F
Fibroptik, UK	SNO 1
	SNO 2

oesophageal wall sclerosis. As Pistocaine (Norgine Ltd, UK) the compound is also available in the UK, but not specifically for sclerotherapy. In the USA combinations of sclerosants and thrombogenic substances are being investigated. However, for practical purposes 5% ethanolamine oleate, 3% sodium tetradecyl sulphate and 75% ethanol are the most effective sclerosants (Jensen, Machicado and Silpa, 1986).

13.6.4 OTHER EQUIPMENT

(a) Tamponade tube

It is essential to have a Sengstaken tube readily available. The four-lumen modification, or Minnesota tube, which allows oesophageal aspiration, is preferable (Figure 13.2). Insertion is easier if the stiffness of the tube is increased by keeping it in a refrigerator before use.

(b) Williams overtube

One of the advantages of the rigid oesophagoscope is that a bleeding varix can be compressed and excluded from the field of vision while others are treated. The Williams tube (KeyMed Ltd, UK) is a semiflexible overtube with an oval hole just short of the distal end (Williams and Dawson, 1979). The design imitates the effect of the rigid oesophagoscope but, while successfully achieving its object, it is difficult to pass and is not widely used (Fig. 13.3).

(c) Compression devices

A number of ingenious devices have been invented to prevent flow into or out of the varices during injection. None is of proven benefit.

(d) Goggles

Although not yet widely worn by endoscopists, it is advisable to consider wearing eye protection. Sclerosant under high pressure not infrequently 'blows out' during injection. If the spray enters the eye and is not washed out immediately, a painful red

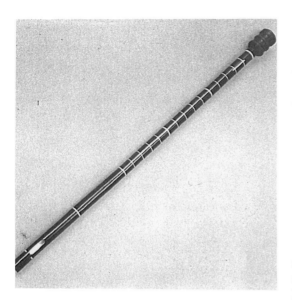

Figure 13.3   Williams overtube.

haemorrhage is not immediately life threatening, injection to stop the bleeding should be attempted. However, in the face of massive bleeding, discretion is the better part of valour and the endoscope should be withdrawn and a Sengstaken balloon inserted. Similarly, massive bleeding from varices on the ward in the middle of the night is best treated by transfusion and tamponade followed by elective injection next day with alert and experienced staff. The balloon is kept inflated until all preparations for injection are ready. The oesophageal and then the gastric balloon are deflated in the endoscopy theatre. A gush of blood at this stage indicates that the balloon should be reinflated and another treatment, such as surgical transection, be considered. In the majority of cases, however, even though bleeding may restart, there is time to insert the endoscope and inject the varices.

'sclerotherapist's eye' results. A fine aerosol of blood and other fluids, which may be infectious, can spurt from the biopsy valve.

Table 13.3 gives a checklist of equipment required.

13.7 TIMING OF SCLEROTHERAPY

It is essential that the source of a bleed, which could be variceal, is identified so that management can proceed logically. This almost invariably involves a diagnostic endoscopy during which active variceal haemorrhage may be found. If the varices can be identified and the

Table 13.3 Additional equipment required for sclerotherapy

Hyoscine butyl bromide or glucagon
Injector needles
Sclerosant
Syringes (2 ml and 5 ml)
Minnesota tube
Goggles

13.8 METHOD

13.8.1 ORIENTATION, GRADING AND RECORDING OF VARICES

It may seem superfluous to orientate oneself within the oesophagus and then grade and record the varices observed before treatment and, on occasions of great emergency, it may be (Figure 13.4). However, a number of practical points relate to each of these procedures. It is advisable to inject the lowest lying varices first, so that any bleeding will not obscure the uninjected varices. The size and number of varices is of prognostic significance. The patient with multiple large varices will require more treatment and is more likely to suffer recurrent haemorrhage than a patient with only small varices. A record of the varices is helpful for the sclerotherapist, who after two or three sessions feels little progress has been made. Reference to the initial description will usually prove encouraging.

With the patient lying in the left lateral position, a drop of water from the end of a

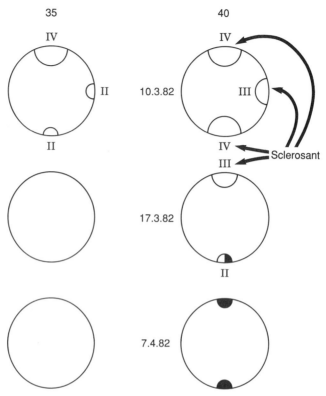

Figure 13.4 Progress of sclerotherapy. Varices recorded and graded to demonstrate thrombosis and reduction in size at 35cm and 40cm (just above oesophagogastric junction).

catheter or injection needle protruding from the biopsy channel will fall 'down' to the left. If this point is considered to be 6 o'clock on a clock-face, then varices and other features can be recorded around the clock. A small pool of secretions may also serve the same purpose, but with less precision.

A number of classifications of variceal size have been made, but grading the varices from I to IV according to the degree of protrusion into the oesophageal lumen has gained acceptance. A grade I varix just protrudes into the lumen and a grade IV varix occupies the whole of its quadrant of the oesophageal lumen (Paquet, 1982). A written record of the varices, their grades and positions can then be made. We record just above the oesophagogastric junction and 5 cm proximally.

13.8.2 SITE OF INJECTION

The lower 5 cm of the oesophagus is almost invariably the site of bleeding and it is here that the injections should be aimed. This area is also rich in large perforating vessels which supply the varices with blood from the perioesophageal plexus (McCormack et al., 1983). Their occlusion is important in obliterating the varices. 'Red blebs' are very thin areas prone to bleeding and should not be needled directly, since they bleed excessively. Injections should also be kept away from any ulceration, and thrombosed varices should not be injected, since further ulceration results.

13.8.3 METHOD OF INJECTION – INTRAVARICEAL

Large varices are easier to inject than small varices so it is sensible to choose the largest varix nearest to 6 o'clock just above the oesophagogastric mucosal junction. The injector with its needle retracted is advanced into the field of view and the needle protruded. The angle of injection to obtain an intravariceal injection is oblique, approximately 45°, and this is achieved by manipulating the flexible distal tip of the endoscope and/or the bridge. The injector is then darted into the varix and sclerosant injected. Bulging and blanching at the site of the injection are signs of extravasation and are to be avoided. The addition to the sclerosant of radiological contrast media (Rose, Crane and Smith, 1983), fluorescein (Hine et al., 1984) or methylene blue (Korula et al., 1985) assists the detection of extravasation. An experienced nurse can often detect an intravariceal injection from the lower resistance felt on compressing the syringe plunger. However, despite these signs, extravasation may still go undetected and it is recommended that no more than 2 ml of sclerosant are injected at any one site. Ulceration is related to the volume injected. If there is any doubt, the injection should be stopped and the varix injected at another site. On withdrawing the needle a little bleeding may occur. If this is troublesome the site can be compressed by the tip of the endoscope for 2 minutes. The varices are then injected in turn until all have been treated. If varices are large, further, more proximal, injection within the 5-cm zone may be required.

13.8.4 PARAVARICEAL METHOD OF INJECTION – OESOPHAGEAL WALL SCLEROSIS

As the aim is to produce fibrosis without ulceration or variceal thrombosis, dilute sclerosant (e.g. 1% polidocanol) is injected in small volumes (0.5 ml) superficially alongside the varices. The injections are placed more obliquely and more superficially than for variceal thrombosis and blanching at the site of injection is expected. Beginning just above the oesophagogastric junction and proceeding in a spiral up the oesophagus, a uniform oedematous sheath surrounds the varices in the distal third of the oesophagus.

As with intravariceal injection, repeat injection and follow-up are required. If a 1% solution is tolerated without severe inflammation or ulceration, a 2% solution may be tried. Some operators inject into the varix to thrombose it and place injections along the side and over the surface for added effect.

13.8.5 GASTRIC VARICES

These may be a continuation of oesophageal varices extending into the stomach. Oesophageal sclerotherapy can be effective, as radiology and Doppler studies have shown blood flow to be from the oesophagus to the stomach (McCormack et al., 1983). Hosking and Johnson (1988) achieved successful sclerotherapy by this technique in 19/23 patients. In contrast, direct injection of fundal varices can lead to serious complications (Trudeau and Prindiville, 1986).

13.8.6 AFTERCARE

It is rarely necessary to place a Sengstaken tube after injection to stop haemorrhage and there is no evidence that this procedure increases thrombosis (Barsoum et al., 1982). Indeed, it is likely that compression aggravates the effect of extravasated sclerosant (Helpap and Bollweg, 1981), and increases the risk of aspiration, which should be treated vigorously if it has occurred. If the patient is sufficiently alert he is sat upright and frequent observations of pulse and blood pressure performed for the next 3–4 hours. Fluids are permitted once the pharyngeal anaesthesia has worn off and food may be given the same day. Patients with small varices and a low risk of bleeding can be safely treated as day cases.

13.8.7 TREATMENT INTERVALS

Since the patient remains at risk of recurrent haemorrhage until the varices are obliterated, frequent treatment is recommended. However, the more serious complication of deep ulceration takes several days to develop and it is prudent not to reinject until any potential ulcers have declared themselves. Weekly injections provide the optimum and can be fitted into regular endoscopy lists. Residual small varices can be treated monthly. After variceal obliteration has been achieved, 3-monthly endoscopic follow-up to check for variceal recurrence is recommended. The great majority of recurrences occur in the first few months and follow-up can be yearly if there has been no recurrence in the first 24 months.

13.9 COMPLICATIONS

Sclerosants are agents which damage tissue. The damage is proportional to the dose, so local complications depend on concentration and volume extravasated. Smaller volumes of sclerosant escape along the track of successful intravariceal injections and produce small ulcers very soon after the injection. These appear to have no clinical significance. Larger volumes injected alongside or into the varix produce extensive necrosis which is not usually observable through the surviving squamous epithelium. On occasions the necrosis extends through the epithelium to produce an oesophageal wall ulcer. Extension into a patent varix can produce iatrogenic haemorrhage. Although transmural necrosis after extravasation occurs, free perforation is rare but can lead to mediastinitis, empyema, oesophagobronchial or oesophagoaortic fistulae (Carr-Locke and Sidky, 1982). The peak time of onset of these more serious complications is from 7 to 10 days and is associated with the development of fever.

Oesophageal strictures develop in a small proportion of cases after multiple injection sessions. They can be safely dilated by the same techniques used for peptic strictures; a single dilatation suffices in most cases. However, as oedema is often a major component, spontaneous resolution can occur.

Distant complications are much less common but acute pulmonary oedema after sclerosant injection has been reported (Monroe et al., 1983). Although the sclerosant undergoes considerable dilution, it should be borne in mind that the next capillary bed it meets is the pulmonary vasculature.

Fortunately, sclerotherapy complications are rarely a cause for major concern, the procedure having a mortality of approximately 1%, usually from recurrent bleeding, perforation, sepsis and respiratory problems. (Schuman et al., 1987). The key to keeping the incidence and severity of complications low is to limit the volume of extravasated sclerosant by careful observation of the site of injection and by injecting no more than 2 ml sclerosant at each site.

13.10 RESULTS OF SCLEROTHERAPY

Terblanche and his colleagues published the first controlled trial of sclerotherapy in 1979. A group of patients with variceal bleeding who underwent intravariceal endoscopic sclerotherapy with a rigid endoscope under general anaesthesia were compared with another group who underwent orthodox medical therapy, but also, for ethical reasons, acute sclerotherapy if active variceal bleeding was diagnosed. The treated group had fewer bleeds than the control group, although the mortality was not improved (Terblanche et al., 1983). However, 37% of the control group had partial or complete eradication of their oesophageal varices, a factor likely to influence the trial's outcome.

The largest controlled trial of sclerotherapy was performed at King's College Hospital, London (Westaby et al., 1985), and was the first to show a reduction in mortality. During a mean follow-up period of 37 months, only five patients of 56 died from variceal bleeding after intravenous sclerotherapy compared with 25 of 60 patients in the control group, a highly significant difference ($P < 0.001$). Sclerotherapy reduced the overall bleeding rate per patient-month threefold, the great majority of haemorrhages occurring before variceal obliteration had been completed. Ten treated patients died from liver failure and one from a hepatoma associated with the underlying cirrhotic process.

The Copenhagen Oesophageal Varices Sclerotherapy Project (1984) compared paravariceal sclerotherapy with medical treatment. One hundred and eighty-seven cirrhotic patients were randomly assigned to either group, and were followed for up to 52 months. Sixty-five per cent of the sclerotherapy group and 78% of the controls died, most of the deaths occurring in the first 2 months before the varices had been obliterated. Thereafter the mortality of the treated patients fell to only 43% of the control group.

The Los Angeles trial (Korula et al., 1985) demonstrated a reduction in variceal bleeding in the sclerotherapy group, but failed to show an improvement in the survival. However, 21% of the patients were lost to follow-up, and in only 28 of the original treatment group of 63 was variceal obliteration achieved.

A Swedish trial (Soderlund and Ihre, 1985) showed no improvement in mortality for those receiving sclerotherapy, both on a long-term basis and on initial control of acute variceal bleeding when compared to balloon tamponade and vasopressin. The risk factor for rebleeds over a period of 25 months was significantly reduced, however, although 15% of the treated patients developed major complications.

All five of these trials have shown a significant reduction in the total number of bleeding episodes with sclerotherapy, whether intravariceal or paravariceal, and the larger two of the four have demonstrated an improved survival rate once variceal obliteration has occurred. Rebleeding during treatment is liable to occur as long as large varices (grade III or IV) persist, usually in the early stages (Rose, Crane and Smith, 1983), but obliteration of varices can be achieved more rapidly by reducing the time interval between courses of treatment to 1 week (Westaby et al., 1984). The addition of propranolol to the treatment regimen during sclerotherapy has no effect on the frequency of recurrent variceal bleeding (Westaby et al., 1986).

Sclerotherapy while the oesophageal varices are actively bleeding can be very difficult, with poor visibility, a shocked patient and the possibility of pulmonary aspiration of blood. Most endoscopists have therefore sought to stop the bleeding with vasoconstrictor therapy or balloon tamponade before attempting sclerotherapy. There have, however, been two controlled trials to compare sclerotherapy with a Sengstaken–Blakemore tube tamponade in controlling acute variceal haemorrhage. In the first of these, Barsoum et al. (1982) were able to control the acute bleeding episode in 74% by sclerotherapy and in only 42% by balloon tamponade, a significant difference.

In another study from Germany, active bleeding was controlled in 19 out of 21 patients with sclerotherapy but in only 12 out of 22 patients by tamponade (Paquet and Feussner, 1985). However, there was an improvement in mortality only in the latter trial. A trial from King's College Hospital compared immediate injection sclerotherapy (intravariceal 5% ethanolamine) with a combination of vasopressin and nitroglycerin in 64 episodes of variceal bleeding in 50 patients actively bleeding at endoscopy. The end point was control of bleeding over twelve hours, assessed by repeat endoscopy or naso-gastric tube aspiration. Bleeding occurred in only 12% at twelve hours in the 33 episodes treated by sclerotherapy, compared to 35% of the 31 episodes treated by drugs (p is less than 0.05). Recurrence of bleeding was observed in 31%

of patients in both trial groups during the same admission. Deaths per admission were 27% in the sclerotherapy group versus 39% in the drugs group, with more deaths attributed to bleeding in the drugs group (Westaby *et al.*, 1989).

All three of these studies support the use of sclerotherapy as the initial treatment of variceal bleeding, but we would prefer to perform sclerotherapy, not an easy procedure in the best of conditions, with as little blood as possible obscuring the varices.

A number of other small trials of sclerotherapy have been published and almost all have confirmed that it is more effective than medical treatment alone, whether the injections were paravariceal or intravariceal. For the actively bleeding patient, however, who still has large varices, and fails to respond to tamponade, vasopressin or sclerotherapy, anastomotic gun transection of the oesophagus may be life-saving (Johnston, 1982). In a comparison of sclerotherapy with transection, there were similar death rates (Huizinga *et al.*, 1985), rebleeding being the major cause of mortality in the sclerotherapy group and liver failure in the surgical group. Varices do reappear after transection, however, the risk increasing with time and endoscopic follow-up is essential. One patient of ours was found at operation to have a longitudinal ulcer involving the full thickness of the oesophageal wall following an injection of sclerosant four days earlier; the necrotic tissue was excised and the varices successfully ligated, but previous sclerotherapy can make transection more difficult.

Cirrhotic patients with bad liver function should not be allowed to have more than one large bleed while undergoing a course of sclerotherapy. Hepatic decompensation, with coma and aspiration pneumonia, may follow haemorrhage, and coagulation problems can follow multiple blood transfusions. For patients like this, oesophageal transection should be considered rather than persisting with sclerotherapy.

A recent small controlled trial compared intravariceal sclerotherapy with portacaval shunting in a group of patients with bleeding varices and Child's grade C cirrhosis. The duration of initial hospitalization and the total amount of blood transfused was slightly less in the patients receiving sclerotherapy, but there was no difference in short-term survival and rebleeding after discharge was commoner in the sclerotherapy group, but in none of them had the varices been obliterated by the time of discharge, and even with outpatient treatment there was variceal persistence in seven of the survivors (Cello *et al.*, 1987).

Because of the high incidence of encephalopathy after portacaval shunting, Rueff and his colleagues (1976) concluded that shunting could no longer be considered suitable treatment for cirrhotic patients with gastrointestinal bleeding. The distal splenorenal shunt (Warren, Zeppa and Fomon, 1967) preserves portal variceal flow, and was originally thought to lead to a reduced incidence of encephalopathy and hepatic failure (Warren *et al.*, 1974). However, in a comparison with sclerotherapy, the distal shunt was found to lead to a lower survival rate, poorer liver function (Warren *et al.*, 1986) and to more encephalopathy (Teres *et al.*, 1986).

13.11 INTRAVARICEAL OR PARAVARICEAL INJECTION

While most British endoscopists try to inject the sclerosant directly into the varix, some European workers have preferred injection into the lamina propria and submucosa along the varix, producing submucosal oedema which will stop bleeding and eventually bury the varix in a protective fibrous coat (Wodak, 1960).

In a comparison of intravariceal with paravariceal sclerotherapy, Rose, Crane and Smith (1983) found that intravariceal injection thrombosed eight out of ten varices and gave rise to no complications, whereas paravariceal injection thrombosed only three out of ten

varices, was significantly less successful
($P<0.05$), and produced an ulcer in one
patient and dysphagia in another. These
results were confirmed in a larger Indian trial,
in which the intravariceal route was more
effective in controlling active bleeding (91%
versus 19%), faster at obliterating varices (15
versus 27 weeks), yet requiring fewer treatment sessions to achieve obliteration (5.1 versus 8.3) (Sarin *et al.*, 1987). Apart from retrosternal pain, which occurred significantly more
often with the paravariceal technique, there
was no difference in the incidence of
complications.

Whatever method is used, most patients
probably end up with a combination of intra-
and para-variceal injections, particularly in
the early stages when haemorrhage may
obscure the varix, and later when the varix
becomes small. Using a mixture of urografin
and sclerosant, 18% of intended intravariceal
injections into large varices were paravariceal,
and 38% of injections into small varices (Rose,
Crane and Smith, 1983). In an American
study, 44% of attempted intravariceal injections resulted in paravariceal extravasation of
contrast (Grobe *et al.*, 1984). It has also been
estimated that 10–15% of paravariceal injections are intravariceal (Conn and Grace, 1985).
Techniques have therefore been devised to
increase the chance of intravariceal injection,
in which various markers are added to the
sclerosant. These include the use of a radiological contrast and X-ray screening (Rose,
Crane and Smith, 1983), fluorescein (Hine *et
al.*, 1984) and methylene blue (Korula *et al.*,
1985).

Large varices require more treatments than
small varices (Rose, Crane and Smith, 1983),
about four to six injections per varix over a 1-
to 3-month period being required for obliteration. Compression devices, such as the
Williams tube (Westaby *et al.*, 1982) or
balloons above (Scott Brookes, 1980) or below
(Lewis, Chung and Allison, 1980), do not give
better results than simple sclerotherapy
(Smith, Jones and Rose, 1982).

13.12 LONG-TERM FOLLOW-UP

Westaby and Williams (1984) followed up 162
patients whose varices had been obliterated
by sclerotherapy. New varices developed in
99, but in only 28 did they bleed, causing three
deaths. Three-quarters of all recurrences took
place in the first year, and required only two
courses of sclerotherapy for obliteration to be
completed. Similar results were obtained in
Cardiff, where 50 patients were followed up
for up to 2 years after eradication of varices
(Rose and Smith, 1984). Varices recurred in 20,
17 of them appearing within the first year.
Only three patients suffered a variceal bleed.
During the period of follow-up, 13 patients
(26%) died, seven from hepatic failure, three
from infection, two from non-variceal bleeding and one from a hepatoma. Continuing
deaths from underlying liver disease were
also recorded at King's College Hospital, 11
patients dying of liver failure and five from a
hepatocellular carcinoma as opposed to only
three from variceal bleeding.

Based on these results, patients should be
followed up after variceal obliteration at 3-
monthly intervals for the first year, at 6-
monthly intervals for the second year and, if
no recurrences have been found, annually
thereafter.

13.13 PROPHYLACTIC SCLEROTHERAPY

Should patients with large varices that have
never bled be treated? Three German trials
have been published, but the answer is still
not clear. Paquet (1982) found that during 3
years of follow-up 29 (8%) of the control
patients had a variceal bleed and 21 died,
whereas after sclerotherapy only three (9%)
patients bled and only six died. A second trial
(Witzel, Wolbergs and Merki, 1985) has also
supported the use of sclerotherapy, but both
these trials are characterized by a higher rate
of variceal bleeding in the control group than
would be expected for British alcoholic cirrhotics. A third control trial (Koch *et al.*, 1986) has
failed to show a decline in mortality with

prophylactic sclerotherapy, 33% of the control group and 37% of the treated group dying over a mean follow-up period of 3 years. The most frequent cause of death was variceal bleeding in the control group and liver failure in the treated group. Three patients had a sclerotherapy-induced ulcer leading to haemorrhage requiring transfusion, three had an oesophageal stricture and one each developed an empyema and pleural effusion.

Three further controlled trials of prophylactic sclerotherapy have been published recently. Neither Sauerbruch (Sauerbruch *et al.*, 1988) or Santangelo (Santangelo *et al.*, 1988) were able to show any improvement in variceal haemorrhage or survival. The large Veterans Administration Cooperative Study (Gregory *et al.*, 1987), including 282 male alcoholics, showed both a significantly higher frequency of first haemorrhage and mortality rate in those treated by prophylactic sclerotherapy. The trial was terminated because of the excess mortality in the sclerotherapy group.

Prophylactic sclerotherapy is probably only justified for large varices in controlled clinical trials until the picture becomes clearer (Terblanche, 1986). For small varices the risk of haemorrhage is slight, the chance of extravasation of sclerosant is fairly high and they should therefore be left alone.

13.14 SUMMARY

Injection sclerotherapy is at present the best available treatment for bleeding varices. It does not require general anaesthesia and does not lead to encephalopathy, unlike the portacaval shunt. Controlled trials have demonstrated that the technique significantly reduces the risk of variceal bleeding, and once the varices have gone, reduces the mortality rate. In the first few weeks, however, while the varices remain large, the rebleeding risk remains high, and oesophageal transection with the anastomotic gun may be life saving if an uncontrollable haemorrhage occurs.

After obliteration, varices can recur, and follow-up sclerotherapy is necessary. In addition, there is a significant death rate from liver failure and hepatoma and continuing treatment of the underlying liver disease will be necessary.

Injection sclerotherapy is sometimes difficult, and should not be attempted by the inexperienced endoscopist. Complications are common, but can be reduced by using small volumes of sclerosant and the intravariceal, rather than the paravariceal, route.

REFERENCES

Barsoum, M. S., Boulas, F. I., El-Rooby, A. A. *et al.* (1982) Tamponade and injection sclerotherapy in the management of bleeding oesophageal varices. *Br. J. Surg.*, **69**, 76–8.

Carr-Locke, D. L. and Sidky, K. (1982) Broncho-oesophageal fistula: a late complication of endoscopic variceal sclerotherapy. *Gut*, **23**, 1005–7.

Cello, J. P., Grendell, J. H., Crass, R. A. *et al.* (1987) Endoscopic sclerotherapy versus portacaval shunt in patients with severe cirrhosis and acute variceal hemorrhage. *N. Engl. J. Med.*, **316**, 11–5.

Conn, H. O. and Grace, N. D. (1985) Portal hypertension and sclerotherapy of esophageal varices. A point of view. *Endosc. Rev.*, **2**, 39–53.

The Copenhagen Oesophageal Varices Sclerotherapy Project (1984) Sclerotherapy after first variceal hemorrhage in cirrhosis. *N. Engl. J. Med.*, **311**, 1594–600.

Crafoord, C. and Frenckner, P. (1939) New surgical treatment of varicose veins of the oesophagus. *Acta Otolaryngol. (Stockh.)*, **27**, 422–9.

Gregory, P., Hartigan, P., Amodeo, D. *et al.* (1987) Prophylactic sclerotherapy for esophageal varices in alcoholic liver disease: results of a VA cooperative randomized trial. *Gastroenterology*, **92**, 1414.

Grobe, J. L., Kozarek, R. A., Sanowski, R. A. *et al.* (1984) Venography during endoscopic injection sclerotherapy of esophageal varices. *Gastrointest. Endosc.*, **30**, 6–8.

Helpap, B. and Bollweg, L. (1981) Morphological changes in the terminal esophagus with varices, following sclerosis of the wall. *Endoscopy*, **13**, 229–33.

Hine, K. R., Morris, D., Toghill, P. and Dykes, P. W. (1984) Fluorescin mixed with sclerosant improves the accuracy of endoscopic injection of oesophageal varices. *Lancet*, **ii**, 322–3.

Hosking, S. W. and Johnson, A. G. (1988) Gastric varices: a proposed classification leading to management. *Br. J. Surg.*, **75**, 195–6.

Huizinga, W. K. J., Angorn, I. B. and Baker, L. W. (1985) Esophageal transection versus injection sclerotherapy in the management of bleeding esophageal varices in patients at high risk. *Surg. Gynecol. Obstet.*, **160**, 539–46.

The Italian Liver Cirrhosis Project (1987) Reliability of endoscopy in the assessment of variceal features. *J. Hepatol.*, **4**, 93–8.

Jensen, D. M., Machicado, G. A. and Silpa, M. (1986) Esophageal varix hemorrhage and sclerotherapy – animal studies. *Endoscopy*, **18**, suppl. 2, 18–22.

Johnston, G. W. (1982) Six years experience of oesophageal transection for oesophageal varices using a circular stapling gun. *Gut*, **23**, 770–3.

Johnston, G. W. and Rodgers, H. W. (1983) A review of 15 years' experience in the use of sclerotherapy in the control of acute haemorrhage for oesophageal varices. *Br. J. Surg.*, **60**, 797–800.

Kahn, D., Jones, B., Bornman, P. C. and Terblanche, J. (1989) Incidence and management of complications after injection sclerotherapy. A ten-year evaluation. *Surgery*, **105**, 160–5.

Koch, H., Henning, H., Grimm, H. and Soehendra, N. (1986) Prophylactic sclerosing of esophageal varices – results of a prospective controlled study. *Endoscopy*, **18**, 40–3.

Korula, J., Balart, L. A., Radvan, G. *et al.* (1985) A prospective randomized controlled trial of chronic esophageal variceal sclerotherapy. *Hepatology*, **5**, 584–9.

Lebrec, D., De Fleury, P., Rueff, B. *et al.* (1980) Portal hypertension, size of esophageal varices and risk of gastrointestinal bleeding in alcoholic cirrhosis. *Gastroenterology*, **179**, 1139–44.

Lewis, J., Chung, R. S. and Allison, J. (1980) Sclerotherapy of esophageal varices. *Arch. Surg.*, **115**, 476–80.

McCormack, T. T., Rose, J. D., Smith, P. M. and Johnson, A. G. (1983) Perforating veins and blood flow in oesophageal varices. *Lancet*, **ii**, 1442–4.

McCormack, T. T., Sims, J., Eyre Brook, J. *et al.* (1985) Gastric lesions in portal hypertension: inflammatory gastritis or congestive gastropathy. *Gut*, **26**, 1226–32.

Monroe, P., Morrow, C. F., Millen, J. E. *et al.* (1983) Acute respiratory failure after sodium morrhuate and esophageal sclerotherapy. *Gastroenterology*, **85**, 693–9.

Paquet, K. J. (1982) Prophylactic endoscopic treatment of the eosophageal wall in varices –

a prospective controlled randomised trial. *Endoscopy*, **14**, 4–5.

Paquet, K. J. and Feussner, H. (1985) Endoscopic sclerosis and esophageal tamponade in acute hemorrhage from esophago-gastric varices. A prospective controlled randomized trial. *Hepatology*, **5**, 580–3.

Rose, J. D. R., Crane, M. D. and Smith, P. M. (1983) Factors affecting successful endoscopic sclerotherapy for oesophageal varices. *Gut*, **24**, 946–9.

Rose, J. D. R. and Smith, P. M. (1984) Factors affecting variceal recurrence after endoscopic sclerotherapy. *Gut*, **25**, A577.

Rueff, B., Pandi, D. and Degos, F. (1976) A controlled study of therapeutic portacaval shunt in alcoholic cirrhosis. *Lancet*, **i**, 655–9.

Santangelo, W. C., Dueno, M. I., Estes, B. L. and Frejs, G. J. (1988) Prophylactic sclerotherapy of large esophageal varices. *New Engl. J. Med.*, **318**, 814–8.

Sarin, S. K., Nanda, R., Sachdev, G. *et al.* (1987) Intravariceal versus paravariceal sclerotherapy. A prospective, controlled, randomised trial. *Gut*, **28**, 657–62.

Sauerbruch, T., Wotzka, R., Kopeke, W. *et al.* (1988) Prophylactic sclerotherapy before the first episode of variceal hemorrhage in patients with cirrhosis. *New Engl. J. Med.*, **319**, 8–15.

Schuman, B. M., Beckman, J. W., Tedesco, F. J. *et al.* (1987) Complications of endoscope injection sclerotherapy; a review. *Am. J. Gastroenterol.*, **82**, 823–9.

Scott Brookes, W. (1980) Adapting flexible endoscopes for sclerosis of oesophageal varices. *Lancet*, **i**, 266.

Smith, P. M., Jones, D. B. and Rose, J. D. R. (1982) Simplified fibre endoscopic sclerotherapy for oesophageal varices. *J. R. Coll. Physicians Lond.*, **16**, 235–6.

Soderlund, C. and Ihre, T. (1985) Endoscopic sclerotherapy versus conservative management of bleeding oesophageal varices. A 5-year prospective controlled trial of emergency and long term treatment. *Acta Chir. Scand.*, **151**, 449–56.

Terblanche, J. (1986) Sclerotherapy for prophylaxis of variceal bleeding. *Lancet*, **i**, 961–3.

Terblanche, J., Bornman, P. C., Kahn, D. *et al.* (1983) Failure of repeated injection sclerotherapy to improve long term survival after oesophageal variceal bleeding. A five year prospective controlled trial. *Lancet*, **ii**, 1328–32.

Terblanche, J., Northover, J. M. A., Bornman, P. *et al.* (1979) A prospective controlled trial of sclerotherapy in the long term management of patients

150   Oesophageal variceal obliteration

after esophageal variceal bleeding. *Surg. Gynecol. Obstet.*, **148**, 323–33.

Teres, J., Bordas, J. M., Bravo, M.D. *et al.* (1986) Endoscopic sclerotherapy vs distal splenorenal shunt in the elective treatment of variceal haemorrhage. A randomized controlled trial. *J. Hepatol.* **3**, suppl. 1, 525.

Trudeau, W. and Prindiville, T. (1986) Endoscopic injection sclerosis in bleeding gastric varices. *Gastrointest. Endosc.*, **32**, 364–8.

Warren, W. D., Galambos, J. T., Riepe, S. P. *et al.* (1986) Distal splenorenal shunt versus endoscopic sclerotherapy for long term management of variceal bleeding. Preliminary report of a prospective randomized trial. *Ann. Surg.*, **203**, 454–63.

Warren, W. D., Salam, A. A., Hutson, D. and Zeppa, R. (1974) Selective distal spleno renal shunt. Technique and results of operation. *Arch. Surg.*, **108**, 306–14.

Warren, W. D., Zeppa, R. and Fomon, J. J. (1967) Selective transplenic decompression of gastroesophageal varices by distal splenorenal shunt. *Ann. Surg.*, **166**, 437–55.

Westaby, D., Melia, W., Hegarty, J. *et al.* (1986) Use of propranolol to reduce the rebleeding rate during injection sclerotherapy prior to variceal obliteration. *Hepatology*, **6**, 673–5.

Westaby, D., Melia, W. M., Macdougall, B. R. D. *et al.* (1984) Injection sclerotherapy for oesophageal varices: a prospective randomized trial of different treatment schedules. *Gut*, **25**, 129–32.

Westaby, D. and Williams, R. (1984) Follow up study after sclerotherapy. *Scand. J. Gastroenterol.*, **19**, suppl. 102, 71–5.

Westaby, D., Macdougall, B. R. D. and Williams, R. (1985) Improved survival following injection sclerotherapy for oesophageal varices: final analysis of a controlled trial. *Hepatology*, **5**, 827–30.

Westaby, D., Hayes, P. C., Gimson, A. E. S. *et al.* (1989) Controlled clinical trial of injection sclerotherapy for active variceal bleeding. *Hepatology*, **9**, 274–7.

Wodak, E. (1960) Osophagusvarizen-bluting bei portaler Hypertension: Therapie und Prophylaxe. *Wien. Med. Wochenschr.*, **110**, 581–3.

Williams, K. G. D. and Dawson, J. L. (1979) Fibreoptic injection of oesophageal varices. *Br. Med. J.*, **2**, 766–7.

Williams, S. W. and Dawson, J. L. (1988) Gastric varices: a proposed fibreoptic injection of oesophageal varices. *Br. Med. J.*, **2**, 766–7.

Witzel, L., Wolbergs, E. and Merki, H. (1985) Prophylactic endoscopic sclerotherapy of oesophageal varices. A prospective controlled trial. *Lancet*, **i**, 733–75.

CHAPTER FOURTEEN

Gastroduodenal haemorrhage: endoscopic diathermy with the BICAP and the heater probe

G. Jiranek, S. English, D. Jensen, D. Auth
and
F. Silverstein

Bleeding from the upper gastrointestinal tract continues to be a significant problem. The incidence of hospital admissions for bleeding is between 50 and 150 per year per 100 000 population. Studies by Allan and Dykes (1976) and Silverstein *et al.* (1981a) have shown that mortality from upper gastrointestinal bleeding has remained at approximately 10% for the past 40 years despite advances in acute care. As noted by Eastwood (1977) and Peterson *et al.* (1981), the advance of diagnostic endoscopy by itself has not been shown to improve the outcome of bleeding patients. Recent trials in the 1980s however have demonstrated that therapeutic interventional endoscopy in selected patients with non-variceal upper gastrointestinal bleeding can improve outcome. This chapter will present the principles, the clinical trials and the techniques pertinent to the bipolar electrocoagulation and the heater probes.

14.1 PRINCIPLES OF ENDOSCOPIC DIATHERMY

There are pharmacological, angiographic, surgical and endoscopic approaches to control upper gastrointestinal bleeding. Although pharmacological therapy might seem to be rational, it has not been proved in controlled clinical trials to reduce further bleeding. The pharmacological approaches studied include H_2 blockers, antacids, sucralfate, vasoconstrictors, prostaglandins and other hormones. Angiographic and surgical therapy are presented in Chapter 16.

Endoscopic therapy was first reported by Youmans *et al.* (1970). Our group and others have investigated a variety of endoscopic haemostatic approaches. Fleischer (1986) has written an excellent review. The most promising techniques include mechanical and thermal methods to achieve haemostasis. Mechanical methods include topical sprays, clips and injections. Injections with vasoconstrictors, alcohol or sclerosing agents have been reported by Soehendra (1984) and Sugawa *et al.* (1984) to have excellent haemostasis and safety. This inexpensive technique was shown by Panes (1987) and Leung *et al.* (1987) in controlled clinical trials to improve outcome with acceptable safety. Injection therapy is covered in detail in Chapter 15.

The most widely investigated approach to endoscopic haemostasis involves the delivery of heat. There are several questions to consider about thermal coagulation. These include: what minimal temperature is necessary to achieve a haemostatic bond; is there a maximum safe temperature; what role does blood flow have as a heat sump; is washing the tissue required; how can these requirements best be achieved; and what is the most cost-effective approach?

Increasing tissue temperature to 42°C causes selective death of cells. At 47°C all cells are killed. At 57°C protein is denatured. At 80°C collagen shrinks. At 250°C carbonization occurs and at 800°C vaporization occurs. It appears that heating a blood vessel to between 100°C and 250°C is associated with a maximal haemostatic bond. Temperatures in excess of this can cause ablation of tissue, resulting in extensive tissue destruction without adding to the strength of the bond. Such destruction could lead to deeper ulcers and to weakening or perforation of the gut wall.

The heat sump caused by blood flowing through vessels can remove heat from the area of coagulation to make a seal more difficult to achieve. Sigel and Dunn (1965) demonstrated that the strength of a vascular thermal bond was increased if the vessel was mechanically closed with a clamp during heating. This increase in strength results from a reduced heat sump effect and placement of the intima of the opposing vessels in physical contact with one another, thereby facilitating the coagulated seal. Closing the vessel during heating is called coaptation.

It is essential to wash the tissue with a stream of gas or water for good vision. If the bleeding point is obscured by blood, therapy is difficult. Further, coaptation can be verified before heating a bleeding point by irrigation to demonstrate cessation of bleeding which implies mechanical compression of the target blood vessel. Heating is more likely to succeed under these circumstances.

Tissue can be heated endoscopically by thermal conversion of electrical energy in the optical frequency (lasers), radiofrequency (electrocautery) or very low frequency (heater probe). The lasers used for photocoagulation include the CO_2 laser, argon ion laser and the Nd–YAG laser. Swain et al. (1986) has shown the Nd–YAG laser to be effective in reducing further bleeding with an acceptable complication rate (Chapter 12). However, lasers have several disadvantages. First, they are costly; equipment starts at US $100 000 (£60 000). Second, most lasers are not portable. This prohibits their use in patients who are too unstable to transport. The lasers generally cannot be used in several locations in one hospital or be moved to other hospitals. Laser installation may be difficult and many hospitals require a special laser room with safeguards against injury to the staff or patient caused by laser failure or stray radiation. Third, traditional lasers do not permit coaptation. There are now contact laser probes but they have not yet been thoroughly tested. Finally, in theory lasers can cause unpredictably deep tissue injury with an increased risk of perforation. Lasers can heat tissue up to and above 1000°C. At this temperature tissue is vaporized. Further, with the Nd–YAG laser, the light intensity persists at about 30% of its surface value at a tissue depth of 2 mm. It persists at about 10% of its surface value at a depth of 4 mm. This implies some penetration of deep heating at depths greater than 4 mm. These disadvantages provided the impetus to develop an equally effective mode of thermal coagulation which is less costly, portable, easy to use, coaptive and safe.

Electrocoagulation can be achieved with monopolar or bipolar systems. The monopolar system can use dry electrodes or a wet electrode with the electrohydrothermal modification of Fruhmorgen and Matek (1986). Sparking can occur with temperatures up to and above 1000°C and the relatively deep penetration of heat into tissue is similar to laser. This can result in unpredictably deep injury into the wall and reports of haemostatic efficacy vary. A European survey revealed five perforations occurring in 314 patients treated with monopolar coagulation. However, Papp (1982) reports excellent efficacy and safety in a small trial. Others have sought better methods to apply electrocoagulation.

Bipolar electrocoagulation allows electric current density to concentrate on superficial aspects of the intestinal wall which produces thermal coagulation with a more acceptable and controllable depth of injury. The BICAP is a bipolar device with three sets of stripe electrodes arranged in a radial pattern around the tip to allow it to work whether it faces the target end-on or tangentially.

An alternative method of coagulation is that of direct heating. A heater probe (Protell, Silverstein and Auth, 1978) converts electrical energy into thermal energy at the probe tip which can be pressed against the tissue to coagulate the bleeding vessel. A non-adherent surface reduces sticking of the device to the coagulum.

The BICAP and heater probes have many favourable characteristics. They are both relatively inexpensive. The cost of US $6000 (£4000) is much less than the laser. These devices are fully portable and can be taken to the patient's bedside. No special installation is required; the devices plug into a standard wall electric socket. No special safeguards are needed for the staff or patient other than attention to the local effects of the probe on tissue. No endoscopic modifications are needed other than an endoscope with a standard size accessory channel. Both devices have wash systems and have the ability for coaptive coagulation. Finally, the BICAP and heater probes have much shallower penetrations of heat into tissue when the surface is heated to 100°C or higher when compared with laser and monopolar therapy. In an animal experimental model of bleeding ulcer reviewed by Johnston (1987), bipolar and heater probes consistently produced less frequent deep injury than monopolar or laser coagulation.

14.2 CLINICAL TRIALS

14.2.1 BIPOLAR ELECTROCOAGULATION

Uncontrolled trials have been reported by Gilbert *et al.* (1982), Winkler *et al.* (1983), Jessen (1983), Hajiro *et al.* (1984) and Jensen *et al.* (1986) using bipolar coagulation (usually BICAP) for gastroduodenal endoscopic haemostasis. The lesions were either actively bleeding or had stigmata of recent bleeding and included ulcers, Mallory–Weiss tears, vascular malformations, oesophagitis, gastritis, duodenitis and neoplasms. In general, active bleeding was stopped in 81% to 100% of cases but rebleeding occurred from 0% to 29% (typically 25%) in those where initial haemostasis was effective. There were no reported deaths or perforations related to therapy but occasionally (0–9%) brisk haemorrhage occurred during probe application to non-bleeding visible vessels.

These generally favourable reports encouraged controlled trials. Two small randomized controlled trials did not show beneficial effects from BICAP therapy. Goudie (1984) randomized 46 patients with solitary peptic ulcers with stigmata of recent bleeding. There was no difference in the rate of rebleeding, rate of surgery or rate of transfusion. There were no deaths or perforations in either group. One patient developed massive bleeding during treatment to a visible vessel. The control group had a rebleeding rate of only 20% and a surgical rate of only 8% – it would take a very large trial to show statistically significant reductions in these two rates. Kernohan *et al.* (1984) randomized 45 patients with peptic ulcers or erosions with active bleeding or stigmata of recent bleeding. No difference in the rates of rebleeding, surgery or transfusion requirements were noted. In this study the probe was applied circumferentially rather than directly to the lesion. This circumferential application was incomplete in 50% of the treated patients. In addition, the control group had a rebleeding rate of only 29%. No complications resulted from therapy in this study.

A third more recent controlled trial reported by Laine (1987) randomized 44 patients with active upper gastrointestinal haemorrhage from an ulcer, a Mallory–Weiss tear or a vascular malformation. The group treated with the BICAP had significantly better haemostasis (90% versus 13%, $P < 0.0001$), less emergency surgery (14% versus 57%, $P = 0.01$), fewer units of blood transfused (2.4 versus 5.4, $P = 0.002$) and fewer hospital days (4.4 versus 7.24, $P = 0.02$) than controls. The inpatient death rate was lower but not statistically significant for the BICAP group (0%) compared with controls (13%). No complications of endoscopy or electrocoagulation therapy were observed.

O'Brien et al. (1986) has reported a large trial which randomized 204 patients with peptic ulcer bleeding that was either active, had a visible vessel or adherent clot to BICAP or sham therapy. The BICAP was applied directly to the point of the lesion with a power setting of 7 with 2-second impulses. The outcome is seen in Table 14.1. Continued or recurrent bleeding was determined by a clinician who did not know if the probe had been used. The BICAP decreased further bleeding in patients with ulcers with visible vessels whether bleeding was active or not.

Table 14.1 BICAP coagulation of bleeding peptic ulcers

	Clinically significant further bleeding			
	BICAP		Control	
	No.	%	No.	%
Visible vessel				
Bleeding	6/40	15	13/21	62*
Not bleeding	7/43	16	16/43	37*
Adherent clot	4/18	22	5/39	12

*$P<0.05$
From O'Brien et al. (1986) with permission: 204 patients.

There was no benefit in treating ulcers that contained clot without an identifiable vessel. Active bleeding was sometimes induced by the probe when treating adherent clots. There were no significant differences in the need for surgery (7/101 treated versus 10/103 untreated) or death associated with bleeding (9/101 treated versus 12/103 untreated). No perforation or death related to the procedure was reported.

Brearley et al. (1987) conducted a randomized controlled trial of 41 patients with peptic ulcers with non-bleeding visible vessels. BICAP therapy did not reduce the rebleeding rate, the need for surgery or the death rate. One patient had a perforation after probe therapy which resolved uneventfully with non-surgical conservative therapy. The perforation may have been due to excessive air insufflation during the difficult endoscopy.

Different results were reported by Laine (1988) in a randomized controlled trial of the BICAP in 74 patients who had non-bleeding visible vessels in peptic ulcers. The BICAP-treated group had significantly less rebleeding (19% versus 54%) and less surgery (8% versus 30), but seven of 37 patients treated with the BICAP developed bleeding during probe application; in one instance, the bleeding required surgical control. No perforation was noted.

14.2.2 HEATER PROBE

The heater probe was developed with three possible advantages over the BICAP probe. First, maximal heating is increased from 100°C to 250°C, which may increase the strength of coagulative bonding of tissue. Second, irrigation proximal to the probe tip allows effective washing during probe apposition. Third, the probe tip tends to stick less to coagulated tissue after coaptive treatment. Most of the published clinical assessment on the heater probe has been in uncontrolled trials.

Storey (1983) applied the heater probe to peptic ulcer patients who were candidates for immediate operative intervention because of severe bleeding or rebleeding. Of 15 patients with a gastric ulcer, one required immediate surgery and one required subsequent surgery to arrest haemorrhage. The other 13 treated patients avoided surgery. However, eight of ten patients with a bleeding duodenal ulcer required an operation. The author attributed the poor result in the duodenum to difficult access with the probe in several cases.

Shorvon et al. (1985) reported an uncontrolled retrospective study using the heater probe to stop peptic ulcer haemorrhage in a group of patients considered to be a poor operative risk. Fifteen of the 16 patients selected had been resuscitated from clinical shock. All six patients with gastric ulcer (four active, one visible vessel, one adherent clot) had no rebleeding after treatment. Ten patients with duodenal ulcer were selected for treatment. However, in four patients the probe was not applied because the lesion was not accessible. The six patients who were treated did well: only one rebled 12 days later. This rebleeding was stopped with a second application of the heater probe.

Jensen et al. (1986) retrospectively assessed their experience with the heater probe in severe ulcer bleeding. Initial haemostasis was achieved in 16 out of 17 patients with active arterial bleeding with probe application. Bleeding was precipitated in one of seven patients who had a non-bleeding visible vessel. Overall, four episodes of rebleeding occurred in the 24 patients.

The largest, published, uncontrolled experience with the heater probe is that of Johnston (1985). Table 14.2 summarizes the results of 74 patients with bleeding peptic ulcers. Most of the patients were aged over 60, had significant concomitant medical disease, and had hypotension. The mean transfusion requirement was 6.8 units before therapy. Bleeding was pumping in 21, oozing in 11 and was inactive with a visible vessel in 42. There were no perforations but arterial bleeding was induced in seven of 53 lesions that were

Table 14.2 Heater probe treatment of bleeding peptic ulcers: consecutive series

	No.	%
Initial haemostasis	72/74	97
Rebleeding	13/72	18
Haemostasis with repeat application	10/12	83
Ultimate haemostasis	69/74	93
Emergency surgery	5/74	7
Induced arterial bleeding	7/53	13
Deaths due to bleeding	1/74	1

From Johnston et al. (1985) with permission: 74 patients.

not pumping before therapy. In six of these further probe application controlled the bleeding. Only one death in the entire group was attributed to bleeding. There were no perforations or deaths related to heater probe coagulation.

The first controlled trial comparing the heater probe with sham treatment was reported by Fullarton et al. (1988). Forty-three patients with peptic ulcer and major stigmata of bleeding were entered. No patient who was treated with the heater probe had further bleeding, surgery or death. Reduction in further bleeding attained statistical significance when compared with the 'placebo' group, and no complication was reported with the heater probe.

14.2.3 COMPARISON OF TECHNIQUES

There have been five randomized trials comparing bipolar electrocoagulation or the heater probe with alternative endoscopic haemostatic techniques. Goff (1986) randomized 19 patients with various upper gastrointestinal bleeding lesions to BICAP versus Nd–YAG laser coagulation. Rebleeding and surgical intervention rates were similar, although physicians were not blinded to the type and details of coagulation when assessing rebleeding and the need for surgery.

Rutgeerts et al. (1987) randomized 100 patients with peptic ulcers which were actively

Table 14.3 Bleeding peptic ulcers: Nd–YAG versus BICAP: randomized controlled trial

	Nd–YAG %	BICAP %
Further bleeding	12	14
Emergency surgery	12	6
Mortality	14	14

From Rutgeerts *et al.* (1987) with permission: 100 patients.

bleeding or had a visible vessel to BICAP versus Nd–YAG laser. All ulcers were injected with adrenaline (epinephrine) before thermal coagulation. The groups were similar with regard to the following factors: age, sex, ratio of gastric to duodenal ulcers, pretreatment blood requirements and activity of bleeding or presence of stigmata. The results are shown in Table 14.3. These authors concluded that the devices were equally effective. In the BICAP-treated group one patient with a prepyloric ulcer sustained a perforation 4 days after therapy. Matthewson *et al.* (1988) reported a trial between the Nd–YAG laser, the BICAP and placebo in 143 patients with peptic ulcers with stigmata of recent bleeding. The rebleeding rate and the surgical rate appeared to favour the laser over the BICAP and placebo but in the randomized portion of the study the results fell short of statistical significance.

Jensen *et al.* (1988) are conducting a large, controlled, randomized, blinded, multicentre trial to compare routine medical care, BICAP coagulation, and heater probe coagulation in ulcer patients with active bleeding or non-bleeding visible vessels. Table 14.4 shows the interim results in this continuing trial. The heater probe has been associated with significantly less rebleeding and surgery. No complication with either probe was reported.

Lin *et al.* (1988) have reported a randomized comparison between the heater probe and alcohol injection therapy in 78 patients with peptic ulcers with signs of bleeding or a non-bleeding visible vessel. The heater probe produced statistically better haemostasis overall, and in the subgroup with spurting arterial haemorrhage.

14.2.4 SUMMARY

The controlled trials have been important in emphasizing the natural history of untreated patients who have gastroduodenal haemorrhage. The majority who have recently bled from non-variceal sources in the upper gastrointestinal tract do not have active bleeding at the time of endoscopy. Endoscopy often reveals ulcers which do not have stigmata of recent or active haemorrhage, or have only flat black spots in their bases. These patients have been shown repeatedly to have a low chance of further bleeding. These patients would be unlikely to benefit from prophylactic endoscopic coagulation therapy. The primary goal of thermal coagulation is to stop active bleeding and to prevent rebleeding. If this goal is fulfilled, the need for surgery, the transfusion requirement, the length of hospital stay and mortality should all be reduced. As shown by Bown (1985) and others, approximately 85% of active bleeding ulcers, 50% of ulcers with non-bleeding visible vessels and 10–40% of ulcers with overlying clot

Table 14.4 BICAP versus heater probe versus control groups for severe ulcer bleeding from active or visible vessel: randomized, controlled, blinded study, preliminary results

	BICAP %	Heater probe %	Control %
Continued bleeding – rebleeding	44	22*	72
Emergency ulcer surgery	33	3*	41
Deaths – 30 days	3	3	9

From Jensen and CURE Haemostasis Study Group: 94 patients.
* $P < 0.05$ versus placebo.

have significant rebleeding. These patients may benefit from thermal coagulation, but better techniques to predict the risk of rebleeding, and the likely outcome of therapeutic intervention are needed.

Three of the six controlled clinical trials demonstrate an improved outcome using BICAP coagulation in patients who have bled from gastroduodenal ulcers. The three favourable trials have had larger numbers of subjects than the three unfavourable trials. In addition, the favourable trials defined patients who had higher rates of further bleeding when not treated. The single placebo-controlled trial with the heater probe was small but promising in similar patients. Comparative trials between the BICAP and the laser have not shown a statistically different outcome. In a threeway comparison between the BICAP, the heater probe and placebo, only the heater probe significantly improved outcome compared with placebo. A single trial showed improved outcome with the heater probe compared with injection therapy with alcohol.

The BICAP and heater probes appear to have low complication rates. There has been no report of death directly related to their use. There have been only two perforations reported in over 500 patients treated with the BICAP and none with the heater probe. Rebleeding may be induced in 10–20% but in the majority this can be stopped by continued coagulation. Clinical trials show that most patients with actively bleeding peptic ulcers benefit from BICAP or heater probe application. Some patients with the following lesions may also be suitable candidates for endoscopic thermal coagulation:

Peptic ulcer with non-bleeding visible vessel.
Active bleeding from Mallory–Weiss tear.
Active bleeding from vascular malformation.
Chronic bleeding from vascular malformation unresponsive to iron therapy.

14.3 PRACTICAL GUIDELINES

14.3.1 EQUIPMENT: BICAP

When activated, the BICAP device allows electric current to flow from negative electrodes in the probe tip into tissue and return to positive electrodes in the probe tip. The need for a distant patient plate is eliminated. The depth of tissue coagulation is limited to no more than 3 mm.

The maximum power is 50 W and the maximum tissue temperature is 100°C. The coagulation dial settings regulate the power output. For example, a dial setting of 1 provides approximately 5 W, while settings of 5 and 7 provide approximately 25 and 35 W respectively. However, the power delivered to tissue is not necessarily equal to the available power output. Instead it is dependent on a functioning probe, effective probe contact to tissue, voltage, tissue resistance (a function of desiccation) and the time duration of the pulse. The coagulation time settings regulate the total amount of energy delivered. For example, a power setting of 5 with a time setting of 2 seconds will deliver a maximum of 25 W × 2 seconds or 50 W-seconds. A time setting of 'continuous' will coagulate until tissue is desiccated and electrical conductivity disappears because water is absent. This usually occurs in between 4 and 12 seconds. The generator and the system costs about US$5600 (£3500).

Two probes are currently available, and the larger one has a diameter of 3.2 mm with a tangential area of 9 mm × 3.2 mm. The smaller probe has a diameter of 2.3 mm and a tangential area of 9 mm × 2.3 mm. There are six longitudinal silver electrodes separated by ceramic insulators in the tip to permit both *en face* and tangential application. There is a central opening in the probe tip for irrigation. Therefore, simultaneous irrigation and coaptation are not possible in the *en face* position. The cost of the small and large probes is about US$185 (£115) each. Probes are readily available.

The probes should be checked for kinks or bends. These can cause decreased current flow and difficulty passing the probe through the endoscope channel. A second set of probes should be checked and always available. The ability to wash should be verified by pressing WASH on the foot pedal and observing a strong jet from the central port. The ability to coagulate should be verified by setting the power dial to 2 and the time dial to 1 second and activating the probe tip in a few drops of saline in a small dish. The saline should bubble or evaporate with a 'frying' sound.

14.3.2 EQUIPMENT: HEATER PROBE

Thermal coagulation is achieved with the heater probe by conduction of heat from the probe tip directly into tissue. The maximum energy delivery is 30 J per pulse. The maximum internal temperature is 250°C. The depth of tissue burn is limited to 3 mm. A silicon chip in the probe tip senses the heat energy delivered and stops heating when a predetermined amount of heat energy has been delivered. A continuous tone is heard when the energy is being delivered. The actual delivery time depends on the size of the contact area of the probe with tissue. Larger contact areas require less time to deliver a given energy. It usually takes 6–8 seconds to deliver 30 J and 3–4 seconds to deliver 20 J. The generator and heater probe system costs about US $6400 (£4000).

There are two heater probes available. The larger one has a diameter of 3.2 mm while the smaller probe has a diameter of 2.4 mm. The heat source (silicon chip) is inside a metal cylinder which has high thermal conductivity. A special outer coating reduces adherence to coagulated tissue. Irrigation occurs proximal to the probe tip and allows for simultaneous irrigation and coaptation. The probe can be applied in the *en face* and tangential positions. The cost per probe is about US $300 (£200), and probes are readily available.

As with the BICAP, the probes should be checked for kinks and bends, and a second set of probes should be immediately available. The wash system should be checked to be certain it is working. The ability to coagulate should be checked by placing the probe tip into a drop of distilled water in a small dish and activating at a power of 15–20 J. A tone should sound for 2–4 seconds and the water should visibly boil.

14.3.3 PATIENT PREPARATION

Candidates for endoscopic thermal coagulation of gastroduodenal bleeding lesions should be resuscitated and stabilized using established techniques. Intravenous access must allow potentially rapid infusions of blood and fluids for volume replacement. Coagulopathies must be identified and treated as rapidly as possible. The portability of the BICAP and heater probes allows therapeutic endoscopy to be performed in the intensive care unit or operating theatre if needed. Effective sedation should be given and special attention directed to reduce the risk of aspiration. Endotracheal intubation should be considered if the patient is at particular risk of aspiration. Informed consent should be obtained before sedation from the patient or relatives.

14.3.4 SETTINGS AND TECHNIQUE

When used properly the BICAP and heater probes are used to weld tissue (i.e. the intima of the artery). This requires firm apposition of the intimal surfaces with pressure and the subsequent application of heat. This approach is similar to the familiar Bovie 'buzzing' of closed artery forceps as a surgical means of vessel closure, except that the probe pushes against the tissue instead of having two forceps arms to apply pressure. When used in this way with adequate heat delivery the result is a thermal 'ligature'. Some researchers have demonstrated anastomosis of blood vessels using only heat energy without any conventional stitches. The BICAP probe and heater probe were designed to be applied for time intervals far exceeding those necessary for good thermal ligature without causing tissue injury beyond a depth of 3–4 mm. Therefore, it is possible to apply heavy doses of coagulation energy with these inherently safe and non-penetrating, non-erosive devices when the clinical goal is certain closure of a large artery and high probability that it will stop rebleeding. Marginal heating implies marginal welding. The highest clinical benefit to risk ratio for major arterial bleeders is usually thorough heating and welding of the target vessel intima without tissue erosion or deep heating. This is only possible with the BICAP and heater probes. Using minimal heat to accomplish threshold coagulation of bleeding arteries can lead to subsequent rebleeding because the thermal ligature was too weak. The clinician should assess in advance the likely size of the vessel being treated and select adequate energy to assure good vessel welding and resistance to rebleeding. Johnston, Jensen and Auth (1987) have recently demonstrated these principles in an animal model.

The endoscopist must understand coagulation theory and alter the specific guidelines as needed to account for the type of patient, the type and location of the lesion and operator experience. These are the guidelines we have found most useful, but they may need modifying as experience accumulates.

For gastric or duodenal ulcers which are actively bleeding or have a visible vessel the larger probes are preferred. For the BICAP with the 50-W generator the power setting is 7 with 2-second pulse. If the heater probe is selected the energy is set at 30 J. Whichever probe is chosen should be placed on the vessel (or bleeding point if active) with firm pressure. With the heater probe, washing can verify coaptation. Heat can then be delivered in a series of two or four pulses in rapid succession without changing the probe's coaptive position. With large arteries of 0.5–1.5 mm in diameter, or if active bleeding occurs when the probe is withdrawn, a further series of similar pulses should be applied. The site of coagulation should show a white-brown colour and should not bleed on gentle washing. Any protruding plug should be flattened by the thermal effect.

For Mallory–Weiss tears with active bleeding, large probes are also preferable. The setting for BICAP is a power of 7 and a 2-second pulse. With the heater probe, the energy is set at 30 J. Coagulation should be initiated after coaptation is achieved on the bleeding point. The tamponade should be firm, but not as firm as for an ulcer. Further pulses should be applied if bleeding continues when the probe is withdrawn.

For actively bleeding vascular abnormalities, small probes are used for lesions smaller than 3 mm, and large probes for lesions larger than 3 mm. For the BICAP, the power should be set at 3–5 with a 1-second pulse. With the heater probe the energy is set at 15–20 J. The focal bleeding point is identified and gentle tamponade applied with the probe. Coagulation is usually achieved with two to three pulses.

For elective treatment of non-bleeding vascular abnormalities the probe size and energy settings are identical to those described for actively bleeding ones. Coagulation should be applied with gentle contact circumferentially starting at the perimeter, and then progressing inward to coagulate the centre.

14.4 CONCLUSION

Gastroduodenal bleeding is an important problem in clinical medicine. Endoscopic diathermy with either the BICAP or the heater probe appears to be an acceptably safe and low-cost method to reduce the risk of further bleeding in selected patients. Optimal use of these devices requires the accurate identification of patients at risk of further bleeding and adequate endoscopic access.

160 BICAP and heater probe

REFERENCES

Allan, R. and Dykes, P. (1976) A study of the factors influencing mortality rates from gastrointestinal haemorrhage. *Q. J. Med.*, **180**, 533.

Bown, S. (1985) Controlled trials of laser therapy for hemorrhage from peptic ulcer. *Acta Endoscopia*, **15**, 1–12.

Brearley, S. *et al.* (1987) Per-endoscopic bipolar diathermy coagulation of visible vessel using a 3.2 mm probe – a randomized clinical trial. *Endoscopy*, **19**, 160–3.

Donahue, P. *et al.* (1984) Endoscopic control of upper gastrointestinal hemorrhage with a bipolar coagulation device. *Surg. Gynecol. Obstet.*, **159**, 113–8.

Eastwood, G. (1977) Does early endoscopy benefit the patient with active upper gastrointestinal bleeding? *Gastroenterology*, **72**, 737–9.

Fleischer, D. (1986) Endoscopic therapy of upper gastrointestinal bleeding in humans. *Gastroenterology*, **90**, 217–34.

Fruhmorgen, P. and Matek, W. (1986) Electro-hydro-thermo and bipolar probes. *Endoscopy*, **18**, suppl. 2, 62–4.

Fullarton, G. *et al.* (1988) Controlled study of heater probe (H.P.) in bleeding peptic ulcers. *Gastroenterology*, **94**, A138.

Gilbert, D. *et al.* (1981) The national ASGE survey on upper gastrointestinal bleeding III: endoscopy in upper gastrointestinal bleeding. *Gastrointest. Endosc.*, **27**, 94–103.

Gilbert, D. *et al.* (1982) A multicenter clinical trial of the BICAP probe for upper gastrointestinal bleeding. *Gastrointest. Endosc.*, **29**, 150A.

Goff, J. (1986) Bipolar electrocoagulation versus Nd–YAG laser photocoagulation for upper gastrointestinal bleeding lesions. *Dig. Dis. Sci.*, **31**, 906–10.

Goudie, B. (1984) Controlled trial of endoscopic bipolar electrocoagulation in the treatment of bleeding peptic ulcers. *Gut*, **25**, 1185A.

Hajiro, K. *et al.* (1984) Endoscopic bipolar electrocoagulation in upper gastrointestinal bleeding. *Endoscopy*, **16**, 6–9.

Jensen, D. *et al.* (1986) Bleeding UGI angioma: endoscopic coagulation and outcome. *Gastrointest. Endosc.*, **32**, 142A.

Jensen, D. *et al.* (1986) BICAP vs. heater probe for hemostasis of severe ulcer bleeding. *Gastrointest. Endosc.*, **32**, 143A.

Jensen, D. *et al.* (1988) Controlled randomized study of heater probe and BICAP for hemostasis of severe ulcer bleeding. *Gastroenterology*, **94**, A208.

Jessen, K. (1983) BICAP control of UGI bleeding. *Gastroenterology*, **21**, 68A.

Johnston, J. (1985) Endoscopic thermal treatment of upper gastrointestinal bleeding. *Endosc. Rev.*, **7/85**, 12–26.

Johnston, J. *et al.* (1985) Comparison of heater probe and YAG laser in endoscopic treatment of major bleeding from peptic ulcers. *Gastrointest. Endosc.*, **31**, 175–80.

Johnston, J., Jensen, D. and Auth, D. (1987) Experimental comparison of endoscopic YAG laser, electrosurgery, and heater probe for canine gut arterial coagulation. Importance of compression and avoidance of erosion. *Gastroenterology*, **92**, 1101–8.

Kernohan, R. *et al.* (1984) A controlled trial of bipolar electrocoagulation in patients with upper gastrointestinal bleeding. *Br. J. Surg.*, **71**, 889–91.

Laine, L. (1987) Multipolar electrocoagulation in the treatment of active upper gastrointestinal tract hemorrhage. A prospective controlled trial. *New Engl. J. Med.*, **316**, 1613–7.

Laine, L. (1988) Multipolar electrocoagulation (MPEC) for the treatment of ulcers with non-bleeding visible vessels (VV): a prospective, controlled trial. *Gastroenterology*, **94**, A246.

Leung, J. *et al.* (1987) Endoscopic injection of adrenalin in bleeding peptic ulcer. *Gastrointest. Endosc.*, **33**, 73–5.

Lin, H. *et al.* (1988) A prospectively randomized trial of heat probe thermocoagulation versus pure alcohol injection in nonvariceal peptic ulcer hemorrhage. *Am. J. Gastroenterol.*, **83**, 283–6.

Matthewson, K. *et al.* (1988) Randomized comparison of Nd–YAG laser, heater probe (HP) and no endoscopic therapy for bleeding peptic ulcer. *Gastroenterology*, **92**, A1522.

O'Brien, J. *et al.* (1986) Controlled trial of small bipolar probe in bleeding peptic ulcers. *Lancet*, **i**, 464–7.

Panes, J. (1987) Controlled trial of endoscopic sclerosis in bleeding peptic ulcers. *Lancet*, **ii**, 1292–4.

Papp, J. (1982) Endoscopic electrocoagulation in the management of upper gastrointestinal tract bleeding. *Surg. Clin. North Am.*, **62**, 5, 797–806.

Peterson, W. *et al.* (1981) Routine early endoscopy in upper gastrointestinal tract bleeding: a randomized, controlled trial. *New Engl. J. Med.*, **304**, 925–30.

Protell, R., Silverstein, F. and Auth, D. (1978) The heater probe – a new endoscopic method for stopping massive gastrointestinal bleeding. *Gastroenterology*, **74**, 257–62.

Rutgeerts, P. *et al.* (1987) Neodynium – YAG laser photocoagulation versus multipolar electrocoagulation for the treatment of severely bleeding ulcers: a randomized comparison. *Gastrointest. Endosc.*, **33**, 199–202.

Shorvon, P. *et al.* (1985) Preliminary clinical experience with the heat probe at endoscopy in acute upper gastrointestinal bleeding. *Gastrointest. Endosc.*, **31**, 364–6.

Sigel, B. and Dunn, M. (1965) The mechanism of blood vessel closure by high frequency electrocoagulation. *Surg. Gynecol. Obstet.*, **121**, 823–31.

Silverstein, F. *et al.* (1981a) The national ASGE survey on upper gastrointestinal bleeding II: clinical prognostic factors. *Gastrointest. Endosc.*, **27**, 80–93.

Silverstein, F. *et al.* (1981b) The national ASGE survey on upper gastrointestinal bleeding I: study design and baseline data. *Gastrointest. Endosc.*, **27**, 73–9.

Soehendra, N. (1984) Results in sclerosing of bleeding ulcers. *Workshop Traunstein.* European Laser Association, Traunstein, Germany.

Storey, D. (1983) Endoscopic control of peptic ulcer hemorrhage using the 'heater probe'. *Gut*, **24**, 967–8A.

Sugawa, C. *et al.* (1984) Endoscopic hemostasis of upper gastrointestinal bleeding by local injection of dehydrated (98%) ethanol. *Gastrointest. Endosc.*, **30**, 152A.

Swain, C. *et al.* (1986) Controlled trial of Nd–YAG laser photocoagulation in bleeding peptic ulcers. *Lancet*, **i**, 1113–6.

Winkler, W. *et al.* (1983) Initial experience with BICAP multipolar electrocautery in the control of upper gastrointestinal hemorrhage. *Gastrointest. Endosc.*, **29**, 169A.

Youmans, C. R. *et al.* (1970) Cystoscopic control of gastric hemorrhage. *Arch. Surg.*, **100**, 721–3.

CHAPTER FIFTEEN

Endoscopic injection techniques for control of gastroduodenal haemorrhage

N. Soehendra

Control of haemorrhage by injection treatment is the simplest endoscopic method of haemostasis. The preparation required is minimal and the only necessary accessory is an injection needle.

15.1 INSTRUMENTATION

Two types of injection probes are available on the market: metal and Teflon probes. The probes made of Teflon (Wilson–Cook) are preferred to metal probes (Olympus) because they are more durable and easier to clean.

The outer diameter of the probe is 1.65 mm or 2.31 mm. The thin probes are for endoscopes with a working channel of less than 2.8 mm and the thicker ones for large-bore endoscopes with a minimum working channel of 3.7 mm. Injecting with a larger catheter is easier. It is desirable that the working channel of the endoscope should be at least 1.2 mm larger than that of the probe, enabling simultaneous suction during the therapeutic procedure.

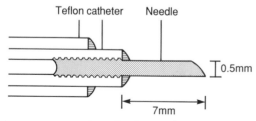

Figure 15.1 Technical data of the injection needle.

An injection cannula with an outer diameter of 0.5 mm is sufficient for low-viscosity solutions. The length should be no longer than 7 mm in order to avoid perforation. The bevel of the needle should be short (Figure 15.1). The use of a high-pressure injector facilitates injection (Figure 15.2), which is especially important when using an oily or more viscous solution.

Patency of the injection needle should always be verified before use (Herlihy and Bozymski, 1982).

15.2 PRINCIPLE

Injection therapy is thought to produce its effect by compression of the submucosal vessels by the infiltrated solution (Figure 15.3). The first agent used was the sclerosant polidocanol 1% alone (Soehendra and Werner, 1976), but some years later the method was modified. In this later technique adrenaline solution (1 : 10 000) was first injected to produce initial haemostasis by its vasoconstrictor effect. This was particularly helpful in cases of arterial bleeding. Sclerosis of the vessel, using polidocanol 1%, could then be used under improved viewing conditions when the bleeding had stopped. This reduced the amount of sclerosant required and therefore the undesirable side-effects.

Initial use of 1 : 10 000 adrenaline is also recommended if substances such as absolute

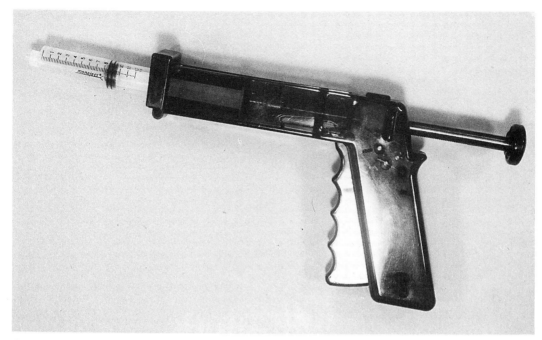

Figure 15.2   High-pressure injector to facilitate injection (Wilson–Cook).

alcohol (Asaki *et al.*, 1983) or hypertonic saline (Hirao *et al.*, 1982) are to be used, as these are known to cause more mucosal necrosis. Another solution which has been used is thrombin which produces submucosal fibrosis without causing mucosal necrosis (Fuchs *et al.*, 1986).

15.3 SCLEROSING SOLUTIONS

The amount of injection solution given depends on the intensity of the bleeding; for example, for arterial bleeding 10 ml adrenaline is usually required and a maximum of 5 ml polidocanol 1% to obliterate the vessel. If absolute alcohol is used only small amounts are required (single doses of 0.2–0.4 ml with no more than 1 ml total). Hypertonic (15–20%) saline is an effective sclerosant but the dose should not exceed a few millilitres. Thrombin solutions consist of 100 iu thrombin (Behringwerke, Fr Germany) made up in 3 ml 0.9% saline. Up to 15 ml are necessary for severe bleeding.

15.4 TECHNIQUE

The advised technique is that the base of the ulcer is first injected by 1 : 10 000 adrenaline. If there is a visible vessel adrenaline can be injected into the lumen and around its circumference. A subsequent sclerosant is injected in the same way – into a visible vessel, or around the bleeding point.

It is desirable to use a tightly connecting catheter with a Luer-lock syringe, as sclerosant, inadvertently sprayed because of disengagement of the syringe, may cause eye injury to the patient and endoscopic staff.

15.5 COMPLICATIONS

Hypertonic saline injections may cause pain. Sclerosing agents cause local necrosis of the mucosa, the extent of which is proportionate to the amount injected. If the recommended dosage is exceeded then extensive necrosis, resulting in perforation at the extreme, is likely. Our own perforation rate is lower than 0.5%. Extensive necrosis of the intestinal wall

164 Endoscopic injection techniques

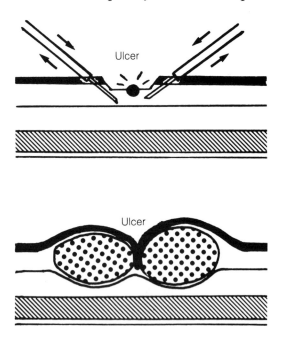

Figure 15.3 Principle of the injection treatment in a case of bleeding ulcer.

causes problems for the surgeon if recurrent bleeding requires surgery.

Certain sclerosing agents can cause systemic side-effects if resorption is rapid (e.g. heavily vascularized, acutely inflamed lesions) or if the injection is by chance intra-arterial. These complications are rare. One should be aware that adrenaline can cause tachycardia and hypertension which may become manifest in patients with shock or high blood pressure.

Pulmonary aspiration is a familiar complication in acute gastrointestinal bleeding. After acute gastrointestinal haemorrhage endoscopy should be performed with minimal premedication. Unconscious patients, or those with respiratory problems, may need airway intubation.

15.6 INDICATIONS AND CONTRAINDICATIONS

Injection treatment is suitable for all localized bleeding lesions which are endoscopically visible and accessible. Indications besides gastroduodenal ulcers include vascular abnormalities, Mallory–Weiss tears, and bleeding after polypectomy or papillotomy.

In the case of Mallory–Weiss bleeding the mucosal tear is infiltrated bilaterally. For bleeding after polypectomy or papillotomy the injection is performed as close as possible around the bleeding vessel into the residual stump or the incised edges. Injection treatment is also suitable to prevent after-bleeding in polyps with thick stalks. Here, the centre of the polyp stalk is injected with a few millilitres of adrenaline and polidocanol before removal of the polyp is begun.

Contraindications for injection treatment include: extensive lesions, such as diffuse haemorrhagic erosions, widespread vascular abnormalities or angiodysplasia in the colon and also large, deep ulcers of the posterior wall with erosion of the gastroduodenal or gastric arteries. These cases are best referred for immediate surgical treatment.

15.7 RESULTS

Most reports of this technique are in uncontrolled trials, but reports indicate that 80–85% of arterial bleeding can be successfully managed by injection treatment. Definite haemostasis can be achieved in 70–75% of cases after single treatments. In a Spanish study in which adrenaline injections were combined with electrocoagulation, haemostasis was obtained in 82% of 28 high-risk patients (Boix et al., 1987). The one published controlled trial (Panés et al., 1987) showed a recurrence rate of 5.5% after endoscopic sclerotherapy compared with 43.1% in controls. The requirement for urgent surgery was also reduced.

Recurrent bleeding occurs in about 30% of patients, usually 3 or 4 days after the initial scleropathy, but repeat injections usually achieve definitive haemostasis (Soehendra, Grimm and Tietze, 1984; Soehendra, Grimm and Stenzel, 1985). Oozing from localized bleeding lesions is usually managed successfully by injection treatment.

15.8 CONCLUSION

The success of injection treatment depends on the appropriate choice of patients and the experience of the endoscopist. Close co-operation with a surgical team is essential for any therapeutic procedure which may be necessary subsequently. Most peptic ulcers can be healed with appropriate drugs after successful haemostasis, however. The goal of endoscopic sclerotherapy is to avoid surgery, especially in high-risk patients.

REFERENCES

Asaki, S., Nishimura, T., Satoh, A. and Goto, Y. (1983) Endoscopic control of gastrointestinal hemorrhage by local injection of absolute ethanol – a basic assessment of the procedure. *Tohoku J. Exp. Med.*, **140**, 339–52.

Boix, J., Planas, R., Humbert, P. *et al.* (1987) Endoscopic hemostasis by injection therapy and electro-hydro-coagulation in high risk patients with active gastroduodenal bleeding ulcer. *Endoscopy*, **19**, 225–7.

Fuchs, K.-H., Wirtz, H.-J., Schaube, H. and Elfeldt, R. (1986) Initial experience with thrombin as injection agent for bleeding gastroduodenal lesions. *Endoscopy*, **18**, 146–8.

Herlihy, K. J. and Bozymski, E. M. (1982) Sclerotherapist's eye. *Gastrointest. Endosc.*, **28**, 42–3.

Hirao, M., Kobayashi, T., Masuda, K. *et al.* (1982) Endoscopic local injection of hypertonic saline epinephrine solution to arrest hemorrhage from the upper digestive tract. II. Clinical application and hemostatic effect. *Gastroenterol. Endosc. Jpn*, **24**, 234–41.

Panés, J., Viver, J., Forné, M. *et al.* (1987) Controlled trial of endoscopic sclerosis in bleeding peptic ulcers. *Lancet*, **ii**, 1292–4.

Soehendra, N., Grimm, H. and Stenzel, M. (1985) Injection of nonvariceal bleeding lesions of the upper gastrointestinal tract. *Endoscopy*, **17**, 129–32.

Soehendra, N., Grimm, H. and Tietze, B. (1984) Gastrointestinale Blutung-Therapeutische Sklerosierung. *Z. Gastroenterol.*, **22**, 102–8.

Soehendra, N. and Werner, B. (1976) New techniques for endoscopic treatment of bleeding gastric ulcer. *Endoscopy*, **8**, 85–7.

CHAPTER SIXTEEN

Angiographic diagnosis and therapy of upper gastrointestinal haemorrhage

T. G. Walker
and
A. C. Waltman

In 1963 Nusbaum and Baum demonstrated active gastrointestinal bleeding in four patients by angiography. It was subsequently shown in 1971, by Rosch, Dotter and Rose, and Baum and Nusbaum, that arterial gastrointestinal bleeding could be controlled with the selective intra-arterial infusion of vasopressin. Other investigators later reported on the control of arterial bleeding by occlusion of the bleeding artery with various embolic agents (Rosch, Dotter and Brown, 1972; Bookstein *et al.*, 1974; White *et al.*, 1974; Gianturco, Anderson and Wallace, 1975). In the succeeding years, a large volume of experience has accumulated with regard to the use of angiography for the diagnosis and treatment of arterial gastrointestinal haemorrhage.

The initial diagnostic procedure in patients with upper gastrointestinal haemorrhage is endoscopy. Angiography should be employed only when endoscopy has failed to demonstrate the bleeding site, or if angiographic therapy is considered necessary. Before angiography, the severity of bleeding should be assessed, as the source of haemorrhage can be demonstrated only when the patient has active, vigorous bleeding. This may be accomplished by placement of a nasogastric tube, followed by saline lavage. If the nasogastric aspirate clears with lavage, the patient generally is not bleeding actively enough to permit angiographic demonstration of the bleeding site.

The angiographic appearance of active arterial bleeding is extravasation of contrast medium at the bleeding site. If the bleeding is rapid, the extravasated contrast will appear dense, whereas very slow bleeding may be difficult to differentiate from a mucosal blush. The minimum bleeding rate that is considered detectable by angiography is about 0.5 ml per minute, based upon animal models studied by Nusbaum and Baum (1963).

Regardless of whether arteriography is done for diagnostic or therapeutic purposes, the patient must be in a haemodynamically stable condition to undergo examination. Although the success rate for angiographic management of gastrointestinal haemorrhage is high, there is always the possibility that the patient's condition may rapidly deteriorate, necessitating emergency surgery. Therefore a 'team management' approach involving consultation with gastrointestinal endoscopy and surgery as well as angiography services should be routine practice. Additionally, the angiography suite should be considered a 'presurgical' area, and should have appropriate monitoring equipment, oxygen and suction capabilities, and nursing cover.

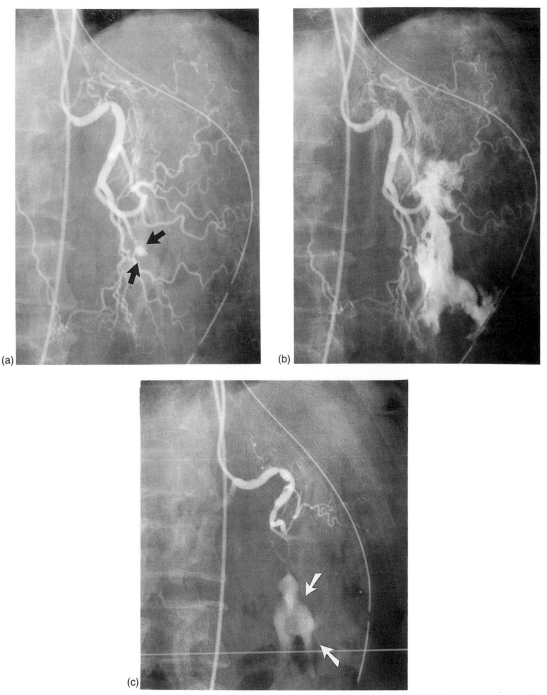

Figure 16.1   (a) Left gastric arteriogram demonstrates focal extravasation (arrows) in lesser curvature. (b) In the later phase of the left gastric arteriogram, extravasation is massive. An attempt to control with intra-arterial vasopressin infusion was unsuccessful. (c) Following gelfoam embolization, the bleeding is controlled, with extravasation no longer present. The contrast collection (arrows) in the lower field is the left renal collecting system.

16.1 OESOPHAGEAL AND GASTRIC HAEMORRHAGE

The source of upper gastrointestinal bleeding can be identified by endoscopy in almost all patients. If angiographic therapy becomes necessary, endoscopic localization can play an important role in directing the sequence of the angiographic procedure. If, for example, endoscopy demonstrates a focal arterial bleeding

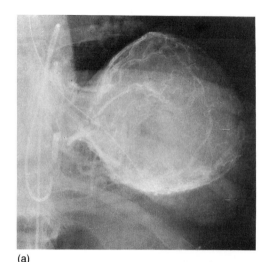

(a)

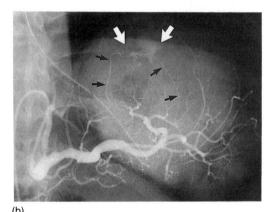

(b)

Figure 16.2 (a) Left gastric arteriogram in a patient with endoscopically visualized gastric bleeding. No extravasation is demonstrated. (b) A splenic arteriogram demonstrates extravasation (white arrows). An arterial supply to the bleeding site is from the short gastric arteries (black arrows).

point in the proximal portion of the stomach, the angiographer should initially catheterize the left gastric artery, as this supplies the arterial bleeding site in 85% of patients (Figure 16.1) (Kelemouridis, Athanasoulis and Waltman, 1983). If no extravasation is identified, and the nasogastric aspirate indicates continued bleeding, other potential arterial sources are sought. These include the short gastric branches of the splenic artery (Figure 16.2), the phrenic, hepatic, gastroduodenal and right gastric arteries. If again no bleeding site is demonstrated, and the patient is still actively bleeding, one may selectively catheterize the left gastric artery, and empirically begin a therapeutic vasopressin infusion.

If endoscopy suggests a diffuse gastritis as the source of bleeding, left gastric arteriography may not demonstrate extravasation, but rather an intense hyperaemic blush of the gastric wall (Figure 16.3). This is considered diagnostic of haemorrhagic erosive gastritis, and warrants vasopressin therapy in the face of continued uncontrolled bleeding.

In a series of 222 patients with gastric bleeding, who were evaluated and treated angiographically, control of haemorrhage was achieved in 75% of patients with left gastric artery vasopressin infusions and in 80% with coeliac artery infusions (Eckstein *et al.*, 1984). Although left gastric infusion did not control haemorrhage in 25% of patients, as demonstrated by the postinfusion arteriogram, catheter position allowed embolotherapy to be added to the vasopressin therapy with an additional 10% clinical success.

If an endoscopic attempt to control gastric bleeding by electrocautery has failed, the bleeding vessel has been thermally injured. The vascular musculature is no longer viable and is unlikely to respond to vasopressin. Therefore, if bleeding continues after attempted endoscopic therapy, embolization is usually necessary. If embolization is attempted without the catheter selectively positioned in either the left gastric artery or the vessel supplying the bleeding site, the success

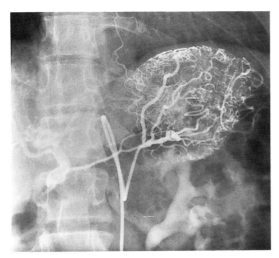

Figure 16.3   Intense hyperaemic blush, characteristic of diffuse haemorrhagic gastritis.

rate is low, and there may be significant associated complications such as splenic infarction (Trojanowski *et al.*, 1980).

16.2 PYLORODUODENAL HAEMORRHAGE

The typical patient with signs and symptoms of duodenal ulcer complicated by bleeding generally does not require either diagnostic or therapeutic angiography. After endoscopic confirmation, the patient is usually treated with either endoscopic intervention, surgery or conservative medical management. In the patient who requires surgical control of bleeding, but is a poor operative risk, angiographic intervention may be considered.

Before initiating angiographic therapy a diagnostic arteriogram is performed to identify the bleeding artery (Figure 16.4). Because the pyloroduodenal region has a dual blood supply, both the coeliac and the superior mesenteric arteries must be evaluated. This dual vascular supply accounts for the lower success rate in angiographic control of pyloroduodenal bleeding, compared with the results achieved in gastric bleeding. The potential for reversal of blood flow within the pancreatico-

duodenal arcades may make therapy ineffective when it is based on occluding flow from only one side of the arcade. Initial therapy should use intra-arterial vasopressin infusion, with subsequent embolization if the infusion fails. With this approach, the overall success rate is 55–65% bleeding control, with a 20–30% incidence of recurrent haemorrhage (Waltman *et al.*, 1979).

16.3 OTHER SITES OF GASTROINTESTINAL HAEMORRHAGE

Angiographic intervention may also be employed in the patient who develops anastomotic bleeding following gastrojejunostomy. In the majority of these patients, the bleeding arises from the jejunal side of the anastomosis, and thus involves a branch of the superior mesenteric artery. Vasopressin infusion may be initiated and, if unsuccessful, may be followed by selective catheterization and embolization of the bleeding jejunal arterial branch.

In patients in whom endoscopy fails to localize the source of gastrointestinal haemorrhage, angiography plays an important primary diagnostic role. In addition, therapeutic intervention is often possible but depends upon the aetiology and source of bleeding.

If there is a clinical suspicion of aortoenteric fistula, as in the patient who has undergone aortic bypass graft, a midstream aortogram is performed. Films are obtained in both the anteroposterior and lateral projections (biplane filming), as the 'beak' or 'nipple' at the site of aortoenteric communication is best seen in the lateral projection (Figure 16.5).

In the absence of suspected aortic pathology, the initial vessel evaluated is the coeliac trunk. If extravasation is seen from one of the branches, the corresponding vessel is then selectively catheterized for further evaluation and therapy if indicated. If there is no extravasation or other pathology identified on the

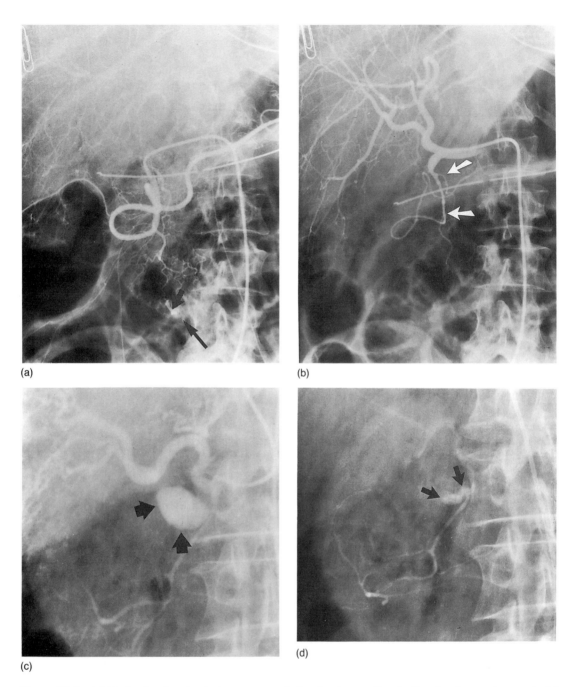

(a)

(b)

(c)

(d)

Figure 16.4 (a) Gastroduodenal arteriogram reveals focal extravasation in the duodenum (arrows). (b) Intra-arterial vasopressin infusion controls bleeding. The vasoconstrictive effect on small vessels is evident (arrows), and extravasation is no longer present. (c) Hepatic arteriogram in another patient with duodenal bleeding reveals a rounded contrast collection (arrows) that corresponds to extravasated contrast that has pooled in an ulcer crater. (d) Successful embolization with isocyanobucrylate (ICB). The contrast collection (arrows) represents the ICB, which was mixed with contrast when injected.

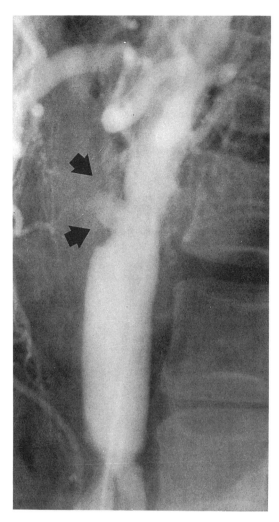

Figure 16.5 Lateral aortogram in a patient who had previously undergone aortic bypass graft. The 'nipple' (arrows) represents the point of communication in an aortoenteric fistula.

Occasionally unusual sources of gastrointestinal haemorrhage are identified. Visceral artery pseudoaneurysms are a well-known complication of acute pancreatitis, and may cause life-threatening gastrointestinal bleeding. Haemorrhage is the major cause of death in over 50% of fatal cases of pancreatitis and is associated with necrosis and infection (Kirby, Howard and Rhoads, 1955). Aggressive therapy is mandatory and may involve arteriography. Surgery alone incurs a 30% mortality (Frey, 1979). Surgical attempts to control the haemorrhage usually precede angiographic intervention. Unlike most types of gastrointestinal bleeding, there is often more than one bleeding site present. The arterial anatomy may be distorted as a result of prior surgery, or because of complications such as pancreatic pseudocyst or abscess. Arteriography is initiated in an attempt to localize the bleeding site(s). In the angiographic evaluation of these patients, aortography may be helpful in delineating the major vascular anatomy as well as possible retroperitoneal sites of extravasation. Selective studies of the coeliac and superior mesenteric arteries are also necessary in the initial assessment. After the bleeding site(s) have been demonstrated by coeliac and superior mesenteric arteriograms, further selective vessel catheterization is necessary to accomplish angiographic control of bleeding (Waltman et al., 1986). The use of directable guide-wires and coaxial catheter systems has further expanded the range of vessels that can be selectively catheterized. These refinements allow for selection and occlusion of only the affected vessel (Figure 16.6), with reduced risk of reflux embolization.

Another unusual category of upper gastrointestinal bleeding is that of haematobilia. This entity may be due to an iatrogenic cause, such as percutaneous biopsy or drainage procedures, or it may occur as a result of penetrating trauma. Once the site of communication between the hepatic arterial and biliary systems has been demonstrated by angiography,

coeliac arteriogram, a left gastric arteriogram is still necessary, because small amounts of contrast extravasation may only be apparent from selective injections (Waltman et al., 1973; Athanasoulis, 1982). If this fails to identify a source, a superior mesenteric arteriogram is then performed. If a source of bleeding is identified, appropriate therapy may then be instituted.

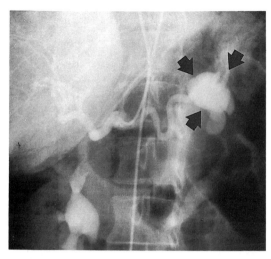

Figure 16.6 Pseudoaneurysm (arrows) of the splenic artery in a patient with haemorrhagic pancreatitis.

selective embolization usually provides effective control (Figure 16.7).

Arteriovenous malformations, aneurysms, and primary small bowel neoplasms constitute other causes of gastrointestinal bleeding that may be effectively evaluated by angiography (Figures 16.8 and 16.9). Because the small bowel is an endoscopic 'blind spot', these patients often present with chronic gastrointestinal bleeding that remains unexplained despite multiple diagnostic examinations. Arteriography may successfully demonstrate the source of haemorrhage, even though these patients may not be actively bleeding. However, the diagnostic angiographic examination must be meticulous and thorough, and often must include multiple projections and magnification views.

16.4 ANGIOGRAPHIC THERAPY IN UPPER GASTROINTESTINAL HAEMORRHAGE

Upper gastrointestinal haemorrhage that requires therapeutic angiographic intervention may be managed by either vasopressin infusion or embolization (Gomes, Lois and

McCoy, 1986). Sometimes a combination of these two therapies is required (Waltman *et al.*, 1979; Eckstein *et al.*, 1984). Except for the treatment of certain specific entities (e.g. haemorrhagic gastritis, pseudoaneurysm), the choice of whether to infuse or embolize is largely a matter of personal preference or experience.

16.4.1 VASOPRESSIN THERAPY

Vasopressin, or antidiuretic hormone (ADH), causes contraction of smooth muscle in the walls of arterioles and capillaries, as well as the intestine. Reabsorption of water in the distal renal tubules is also stimulated. The vasoconstrictive effect is caused by the direct action of vasopressin on vascular smooth muscle. The degree of vasoconstriction is dependent on the particular vascular bed infused.

Systemic intravenous vasopressin infusion is much less effective in controlling arteriocapillary bleeding than an intra-arterial infusion (Athanasoulis *et al.*, 1977). An experimental model demonstrated that intravenous vasopressin controlled only 50% of gastric bleeding, whereas selective left gastric arterial infusion controlled 95% (Athanasoulis, 1982a). Intra-arterial infusions of vasopressin into a given vascular bed achieve high regional levels of the drug and produce effective vasoconstriction. For an intravenous infusion to accomplish comparable vasoconstriction, very high systemic levels of the drug are necessary. These high systemic levels have important adverse effects on other vascular beds, including the myocardium. Severe vasoconstriction, combined with reduced cardiac output may lead to myocardial, bowel, renal or cerebral ischaemic injuries.

It is presumed that vasopressin controls bleeding from arteriocapillary sites by causing both vasoconstriction and bowel wall muscular contraction. The peripheral arteries and arterioles contract and reduce flow to the bleeding site. In addition, contraction of the

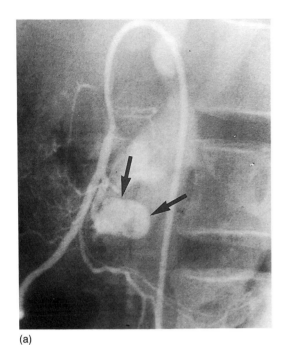

(a)

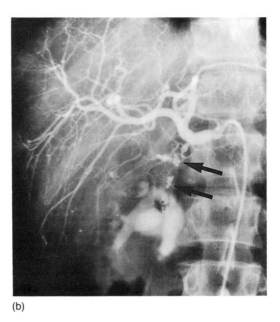

(b)

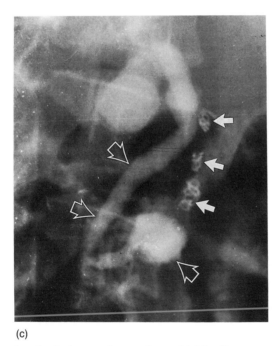

(c)

Figure 16.7 (a) Gastroduodenal arteriogram in a patient with bleeding seen at endoscopy to arise from the ampulla of Vater. A rounded contrast collection of extravasation is present (arrows). (b) The gastroduodenal artery has been embolized successfully with coils (arrows), with control of bleeding. (c) ERCP study following embolization of the gastroduodenal artery with coils (arrows) demonstrates that the rounded contrast collection is a pancreatic pseudocyst in communication with the common bile duct (open arrows).

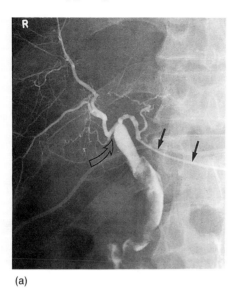

(a)

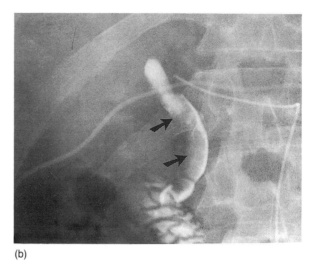

(b)

(c)

Figure 16.8 (a) Catheter (black arrows) in hepatic artery. Injection demonstrates communication (open arrow) between hepatic artery and biliary tree in patient with haematobilia. (b) Later phase of hepatic arteriogram demonstrates thrombus within the common bile duct (arrows), with contrast also opacifying mucosal folds in the duodenum. (c) Following embolization with gelfoam and coils, there is no longer arterial communication with the biliary system (arrow).

muscular structures of the bowel constricts the penetrating blood vessels as they pass through the musculature. Together these effects diminish the blood flow to the mucosa and submucosal tissues, as well as to the point of haemorrhage. Maintaining drug effect allows the formation of a stable thrombus and repair of the mucosal surface. Vasopressin is not able to achieve the same degree of vaso-constriction in larger arteries, unless infused at very high doses. Thus, bleeding from large or named vessels (e.g. gastroduodenal, supra-duodenal, splenic, etc.), or which involves vessels that are not confined to the bowel wall, is unlikely to respond to or be controlled with vasopressin therapy.

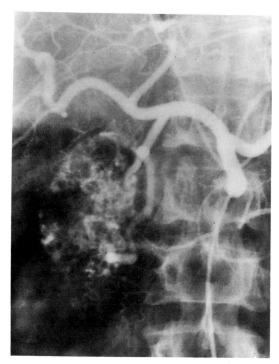

Figure 16.9 Duodenal arteriovenous malformation supplied by the gastroduodenal artery.

Therapeutic protocol for intra-arterial vasopressin infusion (Athanasoulis 1982a, b)

1. Selective arteriography with demonstration of extravasation.
2. Vasopressin infusion: solution is prepared by the addition of 200 u of vasopressin to 500 ml of normal saline or 5% dextrose in water. This is a concentration of 0.4 u/ml. Infusion of 30 ml/h will result in an infusion of 0.2 u/min; a rate of 45 ml/h will be 0.3 u/min; and a rate of 60 ml/h will be 0.4 u/min. Infusion is accomplished with a constant arterial infusion pump (e.g. Sigmamotor, IVAC).
3. Infusion is started at 0.2 u/min for 20 minutes in the angiographic suite, following which a repeat arteriogram is obtained.
4. If there is no extravasation, the catheter is secured in place, and the patient is transferred to an intensive care unit for continuous monitoring while the infusion is continued.
5. If extravasation persists, the infusion is increased to 0.4 u/min and continued for an additional 20 minutes. A repeat arteriogram is performed to confirm arteriographic cessation of extravasation. If there is continued extravasation, then other means (e.g. surgery, embolization) to control the bleeding should be undertaken.
6. After establishing a dose that controls the arteriographic bleeding, this infusion is continued for 16–24 hours. If clinical evaluation confirms that bleeding is controlled, the infusion rate is slowly reduced over an additional 24 hours. The catheter is then infused with saline for an additional 6–12 hours before removal.

If breakthrough or recurrent bleeding is suspected during the course of the infusion and weaning process, there are several possibilities to be considered. It is important first to confirm physically the status of the infusion mixture, lines and the pump when evaluating the rebleeding patient. If these factors are satisfactory, correct catheter tip position must be confirmed. This may be done either with a portable film of the abdomen obtained with contrast injection, or the patient may be returned to the angiography suite. If the catheter has been dislodged, catheter exchange and/or repositioning must be performed.

Vasopressin therapy, whether intravenous or intra-arterial, is potentially hazardous. Minor adverse effects are largely due to the antidiuretic hormone action. These include oliguria, hyponatraemia and pulmonary oedema. The adverse vasopressor effects are those of hypertension, arrhythmias and peripheral vasoconstriction or acrocyanosis. These are reversible and are easily managed symptomatically. Cardiac monitoring and careful attention to fluid and electrolyte balance are mandatory.

Major complications are most often due to the vasoconstrictive aspects of the drug and

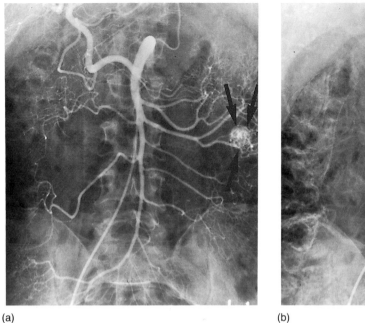
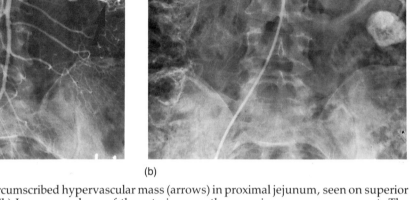

(a)   (b)

Figure 16.10   (a) Well-circumscribed hypervascular mass (arrows) in proximal jejunum, seen on superior mesenteric arteriogram. (b) In venous phase of the arteriogram, the mass is even more apparent. The appearance is characteristic of a leiomyoma.

result in severe hypertension, arrhythmias and tissue (bowel, myocardial or peripheral) ischaemia. These complications may mean cessation of vasopressin therapy.

16.4.2 EMBOLIZATION

When the bleeding vessel cannot be controlled by vasopressin infusion, embolization may be considered as an alternative approach. The choice of embolic materials has expanded to include gelfoam, ivalon particles, liquid adhesives (Bucrylate), detachable balloons and mechanical occlusion coils in a wide range of diameters. Techniques for delivering these materials include standard and coaxial catheter systems. The success of embolization is largely dependent upon selective catherization of the bleeding vessel. A selective catheter position allows one directly to occlude the vessel supplying the bleeding site, and minimizes the potential for reflux of embolic ma-

terial into other vessels. None the less, reflux of emboli into non-target vessels must be recognized as a potential complication of embolotherapy. If this should occur, major complications, such as gallbladder, bowel wall, hepatic or splenic infarction with abscess formation may result (Trojarowski *et al.*, 1980).

Selective embolization of the left gastric artery may occasionally be successful in a patient with endoscopically diagnosed gastric haemorrhage, who does not demonstrate extravasation at arteriography (Eckstein *et al.*, 1984). However, in the pyloroduodenal region, embolization should not be performed in the absence of arteriographically demonstrated extravasation (Waltman *et al.*, 1979).

16.5   SUMMARY AND CONCLUSIONS

We have considered the role of diagnostic and therapeutic angiography in the management of patients with upper gastrointestinal bleeding. Diagnostic angiography should be performed only when endoscopy is unavailable or is non-diagnostic. Angiography for therapeutic purposes may become necessary in the patient who fails to respond to medical management, is a poor surgical candidate, or who continues bleeding following surgery. The available therapeutic interventions include intra-arterial vasopressin infusion, transcatheter embolization, or a combination of these modalities. The results of angiographic therapy are dependent upon the aetiology as well as the source of bleeding.

REFERENCES

Athanasoulis, C. A. (1982a) Upper gastrointestinal bleeding of arteriocapillary origin, in *Interventional Radiology*, ch. 6, (eds C. A. Athanasoulis, R. Pfister, R. Greene and G. Roberson), W. B. Saunders, Philadelphia, p. 55.

Athanasoulis, C. A. (1982b) Lower gastrointestinal bleeding, in *Interventional Radiology*, ch. 8 (eds C. A. Athanasoulis, R. Pfister, R. Greene and G. Roberson), W. B. Saunders, Philadelphia, p. 115.

Athanasoulis, C. A., Simmons, J. T., Sheehan, B. *et al.* (1977) Gastric blood flow alterations during intraarterial and systemic infusion of vasopressin. Presented at Association of University Radiologists Meeting, Kansas City (abstr.).

Baum, S. and Nusbaum, M. (1971) The control of gastrointestinal haemorrhage by selective mesenteric arterial infusion of vasopressin. *Radiology*, **98**, 497.

Bookstein, J. J., Chlosta, E., Foley, D. *et al.* (1974) Transcatheter hemostasis of gastrointestinal bleeding using modified autogenous clot. *Radiology*, **113**, 277.

Eckstein, M. R., Kelemouridis, V., Athanasoulis, C. A. *et al.* (1984) Gastric bleeding: therapy with intraarterial vasopressin and transcatheter embolization. *Radiology*, **152**, 643.

Frey, F. (1979) Hemorrhagic pancreatitis. *Am. J. Surg.*, **137**, 616.

Gianturco, C., Anderson, J. H. and Wallace, S. (1975) Mechanical devices for arterial occlusion. *Am. J. Roentgenol.*, **124**, 428.

Gomes, A. S., Lois, J. F. and McCoy, R. D. (1986) Angiographic treatment of gastrointestinal hemorrhage: comparison of vasopressin infusion and embolization. *A.J.R.*, **146**, 1031.

Kelemouridis, V., Athanasoulis, C. A. and Waltman, A. C. (1983) Gastric bleeding sites: an angiographic study. *Radiology*, **149**, 643.

Kirby, C. K., Howard, J. M. and Rhoads, J. E. (1955) Death due to delayed hemorrhage in acute pancreatitis. *Surg. Gynecol. Obstet.*, **100**, 458.

Nusbaum, M. and Baum, S. (1963) Radiographic demonstration of unknown sites of gastrointestinal bleeding. *Surg. Forum*, **14**, 374.

Rosch, J., Dotter, C. T. and Brown, M. J. (1972) Selective arterial embolization. A new method for control of acute gastrointestinal bleeding. *Radiology*, **102**, 303.

Rosch, J., Dotter, C. T. and Rose, R. W. (1971) Selective arterial infusions of vasoconstrictors in acute gastrointestinal bleeding. *Radiology*, **99**, 27.

Trojanowski, J. Q., Harrist, T. J., Athanasoulis, C. A. *et al.* (1980) Hepatic and splenic infarctions: complications of therapeutic transcatheter embolization. *Am. J. Surg.*, **139**, 272.

Waltman, A. C., Courey, W. R., Athanasoulis, C. A. *et al.* (1973) Technique for left gastric artery catheterization. *Radiology*, **109**, 732.

Waltman, A. C., Greenfield, A. J., Novelline, R. A. *et al.* (1979) Pyloroduodenal bleeding and intraarterial vasopressin: clinical results. *A.J.R.*, **133**, 643.

Waltman, A. C., Luers, P. R., Athanasoulis, C. A. *et al.* (1986) Massive arterial hemorrhage in patients with pancreatitis: complementary roles of surgery and transcatheter occlusive techniques. *Arch. Surg.*, **121**, 439.

White, R. I., Giargiana, F. A. Jr and Bell, W. (1974) Bleeding duodenal ulcer control. Selective arterial embolization with autologous blood clot. *JAMA*, **229**, 546.

CHAPTER SEVENTEEN

Angiodysplasia of the gut

R. H. Hunt

Vascular abnormalities of the gastrointestinal tract are attracting increasing interest and there have been numerous isolated reports in the literature since the first description by Phillips in 1839 of an erectile vascular tumour of the rectum. However, few reported series of gastrointestinal bleeding have identified vascular malformations as a source of haemorrhage, and almost 25% of patients with gastrointestinal bleeding may go undiagnosed (Catem and Jiminez, 1963).

The classification of gastrointestinal tract vascular abnormalities has become confused by the variety of synonymous terms which have been used. Problems of terminology have been compounded by a lack of conformity both within and between disciplines. Radiologists and endoscopists have often used terminology usually reserved for histopathology. Vascular lesions cause gastrointestinal bleeding when they involve the mucosa, but the abnormality may extend through the submucosa so that the term 'mucosal vascular abnormality' is open to criticism. The general term 'vascular abnormality' should probably be used as an endoscopic or radiological description, reserving all others for confirmed histological diagnosis.

Some classifications refer to angiodysplasia as 'non-hereditary telangiectasia' (Gentry, Dockerty and Clagett, 1949) and mention will also be made of hereditary telangiectasia and haemangiomas, since these may present in an identical fashion.

True angiomas are relatively rare in the gastrointestinal tract while telangiectases are more common and often multiple. The most frequently recognized telangiectatic lesion is found in the right colon and commonly described as angiodysplasia (Boley *et al.*, 1977a; Rogers, 1980; Howard, Buchanan and Hunt, 1982; Hunt, 1984a), arteriovenous malformation or vascular dysplasia. These colonic lesions appear to be degenerative and the term 'vascular ectasia' has been suggested by Mitsudo *et al.* (1979). In contrast, Weaver *et al.* (1979) proposed a spectrum of abnormalities ranging from hereditary haemorrhagic telangiectasia (HHT) through angiodysplasia to radiation-associated telangiectasia. Mucosal vessels in angiodysplasia are small, ectatic and dilated, and similar to those seen in HHT, while haemangiomas show neovascularization with vessels of varying size displacing adjacent tissue.

The distribution of vascular abnormalities in angiodysplasia will be detailed below.

17.1 OESOPHAGUS

Haemangiomas rarely occur in the oesophagus, and accounted for about 2% of all benign oesophageal lesions in one series (10), but only 29 cases are recorded in the literature. The lesions of hereditary haemorrhagic telangiectasia may be found in the oesophagus, but less commonly than in the stomach or small and large bowel. It is wise not to attempt biopsy of a suspected vascular lesion in the oesophagus (Foster, Yomehiro and Benjamin, 1978).

17.2 STOMACH

Vascular lesions in the stomach are increasingly recognized and may be localized or diffuse. A recent study has suggested a frequency of up to 1 and 285 upper gastrointestinal endoscopies (Blankenstein, Van Dees and Tenkate, 1978). Apart from the lesions seen in hereditary haemorrhagic telangiectasia, an association has been suggested with previous abdominal radiation (Boley *et al.*, 1977b), with the CRST (calcinosis, Raynaud's syndrome, sclerodactyly and telangiectasia) syndrome, and with von Willebrand's disease (Posner and Sampliner, 1978; McGrath, Johnson and Stuart, 1979; Cass *et al.*, 1980).

17.2.1 DIFFUSE GASTRIC ANTRAL VASCULAR ABNORMALITY

Several reports have appeared in the past 5 years describing an antral vascular abnormality radiating from the pylorus (Lewis, Laufer and Goodacre, 1978; Wheeler *et al.*, 1979, Calam and Walker, 1980; Colin-Jones, 1984; Hunt, 1984b). To the inexperienced endoscopist this may appear as a linear gastritis with apparently normal gastric mucosa in between (Figure 17.1). Histology reveals a mass of tortuous dilated vessels.

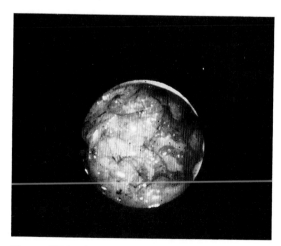

Figure 17.1 A gastric antral angioma of the watermelon type radiating from the pylorus and involving the entire antrum.

Patients invariably present with recurrent anaemia, sometimes over many years, and some are women with chronic liver disease. Patients may stop bleeding after oral corticosteroid therapy (Calam and Walker, 1980; Hunt, 1984b), but as partial gastrectomy is usually curative, this observation requires confirmation.

17.2.2 GASTROPATHY OF PORTAL HYPERTENSION

A particular vascular abnormality occurring in patients with cirrhosis has recently been reviewed by two groups (McCormack *et al.*, 1985; Quintero *et al.*, 1987) who describe small flat red spots in the gastric mucosa of cirrhotic patients. These small red lesions are 2–5 mm in diameter, usually close to one another but not confluent, and cover the major part of the gastric antrum. Histology shows a diffuse vascular ectasia with little or no inflammation. An association was demonstrated with raised gastrin levels and low serum pepsinogen 1 (Quintero *et al.*, 1987). Following shunt surgery bleeding from this lesion decreases, as does variceal bleeding.

17.2.3 GASTRIC HAEMANGIOMA

Gastric haemangiomas are rare; less than 50 cases have been published in the world literature. They usually present with chronic bleeding and may be polypoid in appearance, making differential diagnosis from other lesions difficult.

17.3 DUODENUM AND SMALL BOWEL

Vascular abnormalities affecting the duodenal mucosa may be seen at endoscopy, but small bowel lesions beyond the descending duodenum are beyond the range of conventional endoscopy. Hereditary haemorrhagic telangiectasia usually affects the duodenum (Moore *et al.*, 1978; Lewis and Waye, 1988) and frequently the small bowel. Non-hereditary telangiectases and haemangiomas are also relatively common at these sites.

Blood loss may be mild, moderate or exsanguinating, and is more common from sessile lesions; polypoid haemangiomas more commonly produce partial or complete intestinal obstruction.

Developments in selective angiography and peroperative endoscopy have provided major clinical advances in the management of patients with bleeding from suspected vascular abnormalities in the small intestine. More recently the introduction of an experimental transnasal enteroscope has made the whole small bowel potentially accessible (Lewis and Waye, 1988) (Figure 17.2).

17.4 COLON

Angiodysplasia of the right colon and caecum is the most commonly encountered vascular abnormality in the gastrointestinal tract.

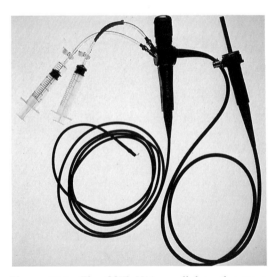

Figure 17.2 The SSIF V11 small bowel enteroscope. The instrument is 5 mm in diameter with a working length of 2750 mm, has an angle of vision of 90°. The instrument has two channels, one for air insufflation, and the other to inflate the Sonde balloon at the tip of the instrument which aids passage through the small bowel with intestinal peristalsis.

Lesions have been recognized by radiologists since the initial report by Margulis, Heinbecker and Bernard (1960) and the development of selective mesenteric angiography (Baum *et al.*, 1965; Tarin *et al.*, 1978; Giacchino *et al.*, 1979; Allison, Hemingway and Cunningham, 1982). Colonoscopic diagnosis of the lesions of angiodysplasia were first reported in 1976 by Skibba *et al.* (1976) and by Rogers and Adler (1976), and are now recognized as an important cause of colonic bleeding which should be exhaustively sought by the colonoscopist (Howard, Buchanan and Hunt, 1982), although the frequency with which this diagnosis is made has recently been questioned (Danesh *et al.*, 1987). Meticulous cleansing of the colon is essential when colonoscopy is performed in cases where angiodysplasia is suspected (Nagy, 1981), and since this lesion represents a low-pressure arteriolar-venous communication (see below), excessive inflation of the caecum and right colon by the introduction of air from the colonoscope can result in the blanching of the lesion which then becomes invisible. It may take several minutes for the lesion to refill and the endoscopist should deflate the right colon periodically during the examination. Diagnosis of angiodysplasia may be made at operation if a careful examination of the mucosal surface of the colon is made immediately after segmental resection (Heald and Ray, 1974); although angiomatous lesions may produce changes on the serosal surface of the colon at surgery, this is not the case with angiodysplasia. This emphasizes the importance of defining the extent of angiodysplasia by both colonoscopy and angiography when surgery is contemplated.

17.4.1 AETIOLOGY AND PATHOLOGY OF ANGIODYSPLASIA OF THE COLON

Angiodysplasia (Figures 17.3 and 17.4) is most commonly seen in the caecum and ascending

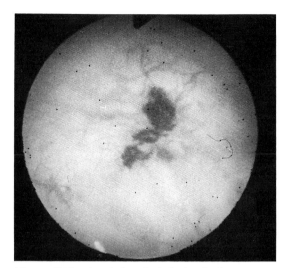

Figure 17.3 Angiodysplasia lesion in the caecum. This lesion is cherry red in colour with dilated and irregular superficial capillaries.

colon but the frequency in the population is not known. Some workers believe that the lesions are unique to the right colon (Boley *et al.* (1977a), although others have reported similar lesions elsewhere in the colon (Miller *et al.*, 1979) and in the stomach (Bourdette and Greenberg, 1979; Weaver *et al.*, 1979, Rogers, 1980; Roberts *et al.*, 1981; Colin-James, 1984).

Baum, Athanasoulis and Waltman (1977) suggest that angiodysplasia is an acquired lesion resulting from mucosal ischaemia, secondary to arteriovenous shunting in the mucosa which occurs with changes in intracolonic pressure.

Galloway, Casarella and Waltman (1977) confirmed earlier reports of an association with aortic stenosis, and believe lesions develop as a consequence of decreased perfusion pressure in the terminal branches of the superior mesenteric artery, which is secondary to a decreased left ventricular output. A similar association with aortic valve disease and also chronic lung disease was noted by Rogers (1980) whose patients were all diagnosed at colonoscopy. He suggested that a lowered oxygen tension in the end-arterial

vessels of the superior mesenteric artery results in capillary dilatation and proliferation, eventually leading to a vascular abnormality.

Boley *et al.* (Boley *et al.* 1977a, b; Mitsudo *et al.*, 1979) believe that lesions in the right colon and caecum represent a unique entity, separate from other vascular lesions of the gastrointestinal tract. They base their conclusions on evidence obtained from elegant injection techniques and painstaking study of the histopathology. They suggest a chronic intermittent partial obstruction of the low-pressure submucosal veins, at the point where they pass through the longitudinal and circular muscle of the bowel, not affecting the higher pressure arterial inflow. The resulting pressure differential causes capillary vessel and later capillary ring dilatation with subsequent precapillary sphincter incompetence. Small arteriovenous malformations thus develop at the level of the mucosal capillaries. They attribute the frequency of this lesion in the right colon to Laplace's law, the effect of which implies that the tension in the bowel wall will

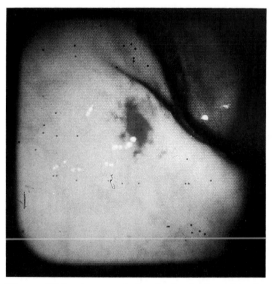

Figure 17.4 An angiodysplasia lesion in the caecum on the superior aspect of the ileocaecal valve. The lesion is bright red in colour, and the dilated central capillary is seen with radiating peripheral mucosal vessels.

be highest where the colon has the greatest diameter (Wangensteen, 1955). Boley *et al.* (1977a, b) suggested that if angiodysplasia were due to ageing, lesions should be present in the colon of elderly patients who had not yet bled, and by injection and histopathological studies of the colon in a control group of 15 patients identified mucosal ectasia in 27% and a large dilated submucosal vein in 53%.

The pathology of angiodysplasia of the right colon shows a spectrum from small early focal lesions to multiple large lesions (Mitsudo *et al.*, 1979). Sometimes superficial mucosal capillaries are dilated, mildly compress the lamina propria and communicate with a tortuous dilated submucosal vein. In more advanced cases, submucosal changes are more

apparent, there is marked ectasia of mucosal vessels and the submucosal veins become increasingly tortuous and dilated while the arteries remain normal. The submucosal veins communicate with mucosal capillaries which are continuous with large or small groups of dilated vessels compressing the surrounding crypts. In severe cases, the capillary wall and attenuated epithelium are all that separate the capillary lumen from the colonic lumen (Figure 17.5). It is clear from these observations how easily the wall may rupture and result in severe colonic bleeding. A careful search by the histopathologist often reveals the site of bleeding (Figure 17.6).

17.5 CLINICAL FEATURES

Vascular abnormalities of the gut may affect patients of all ages, hereditary telangiectasia and angiomas being more common in younger patients and degenerative vascular ectasias almost exclusively in the elderly. Sex incidence appears to be almost equal.

Patients usually present with anaemia which may be marked and many, especially those with mucosal lesions of angiodysplasia, will often have experienced one or more episodes of overt gastrointestinal bleeding. This may vary from slow occult blood loss to massive haemorrhage with hypovolaemic shock (Hunt, 1984a). The pattern of bleeding may vary both within and between individuals but, even when severe, each episode is usually self limiting. Bleeding is often bright red or maroon coloured from colonic or small bowel lesions, but a history of tarry stools may also be obtained. Some patients with colonic vascular ectasias give a history of one or more operations for a diagnosis such as duodenal ulcer or diverticular disease which had been considered the site of blood loss (Hunt, 1984).

A careful history and physical examination should be taken in order to exclude the Osler–Weber–Rendu syndrome or von Willebrand's disease (Ramsay *et al.*, 1976; Rogers and Adler, 1976; Weaver *et al.*, 1979; Rogers, 1980).

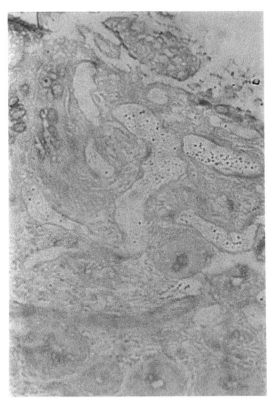

Figure 17.5 Dilated ectatic thin-walled superficial capillaries are seen in this coagulation biopsy specimen. Here the thin vessel wall has no overlying mucosa to protect it from the colonic lumen (× 250).

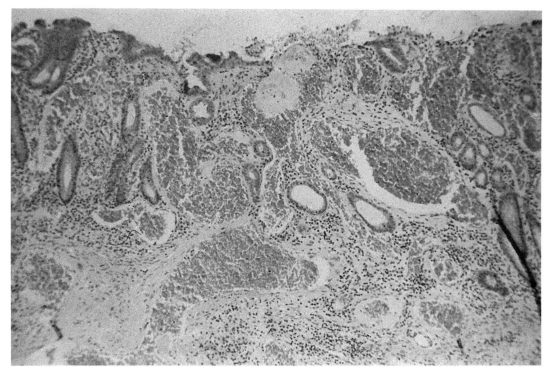

Figure 17.6   Tortuous dilated submucosal vessels are seen communicating with ruptured superficial capillaries and a platelet thrombus can be seen at the site of bleeding (× 212.5).

It is not yet clear if the pathology of the vascular lesions associated with von Willebrand's disease correlates with the angiodysplasia lesions described by Mitsudo *et al.* (1979).

Vascular abnormalities in the colon may be associated with aortic valve stenosis (Williams, 1961; Boss and Rosenbaum, 1971; Boley *et al.*, 1977b; Rogers, 1980), although few cases have been confirmed by cardiac catheterization. Aortic sclerosis, hypertension and other cardiovascular disorders are also common, although they may be chance associations due to ageing. Hence the association of angiodysplasia with aortic stenosis has recently been questioned (Imperiale and Ransohoff, 1988).

17.6 DIAGNOSIS

Until recent years, vascular abnormalities in the gastrointestinal tract have been diagnosed almost exclusively by radiological means. With the widespread use of fibreoptic endoscopy, more lesions are now diagnosed at routine upper gastrointestinal endoscopy or at colonoscopy.

A plain film of the abdomen may occasionally reveal calcification in a large angioma. Barium studies are usually not helpful since most vascular abnormalities are flat or have a low profile extending within the submucosa, making them invisible to these conventional investigations. The development of selective three-vessel angiography (Baum *et al.*, 1965; Baum, Athanasoulis and Waltman, 1977; Tarin *et al.*, 1978; Giacchino *et al.*, 1979; Allison, Hemingway and Cunningham, 1982) has enabled the radiologist to identify the site and cause of bleeding in many cases. Further experience using subtraction film techniques has defined important radiological criteria for diagnosis which include a vascular tuft, an

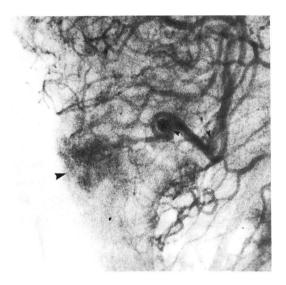

Figure 17.7 Arteriography showing the superior mesenteric angiogram in the arterial phase with a vascular tuft, and a dilated and early draining vein indicated by the arrows.

early filling vein and a dense, slowly emptying vein (Figure 17.7) (Galloway, Casarella and Shimkin, 1974; Boley *et al.*, 1977b) and these features may be present individually or in any combination.

In patients with a history of gastrointestinal bleeding, fibreoptic endoscopy should be undertaken before selective angiography is considered and this will often lead to the diagnosis, especially when the endoscopist makes a meticulous search for a lesion. Selective angiography may still be useful as a complementary investigation to confirm the extent of a lesion and exclude any additional lesions.

The endoscopic appearance of a vascular abnormality depends upon its nature. In the stomach, a diffuse antral vascular abnormality has been likened to a water melon (Lewis, Laufer and Goodacre, 1978; Wheeler *et al.*, 1979; Colin-Jones, 1984; Jabbari *et al.*, 1984) or to an octopus with limbs which radiate from the pylorus. The surface is nodular with tortuous vessels which blanch on pressure with the biopsy forceps (Figure 17.1). Telangiec-

tases in the stomach are more common in the body or fundus as discrete, bright red lesions about 5 mm in diameter with a raised central bleb; they may sometimes be confused with the Dieulefoy lesion (Dieulefoy, 1912; Van-Zanten *et al.*, 1986).

Angiodysplasia lesions in the right colon are cherry-red in colour and usually about 5 mm in size (Figures 17.3 and 17.4), although they can be larger and more extensive (Figure 17.9). There is usually an elevated dilated central vessel which, to the endoscopist, is visibly distended with radiating peripheral vessels.

Radionuclide studies are usually unhelpful in the diagnosis of vascular abnormalities unless there is active bleeding at the time of the study. $^{99}Tc^m$-labelled sulphur colloid or $^{99}Tc^m$-labelled red cells (McKusick *et al.*, 1981) may be used as a screening test to see if the patient is bleeding rapidly enough for formal angiography to identify the site of bleeding, and $^{99}Tc^m$-labelled sodium pertechnetate may be used to confirm a Meckel's diverticulum (Jewett, Duszinski and Allen, 1970).

If these investigations do not provide a diagnosis, laparotomy may be considered in the patient who continues to bleed but a positive diagnosis was made at laparotomy in only half the cases in a paediatric series (Shandling, 1965). With the variety of diagnostic methods now available, most lesions may be detected without the necessity for surgery. Laparotomy is best reserved to manage life-threatening haemorrhage rather than to identify an otherwise undetected lesion (Boley, Brandt and Frank, 1981). If diagnostic laparotomy is performed, it is wise to consider the use of intraoperative endoscopy. Perioperative colonoscopy of the large bowel extended through to the small bowel or the use of a long colonoscope or enteroscope through the small bowel from above may be valuable to transilluminate the intestinal wall in a search for vascular abnormalities. The surgeon views from the serosal aspect and pleats the bowel segments over the colonoscope, which is

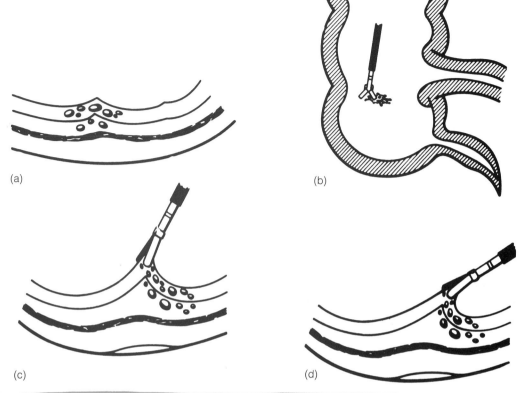

(a)

(b)

(c)

(d)

Figure 17.8   Coagulation of angiodysplasia using the technique with the hot biopsy forceps. (a) The superficial nature of the lesion in the mucosa and submucosa is seen. (b) The forceps are placed at the periphery of the lesion. The mucosa is grasped and pulled into the lumen and 'tented' over itself (d) as a short burst of low power current is applied.

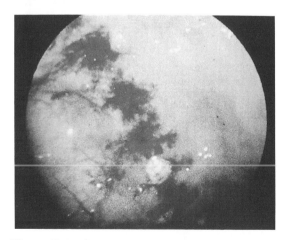

Figure 17.9   An extensive angiodysplasia lesion in the caecum with an area of ulceration seen at the lower part of the field of view.

passed under direct vision by the endoscopist (Bowden, Hooks and Mansberger, 1979; Forde, 1981).

17.7 TREATMENT

When bleeding is severe, initial efforts are directed towards resuscitation before identifying the site and cause of bleeding. Although most vascular abnormalities can present as gastrointestinal bleeding, many episodes are self limiting or lead to chronic blood loss. Emergency surgery may be necessary for life-threatening haemorrhage, but has an increased morbidity and mortality, therefore every attempt should be made to establish a diagnosis so that definitive elective surgery can be planned.

Limited angiodysplasia lesions in the caecum and right colon (Rogers, 1980; Howard, Buchanan and Hunt, 1982), and telangiectasia in the stomach (Weaver *et al.*, 1979; Farup *et al.*, 1981; Colin-Jones, 1984) have been treated at endoscopy by electrocoagulation using the William's coagulation forceps (Williams, 1973; Rogers, 1980; Howard, Buchanan and Hunt, 1982; Hunt, 1984a), a monopolar button electrode (Colin-Jones, 1984), the BICAP (Jensen, Machicado and Slipa, 1984; Johnston, Rawson and Namihira, 1985), the heater probe (Jensen, Machicado and Slipa, 1984; Johnston, Rawson and Namihira, 1985) or laser therapy (Fruhmorgen *et al.*, 1976; Kiefhaber *et al.*, 1977; Rutgeerts *et al.*, 1983; Bown *et al.*, 1985; Rutgeers *et al.*, 1985; Marcon *et al.*, 1985; Marcon, 1987; Jensen *et al.*, 1989; Marcon, 1989). However, most extensive vascular abnormalities will require resection.

Results of these less involved methods have been promising (Rogers, 1980; Howard, Buchanan and Hunt, 1982; Colin-Jones, 1984; Hunt, 1984a, b, Hunt *et al.*, 1984; Marcon, 1987), especially for angiodysplasia of the right colon and caecum, obviating the need for major surgery in an elderly high-risk population. For these lesions the coagulation forceps (Williams, 1973; Rogers, 1980; Howard, Buchanan and Hunt, 1982; Hunt, 1984a; Rogers, 1985) are preferable to the button electrode which is more likely to result in perforation of the thin-walled caecum. Several authors report their experience with the hot biopsy forceps with good results and a low complication rate (Rogers, 1980; Howard, Buchanan and Hunt, 1982; Hunt, 1984a; Marcon *et al.*, 1985; Rogers, 1985; Marcon, 1987). The coagulation biopsy forceps are placed at the periphery of the lesion and gently withdrawn until the mucosa is 'tented' towards the lumen of the colon (Howard, Buchanan and Hunt, 1982; Hunt, 1984a). This pulls the mucosa and submucosa away from the deeper layer of the colonic wall which is especially thin in the caecum and right colon, and decrease the very real risk of transmural coagulation or perforation. The apex of the 'tent' is then pulled asymmetrically over the centre of the lesion to enhance coagulation in the mucosa and submucosa at the site of angiodysplasia. Coagulation is usually performed at no more than 25 W applied in very short bursts to produce a well-controlled, small and superficial coagulation (Figure 17.10). Biopsies may be taken, and may confirm the diagnosis histologically. However, this may increase the risk of immediate or delayed perforation (Rogers, 1980; Hunt, 1984a) and photographic documentation is probably sufficient confirmation of the endoscopic diagnosis.

The heater probe and the BICAP are two new, portable and economical ways to achieve thermal coagulation by contact (Jensen, Machicado and Slipa, 1984; Johnston, Rawson and Namihira, 1985). The 10-Fr heater probe provides a larger surface and better coagulation effect. Gentle pressure is applied to the

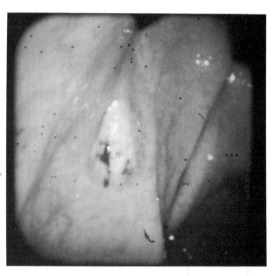

Figure 17.10 The effect of initial coagulation is seen following application of a short burst of low power currrent to the angiodysplasia lesion seen in Figure 17.4. A further limited burst of coagulation should be applied with the hot biopsy forceps placed at the 7 o'clock position to this lesion.

periphery of the lesion until blanching is seen and then subsequently greater pressure can be applied to the central vessels. The coaptive properties of these devices favours coagulation and sealing of the small vessels as they are compressed.

Laser photocoagulation with the argon ion or Nd–YAG has been widely used (Kiefhaber, Nath and Maritz, 1977; Rutgeerts et al., 1983; Bown et al., 1985; Rutgeerts et al., 1985; Jensen, Machicado and Slipa, 1984; Marcon, 1987) and general experience has shown that the Nd–YAG at a power setting of 70–85 W should be used for vascular lesions with the light guide 1–1.5 cm from the lesion with power delivered in short and rapid bursts, with up to 15 pulses for larger lesions to produce blanching around the lesion without vaporization. The coagulation should be just around the periphery of the lesion before the central area is coagulated. Particular difficulties may rise with access to lesions in the duodenum or in the colon when they lie on folds distal to the endoscope and these may be missed altogether or inadequately coagulated. Additional concerns with laser therapy have been complications and cost. Rutgeerts reported a complication rate of 6% in central lesions which may be related to distension of the right colon due to CO_2 insufflation (Rutgeerts et al., 1985). Jensen believes that coaptive electrocautery probes are as effective as argon ion laser for gastric angiodysplasia – and are cheaper (Jensen, Machicado and Slipa, 1984). Contact microprobes have recently been developed for the Nd–YAG laser (Tsunekawa et al., 1985) which reduce the power requirements to between 5 and 15 W and require little CO_2, thus potentially reducing the costs of laser therapy and in one early report suggesting better results for lesions which are otherwise inaccessible (Marcon, 1987). With all the methods discussed many patients will require more than a single treatment session (Howard, Buchanan and Hunt, 1982; Hunt, 1984a; Bown et al., 1985; Rutgeers et al., 1985; Marcon, 1987).

When vascular abnormalities are too numerous or extensive, patients should undergo upper gastrointestinal endoscopy, colonoscopy and triple vessel angiography prior to surgery to assess the full extent of the lesion, and peroperative endoscopy may be useful to define the point of resection.

REFERENCES

Allison, D. J., Hemingway, A. P. and Cunningham, D. A. (1982) Angiography in gastrointestinal bleeding. Lancet, ii, 30–3.

Baum, S., Athanasoulis, C. A. and Waltman, A. C. (1977) Angiodysplasia of the right colon: a cause of gastrointestinal bleeding. Am. J. Roentgenol., 129, 789–94.

Baum, S., Nusbaum, M., Blakemore, W. S. and Finkelstein, A. K. (1965) The preoperative radiographic demonstration of intra-abdominal bleeding from undetermined sites by percutaneous selective celiac and superior mesenteric arteriography. Surgery, 58, 797–805.

Blankenstein, M., Van Dees, J. and Tenkate, F. J. W. (1978) Bleeding arteriovenous malformations diagnosed by endoscopy. Gut, 19, 432.

Boley, S. J., Brandt, L. J. and Frank, M. S. (1981) Severe lower intestinal bleeding. Clin. Gastroenterol., 10, (1), 65–91.

Boley, S. J., Sammartano, R., Adamas, A. et al. (1977a) On the nature and aetiology of vascular ectasias of the colon: degenerative lesions of aging. Gastroenterology, 72, 650–60.

Boley, S. J., Sprayregan, S., Sammartano, R. J. et al. (1977b) The pathophysiologic basis for the angiographic signs of vascular ectasias of the colon. Diagn. Radiol., 125, 615–21.

Boss, E. G. and Rosenbaum, J. M. (1971) Bleeding from the right colon associated with aortic stenosis. Am. J. Dig. Dis., 16, 269–75.

Bourdette, D. and Greenberg, B. (1979) Twelve year history of gastrointestinal bleeding in a patient with calcific aortic stenosis and haemorrhagic telangiectasia. Dig. Dis. Sci., 24, 77–82.

Bowden, T. A., Hooks, V. H. and Mansberger, A. R. (1979) Intraoperative gastrointestinal endoscopy. Ann. Surg., 191, 680–7.

Bown, S. G., Swain, C. P., Storey, D. W. et al. (1985) Endoscopic laser treatment of vascular abnormalities of the upper gastrointestinal tract. Gut, 26, 1338–48.

Calam, J. and Walker, R. J. (1980) Antral vascular lesion, achlorhydria and chronic gastrointestinal blood loss. Dig. Dis. Sci., 25, 236–9.

Cass, A. J., Bliss, B. P., Bolton, R. P. and Cooper, B.

T. (1980) Gastrointestinal bleeding, angiodysplasia of the colon and acquired Von Willebrand's disease. *Br. J. Surg.*, **67**, 639–41.

Catem, W. S. and Jiminez, F. A. (1963) Vascular malformations of the intestines: their role as a source of haemorrhage. *Arch. Surg.*, **85**, 571–9.

Colin-Jones, D. G. (1984) Vascular malformations of the upper G.I. tract, in *Advances in Gastrointestinal Endoscopy* (ed. P. R. Salmon), Chapman and Hall, London.

Danesh, B. J. Z., Spiliadis, C., Williams, C. B. and Zambamtas, C. M. (1987) Angiodysplasia – an uncommon cause of colonic bleeding: colonoscopic evaluation of 1050 patients with rectal bleeding and anemia. *Int. J. Colorectal.*, **2**, 218–22.

Dieulefoy, G. (1912) *A Textbook of Medicine* (English translation by V. E. Collins and J. A. Liebman), Appleton, New York, pp. 666–80.

Farup, P. G., Roseland, A., Stray, N. *et al.* (1981) Localised telangiopathy of the stomach and duodenum diagnosed and treated endoscopically. *Endoscopy*, **12**, 1–6.

Forde, K. A. (1981) Intraoperative colonoscopy, in *Colonoscopy Techniques, Clinical Practice and Colour Atlas* (eds) (R. H. Hunt and J. D. Waye), Chapman and Hall, London, pp. 189–98.

Foster, C. A., Yomehiro, E. G. and Benjamin, R. B. (1978) Oesophageal haemangioma. *Ear, Nose Throat J.*, **57**, 455–9.

Fruhmorgen, P., Bodem, F., Reidenbach, H. D. *et al.* (1976) Endoscopic laser coagulation of bleeding gastrointestinal lesions with report of the first therapeutic application in man. *Gastrointest. Endosc.*, **23**, 73–5.

Galloway, S. J., Casarella, W. J. and Shimkin, P. M. (1974) Vascular malformations of the right colon as a cause of bleeding in patients with aortic stenosis. *Radiology*, **113**, 11–15.

Gentry, R. W., Dockerty, M. B. and Clagett, O. T. (1949) Vascular malformations and vascular tumours of the gastrointestinal tract. *Int. Abstr. Surg.*, **88**, 281–323.

Giacchino, J. L., Geis, W. P., Pickleman, J. R. *et al.* (1979) Changing perspectives in massive lower intestinal haemorrhage. *Surgery*, **86**, 368–76.

Heald, R. J. and Ray, J. E. (1974) Vascular malformations of the intestine: an important cause of obscure gastrointestinal haemorrhage. *South. Med. J.*, **67**, 33–8.

Howard, O. M., Buchanan, J. D. and Hunt, R. H. (1982) Angiodysplasia of the colon: experience of 26 cases. *Lancet*, **ii**, 16–19.

Hunt, R. H. (1984) Angiodysplasia of the colon, in *Advances in Gastrointestinal Endoscopy* (ed. P. R.

Salmon), Chapman and Hall, London, pp. 97–114.

Hunt, R. H. (1984) Angiodysplasia of the gut, in *Textbook of Gastroenterology* (eds I. A. D. Bouchier, R. N. Allan, H. J. F. Hodgson and M. R. B. Keighley), Ballière Tindall, London, pp. 259–66.

Imperiale, T. F. and Ransohoff, D. F. (1988) Aortic stenosis, idiopathic gastrointestinal bleeding and angiodysplasia: is there an association? *Gastroenterol.*, **95**, 1670–6.

Jabbari, M., Cherry, R., Lough, J. O. *et al.* (1984) Gastric antral vascular ectasia: the watermelon stomach. *Gastroenterology.*, **87**, 1165.

Jensen, D. M., Machicado, G. A. and Slipa, M. L. (1984) Argon laser vs heater probe on BICAP for control of severe ulcer bleeding. *Gastrointest. Endosc.*, **30**, 134.

Jensen, D., Machicada, G., Kovacs, T., Randall, G. and Reedy, T. (1989) Diagnosis and treatment of severe UGI bleeding from angiomata. *Gastroenterol.*, **96**, 5, A238.

Jewett, T. C., Duszinski, D. O. and Allen, J. F. (1970) The visualization of Meckel's diverticulum with ^{99m}Tc pertechnetate. *Surgery*, **68**, 567–70.

Johnston, J., Rawson, S. and Namihira, Y. (1985) Experimental comparison of heater probe and BICAP for endoscopic treatment of gastrointestinal bleeding. *Gastrointest. Endosc.*, **31**, 155–6.

Kiefhaber, P., Nath, G. and Maritz, K. (1977) Endoscopical control of massive gastrointestinal hemorrhage by irradiation with a high power Nd-YAG laser. *Prog. Surg.*, **15**, 140.

Lewis, T. D., Laufer, I. and Goodacre, R. L. (1978) Arteriovenous malformation of the stomach. *Dig. Dis.*, **23**, 467–71.

Lewis, B. S. and Waye, J. D. (1988) Total small bowel enteroscopy. *Gastrointest. Endosc.*, **33**, 435–8.

McCormack, T. T., Sims, J., Eyre Brook, I. *et al.* (1985) Gastric lesions in portal hypertension: inflammatory gastritis or congestive gastropathy. *Gut*, **26**, 1226–32.

McGrath, K. M., Johnson, C. A. and Stuart, J. J. (1979) Acquired von Willebrand disease associated with an inhibitor to factor VIII antigen and gastrointestinal telangiectasis. *Am. J. Med.*, **67**, 693–6.

McKusick, K. A., Froelich, J., Callahan, R. J. *et al.* (1981) ^{99m}Tc red blood cells for detection of gastrointestinal bleeding: experience with 80 patients. *Am. J. Roentgenol.*, **137**, 1113–8.

Marcon, N. E. (1987) The endoscopic management of angiodysplasia. *Acta Endoscopica*, **17**, (3), 109–19.

Marcon, N. E., Haber, G. B., Kortan, P. P. and Cohen, L. (1985) Gastroduodenal angiodysplasia

– an under diagnosed cause of upper gastrointestinal bleeding. *Gastrointest. Endosc.*, **31**, 167.

Margulis, A. R., Heinbecker, P. and Bernard, H. R. (1960) Operative mesenteric arteriography in the search for the site of bleeding in unexplained gastrointestinal bleeding. *Surgery*, **48**, 534–9.

Marnon, N. E. (1990) Lasers in Gastrointestinal Haemorrhage. *European J. Gastroenterol. and Hepatol.* **2** (in press).

Miller, K. D., Tutton, R. H., Bell, K. A. and Simon, B. K. (1979) Angiodysplasia of the colon. *Radiology*, **132**, 309–13.

Mitsudo, S. M., Boley, S. J., Brandt, L. J. *et al.* (1979) Vascular ectasias of the right colon in the elderly: a district pathological entity. *Hum. Pathol.*, **10**, 585–600.

Moore, J. D., Thompson, N. W., Appelman, H. D. and Foley, D. (1978) Arteriovenous malformations of the gastrointestinal tract. *Arch. Surg.*, **111**, 381–9.

Nagy, G. S. (1981) Preparing the patient, in *Colonoscopy, Techniques, Clinical Practice and Colour Atlas* (eds R. H. Hunt and J. D. Wayne), Chapman and Hall, London, pp. 19–26.

Phillips, B. (1839) Surgical cases. *Lond. Med. Gaz.*, **23**, 514–7.

Posner, D. E. and Sampliner, R. E. (1978) Hereditary haemorrhagic telangiectasis in three black men. *Am. J. Gastroenterol.*, **70**, 389–92.

Quintero, E., Pigne, J. M., Bombi, J. A. *et al.* (1987) Gastric mucosal vascular ectasias causing bleeding in cirrhosis. *Gastroenterology*, **93**, 1054–61.

Ramsay, D. J., MacLeod, D. A. D., Buist, T. A. S. and Heading, R. C. (1976) Persistent gastrointestinal bleeding due to angiodysplasia of the gut in Von Willebrand's disease. *Lancet*, **ii**, 275–8.

Roberts, L. K., Gold, R. E. and Routt, W. E. (1981) Gastric angiodysplasia. *Radiology*, **139**, 355–9.

Rogers, B. H. G. (1980) Endoscopic diagnosis and therapy of mucosal vascular abnormality of the gastrointestinal tract occurring in elderly patients and associated with cardiac, vascular and pulmonary disease. *Gastrointest. Endosc.*, **26**, 134–8.

Rogers, B. H. G. (1985) The electrocoagulation forceps is ideal for the diagnosis and management of small vascular abnormalities of the cecal area. *Gastrointest. Endosc.*, **31**, 222–4.

Rogers, B. H. G. and Adler, F. (1976) Hemangiomas of the caecum. *Gastroenterology*, **71**, 1079 –82.

Rutgeerts, P., Van Gompel, F., Geboes, K. *et al.* (1985) Long term results of treatment of vascular malformations of the gastrointestinal tract by Nd–YAG laser photocoagulation. *Gut*, **26**, 586 –93.

Rutgeerts, P., Vantrappen, G., Geboes, K. and Broeckaerk, L. (1983) Nd–YAG laser photocoagulation for hemostasis of gastrointestinal non-variceal hemorrhage. *Gastroenterology*, **21**, 263–7.

Shandling, B. (1965) Laparotomy for rectal bleeding. *Pediatrics*, **35**, 787–93.

Skibba, R. M., Hartong, W. A., Mantz, F. A. *et al.* (1976) Angiodysplasia of the caecum: colonoscopic diagnosis. *Gastrointest. Endosc.*, **22**, 177–9.

Tarin, D., Allison, D. J., Modlin, I. M. and Neale, G. (1978) Diagnosis and management of obscure gastrointestinal bleeding. *Br. Med. J.*, **2**, 751–4.

Tradel, J. L., Fazio, V. F. and Sivak, M. V. (1988) Colonoscopic diagnosis and treatment of arteriovenous malformations in chronic lower gastrointestinal bleeding. *Dis Colon. Rect.*, **31**, 107–10.

Tsunekawa, H., Morise, K., Ilzuka, A. *et al.* (1985) Studies on the application of the newly developed laser microprobes for the Nd–YAG laser, in *Proceedings of the 7th International Congress with 2nd International Nd–YAG Laser Conference* (eds W. Waidelich and P. Kiefhaber), Springer-Verlag, New York, pp. 360–6.

VanZanten, V., Bartelsman, J. F. W. M., Schipper, M. E. J. and Tytgat, G. N. J. (1986) Recurrent massive hematemasis from Dieulofoy vascular malformations – a review of 101 cases. *Gut*, **27**, 213–22.

Wangensteen, O. H. (1955) *Intestinal Obstruction*, 3rd edn, C. C. Thomas, Springfield, Illinois.

Weaver, G. A., Alpern, H. D., Davis, J. S. *et al.* (1979) Gastrointestinal angiodysplasia associated with aortic valve disease: part of a spectrum of angiodysplasia of the gut. *Gastroenterology*, **77**, 1–11.

Wheeler, M. H., Smith, P. M., Cotton, P. B. *et al.* (1979) Abnormal blood vessels in the gastric antrum. *Dig. Dis. Sci.*, **24**, 155–8.

Williams, C. B. (1973) Diathermy-biopsy: a technique of endoscopic management of small polyps. *Endoscopy*, **5**, 215–8.

Williams, R. C. Jr (1961) Aortic stenosis and unexplained gastrointestinal bleeding. *Arch. Intern. Med.*, **108**, 859–63.

CHAPTER EIGHTEEN

Colonic angiodysplasia: radiology

D. J. Allison
and
A. P. Hemingway

18.1 INTRODUCTION

Angiodysplasia is the term used to describe a condition of unknown aetiology in which microvascular abnormalities are found in the mucosa and submucosa of the bowel wall. The lesions which are usually found in the caecum and right side of the colon are frequently associated with either intermittent acute or chronic intestinal blood loss. There is no recognized association with vascular abnormalities in other organs, and no known hereditary factors exist.

The lesions of angiodysplasia are very small (less than 5 mm in diameter), often multiple and can be diagnosed by either endoscopy or angiography. They cannot be detected on barium studies and are invisible to the naked eye at laparotomy. The pathologist has great difficulty in localizing the lesions in a resected specimen unless it has been subjected to special injection techniques (see below) prior to fixation and sectioning. The lesions are thought to represent a distinct benign pathological entity, characterized in their early stage by dilated tortuous submucosal veins. In more advanced stages of the disorder further dilatation of the submucosal veins, venules and capillaries occurs (Mitsudo *et al.*, 1979); these characteristic features corresponding to the definition given by Gentry, Dockerty and Claggert (1949) of telangiectasias, i.e. dilatation of pre-existing vascular structures. Galdibini in 1974 first used the term 'angiodysplasia' to describe the pathological

abnormality found in a patient who presented with what is now recognized as a characteristic history and the angiographic features of the condition described above.

Angiodysplasia is thought to represent the commonest single cause of obscure gastrointestinal bleeding in the elderly population (Boley *et al.*, 1977). A number of published series have established that in patients undergoing visceral angiography for the investigation of obscure gastrointestinal blood loss, the most commonly detected abnormality is angiodysplasia (Sheedy, Fulton and Atwell, 1975; Allison, Hemingway and Cunningham, 1982). It must be remembered, however, that these patients undergoing angiography represent a highly selected group; the cause of gastrointestinal bleeding is identified by other routine investigations in between 80% and 95% of cases (Spiller and Parkins, 1983), which means that only a small proportion of all patients with bleeding come to angiography (Hemingway, 1988).

Angiography was for many years the only method of making the diagnosis of angiodysplasia and remains the yardstick against which other diagnostic methods are measured. Endoscopy has acquired an increasingly important role in the management of the disease, being useful not only in diagnosis, but also in therapy. Which of the two methods of investigation should be performed in an individual patient depends to a large extent on local expertise. It is our opinion that the highest diagnostic yield and accuracy of determination of the extent of disease are achieved when both techniques are employed in all patients. A negative angiogram or endoscopy examination in isolation does not exclude the condition, and both techniques are capable of diagnosing other diseases related or unrelated to the patient's presenting symptoms.

This account will discuss the following questions about angiography in the management of angiodysplasia:

1. Which patients should have angiography and when should it be performed?
2. Who should undertake the study and where?
3. How should the study be carried out?
4. What features suggest the diagnosis of angiodysplasia?
5. What are the hazards and complications of angiography?
6. How successful and accurate is the procedure?
7. What is the role of specimen angiography?

18.2 PATIENTS SUITABLE FOR ANGIOGRAPHY

Patients who are referred for angiography fall into two categories: those bleeding rapidly and acutely, and those who have a history of intermittent acute or chronic bleeding. Angiography should only be performed in the 'acute' situation if the patient is clearly bleeding at the time of the study. There is very little virtue in mobilizing an angiographic team at 2.00 a.m. to perform a study on a patient who bled at 10.00 p.m. but 4 hours later is haemodynamically stable and exhibits no clinical features to suggest continued bleeding. This patient should first be investigated with less invasive techniques. In a patient with active bleeding emergency angiography is often successful in localizing the site of haemorrhage and a small percentage of patients with angiodysplasia (about 12%) present in this manner. The vast majority however suffer from chronic blood loss and come to elective angiography only when other investigations have failed to localize a source of bleeding, or when another abnormality has already been treated but the blood loss continues. Patients in this 'chronic' category referred for angiography should previously have undergone upper gastrointestinal endoscopy, colonoscopy, and small intestinal barium studies to exclude causes of bleeding such as peptic ulcers, tumours, diverticula, parasitic infestation, haemorrhoids, blood dyscrasias, etc. Logistically a visceral angiogram cannot be performed for several days following a barium study as residual barium in the abdomen obscures fine vascular detail. This factor must be borne in mind when arranging sequential investigations and it should also be remembered that a computerized tomographic scan with bowel enhancement also precludes subsequent angiography for between 3 and 5 days.

18.3 OPERATORS AND EQUIPMENT NEEDED FOR ANGIOGRAPHY

Selective visceral angiography should only be performed by radiologists experienced in arteriographic techniques and their interpretation. Moderately sophisticated angiographic equipment is essential to allow an appropriate sequence of high-quality images to be acquired. A wide range of catheters and guide-wires should be available to enable the radiologist to deal with variable or difficult anatomy. Although it may be possible to obtain a three-vessel study in many institutions (see below), the ability to perform superselective examinations and, more importantly, expertise in interpretation of the studies may not be available. The abnormal angiographic features of some conditions including angiodysplasia are very subtle and may be missed by an inexperienced observer.

18.4 TECHNIQUE OF ANGIOGRAPHY

Having considered that visceral angiography is appropriate in a particular case the procedure is discussed with the patient and informed consent obtained. It is important to elicit any history of severe allergy or asthma so that steroid prophylaxis may be instituted if it is deemed essential to proceed with the examination. A history of previous intestinal or vascular surgery is important as this may considerably alter the vascular anatomy. Examination of peripheral pulses is essential as absence of the femoral pulses will entail a brachial or axillary approach for which it is prudent to obtain specific consent from the patient. The patient should shave both groins prior to the study and should not be dehydrated. Adequate premedication is very important as the procedure may prove to be long and uncomfortable. Five milligrams of diazepam orally is NOT sufficient. Patients should receive an analgesic (e.g. omnopon) and a sedative (e.g. lorazepam) in doses appropriate for weight and age, about 1 hour prior to the procedure. On arrival in the angiographic suite the radiographic staff should take a preliminary radiograph of the abdominal area to assess the correct exposure factors and identify any pre-existing radiopaque areas. Visceral angiography is almost invariably performed under local anaesthesia. Five to ten millilitres of 2% lignocaine is infiltrated into the soft tissues around the femoral artery in the groin. The correct anatomical site for anaesthesia (and subsequent puncture) is the point at which the artery can be felt most easily and this is also the point at which it can usually be most effectively compressed against bone at the end of the examination. The femoral artery is punctured using the Seldinger needle/guide-wire/catheter exchange technique described in standard texts (Allison, 1986). In adults 5–7 Fr torque control catheters are most commonly used and a wide variety of shapes of catheter is available. The most useful for selective visceral studies are the femorocerebral B (sidewinder) I, II or III and the femorovisceral (cobra) I, II or III. For diagnostic studies catheters with both end- and side-ports should be used.

There is some controversy over the requirement for performing a flush aortogram routinely as part of mesenteric arteriography. On the positive side an aortogram defines the approximate position, condition and course of the principal mesenteric vessels which may assist in their subsequent catheterization, will allow evaluation of any abnormality of the aorta itself, and reveal unexpected retroperitoneal pathology that could be responsible for the patient's bleeding (or even if not, might nevertheless still have relevance to their subsequent management). In addition there are certain disorders responsible for gastrointestinal bleeding such as an aortoduodenal fistula or an aortodiverticular communication that may only be demonstrated by an aortic study and give apparently normal appearances on selective vascular studies. On the negative side it is rare in practice for any significant contribution to be made by an aortic flush, and the examination (which to be done properly entails both anteroposterior and lateral studies) imposes delay, additional radiation, additional contrast load and an extra catheter exchange in an already lengthy examination.

The decision to perform general aortic studies is one that needs to be taken in the light of the circumstances obtaining in each individual case, but it seems reasonable to suggest that relatively inexperienced operators should always include them in their examination as there is little to lose and potentially information to be gained by doing so.

When the preliminary aortic studies (if indicated) have been completed, an appropriately shaped catheter is introduced selectively into the visceral vessels under fluoroscopic control. In patients with a history of chronic intestinal blood loss all three main visceral vessels should be examined, as clinical assessment of the level of bleeding in the alimentary tract is at best unreliable and at worst misleading. In order to avoid unnecessary catheterization of the urinary bladder it is advisable to study the inferior mesenteric artery (IMA) first before contrast medium accumulates in the bladder and obscures vascular detail in the rectum and sigmoid. It is usually necessary to examine the lower and upper IMA by two separate injections of contrast medium to ensure that the entire territory is examined. The lower IMA is studied with the patient in a 35° right anterior oblique projection to 'unwind' the sigmoid; the upper end is examined in a 35–65° left anterior oblique projection to unfold the splenic flexure.

The radiographic contrast medium is injected by hand into the IMA using a 10-ml syringe. It is important to have the tip of the catheter well enough into the vessel so that no contrast medium refluxes into the aorta. At the same time the catheter must not be so far in as to pass the origin of the left colic artery. The IMA is a small and sensitive vessel which readily goes into spasm, so care must be taken with catheterization. It is advisable to employ a low-osmolar or non-ionic contrast medium for examination of the IMA to minimize discomfort.

An image is obtained immediately before contrast medium injection (to act as a mask for subtraction). Further images should then be obtained during the arterial, capillary and venous phases, up to 20 seconds after the beginning of contrast injection (e.g. 2 f.p.s. (films per second) for 4 s, 0.5 f.p.s. for 12 s, 1 f.p.s. for 5 seconds). It is advisable to leave the catheter in place until the radiographs have been developed and reviewed. If the images are technically satisfactory and no further pictures are required the catheter is repositioned in either the coeliac axis or superior mesenteric artery (SMA). If angiodysplasia is suspected clinically it is sensible to study the coeliac axis next to exclude pathology in this region before concentrating one's efforts on the SMA territory where superselective studies, possibly requiring a catheter change,

may be required. It is desirable to opacify the splenic artery, left gastric artery, hepatic vessels and gastroduodenal artery. The catheter is lodged securely in the main coeliac trunk and 30–50 ml of contrast medium delivered at 6–8 ml/s using a mechanical pump. Images are acquired in a similar sequence to that described for the IMA. It is important to demonstrate the splenic and portal venous phases of the study to exclude varices.

The catheter can then be positioned in the SMA. As with the IMA it is almost always necessary to study the SMA with two separate injections, to ensure demonstration of the entire vascular territory. The filming sequence is the same; 40 ml at 6–8 ml/s is an appropriate contrast volume and delivery rate (although this may require modification if digital vascular imaging equipment is being used).

It may prove necessary to perform superselective studies of branches of one of the major vessels to clarify a suspected abnormality seen on a general study of the parent vessel. This occasionally requires a change of catheter but more often than not the original catheter will suffice. The filming sequence, contrast volume and rate of injection will depend on the nature of the lesion and size of the vessel selected.

All images should be reviewed before the catheter is withdrawn from the body. As a general guide the total volume of radiographic contrast medium used in a single elective angiogram in a patient with normal renal function should not exceed 3 ml/kg body weight (1100 mg iodine/kg) with an absolute maximum of 4 ml/kg body weight (i.e. a total of 103 gm iodine in a 70-kg man).

At the completion of the study the catheter is withdrawn from the femoral artery and firm digital pressure applied to produce haemostasis. This usually takes about 10 minutes, but in elderly and hypertensive patients may take longer. It is essential that proper haemostasis is secured before the patient leaves the angiographic suite. A significant groin haematoma should never occur if appropriate care is taken; in patients on anticoagulants, or in whom multiple catheter exchanges have been necessary, particular care is required.

It is customary for the patient to remain in bed for 12 hours after the procedure while the groin puncture site is observed frequently. With the smaller calibre catheters being used for digital subtraction angiography (DSA) systems, however, modifications in this regimen are now occurring with shortening of the period of close observation. The procedures are also performed in outpatients in some institutions. Adequate hydration to ensure excretion of contrast medium is essential.

18.5 ARTERIOGRAPHIC FEATURES SUGGESTING THE DIAGNOSIS (Hemingway, 1988)

Angiodysplasia usually occurs in the caecum and right colon in the territory supplied by the ileocolic and right colic arteries, although it may be demonstrated in the transverse or descending colon. The characteristic features of angiodysplasia include vascular tufts on the antimesenteric border of the colon during the arterial phase; an early filling and slowly emptying draining vein and a dilated tortuous 'intramural' vein (Figure 18.1). In our institutions we normally require at least two of these

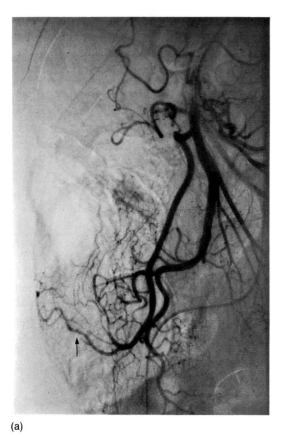
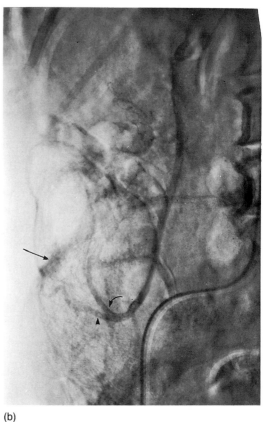

(a)   (b)

Figure 18.1   A selective ileocolic subtraction arteriogram. In the arterial phase (a) a prominent vessel is seen supplying the antimesenteric border of the caecum (arrow). In the venous phase (b) vascular lakes can be seen on the antimesenteric border (arrow); there is a prominent 'intramural' vein (arrowhead) and a large draining vein (curved arrow).

three features to be present before the diagnosis is suggested. Angiodysplasia can only definitely be implicated as the cause of blood loss if the lesions are seen to be actively bleeding at the time of the angiogram. Some radiologists advocate that the colon should be distended with air during the study and that direct serial magnification radiography should be used to improve the chances of detection of angiodysplasia. We have not used these techniques, finding that selective catheterization, the use of adequate volumes of contrast medium and high-quality radiography are the most important factors.

The angiographic features of angiodysplasia may be mimicked by other conditions including malignancy and inflammatory bowel disease (e.g. Crohn's disease). These other diseases must be excluded by colonoscopy, barium enema or, if appropriate, even laparotomy, before the diagnosis of angiodysplasia is accepted.

18.6 HAZARDS AND COMPLICATIONS OF ANGIOGRAPHY

In *experienced* hands the risks of diagnostic angiography are low, but nevertheless it is an invasive procedure and should not be undertaken lightly. A variety of complications (Table 18.1) have been reported; some are related to any angiographic procedure, others are specific to visceral studies.

18.7 SUCCESS AND ACCURACY OF ANGIOGRAPHY

The success of the procedure depends on a number of factors including technical expertise, good radiography (adequate exposure, centring and collimation, etc.), the use of correct contrast volumes, and the ability to interpret the images.

In acute haemorrhage the success rate of angiography in demonstrating an actively bleeding site exceeds 90% (Allison, Hemingway and Cunningham, 1982).

Table 18.1 Potential complications of visceral angiography

Vessel dissection	– at puncture site
	– selective vessels
Haematoma	– at puncture site
Distal embolization	– leg or gut vessels
Contrast medium reactions and overload radiation	
Carotid/vertebral damage/embolus, from catheter manipulation in the aortic arch	

In chronic bleeding an abnormality is detected at angiography which could be responsible for the patient's symptoms in approximately 70% of cases (Allison, Hemingway and Cunningham, 1982). It can only be presumed that this is the causative lesion unless active bleeding is demonstrated. Within this group angiodysplasia represents the single most common lesion detected: in one published series (Allison, Hemingway and Cunningham, 1982) angiodysplasia was diagnosed in 40% of patients examined. The accuracy of angiography is clearly difficult to determine, since the diagnosis can only be regarded as confirmed if the lesions are seen at colonoscopy, or if the symptoms are cured following resection of the affected segment of bowel and there is pathological confirmation of the angiodysplasia condition. Using these criteria in our own studies the accuracy of angiography in diagnosing angiodysplasia exceeds 90%.

18.8 ROLE OF SPECIMEN ANGIOGRAPHY

The lesions of angiodysplasia are small, invisible to the naked eye on examination of the mucosa. It is neither possible nor practicable for the pathologist to section an entire right hemicolectomy specimen and so the diagnosis may not be confirmed unless special localization methods are employed. Injection of the specimen (after resection) with a barium gelatine mixture considerably facilitates pathological confirmation (Allison and Hemingway, 1981).

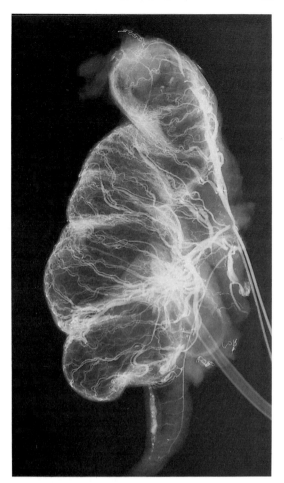

Figure 18.2 Radiograph of a resected colonic specimen in which the vessels have been perfused with a barium gelatine mixture.

The specimen is collected fresh from the operating theatre and the vessels cannulated and flushed through with a warm heparin-saline solution. The vessels are then perfused with a warm barium gelatine mixture (Figure 18.2) until the mixture is seen to exude from the cut ends of the specimen and the veins. The inside of the specimen is then washed with saline and the cut ends tied. The specimen is distended with formalin and fixed for 24 hours before dissecting microscope and pathological examination. It is important to cut the specimen along the mesenteric border to avoid destroying the lesions of angiodysplasia which are usually located on the anti-mesenteric border and may be readily identified on the mucosal surface filled with barium (Figures 18.3 and 18.4). Appropriate areas can then be subjected to histological examination.

18.9 ROLE OF EMBOLIZATION

Percutaneous therapeutic vascular embolization techniques have been widely employed in a variety of conditions including gastrointestinal haemorrhage (Chapter 16). The technique has been used safely and successfully in the upper gastrointestinal tract in both acute and chronic haemorrhage, but its role in

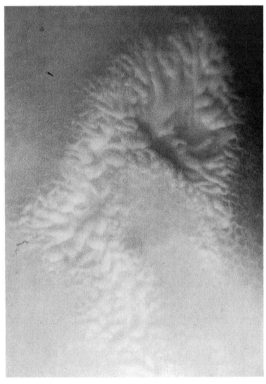

Figure 18.3 The dissecting microscope appearances of angiodysplasia in a resected specimen that has been injected with a barium gelatine mixture. The normal honeycomb mucosal pattern is seen to be disrupted by enlarged tortuous vessels which have filled with barium.

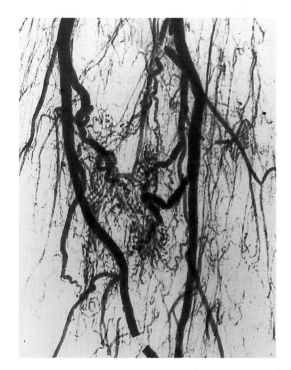

Figure 18.4 Microradiograph of an area of angiodysplasia. The cluster of abnormal vessels is clearly seen and the very large draining veins can be identified.

the management of lesions in the small and large bowel is less clearly defined and potentially more hazardous, for several reasons. In the stomach and duodenum, provided that there has been no surgery, it is possible to embolize, say, the left gastric artery or the gastroduodenal artery with particulate emboli with little risk of organ necrosis. In the small bowel the vascular anastomoses are so rich that an attempt to occlude a bleeding point would require the embolization of numerous vessels which would carry an unacceptably high risk of bowel infarction. In the large bowel individual colonic vessels supply fairly well defined and distinct areas. In a patient with angiodysplasia of the caecum and ascending colon successful obliteration of the bleeding points would require the complete occlusion of the ileocolic, and possibly the right colic, arteries. This would at best result

in ischaemia and stricture formation and at worst infarction and bowel perforation. The two other forms of treatment (surgery and colonoscopic fulguration) are less hazardous, and therefore are to be preferred. In the rare instance of a patient who is actively bleeding from colonic angiodysplasia, where neither of the above treatment options is available or suitable, then embolization with a temporary agent such as sterispon can be considered, provided that the potential complications have been considered and accepted by all parties involved.

18.10 CONCLUSION

Angiodysplasia is a common cause of obscure gastrointestinal bleeding, a major and expensive cause of morbidity. Colonoscopy, if available expertise exists, is the first line of investigation. However it is not always possible to view the entire colon due to tortuosity or faecal contamination. Angiography is an accurate means of making the diagnosis, but is more invasive and requires more sophisticated equipment and greater expertise than colonoscopy. In some institutions angiography will be used as a first-line investigation, but is probably best reserved for those in whom endoscopy has failed, is negative or equivocal. The use of both techniques in a complementary fashion gives the highest diagnostic yield.

REFERENCES

Allison, D. J. (1986) Angiography, in *Diagnostic Radiology: An Anglo-American Textbook of Organ Imaging*, vol. III (eds R. G. Grainger and D. J. Allison), Churchill Livingstone, Edinburgh.

Allison, D. J. and Hemingway, A. P. (1981) Angiodysplasia: does old age begin at nineteen? *Lancet*, ii, 979–80.

Allison, D. J., Hemingway, A. P. and Cunningham, D. A. (1982) Angiography in gastrointestinal bleeding. *Lancet*, ii, 30–3.

Boley, S. J., Sammartano, R., Adams, A. *et al.* (1977) On the nature and etiology of vascular ectasias of the colon: degenerative lesions of ageing. *Gastroenterology*, **72**, 650–60.

Galdibini (1974) Case records of the Massachusetts General Hospital 1974. Case 36. *N. Engl. J. Med.*, **291**, 569–75.

Gentry, R. W., Dockerty, M. B. and Claggett, O. T. (1949) Vascular malformations and vascular tumours of the gastrointestinal tract. *Int. Abstr. Surg.*, **88**, 281–323.

Hemingway, A. P. (1988) Angiodysplasia: current concepts. *Postgrad. Med. J.*, **64**, 259–63.

Mitsudo, S. M., Boley S. J., Brandt, L. J. *et al.* (1979) Vascular ectasias of the right colon in the elderly: a distinct pathological entity. *Hum. Pathol.*, **10**, 585–600.

Sheedy, P. F., Fulton, R. E. and Atwell, D. T. (1975) Angiographic evaluation of patients with chronic gastrointestinal bleeding. *A.J.R.*, **123**, 338–47.

Spiller, R. C. and Parkins, R. A. (1983) Recurrent gastrointestinal bleeding of obscure origin: report of 17 cases and a guide to logical management. *Br. J. Surg.*, **70**, 489–93.

CHAPTER NINETEEN

Gastroduodenal polyps

A. Ghazi

19.1 HISTORY

A gastric polyp was first described by Amatus Lusitanus in 1557 and later Morgagni (1761) reported the first duodenal polyp. The first fluoroscopic documentation of a gastric polyp is attributed to Heinz (1911) and this was followed by radiographic delineation of a gastric polyp by Myer (1912). Endoscopic visualization of a gastric polyp was described at examination with a rigid gastroscope passed by Schindler (1922). Until recently the management of gastroduodenal polyps was by radiological follow-up (Marshak and Feldman, 1965) or surgical removal (Brunn and Pearl, 1926), either by gastrotomy and local excision or by gastric resection.

Tsuneoka *et al.* (1968) published the first report of gastric polypectomy by the endoscopic route, using a fibreoptic scope, and this was shortly followed by numerous similar reports such as those by Aper *et al.* (1975), Minzuno, Kobayashi and Kasugai (1975) and Seifert and Elster (1975). This technique represents a notable departure and advance from the classical surgical approach.

19.2 CLINICAL MATERIAL

We began doing fibreoptic endoscopic gastroduodenal polypectomy in 1973. Over the ensuing years, fibreoptic endoscopic gastroduodenal polypectomy has gradually become routine. In the past 13 years over 850 gastroduodenal polyps have been removed at our institution. On occasions when an invasive carcinoma was found in an otherwise benign-appearing polyp, the patient was treated by surgery. We have previously reported on part of our own experience (Ghazi, Ferstenberg and Shinya, 1984).

During a 6-year period, starting in 1976 and ending in 1982, we treated 257 patients for gastroduodenal polyps, from whom a total of 443 polyps were removed. Of these 399 were gastric and 44 were duodenal. One hundred and eighty-five of these patients (72.3%) had a single polyp; the remainder had two or more. Polyps occurred with the same frequency in male and female patients. Polyp sizes ranged from 0.3 cm to 6.0 cm in diameter. Grossly, 63% of the polyps were sessile and 37% appeared pedunculated. The group included seven patients with Peutz–Jeghers syndrome.

19.3 SYMPTOMS

Epigastric pain was the major complaint in the majority of the patients, and ranged in intensity from mild epigastric discomfort to severe ulcer-type pain. Endoscopy frequently revealed one or more associated conditions such as reflux oesophagitis, gastroduodenitis, superficial gastroduodenal erosions or ulcer which could have contributed to the pain. Infrequently, partial obstruction of either the pylorus or the duodenum may have been contributory. Marshak and Feldman (1965) have suggested that ulceration of a polyp might account for both anaemia and pain. Nausea was present in 14% of cases but vomiting was rare. Anaemia from chronic blood loss was observed in 13% of patients but haematemesis or melaena was rare. Twenty-three patients (8.9%) had no symptoms, their polyps being discovered in the course of study for an unrelated surgical or medical condition.

19.4 HISTOLOGICAL CLASSIFICATION

Our pathologists utilize the World Health Organization (WHO) classification described by Oota and Sobin (1977) (Table 19.1). More recent and more detailed classifications have been suggested by Hattori (1985) and by Nakamura and Nakano (1985). Their worth remains to be established.

19.5 GASTRIC POLYPS

In the stomach, the most common type of polyp encountered was the hyperplastic variety. These were located principally in the body and antral portions of the stomach. In contrast, hyperplastic polyps are rarely found in the duodenum (two out of 272). In terms of gross configuration, hyperplastic polyps are round or oval in shape, have a smooth or

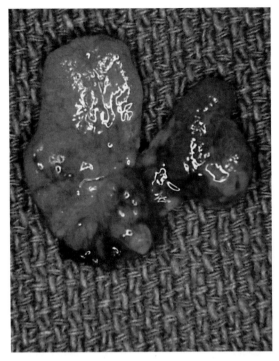

Figure 19.1 A large benign hyperplastic polyp of the antrum which was presumed to be the cause of acute upper gastrointestinal bleeding.

Table 19.1 Histological classifications of gastric tumour (WHO)

 I. Epithelial tumours
    A. Benign (adenoma)
    B. Malignant (carcinoma)
 II. Carcinoid tumours
 III. Non-epithelial tumours
 IV. Haematopoietic and lymphoid neoplasm
 V. Miscellaneous Tumours
 VI. Secondary tumours
 VII. Unclassified tumours
 VIII. Tumour-like lesions
    A. Hyperplastic polyps
    B. Inflammatory fibroid polyps
    C. Lymphoid hyperplasia
    D. Heterotopia
    E. Hamartoma
       1. Peutz–Jeghers polyp
       2. Others
    F. Juvenile polyp
    G. Giant rugal hypertrophy
    H. Others

---

slightly nodular surface and may be lobulated (Figure 19.1). In colour, they appear very similar to the adjacent normal gastric mucosa. Histologically, one sees cystic and pyloric-type glands lined by normal gastric mucosa (Figure 19.2). Malignant degeneration is rare. Hattori (1985) found three of a series of 67 hyperplastic polyps to contain carcinoma. In our series, only one hyperplastic polyp contained carcinoma: this occurred in a 6.0-cm polyp containing both hyperplastic and adenomatous elements with the malignant change confined to the region of adenomatous change. There was no evidence of any dysplasia in the hyperplastic portion.

Adenomatous gastric polyps, on the other hand, have a definite tendency toward carcinomatous degeneration. Characteristically, they contain intestinal-type epithelium displaying varying degrees of dysplasia, in-situ

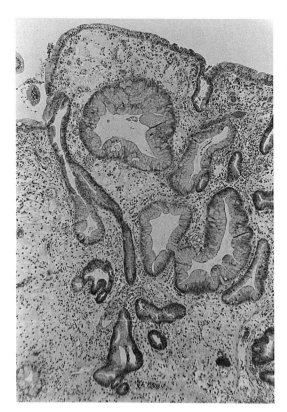

Figure 19.2 Microscopic photograph of a hyperplastic polyp. It is composed of mature, hyperplastic faveolar mucous cells with cyst formation and mild, chronic inflammatory cells.

carcinoma and/or invasive adenocarcinoma. We previously reported on 95 adenomatous polyps, removed from 67 patients (Ghazi, Ferstenberg and Shinya, 1984), among which nine polyps (9.6%) showed *in situ* carcinoma (Figure 19.4). Adenomatous polyps are usually sessile and present in various shapes and sizes (Figure 19.3). They are found most commonly in the antrum, and may ulcerate and cause bleeding. Histologically, these adenomas may be categorized under three headings – tubular, tubulo-villous or villous.

19.6 DUODENAL POLYPS

Duodenal polyps are an uncommon entity, usually being found as part of either Peutz–Jegher syndrome or Gardner's syndrome. In Gardner's syndrome they exist as adenomatous polyps and, consequently, should be totally excised to forestall carcinomatous degeneration (Sinha and Williamson, 1988). In our series only one polyp among 44 was found to harbour invasive carcinoma. This polyp was located in the second portion of the duodenum and arose in a patient with Gardner's syndrome. Polyps found in association with Peutz–Jegher's syndrome are usually hamartomas and solitary hamartomas of the duodenum have been reported (Figures 19.5, 19.6, 19.7 and 19.8).

19.7 MORTALITY AND MORBIDITY

We have had no deaths resulting from endoscopic gastroduodenal polypectomy in our 13-year experience. Morbidity consisted only of two postpolypectomy episodes of haemorrhage. One patient bled from the base of the polyp and responded to blood transfusion alone and was discharged on the third postpolypectomy day. The second patient, on corticosteroid therapy for asthma, bled from a duodenal ulcer which was not seen at the time of polypectomy. This bleeding did not respond to blood transfusion and required operative intervention with antrectomy and vagotomy.

19.8 ENDOSCOPIC TECHNIQUE

Our preparation for endoscopic polypectomy in the upper gastrointestinal tract is as follows. The patient is asked to fast for a period of 8–10 hours prior to the procedure. An intravenous line is inserted in order to ensure adequate hydration. Preparatory studies should include a complete blood count, platelet count, prothrombin time, partial thromboplastin time and bleeding time, serum electrolytes and an electrocardiogram. Any baseline deficiency is corrected. Blood should be typed and cross-matched in advance in the event that transfusion becomes necessary. If the initial haemoglobin level is

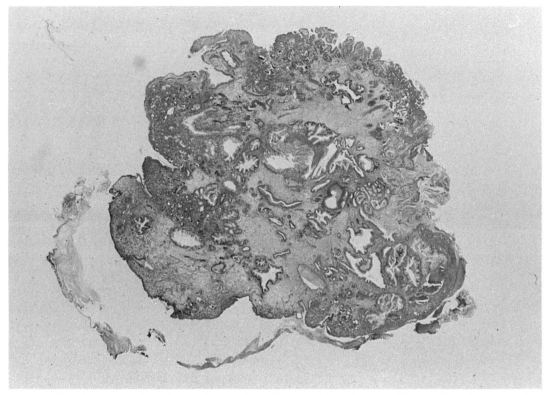

Figure 19.3   A large sessile adenomatous polyp of body of the stomach. Hypercellularity at the right upper corner is worth noting.

below 10 g/100 cm^3 the patient should be transfused prior to the procedure.

Pharyngeal anaesthesia is obtained with a 3-cm^3 mixture of xylocaine 4% and a few drops of simethicone (Mylicon-Stewart Pharmaceuticals). The patient gargles and swallows this admixture, after which he is placed in the left lateral decubitus position. A mouthpiece is inserted to keep the mouth open and to prevent the patient from biting the instrument. Sedation is accomplished by intravenous injections of pethidine (meperidine) 50–75 mg and diazepam 5–10 mg. All medications are given intravenously immediately prior to commencing the endoscopic procedure. The dosage of all the medications should be adjusted according to the patient's age and anxiety level.

If active peristalsis is present, glucagon in 1-mg increments is administered intravenously as required.

The instrument we prefer for upper gastrointestinal polypectomy is an end-viewing pan-endoscope but, on occasion, a side-viewing instrument may prove useful for dealing with a duodenal polyp. Coagulation current alone is used for all electrosurgical transections of the pedicle or the base of a polyp. The power source we customarily employ is a Valley Lab Unit (SSEK or SSE2K) set at a reading to 3–3.5 pure coagulation current. Most commercial snares used for colonic polypectomy can also be employed for gastroduodenal polypectomy.

Once administration of the intravenous sedatives had produced a light, relaxed, somnolent state, the endoscope is introduced through the mouth and examination of the

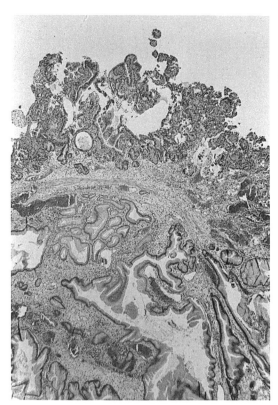

Figure 19.4 Higher magnification of the polyp in Figure 19.3 revealed a focus of in-situ carcinoma. The muscularis mucosae separates the carcinoma from underlying structures.

oesophagus, stomach and duodenum is carried out in a meticulous, disciplined fashion. When the polyp is seen *en face* it is snared and excised by the application of appropriate coagulation current once the snare is tightened. All pedunculated polyps, no matter how large, can be removed in one piece. Since commercially available snares do not open beyond a certain diameter, very large polyps may require the use of the homemade snare as described by Shinya (Wolff and Shinya, 1978). The majority of sessile polyps, especially those of under 1.5 cm diameter, can be excised through the base in one piece. Larger sessile polyps, those 2.0 cm in diameter or greater, were removed in piecemeal fashion (Ghazi, Ferstenberg and Shinya, 1984). Sessile polyps

over 3.0 cm in diameter required, on occasion, more than one session for complete excision. An appropriate interval between sessions is 4–6 weeks.

After polypectomy, patients are not fed overnight. Oral intake is recommended with a liquid diet, advancing to a soft diet by the second day. Antacid therapy and a bland diet are continued for a period of 3–4 weeks.

19.9 DISCUSSION

Compared with colonic polyps, gastroduodenal polyps are rare. The incidence of gastroduodenal polyps in 18 200 autopsy specimens was reported by Brunn and Pearl (1926) to be 0.003%. Their aetiology is not definitely known. There are reports of an increased incidence of gastric polyps of the order of 5–8% in patients with pernicious anaemia, where mucosal atrophy is a consistent finding (Rigler and Kaplan, 1946; Sivak, 1984). Hypochlorhydria and achlorhydria with hypergastrinaemia have been suggested as possible aetiological factors. An increased incidence of carcinoma after 10–15 years of hypochlorhydria in postgastrectomy patients is also a possible factor. Therefore, one may speculate that the presence of acid in the gastroduodenal lumen may have a preventive effect in formation of the polyps.

Bile acids have been incriminated in the formation of colonic polyps and a direct relationship between polyps and cancer is known to exist in the colon. The absence of bile in the stomach could conceivably be a factor related to the regional differences in polyp occurrence.

Once the presence of a gastroduodenal polyp is documented, the likelihood is that this is benign, since about two-thirds of gastric polyps are hyperplastic and, as previously noted, hyperplastic polyps are rarely malignant. In contrast, Hattori (1985) in his study of 67 hyperplastic polyps stated that the incidence of adenocarcinoma was 3/67 patients, which is an incidence of approximately 4.5%.

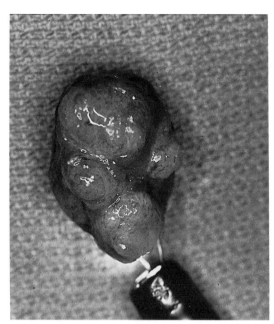

Figure 19.5 A large multilobulated hamartoma of duodenum. After excision of the polyp, due to its large size, it was grasped with a snare and extracted from the duodenal lumen.

We found an incidence of 9.6% of in-situ carcinoma and very rarely an invasive adenocarcinoma among our adenomatous polyp subgroup.

Polyp size as well as histology relates to the presence or absence of cancer. In our series, no polyps under 1.5 cm in diameter contained cancer. Once the polyp attains a 2.0 cm size, the possibility of malignant change or of the lesion being a polypoid carcinoma increases. Minzuno, Kobayashi and Kasugai (1975) reported on follow-up of 118 cases of gastric polyp that seven polyps increased in size, four decreased in size, and four were proven to contain adenocarcinoma (Ghazi, Ferstenberg and Shinya, 1984).

Recognizing the low overall incidence of malignancy among gastroduodenal polyps, one may ask why they should be removed at all. Marshak and Feldman (1965) recommended only radiological follow-up studies of polyps over 6–12-month intervals by gastrointestinal series. This was an appropriate recommendation at that time when the only alternative was major surgery. Fibreoptic endoscopic polypectomy is now a readily accomplished and safe procedure, and there is no reason to submit patients to repeated radiation exposure over the years. In our view endoscopic polypectomy is the procedure of choice, especially if the patient is suffering from anaemia or abdominal pain. Removal of a gastric polyp not only provides cure but it provides a tissue diagnosis and gives the examiner the opportunity to examine the gastroduodenal mucosa for associated conditions such as ulceration, reflux oesophagitis, gastroduodenitis or superficial gastric or duodenal erosions.

The need for, and frequency of, follow-up examinations after removal of a gastric or duodenal polyp depend on the histology of the original polyp and whether the polyp was pedunculated or sessile. For the totally excised pedunculated polyp, which is histologically 'benign', the patient should be re-examined once a year. On the other hand if the polyp is sessile, was removed in piecemeal fashion and, particularly, if it contained dysplastic tissue or changes of carcinoma in-situ, the immediate follow-up examination interval might be as short as 3 months. In general, we feel that all patients with adenomatous polyps should be followed for a minimal period of 5 years but firm statistical documentation is not yet available to determine optimal follow-up.

In conclusion, our recommendations are as follows: Gastroduodenal polyps should be endoscopically excised wherever feasible (Brunn and Pearl, 1926). In the absence of invasive carcinoma such removal should be followed by periodic endoscopic re-examination (Ghazi, Ferstenberg and Shinya, 1984). Malignant neoplastic polyps or polypoid carcinomas, both infrequent polyp forms should be treated when the patient's condition permits, by definitive gastric resection following endoscopic documentation of the pathological process.

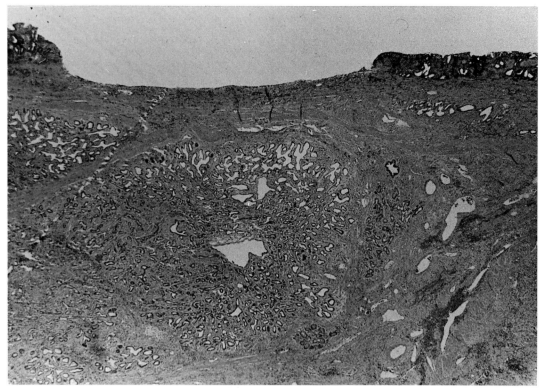

Figure 19.6 Photomicrograph of the hamartoma in Figure 19.5 demonstrating a small, superficial ulcer which is presumed to be the site of the bleeding.

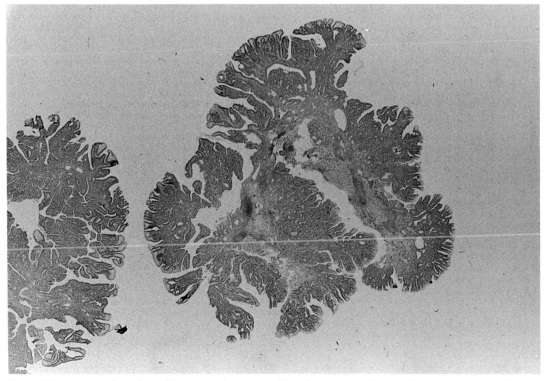

Figure 19.7 A sessile polyp of the second portion of the duodenum. Grossly it appeared to be villous in nature.

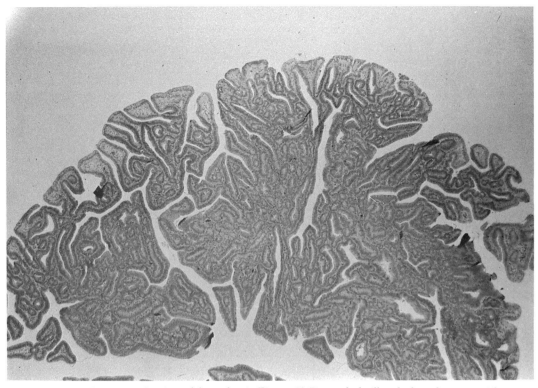

Figure 19.8   Higher magnification of the polyp in Figure 19.7 revealed villotubular adenoma without any evidence of dysplasia.

REFERENCES

Aper, E. I., Foroozan, P., Johnson, R. B. and Haubrich, W. W. (1975) Endoscopic polypectomy in the duodenum. *Gastrointest. Endosc.*, **21**, 119–23.

Brunn, H. and Pearl, F. (1926) Diffuse gastric polyposis – adenopapillomatosis gastric. *Surg. Gynecol. Obstet.*, **43**, 559–98.

Ghazi, A., Ferstenberg, H. and Shinya, H. (1984) Endoscopic gastroduodenal polypectomy. *Ann. Surg.*, **200**, 175–80.

Hattori, T. (1985) Morphological range of hyperplastic polyps and carcinomas arising in hyperplastic polyps of the stomach. *J. Clin. Pathol.*, **38**, 622–30.

Marshak, R. H. and Feldman, F. (1965) Gastric polyps. *Am. J. Dig. Dis.*, **10**, 909–35.

Minzuno, H., Kobayashi, S. and Kasugai, T. (1975) Endoscopic follow-up of gastric polyps. *Gastrointest. Endosc.*, **21**, 112–5.

Nakamura, T. and Nakano, G. (1985) Histopathological classification and malignant change in gastric polyps. *J. Clin. Pathol.*, **38**, 754–64.

Oota, K. and Sobin, L. H. (1977) *Histological Typing of Gastric and Esophageal Tumors*, Vol. 18, WHO, Geneva, pp. 37–46.

Rigler, L. G. and Kaplan, H. C. (1946) Pernicious anemia and tumors of the stomach. *J. Natl. Cancer Inst.*, **7**, 327.

Seifert, E. and Elster, K. (1975) Gastric polypectomy. *Am. J. Gastroenterol.*, **63**, 451–6.

Sinha, J. and Williamson, R. C. (1988) Villous adenomas and carcinoma of the duodenum in Gardner's syndrome. *Postgrad. Med. J.*, **64**, 899–902.

Sivak, V. M. Jr (1984) Gastrointestinal endoscopy in clinical practice. *Gastrointest. Endosc.*, **30**, 101–6.

Tsuneoka, K., Watanabe, N., Uchida, T. *et al.* (1968) Fibergastroscopic polypectomy with snare method. The Third Asian Pacific Congress of Gastroenterology, F-129.

Wolff, W. I. and Shinya, H. (1978) The Impact of Colonoscopy on the Problem of Colorectal Cancer. *Prog. Clin. Can.* **7**, 51–9.

CHAPTER TWENTY

Percutaneous endoscopic gastrostomy

M. D. McKay
and
F. J. Tedesco

20.1 INTRODUCTION

Over the past decade tremendous advances have been made in the area of supportive nutrition. Patients now can be maintained for indefinite periods on total parenteral feeding. However, the enteral route is still the preferred way to provide long-term nutritional support in a patient whose gastrointestinal tract is intact. Before 1980 enteral feeding was achieved by nasogastric, nasojejunal or surgically placed feeding gastrostomy tubes. In 1980, Gauderer, Ponsky and Izant reported their experience of placing percutaneous endoscopic gastrostomy (PEG) feeding tubes, since when the technique has gained wide acceptance as a means of providing long-term enteral feeding for debilitated or comatose patients.

A review of accumulated experience (Foutch *et al.*, 1984) showed that percutaneous endoscopic gastrostomy was technically successful in 98% of cases, with an average time for insertion of 15–30 minutes; the complication rate was low, with no reported mortality. The cost of surgical gastrostomy was three to four times greater than percutaneous endoscopic gastrostomy. Farca *et al.* (1985) reported a decreased incidence of oesophageal damage in patients fed by percutaneous endoscopic gastrostomy compared with patients fed by the nasogastric route.

Modifications to the original procedure of Gauderer, Ponsky and Izant (1980) have been described by Russell, Brotman and Norris (1984) who devised a percutaneous gastrostomy utilizing a guide-wire and dilator with a push technique. The Sach's–Vine gastrostomy technique uses a 300-cm flexible-tipped guide-wire and the feeding tube is pushed over the wire. The pull-string technique has been compared to the push-over-wire technique in randomized studies. Hogan *et al.* (1986) and Kozarek, Ball and Ryan (1986) compared the two techniques and found the pull-string and the 'push' technique had a similar proportion of technically successful procedures and the complication rates were also comparable. Percutaneous endoscopic gastrostomy has proven to be a safe, effective means of providing long-term nutritional therapy.

20.2 PATIENT SELECTION

Any patient who is unable or unwilling to meet his required caloric needs by normal feeding is a candidate for percutaneous endoscopic gastrostomy. The common indications are:

Cerebrovascular accidents.
Head and neck cancers.
Any neurological disease with deglutition problems.
Anoxic encephalopathy.
Huntington's chorea.

Alzheimer's disease.
Recurrent aspiration secondary to nasogastric feedings.
Oral-pharyngeal cancer.
Oesophageal cancer.
Comatose patients.

Advanced neurological disease, partial obstruction of the gastrointestinal tract, impaired deglutition of any aetiology are common reasons for percutaneous endoscopic gastrostomy placement. Patients with oesophageal cancer can undergo endoscopic gastrostomy after dilatation if necessary. The procedure can be performed safely on infants, children and adults. Previous abdominal surgery does not necessarily rule out the procedure.

A technically successful procedure depends on obtaining adequate insufflation of the stomach with displacement of the liver and colon, good transillumination through the abdominal wall and endoscopic visualization of finger ballotment and compression on the anterior wall of the stomach. Relative contraindications to the procedure are:

Obstruction of pharynx or oesophagus secondary to malignancy refractory to dilation.
Ascites.
Massive hepatomegaly.
Gastric malignancy or ulcer involving anterior wall.
Gastrointestinal obstruction.
Massive obesity.
Severe coagulopathy.
Oesophageal varices.

The anterior abdominal wall must be intact in order to promote adequate healing. Massive ascites and obesity will usually preclude good transillumination through the abdominal wall. Patients with a coagulation defect require correction of clotting factors before the procedure and patients with oesophageal varices may need them obliterating by sclerotherapy prior to percutaneous endoscopic gastrostomy.

Aspirin or non-steroidal anti-inflammatory drugs usually are discontinued 7–10 days before the procedure (Cohen, Berman and Bojarski, 1985). Corticosteroids may inhibit the fibrous union of the anterior abdominal wall to the serosal surface of the stomach, so that corticosteroid therapy is a contraindication (Cohen, 1985). Efrusy et al. (1984), who reported higher morbidity and significant mortality in the elderly, recommends caution in elderly patients with multisystem disease.

20.3 PREPARING THE PATIENT

Informed consent must be obtained from the patient or legal guardian. The patient is given nothing by mouth for 12 hours before the procedure. A second-generation cephalosporin is given intravenously or intramuscularly 1 hour prior to the procedure with four further doses at 6-hour intervals. When a gag reflex is present, topical anaesthetic spray is applied to the posterior pharynx. At the time of the procedure the patient is usually sedated with pethidine (meperidine) and diazepam. If required, the left upper quadrant of the abdomen is shaved before the procedure. Patients with a previous history of endocarditis or prosthetic placement of a cardiac valve should receive antibiotic prophylaxis.

20.4 PROCEDURE

With the patient supine, the endoscope is introduced under direct vision into the stomach. Upper gastrointestinal endoscopy is quickly performed to rule out a gastric wall abnormality or gastric outlet obstruction. The skin of the upper abdomen is sterilized with a providine-iodine preparation and the abdomen is draped by the assistant using a sterile technique. The endoscope is then placed in the midbody of the stomach. The stomach is maximally insufflated to allow apposition of the stomach to the abdominal wall. The endoscopy room lights are lowered to allow the assistant to see light from the endoscope

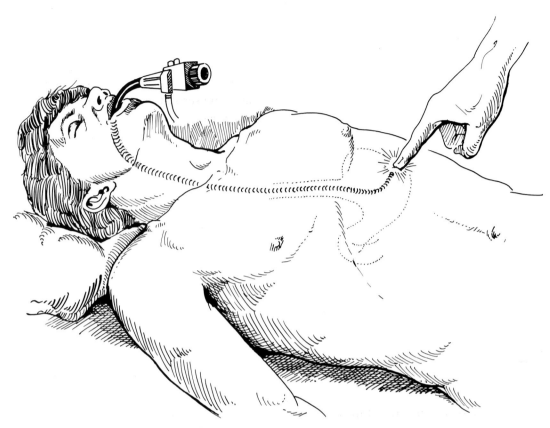

Figure 20.1 Site for placement located on anterior wall.

through the abdominal wall. The assistant locates the site of transillumination. In the left upper quadrant, approximately two-thirds of the distance from the umbilicus to the costal margin, the assistant indents the abdominal wall with his index finger. The endoscopist locates the point of maximal ballotment compression (Figure 20.1 and Plate 4), which, ideally, should be located proximal to the angularis on the anterior wall of the stomach. It is important to identify good finger indentation and not be deceived by transmural compression. The site is infiltrated with 2% lignocaine (lidocaine). A 21-gauge needle is advanced into the stomach until air is aspirated. The needle can usually be seen protruding through the gastric wall by the endoscopist. Using a scalpel blade an incision is made on the skin 0.5–0.75 cm long. A 16-gauge Medicut catheter is inserted through the incision into the stomach (Figure 20.2). The endoscopist loosely places a snare around the Medicut catheter. The stylet is removed by the assistant leaving the catheter in place. The tip of a 150-cm length of black silk is passed through the catheter into the stomach. The thread is snared by the endoscopist (Figure 20.3 and Plate 5). Suture and snare are withdrawn into the endoscope, and the endoscope is removed. The suture now passes through the abdominal wall and the stomach, up the oesophagus and pharynx, exiting from the mouth. The thread from the mouth is tied securely to the tapered suture end of the feeding tube. A second suture is inserted through the holes of the mushroom of the feeding tube

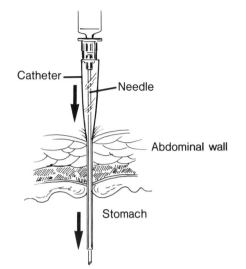

Figure 20.2 Medicut catheter inserted into stomach.

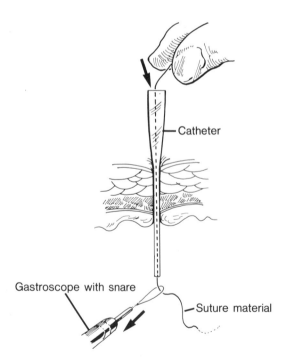

Figure 20.3 Silk threaded through catheter and grasped by snare.

tip as a safety line. (In the event that the catheter becomes lodged in the pharynx, or the pull-string breaks, the safety line allows the feeding tube to be quickly removed.) The mushroom end of the feeding tube is well lubricated with water-soluble jelly and guided over the patient's tongue with a tongue depressor. The assistant provides steady traction on the silk thread at the abdominal wall. The feeding tube is pulled downwards through the pharynx and oesophagus into the stomach, and out through the abdominal wall (Figure 20.4). The endoscope is reinserted to ensure that the rubber bumper of the feeding tube is snug against the stomach wall (Figure 20.5 and Plate 6). Excessive tension should be avoided as this may cause necrosis, ulceration and bleeding. The safety line is cut and removed through the mouth. An external bumper or baby bottle nipple is used to hold the catheter in position on the abdominal wall (Figure 20.6). The dilator end of the tube is cut away and a flared tip adapter fitted to the tube.

20.5 POSTPROCEDURE

The patient is given nothing by mouth for 24 hours after the procedure. Additional doses of cephalosporin are given for 24 hours. The wound site is checked daily for infection and cleaned with hydrogen peroxide and dressed with a topical antibiotic ointment. Feeding is begun with a half-strength osmotic solution at 25 ml per hour and the stomach is aspirated (to measure any residue) after 4 hours. If little or no residue is found, feeding volume is increased as rapidly as can be tolerated to meet the patient's caloric needs.

The gastrostomy tube may need to be removed for a number of reasons. The tube may become worn or cracked, or the patient's condition may improve and allow resumption of oral feeding. Tube removal is accomplished by steady traction at the abdominal wall. When the feeding tube is removed, the inner crossbar remains in the stomach and will pass on uneventfully through the bowel.

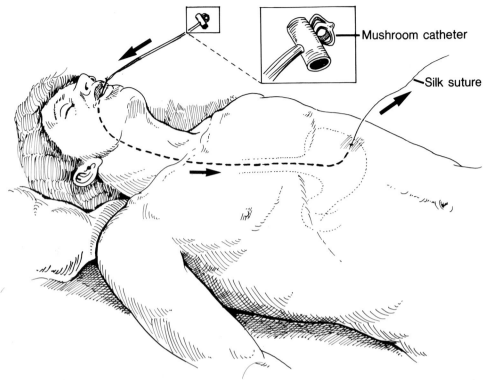

Mushroom catheter

Silk suture

Figure 20.4   Retrograde advancement of mushroom catheter into stomach.

If the tube becomes dislodged during the initial 24 hours, the procedure usually has to be repeated because the gastrostomy tract has not matured and will almost immediately close. In the case of dislodgement after 48 hours a Foley catheter may be inserted if done within 4–6 hours. Prior to insertion the tract may require gentle dilatation with bougie dilators to approximately 27 Fr (9 mm).

20.6 CONVERSION TO JEJUNAL FEEDING TUBE

If the patient develops recurrent aspiration pneumonia or symptoms of severe oeso-phageal reflux the gastrostomy tube may be converted to a jejunostomy tube. The gastros-tomy tube is removed, and the tract dilated to 9 mm using either Savary or other bougies. The distal end of a 20-Fr Foley catheter is cut.

A small-bowel feeding tube is inserted through the Foley catheter until the weighted distal end is just protruding. This is then placed through the dilated tract into the sto-mach. The endoscope is then inserted into the stomach and the distal end of the jejunal feed-ing tube is snared and pulled through the Foley and carried into the second portion of the duodenum. The Foley balloon is inflated and pulled snugly against the stomach wall. The external portion of the tube may be secured with a bottle nipple.

20.7 COMPLICATIONS

Ponsky *et al.* (1985) reported a complication rate of 5.9% and one mortality in 307 percu-taneous gastrostomies. Foutch *et al.* (1986) reviewed the cumulative morbidity and mor-tality of 324 patients reported in the literature:

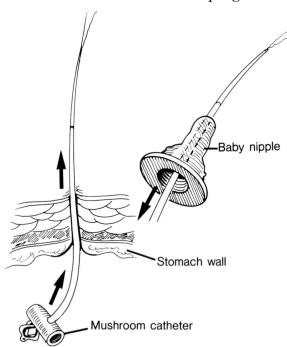

Figure 20.5   Terminal passage through stomach wall.

the minor complication rate was 14%, the major complication rate was 3%; there was no mortality. Twelve patients (4%) required laparotomy for wound infection (three), stomal leak (three), gastrocolic fistula (three), and pneumoperitoneum (three).

The major and minor complications reported are:

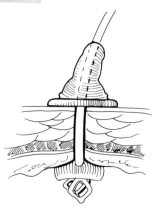

Figure 20.6   Final position of mushroom catheter on abdominal wall.

Wound infection.
Gastrocolic fistula.
Stomal leak.
Necrotizing fasciitis.
Aspiration pneumonitis.
Pneumoperitoneum.
Tube dislodgment.
Bleeding, usually minor.

Wound infection is usually minor and is evident by mild erythema at the incision site. It is probably induced by the indwelling mushroom feeding tube which has been contaminated by oral flora. More extensive wound infections require treatment by antibiotics intravenously and local incision and drainage. Gastrocolic fistula (Gossum, Des Marez and Cremer, 1988) and intraperitoneal leak are usually managed by removal of the feeding tube and exploratory laparotomy. Gottfried, Plummer and Clain (1986) prospectively evaluated the frequency of pneumoperitoneum following percutaneous endoscopic gastrostomy. They found nine of 24 patients developed a pneumoperitoneum postprocedure. These patients were managed by observation alone with no sequelae. In the absence of fever, leucocytosis, or abdominal pain, postprocedural pneumoperitoneum can be handled by close observation. Greif *et al.* (1986) reported one case of fatal necrotizing fasciitis, but several subsequent cases have been successfully treated with surgical débridement and antibiotics parenterally.

20.8 PERCUTANEOUS ENDOSCOPIC JEJUNOSTOMY

In patients with recurrent aspiration pneumonia or symptomatic gastrointestinal reflux, jejunal feeding is preferable to gastric feeding. Ponsky and Aszodi (1984) described the technique of percutaneous endoscopic jejunostomy. The advantage of this technique is that a tube is placed in the small bowel for feeding and an additional gastric tube allows decompression and diminishes reflux.

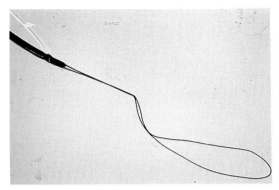

Figure 20.7 The gastrostomy and jejunal tube sutured together proximal to tapered tip.

20.8.1 PRIOR TO PROCEDURE

The mushroom-tipped feeding tube used for gastrostomy must be modified. A hole is cut in the head of the mushroom-tipped feeding tube and another hole is cut just proximal to the tapered tip of the feeding tube. Using haemostat forceps the non-weighted end of the small bowel feeding tube is passed through the head of the gastric mushroom feeding tube and inserted into the hole of the

gastrostomy tube just proximal to the tapered portion of the tube. The tubes are sutured together at that site (Figure 20.7). The tube assembly now consists of a feeding gastrostomy tube and the longer small-bowel feeding tube (Figure 20.8). The patient is prepared in the same manner as for percutaneous gastrostomy.

20.8.2 PROCEDURE

The procedure for percutaneous endoscopic jejunostomy is identical to that of percutaneous endoscopic gastrostomy. When the gastrostomy tube has been pulled down the oesophagus into the stomach and out through the abdominal wall, the longer jejunal tube will be emerging from the patient's mouth. Biopsy forceps are passed through the biopsy channel of the endoscope and the feeding jejunal tube is grasped just proximal to the weighted end by means of a suture previously tied around the feeding tube. The endoscope is reinserted with the jejunal feeding tube held by the forceps. The jejunal feeding tube is pulled into the second portion of the duodenum. The endoscopist ensures that the

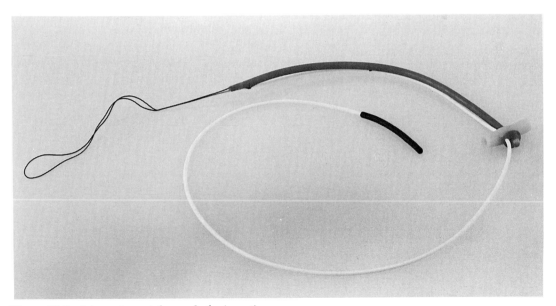

Figure 20.8 Jejunostomy tube ready for insertion.

internal bumper is snug on the stomach wall. The assistant then cuts the two tubes proximal to the suture and inserts the adapters into the two tubes. An abdominal radiograph is obtained to ensure that the jejunal feeding tube is in its proper position. The patient now has a small-bowel tube for feeding, and a gastric tube for decompression which will prevent reflux and aspiration. During feeding the gastric tube can be on low intermittent suction to prevent aspiration.

REFERENCES

Cohen, N. N., Berman A. and Bojarski M. (1985) Complication from steroid use in percutaneous endoscopic gastrostomy (PEG). *Gastrointest. Endosc.*, **31**, 163.

Efrusy, M., Schneider, H., Walter, R. and Kniaz, J. L. (1984) Percutaneous endoscopic gastrostomy tube feedings: the experience in a geriatric population. *Gastrointest. Endosc.*, **30**, (abstr.), 32.

Farca, A., Vargas, E., Gileard, C. *et al.* (1985) Superiority of percutaneous endoscopic gastrostomy to nasogastric intubation for enteral alimentation. *Gastrointest. Endosc.*, **31**, (abstr.), 128.

Foutch, P., Gregory, H., Williams, C. *et al.* (1984) Percutaneous endoscopic gastrostomy (PEG): a new procedure comes of age. *J. Clin. Gastroenterol.*, **8**, (11), 10–5.

Gauderer, M. W. L., Ponsky, J. L. and Izant, R. J. (1980) Gastrostomy without laparotomy: a percutaneous endoscopic technique. *J. Pediatr. Surg.*, **15**, 872.

Gossum, A. V., Des Marez, B. and Cremer, M. (1988). A colo-cutaneous-gastric fistula in a silent and unusual complication of percutaneous endoscopic gastrostomy. *Endoscopy*, **20**, 161.

Gottfried, E. B., Plummer, A. B. and Clain, M. R. (1986) Pneumoperitoneum following percutaneous endoscopic gastrostomy. *Gastrointest. Endosc.*, **32**, 397–9.

Greif, J. M., Ragland, J. J., Ochsner, M. G. and Riding, R. (1986) Fatal necrotizing fascitiis complicating percutaneous endoscopic gastrostomy. *Gastrointest. Endosc.*, **32**, 292–4.

Hogan, R. B., DeMarco, D. C., Hamilton, J. K. *et al.* (1986) Percutaneous endoscopic gastrostomy – to push or pull. *Gastrointest. Endosc.*, **32**, 253–8.

Kozarek, R. A., Ball, T. and Ryan, J. Jr (1985) Percutaneous endoscopic gastrostomy (PEG): when push comes to shove. A comparison of two insertion methods. *Gastrointest. Endosc.*, **31**, (abstr.), 131.

Ponsky, J. L. and Aszodi A. (1984) Percutaneous endoscopic jejunostomy. *Am. J. Gastroenterol.*, **79**, 113–6.

CHAPTER TWENTY-ONE

Percutaneous gastrostomy by radiological technique

Chia-sing Ho

21.1 INTRODUCTION

In a patient malnourished because of dysphagia, an alternative route of nutrient delivery may be indicated. This usually means a choice between parenteral or enteral nutrition. Major metabolic and septic complications have occurred with long-term parenteral nutrition (Bernard, Stahl and Chase, 1971), and it requires much closer medical surveillance and nursing care than enteral feeding and is also expensive. In view of these considerations, enteral feeding is preferred in patients who have dysphagia, obstructive oesophageal lesions, etc. and patients with functional small intestines (Heymsfield *et al.*, 1979).

Enteral diet is conventionally delivered either through nasogastric intubation or surgical gastrostomy. Prolonged nasogastric intubation may cause oesophageal stricture due to reflux oesophagitis and is poorly tolerated by some patients because of pharyngeal irritation. Surgical gastrostomy was proposed by Egbers in 1841 and first performed by Sedillot in 1893. Although it is technically simple, it is associated with significant mortality and morbidity (Heimbach, 1970; Meguid and Williams, 1979; Wasiljew, Ujiki and Beal, 1982). Malnutrition contributes to poor wound healing and other serious complications such as wound dehiscence, bleeding and intraperitoneal leakage. General anaesthesia is required for gastrostomy and post-operative aspiration may lead to pulmonary complications.

In the late 1970s, Ponsky and Gauderer introduced an alternative technique of endoscopic gastrostomy (Chapter 20). However, the need for endoscopic skill and its impossibility in patients with oesophageal or pharyngeal obstruction has promoted the emergence of another non-operative alternative to surgical gastrostomy.

In 1983, several radiologists independently described a non-operative radiological method of percutaneous gastrostomy using the Seldinger technique with fluoroscopic control (Ho, 1983; Sacks *et al.*, 1983; Tao and Gillies, 1983; Wills and Oglesby, 1983). In one modification Ho (1983) suggested placing the gastrostomy tube through the pylorus into the small bowel for direct jejunal feeding. This concept has been gradually accepted as the most desirable method of enteral feeding since, unlike surgical or endoscopic gastrostomies, pulmonary aspiration of enteral feeds is avoided. At the Toronto General Hospital, where the method was first introduced, the percutaneous radiological procedure has largely replaced surgical gastrostomy when long-term enteral feeding is indicated.

21.2 EQUIPMENT

1. 20-gauge Teflon sheathed, 23-gauge Longwell needle (Becton-Dickinson).
2. 70 cm 0.64 mm (0.025 in) Lunderquist type, Ho 060580 (Cook).

3. 6 Fr, 9 Fr Teflon dilators (Cook).
4. 9 Fr Kifa or equivalent polyethylene catheter.
5. 145 cm 0.97 mm (0.038 in) guide-wire (Cook).
6. 10 Fr Nephrostomy catheter with Cope loop and metallic cannula (Cook).
7. 3 0' silk suture with curved needle (Ethicon).
8. 0 silk suture with straight cutting needle (Ethicon).
9. Elastoplast tape.
10. 10 cm × 14 cm Opsite (Smith & Nephew).

21.3 TECHNIQUE

Percutaneous non-endoscopic gastrostomy is performed only if the distended stomach is situated below the costal margin, and there is no interposition of liver or colon between the stomach and anterior abdominal wall. Each patient is carefully evaluated prior to the procedure to ensure these anatomical criteria are satisfied. The inferior liver margin is outlined by ultrasonography. The stomach is distended with air via a nasogastric tube and its position relative to the colon assessed by fluoroscopy. Lateral C-arm fluoroscopy is helpful in confirming the direct apposition of the anterior gastric wall to the anterior abdominal wall. Patients with partial gastrectomy or gastric pull-up operations are excluded because the stomach remnant invariably lies high above the costal margin, making direct puncture of the stomach unpredictable. A skin entry in the epigastrium is selected over the body of the stomach, this avoids the colon and liver. Puncturing of the gastric body is preferred to the antrum as the latter is more contractile and may present more difficulty during subsequent manipulations.

The procedure is performed from the patient's left. The skin entry site is infiltrated with local anaesthetic and puncture into the stomach is made with a 20-gauge Teflon-sheathed skinny needle (Becton-Dickinson). When the stomach is fully air distended the needle is advanced with a sharp forward thrust (Figure 21.1(a)). The puncture is directed towards the antrum to facilitate subsequent cannulation of the duodenum. The sheath is advanced well into the stomach prior to withdrawal of the needle, and its intra-gastric position confirmed with injection of a small amount of water-soluble contrast. A 0.064-cm (0.025-in) guide-wire (Cook) with a short flexible tip and a stainless-steel shaft is then introduced into the stomach through the sheath (Figure 21.1(b)). After withdrawal of the sheath the needle tract is dilated to 9 Fr (3 mm) in size by passing Teflon dilators over the guide-wire.

To cannulate the duodenum, a 9-Fr Kifa catheter with a slight curve at its distal tip is inserted into the stomach and the original guide-wire is replaced by a 145-cm, 0.097-cm (0.038-in) Teflon-coated guide-wire (Cook). Under fluoroscopy, the catheter and the guide-wire are manipulated through the pylorus into the duodenum until it reaches the duodenojejunal flexure. During manipulation, advancement of the catheter or guide-wire may be impeded causing either or both to curl up within the stomach. If unchecked, this may lead to buckling of the catheter out of the gastric lumen into the peritoneum. To prevent this, a metallic cannula, available with the percutaneous nephrostomy catheter (Cook), is inserted co-axially within the catheter over the guide-wire (Figure 21.1(c)). This stiffens the catheter and greatly enhances its manoeuvrability.

To anchor the feeding catheter better within the gastrointestinal lumen, a Cope loop is preferably fashioned to its distal end (Figure 21.1(d)). Such a catheter is available commercially, e.g. 10-Fr percutaneous nephrostomy tube (Cook). Alternately it can be made by first curving the tapering end of a 9-Fr Kifa catheter with hot water. Three- to four-sided holes are cut along its curved portion. A 3 '0' silk suture with a straight cutting needle (Ethicon) is then threaded through and tied to its distal end about 5 mm from its tip. The needle and silk

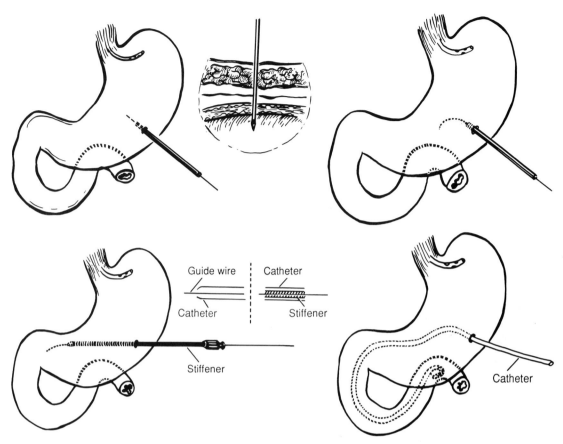

Figure 21.1 Diagrams to show the essential percutaneous gastrostomy. (a) Direct puncture with a 20-gauge Teflon sheath Longwell needle. (b) The skinny needle has been withdrawn and a 0.063-cm (0.025-in) guide-wire placed through the sheath into the stomach. This wire allows dilatation of the tract to 9 Fr in size. (c) Cannulation of the duodenum with a 9-Fr Kifa catheter, supported by a coaxially inserted metallic cannula to prevent buckling. A 0.096-cm (0.038-in) guide-wire is used for this purpose. (d) Final placement of the feeding catheter with a 'Cope loop' fashioned to its distal end.

are threaded into the lumen of the catheter, 6 cm from its tip, and are pushed within the lumen by means of a metallic cannula introduced through one of the side holes, to emerge from its open end (Figure 21.2). Over the guide-wire, the feeding catheter is exchanged for the cannulating catheter and its tip positioned to the duodenojejunal flexure. After removal of the guide-wire, the 'Cope loop' is formed by tightening and securing the silk to the external portion of the feeding catheter (Figure 21.2).

The feeding catheter is tied with a '0' silk

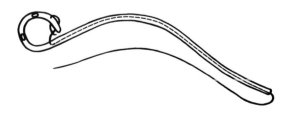

Figure 21.2 Constructing a 'Cope loop' to the feeding catheter. The 3 '0' silk suture is tied to the distal end of the catheter and brought into the lumen 6 cm from the catheter tip, to emerge from its open end.

suture sewn to a 6 cm^2 piece of Elastoplast which is applied to the skin above the catheter exit. A 10 × 14 cm piece of Opsite is then applied to the skin below the catheter exit and the catheter is sandwiched between it and another piece of Opsite.

Enteral feeding is started on the same day as the procedure and the nasogastric tube removed 24 hours later unless the patient complains of abdominal pain or catheter displacement is noted. In the latter event, a plain abdominal film is obtained to assess the catheter position.

21.4 COMPLICATIONS

One of the most serious complications of any gastrostomy is intraperitoneal leakage of gastric contents leading to generalized peritonitis (Torosian and Rombeau, 1980), and in debilitated patients this is potentially fatal. Despite apposition of the anterior gastric wall to the anterior abdominal wall, intraperitoneal leakage still occurs in surgical gastrostomy with an incidence of 1.5–2.0% (Wasiljew, 1982; Swartzendruber and Laws, 1982).

The published literature does not record any case of intraperitoneal leak after percutaneous gastrostomy and none of our patients had leakage after a first percutaneous procedure. In one of 200 patients (0.5%) a leak occurred after a second gastrostomy, necessitated by tube displacement. The fibrous tract found after the first gastrostomy was probably disrupted. The leak was repaired at laparotomy.

The low incidence of intraperitoneal leakage results because the gastrostomy opening is the same size as the catheter which functions as a plug. Even if the catheter is dislodged the small gastrostomy (9 Fr or 3 mm) is effectively sealed off by the thick muscular wall of the stomach. On several occasions catheter dislodgement has happened with no ill effects in our patients, during or immediately after the procedure. After 1 week, a fibrous tract is formed around the gastrostomy tube and leak-

age is even less likely (VanSonnenberg et al., 1986a).

Another serious complication is intraperitoneal infusion of enteral diet. Two of our patients (1%) had this complication due to partial intraperitoneal migration of the feeding catheter from the stomach. One died of respiratory failure after surgical laparotomy while the other survived. Since we have properly fashioned a 'Cope loop' at the end of the feeding catheter in all patients, this complication has not occurred; nor has it occurred in other studies using the Cope loop for anchorage in the stomach (Willis and Oglesby, 1985).

Immediate or delayed haemorrhage from the gastrotomy site may occur following percutaneous or surgical gastrostomy. After surgical gastrostomy the incidence of gastrointestinal bleeding varies from 0.9% to 2% (Wasiljew, Ujiki and Beal, 1982; Shellito and Malt, 1985). In our experience, immediate bleeding following percutaneous gastrostomy is insignificant and self limiting. Delayed, severe life-threatening bleeding from the gastrostomy site occurred in one of our patients 10 days after the procedure, requiring blood transfusion and balloon tamponade through the gastrostomy (Rose, Wolman and Ho, 1986). (Bleeding was probably due to gradual erosion by the feeding catheter into an adjacent vessel in the gastric wall.) No other similar reports have appeared in the literature.

Postoperative aspiration, with its serious sequelae, often accompanies surgical gastrostomy performed under general anaesthesia, and it has been suggested (Raventos, Kraleman and Gray, 1982) that surgical gastrostomy is contraindicated in patients with gastro-oesophageal reflux which might lead to aspiration of enteral fluid. In the percutaneous gastrostomy procedure described the feeding tube is placed in or beyond the duodenojejunal flexure (Figure 21.3). Gastro-oesophageal reflux of enteral nutrient has not occurred in our patients.

Pericatheter leakage and skin infection

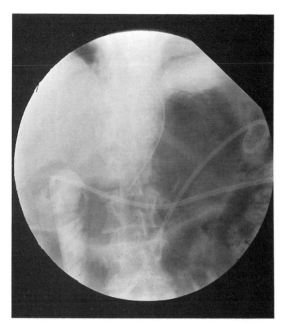

Figure 21.3 Radiograph percutaneous gastrostomy with the feeding tube placed just beyond the dueodenojejunal flexure.

around the gastrotomy site pose problems of varying severity (Gasson, 1982). They may lead to severe wound infection and dehiscence requiring surgical treatment; even in its mild form, frequent nursing care of the wound is necessary. Peristomal problems are uncommon in patients after percutaneous gastrostomy. We have encountered it only once, in a patient with dysgammaglobulinaemia whose impaired immune response probably contributed to poor healing around the gastrostomy site.

Catheter clogging, migration and dislodgement may occur in any tube enterostomy and the actual incidence is difficult to assess as it often goes unrecorded. We take the view that these problems are inherent with tubes and should not be considered as complications. The more conscientiously nursing care is exercised, the less frequently they occur.

One of 200 patients (0.5%) died of myocardial infarction several hours after percutaneous gastrostomy (he had several previous episodes of myocardial infarction). A number of patients had uneventful gastrostomy within 2 weeks of myocardial infarction without complication.

21.5 MANAGEMENT OF PERCUTANEOUS FEEDING TUBES

Peristomal skin infection is uncommon in patients with percutaneous gastrostomy and is usually due to leakage through the gastrostomy tract. It can be controlled by keeping the peristomal skin clean and dry. Frequent change of dressings around the catheter and application of calamine lotion to the skin may be required. If possible, the skin should be cleaned and blown dry once or twice daily with a hairdryer set on low heat. If the skin infection becomes uncontrollable, the catheter may have to be removed entirely.

Tube blockage or dislodgement, however, occurs not infrequently and may require replacement or reinsertion under fluoroscopy by the radiologist. However, the desired aim is to *prevent* clogging of feeding tubes. Antacids, crushed pills and other solid material should not be infused through the tubes. Routine irrigation of the tube with 30 ml of cranberry juice followed by 150 ml of water after infusion of nutrient is discontinued helps to maintain patency (Ramos and Lindine, 1986). When the catheter becomes clogged, instillation of a few millilitres of cranberry juice followed by irrigation half an hour later may unclog it. Should this fail, replacement over a 0.97-mm (0.038-in) guide-wire under fluoroscopy with a larger feeding tube is necessary. A 12-Fr or 14-Fr nasogastric feeding tube (Argyle) is usually adequate for long-term enteral feeding without blockage. Catheter dislodgment is more often related to poor patient restraint in restless or confused patients. Reinsertion of another catheter can often be achieved through the same percutaneous gastrostomy tract provided it is not disrupted during recannulation. Successful reinsertion is often accomplished if attempted within 24–28 hours of catheter dislodgment. After this period, reinsertion may be more difficult, or even impossible as the tract is obliterated completely.

It is imperative that the radiologist performing the procedure should be responsible for catheter replacement or reinsertion.

21.6 INDICATIONS

Patients requiring enteral nutritional therapy fall into three different categories: dysphagia, anorexia and small-bowel dysfunction or disease. The majority (85%) of our patients fall into the dysphagia group, the most common causes being neurological disorders or recurrent head and neck tumours. Less commonly, oesophageal malignancy is managed with percutaneous gastrostomy, intubation being preferred, palliative bypass or intubation.

We have managed, without significant morbidity, a small number of patients with anorexia nervosa, severe psychiatric depression, advanced malignancy and AIDS. In two patients with AIDS, however, there was peritoneal irritation or infection, unrelated to gastric leakage or intraperitoneal infusion of enteral diet. They responded to antibiotic treatment and were able to use the feeding tube subsequently.

A third group are patients who suffer from small-bowel dysfunction or disease: for example, scleroderma, pancreatitis, Crohn's disease, and radiation enteritis, who are unable to eat normal meals without abdominal pain, diarrhoea or vomiting, but tolerate enteral diet delivered slowly at regulated rates through a nasogastric tube placed in the small bowel. Percutaneous gastrostomy rather than long-term parenteral nutrition is a logical and effective solution for their nutritional problem. Currently, the few patients who have been treated this way have responded well, and long-term parenteral nutrition was avoided in all.

REFERENCES

Bernard, R. W., Stahl, W. H. and Chase, R. M. (1971) Subclavian vein catheterization: a prospective study II, infection and complications. *Ann. Surg.* **173**, 184–90.

Gasson, J. E. (1982) Feeding stomas: gastrostomy and jejunostomy. Part I: surgical procedure and complications. *Clin. Gastroenterol.*, **2**, 337–44.

Heimbach, D. M. (1970) Surgical feeding procedures in patients with neurological disorders. *Ann. Surg.*, **172**, 311–4.

Heymsfield, S. B., Bethel, R. A. and Ansley, J. D. *et al.* (1979) Enteral hyperalimentation: an alternative to central venous hyperalimentation. *Ann. Intern. Med.*, **90**, 63–71.

Ho, C. S. (1983) Percutaneous gastrostomy for jejunal feeding, *Radiology*, **149**, 595–6.

Ho, C. S., Gray, R. R. and Goldfinger, M. *et al.* (1985) Percutaneous gastrostomy for enteral feeding. *Radiology*, **156**, 349–51.

Meguid, M. M. and Williams, L. F. (1979) The use of gastrostomy to correct malnutrition. *Surg. Gynecol. Obstet.*, **149**, 27–32.

Ramos, S. M. and Lindine, P. (1986) Inexpensive, safe and simple nasoenteral intubation – an alternative for the cost conscious. *J. Parentr. Entr. Nutr.*, **10**, 78–81.

Raventos, J. M., Kralemann, H. and Gray, D. B. (1982) Mortality risks of mentally ill patients after a feeding gastrostomy. *Am. J. Ment. Defic.*, **86**, 439–44.

Rose, D. B., Wolman, S. L. and Ho, C. S. (1986) Gastric hemorrhage complicating percutaneous transgastric jejunostomy. *Radiology*, **161**, 835–6.

Sacks, B. A., Vines, H. S. and Palestrant, A. M. *et al.* (1983) A non-operative technique for establishment of a gastrostomy in the dog. *Invest. Radiol.*, **18**, 485–7.

Shellito, P. C. and Malt, R. A. (1985) Tube gastrostomy: techniques and complications. *Ann. Surg.*, **201**, 180–95.

Swartzendruber, F. D. and Laws, H. L. (1982) The superior feeding gastrostomy. *Am. Surg.*, **48**, 276–8.

Tao, H. H. and Gillies, R. R. (1983) Percutaneous feeding gastrostomy. *A.J.R.*, **141**, 793–4.

Torosian, M. H. and Rombeau, J. L. (1980) Feeding by tube enterostomy. *Surg. Gynecol. Obstet.*, **150**, 918–27.

VanSonnenberg, E., Wittich, G. R. and Brown, L. K. (1986a) Percutaneous gastrostomy and gastroenterostomy technique derived from laboratory evaluation. *A.J.R.*, **146**, 577–80.

VanSonnenberg, E., Wittich, R. G. and Cabera, O. A. *et al.* (1986b) Percutaneous gastrostomy and gastroenterostomy: 2 clinical experiences. *A.J.R.*, **146**, 581–6.

Wasiljew, B. K., Ujiki, G. T. and Beal, J. M. (1982) Feeding gastrostomy: complications and mortality. *Am. J. Surg.*, **143**, 194–5.

Wills, J. S. and Oglesby, J. T. (1983) Percutaneous gastrostomy. *Radiology*, **139**, 449–53.

Wills, J. S. and Oglesby, J. T. (1985) Percutaneous gastrostomy: further experience. *Radiology*, **154**, 71–4.

CHAPTER TWENTY-TWO

Endoscopic papillotomy and stone removal

L. Safrany
and
M. Stenzel

22.1 INTRODUCTION

The classical clinical presentation of choledocholithiasis is biliary-type pain, fever and jaundice (Charcot's triad). However, even when very large stones are present, any one or all of these symptoms may be missing. In recent years abdominal ultrasound has had an enormous impact on the diagnosis of choledocholithiasis. Using newer scanning techniques, the sensitivity of sonography for detecting choledocholithiasis has improved so that common bile duct stones can now be visualized in 75–80% of patients (Laing, 1987). Small stones often cannot be demonstrated, especially when located in the distal common duct, so endoscopic retrograde cholangiopancreatography (ERCP) has maintained an important place in diagnosis.

Therapeutic ERCP developed as an extension of diagnostic ERCP; the first endoscopic papillotomies (EPTs) were used to remove stones from the common bile duct (Classen and Demling, 1974; Kawai *et al.*, 1974). As the risks of EPT were virtually unknown at that time, only those patients thought to be at high risk were treated endoscopically.

Over the ensuing years the following indications for treating stones in the common bile duct have evolved:

1. Postcholecystectomy patients; originally only in patients with a high operative risk, but now in any patient over age 65.
2. Stones in the common bile duct in high

operative risk patients with an intact gallbladder.
3. Septic cholangitis in patients with or without a gallbladder at any age.
4. Acute biliary pancreatitis at any age.

There are few contraindications, all are relative:

1. Severe coagulopathy.
2. Large stones, or stones above a true narrowing or stricture (i.e. tapered common bile duct).

22.2 TECHNICAL ASPECTS OF ENDOSCOPIC PAPILLOTOMY

Typically, the patient is admitted one day before ERCP/EPT; laboratory data, including coagulation indices, are measured, and informed consent is obtained. We do not give prophylactic antibiotics routinely, but one may choose to do so if the gallbladder is still in place. For sedation and immobilization of the duodenum we prefer pethidine (meperidine) 100 mg i.v. and hyoscine-*N*-butylbromide (Buscopan) 20 mg i.v. Glucagon 0.25 mg i.v. will also produce immobilization, but has a somewhat shorter effect. Atropine in increments of 0.2 mg i.v. may be added.

The patient is placed on the X-ray table with the left arm behind the body which enables rotation into a prone position once the

(a)

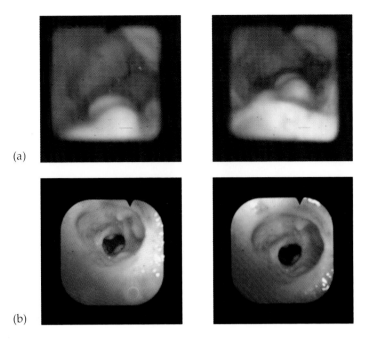

(b)

Plate 1 Oesophageal varices (a) before sclerotherapy, to show Grade III varix and (b) after sclerotherapy, demonstrating a stricture.

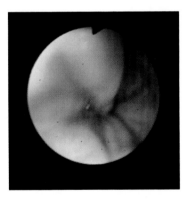

Plate 2 Grade IV varix prior to treatment.

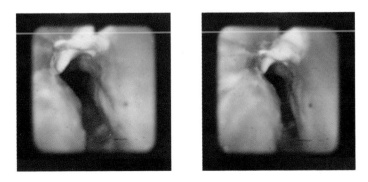

Plate 3 Post sclerotherapy ulcer.

Plates 1–3 refer to chapter 13

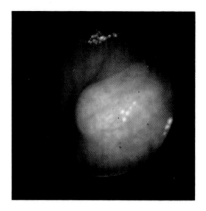

Plate 4 Endoscopic view of finger compression on stomach wall.

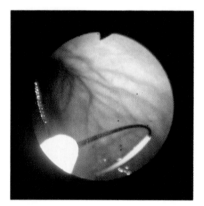

Plate 5 Snare grasping suture as it exits the catheter.

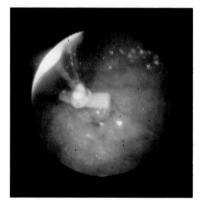

Plate 6 Internal bumper snug against abdominal wall prior to removal of safety line.

Plates 4–6 refer to chapter 20

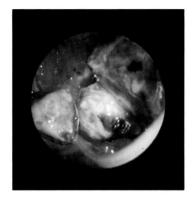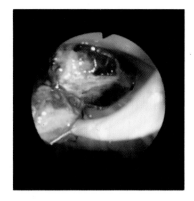

Plate 7 Extracted stones – extraction with dormia basket.

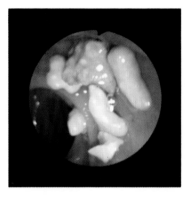

Plate 8 Spontaneously passed stone fragments
from the common bile duct.

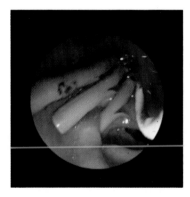

Plate 9 Multiple stents in extremely large
stones that could not be extracted
in a 94-year old patient.

Plates 7–14 refer to chapter 22

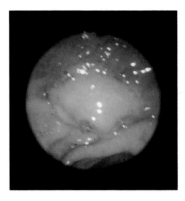

Plate 10   Mildy inflamed, reddened orifice and
haemorrhagic educatous inflammation of
the duodenal mucosa in acute pancreatitis.

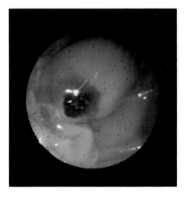

Plate 11   Haemorrhagic, necrotizing orifice in bulging
papilla with incarcerated stone in severe
biliary pancreatitis.

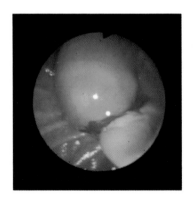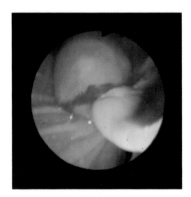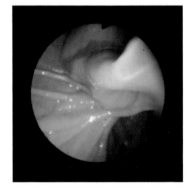

Plate 12   Severe cholangitis with drainage of pus from the papilla.

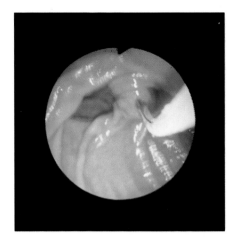

Plate 13 EPT in juxtapapillary diverticulum.

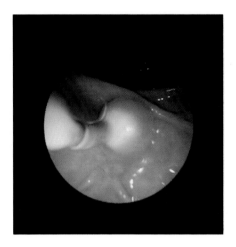

Plate 14 Balloon dilatation of the papilla;
a method that cannot be recommended.

duodenal bulb is passed. With the patient's abdomen flat on the table one can better separate the common bile duct from the pancreatic duct on the fluoroscopic screen and technically this position enhances the chances of selective cannulation of the common bile duct. The radiologist must understand the objectives of the ERCP/EPT, as well as magnification, coning down, etc., as good imaging is a key factor in reducing radiation exposure of health care personnel and patients.

The ERCP is performed using a standard side-viewing duodenoscope with an instrumentation channel of 2.8 mm. We use Hypaque 60% as contrast material. The initial filling phase of the common bile duct is of great importance, as small stones can only be seen with a small amount of contrast material in the duct. Once filling of the biliary tree begins, small stones may be carried with the flow of contrast material toward the bifurcation and then into the hepatic ducts making them difficult, if not impossible, to identify by the time full filling of the biliary tree occurs. Visualization of the entire biliary ductal system, including the gallbladder, should be achieved.

Rarely one may have to turn the patient into a supine position for homogeneous distribution of the contrast material and better filling of the right lobe of the liver. In searching for small stones that are difficult to find, many radiographs may be needed; in one extreme case, 16 films were required to demonstrate the stone.

For routine EPT, we use a standard papillotome with a 30-mm cutting wire and a short insulated and radiopaque tip. Selective, and if possible deep, cannulation of the common bile duct should be achieved. Fluoroscopic control of wire position is mandatory, because inadvertent cannulation of the pancreatic duct may occur and cutting into the pancreas can be disastrous. The wire is then bowed gently, and then the papillotome is pulled back until about half of the wire length is outside the papilla. Looking at the papilla *en face* the wire

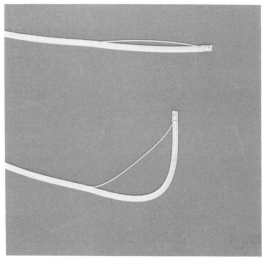

Figure 22.1   Papillotome in straight and taut position.

should point upwards into a sector between 10 and 12 o'clock (Figure 22.1). With the endoscopic picture of the size of the papilla and the length of the intramural segment, plus the information obtained from the radiograph about the width and insertion angle of the distal common bile duct, one obtains a mental picture of the desirable length of the papillotomy cut. In the presence of small stones, or in the case of a small papilla, the cut will be short; with larger stones, one often is forced to cut the full length of about 15 mm (Figure 22.2). If the above variables are straightforward, it is safe to cut in a zipper fashion for the predetermined length. It is important to realize that the transverse or first duodenal fold (omega fold) cannot be used as an anatomical criterion of how far the papillotomy may be cut, as the transverse fold's location is not indicative of the length of the intramural segment. Often, we find it necessary to cut through the fold in order to achieve an adequate papillotomy.

Most papillotomes tend to pull a little to the right, close to or beyond the 2 o'clock position.

cm |1| |2| |3| |4| |5| |6| |7| |8| |9| |10| |1|1|

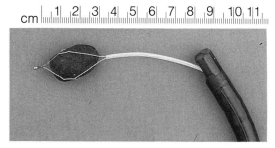

Figure 22.2   Extracted stone in dormia basket.

To counteract this a counterclockwise rotation of the tip of the endoscope during the cutting manoeuvre will direct the wire more towards 12 o'clock (Figures 22.3 and 22.4).

It is not possible to give a standard recommendation about the power setting, as there

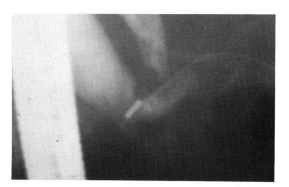

Figure 22.4   Correct positioning of the papillotome in the common bile duct.

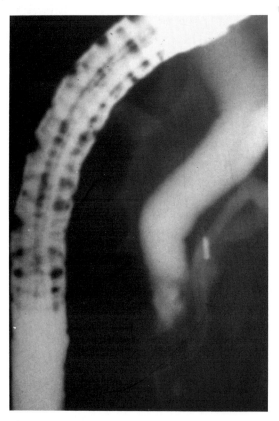

Figure 22.3   Wrong position of the papillotome – pancreatic duct, radiopaque tip of the papillotome can be easily identified.

are various power units available with different wattage output. On our Olympus VES-2 unit we set the dial for cutting and coagulation current to three or four, which provides an equal 50/50 blend. When there is a lot of wire in contact with overlying tissue, the monopolar current is not dense enough and it may take a few seconds until the initial whitening of the tissue which signals the beginning of the cutting action. The ensuing zipper effect may be quite rapid.

If even partial selective cannulation of the common bile duct cannot be achieved with the papillotome, the precutting technique can be employed. We have had to resort to a special precut papillotome in only about 5% of precuts. We do not change the blend from the 50/50 setting for precutting. The precut should have a minimum length of 5 mm in order to cut through the muscle layers of the common channel, the ampullary sphincter, thus aiming for a better cannulation angle of the common bile duct. If cannulation of the common bile duct cannot be achieved even after an adequate precut, we often exchange the papillotome for a diagnostic ERCP catheter to facilitate identification of the access to the duct. If we still fail in our search for the common bile duct, we prefer to discontinue the procedure, and bring the patient back in 2 or 3 days. By then tissue necrosis will have sloughed off and often the tiny opening of the common bile duct can be identified by a slight protrusion of yellowish mucosa. With this approach, our success rate for precutting is close to 100%.

Impacted stones in the prepapillary ampullary segment are not a contraindication to EPT, although it is often difficult to cannulate the orifice of the papilla, due to severe bulging close to the impaction. It is then necessary to create a fistula into the intramural segment using a needle knife papillotome. Once access to the common bile duct has been gained, the fistulotomy is extended with a standard papillotome. Prerequisites for this approach are the unequivocal identification of the stone with contrast material, detailed knowledge of the anatomy of the ampullary region, and experience in performing EPTs.

22.2.1 PARTICULAR HAZARDS

ERCP and EPT after (Billroth II) partial gastrectomy can be technically difficult as the instrument is under increased tension, making control of the cutting length and direction difficult, thus increasing the likelihood of perforation (Figures 22.5a,b).

In the presence of juxtapapillary diverticula, the papilla is often located at the 4 o'clock position and makes cannulation of the common bile duct easier. However, EPT carries an inherent risk if the papilla is located deep within a diverticulum, which is rarely the case.

If emergency decompression of the common bile duct becomes necessary (e.g. when

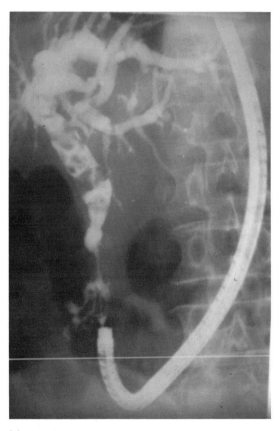

(a)

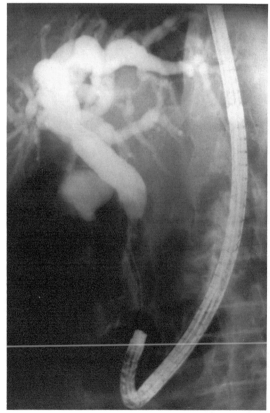

(b)

Figure 22.5   (a) EPT in billroth II stomach common bile duct with stones before EPT and status post EPT and stone extraction (b).

septic cholangitis is complicated by disseminated intravascular coagulation), a nasobiliary drainage catheter can be placed, for which a short EPT often becomes necessary. In the case of incorrectable severe coagulopathy we attempt to minimize the risk of haemorrhage by adjusting the current to 100% coagulation.

In the case of stone formation above a true stricture, stones cannot be extracted without prior lithotripsy. If large stones cannot be removed immediately, due to size and/or number, adequate drainage must be achieved. We use a nasobiliary drainage catheter to minimize the immediate risk of cholangitis and to make possible fluoroscopic checks of stone(s) at any time without ERCP (Cotton, Burney and Mason, 1979).

After routine EPT with successful removal of all stones, a patient observation period of 3–4 hours is required. We give the patient nothing by mouth for the rest of the day and resume feeding next morning. The patient may be discharged 48 hours after papillotomy.

Attempts have been made to extract stones from the common bile duct without the complication of EPT by dilatation of the papilla with balloons, or pharmacodynamically with nitroglycerine, thus preserving the physiological sphincter mechanism. The number of patients treated that way is quite small. Staritz et al. (1985) did not report major complications, but we have seen several cases of severe pancreatitis and cholangitis in the 12 patients we have treated in this manner. We abandoned the method as its complication rate far exceeds our complication rate for EPT.

In postcholecystectomy patients with retained stones but a T-tube still in place, the Burhenne catheter technique is a possibility for stone extraction (Chapter 24). However, a 6-week period is required for maturation of a fistulous T-tube tract, and we no longer use the technique.

22.3 COMPLICATIONS

Most procedure-related complications occur within the first 24 hours and their likelihood can often be predicted during the procedure. In over 3500 EPTs, our complication rate is approximately 7%; the commonest complications being bleeding, retroperitoneal perforation, and pancreatitis, in that order. Cholangitis used to be the second most frequent complication of ERCP/EPT, but has all but disappeared since the introduction of the nasobiliary drainage catheter. Impacted stones occurred as a complication of ERCP/EPT before adequate lithotriptors became available; we no longer encounter this complication. After a routine EPT there is often a little bleeding; it will usually stop even before the procedure is finished. If a significant bleed obliterates vision near the cut papilla, the edges of the cut may be injected with 3–5 ml of adrenaline (epinephrine) 1:10 000, followed by any of the commonly used sclerosants injected in amounts not exceeding 3 ml, but the need for sclerotherapy after EPT arises rarely. However, one has to be able to recognize the intensity of an arterial bleed – when cut into, a branch of the retroduodenal artery will fill the duodenum with blood instantly. In this rare, but life-threatening, emergency, immediate surgical intervention is essential.

Most retroperitoneal perforations can be managed conservatively with a nasogastric tube and antibiotics. Our emergency surgery rate of 2.3% published 10 years ago (Safrany, 1978) has been approximately halved by increased experience, including knowledge of safe, conservative management of retroduodenal perforations. It is now similar to that in other published series (Cotton, 1984; Escourrou et al., 1984).

Mortality hovers in most series around 1% (Cotton, 1984), and we have lowered our mortality figure from the 1.4% published in 1978. The possibility of a near zero complication rate exists, but we accept a higher risk in difficult cases, such as in the elderly, in whom surgery is hazardous. Even with such factors our mortality today is under 1%.

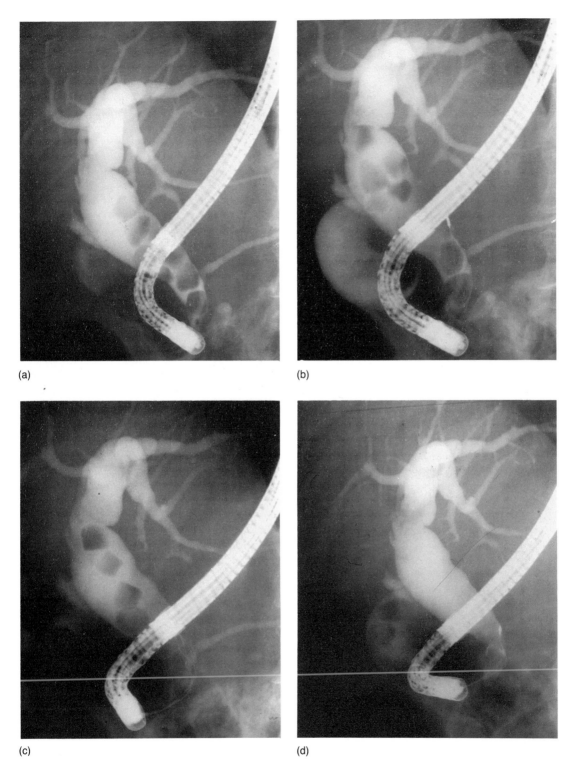

(a)   (b)

(c)   (d)

Figure 22.6 (a), (b), (c), (d) Multiple stones. Ductal clearance achieved by removal of all stones starting with the most distal one.

22.4 SUCCESS RATE OF EPT AND STONE REMOVAL

The success rate of EPT is over 95% and we are able to remove all stones in over 93% of the cases (Cotton, 1984) often clearing the duct completely (Fig. 22.6a,b,c,d). For stone extraction, we prefer the Dormia basket, resorting to the balloon only occasionally, for small and multiple stones that may be difficult to catch with the basket (Fig. 22.7). Stones of any size in a relatively narrower duct which does not permit the basket to expand beyond the dimensions of the stone is another difficult situation. Very large stones or multiple large stones present a true challenge, even for the experienced papillotomist. The decisive factor is the relationship between stone size and length of the EPT. If this relationship makes extraction of a stone impossible one has to resort to lithotripsy (Fig. 22.8). Preferably, one should try to crush the stone high in the common bile duct (Fig. 22.9) before encountering impaction in the distal common bile duct. With multiple stones, one should aim for the most distal one first because of the inherent risk of impaction if one tries also to extract more proximal stones with one sweep (Fig. 22.10).

We use mechanical lithotripsy, as other methods such as electrohydraulic shock wave lithotripsy and laser-lithotripsy are still relatively untried.

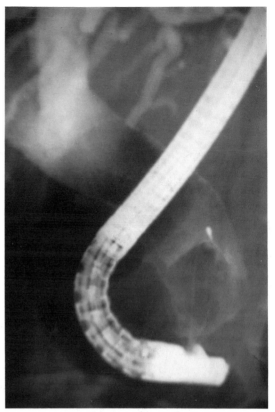

Figure 22.8   Lithotripsy in very large stone.

More than 80% of large stones, which we were once unable to extract, can be removed since the advent of lithotripsy. The remaining 20% of large stones are either too large to be grasped or too hard to be crushed (Fig. 22.11). In this situation, we place a nasobiliary drainage catheter and perfuse the common bile duct with monoocotanoin (Capmul), a semi-synthetic vegetable oil which is a solvent of cholesterol, the major component of most stones in the common bile duct. To enhance the dissolution of calcium salt, we perfuse with EDTA 1% following the monooctanoin in a cycle of 6 hours each. Side-effects are biliary-type pain (which responds readily to lowering the perfusion rate), occasional nausea, diarrhoea or vomiting.

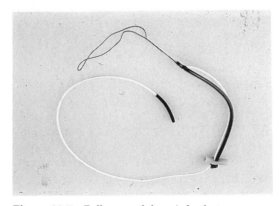

Figure 22.7   Balloon and dormia basket.

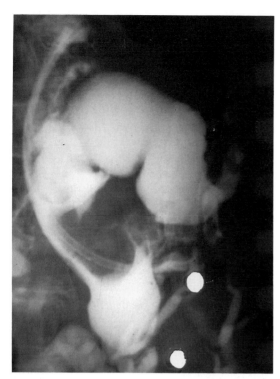

Figure 22.9   After crushing fragments still in the CBD.

The literature claims total dissolution of only 25–50% of stones, and a substantial reduction in size in another 20% (Palmer and Hofman, 1986). In our experience, even these figures are too optimistic. However, even a small reduction in size is an advantage, as the concomitant softening of the surface after perfusion for about 7 days usually makes grasping and even partial fragmentation of the stone possible. In high operative risk patients, we may repeat the perfusion cycle a second or third time, until stone extraction becomes possible.

Rarely, in extremely high operative risk patients in whom large stones cannot be removed by lithotripsy, one may choose to insert a biliary endoprosthesis as a palliative measure (Siegel and Yatto, 1984) (Fig. 22.12). There is also an evolving experience of treating common bile duct stones that cannot be removed endoscopically by extracorporeal shockwave lithotripsy, as an alternative to surgery (Sauerbruch *et al.*, 1987; Sauerbruch and Stern, 1988).

22.5 FOLLOW-UP AFTER ENDOSCOPIC PAPILLOTOMY IN POSTCHOLECYSTECTOMY PATIENTS

About 10% of patients with postcholecystectomy EPT develop recurrent symptoms, and of these 4.4–9.8% develop stenosis, new stones or both. The longest follow-up to date included 163 postcholecystectomy patients (Hawes *et al.*, 1987). At follow-up *ERCP* in 45 patients (10 of the 15 symptomatic patients and 35 asymptomatic), six had abnormal biliary findings – two sphincter stenosis without stones, three stenosis with stones, and one with stones despite a patent papillotomy. All but one patient with abnormal biliary tract findings at ERCP had a history of recurrent biliary pain or cholangitis. Symptoms tended to occur within the first 1–2 years post-EPT. No ductal abnormalities were identified other than sphincter stenosis.

22.6 FOLLOW-UP POST EPT IN PATIENTS WITH GALLBLADDER *IN SITU*

About half of all patients undergoing EPT for removal of stones in the common duct have their gallbladder in place (Cotton, 1984). There are two groups; patients with acute biliary disease (jaundice, acute cholangitis or biliary pancreatitis) treated initially with endoscopic duct decompression with cholecystectomy later; and elderly patients with concomitant medical conditions and a short life-expectancy who never undergo cholecystectomy at all. Only 10% of our 266 patients (mean age 76 years) required cholecystectomy for biliary pain or cholecystitis during a follow-up of 1–6 years (Safrany and Cotton, 1982). Escourrou *et al.* (1984) followed 130

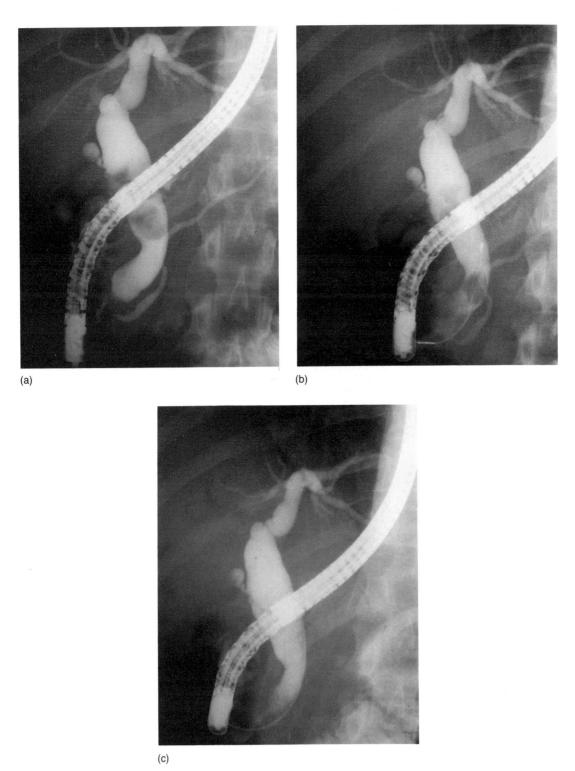

Figure 22.10 (a), (b), (c) A series of stone extractions; three stones were pulled from the common bile duct.

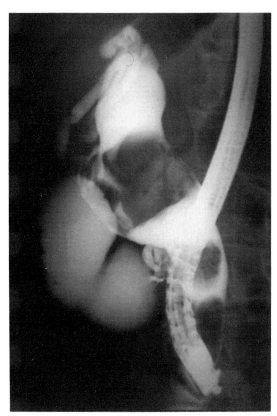

Figure 22.11 Large stone in 94-year old patient that could not be extracted.

22.7 INDICATIONS FOR ENDOSCOPIC PAPILLOTOMY VERSUS SURGERY

Although there are no randomized studies specifically in the elderly patient population, the choice of treatment for common bile duct stones in patients with a high operative risk clearly favours an endoscopic approach. Healthy patients under the age of 60 should go for surgery; with increasing age mortality quickly exceeds 5% (Vellacott and Powell, 1979; McSherry and Glenn, 1980).

The mortality rate for cholecystectomy with choledochostomy is three to four times higher than that for cholecystectomy alone (Doyle, Ward-McQuaid and McEwen-Smith, 1982). It has been proposed that in patients with gall-bladder and duct stones that require surgery,

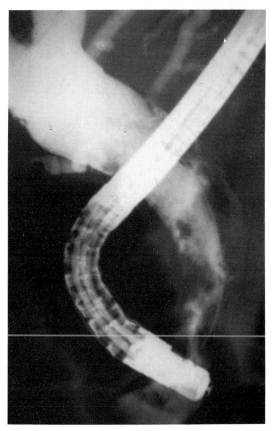

Figure 22.12 Palliative placement of multiple stents.

patients between 6 and 78 months and showed late cholecystitis in only 6.2%. Based on our experience, Siegel *et al.* (1988) published data on 1272 patients followed for up to 11 years. Post-EPT cholecystitis occurred in only 109 patients; in 23 of these (8.6%), it occurred within 1–2 days, in 86 in 7–10 days. Eighty-four patients were treated medically and 25 required surgery. Two deaths occurred within 30 days of papillotomy (0.15%), both in elderly patients after emergency cholecystectomy. In all 108 patients underwent elective cholecystectomy within 3 years of EPT. Our indications for cholecystectomy are the same as in patients without an endoscopic papillotomy.

preoperative EPT and stone removal might be better than surgery alone. The first prospective randomized study of EPT before surgery for common bile duct stones in patients with intact gallbladder failed to show a reduction of morbidity and mortality compared with a conventional surgical approach. Mortality was 1.7% in the group treated surgically alone, but patients unfit for surgery were not included (Neoptolemos, Carr-Locke and Fossard, 1987).

It has been our policy to perform prophylactic papillotomy at the time of ERCP in high operative risk patients with stones in the gallbladder but without proof of stones in the common bile duct if the patient has a history of jaundice, cholangitis or pancreatis with obvious spontaneous stone passage.

22.8 ENDOSCOPIC TREATMENT OF ACUTE SEPTIC CHOLANGITIS

In published literature the role of the endoscopic approach to septic cholangitis is unclear; one publication actually condemned endoscopic papillotomy (Chock, Wolfe and Matolo, 1981). The mortality figures in two series of relatively young patients who underwent emergency operations for acute cholangitis are 12% and 14% (Boey and Way, 1980; Thompson, Tompkins and Longmire, 1982). The evolving endoscopic literature clearly shows a benefit to patients with septic cholangitis treated by early EPT (Leese et al., 1986; Leung, Chung and Li, 1987; Gogel et al., 1987). Treating septic cholangitis by urgent EPT has been our policy for several years, and our experience with several hundred cases indicates a dramatic improvement.

22.9 ENDOSCOPIC TREATMENT OF ACUTE BILIARY PANCREATITIS

Obstruction of the papilla of Vater with reflux of bile into the pancreatic duct and retention of pancreatic juice is the supposed cause of biliary pancreatitis (Opie, 1901; Acosta and Ledesma, 1974). Incarcerated papillary stones

are rarely encountered, as the majority obstruct transiently while passing through the papilla (Kelly, 1980) and will only be seen if operation is done early (Kelly, 1980; Spuy, 1981), but stones can often be identified in the faeces (Acosta and Ledesma, 1974).

Non-invasive imaging techniques are of dubious value for detecting common bile duct stones (Stone, Fabian and Dunlop, 1981; Neoptolemos et al., 1984; Lux, Riemann and Demling, 1984) and clinical criteria for the assumption of a biliary aetiology of pancreatitis are usually sufficient.

The therapeutic concept in acute biliary pancreatitis is early removal of ampullary obstruction to prevent the development of severe pancreatitis. As surgical treatment in the acute phase carries a high risk (Acosta et al., 1978; Kelly, 1980), urgent ERCP/EPT has established itself as an alternative approach (Safrany et al., 1980; Safrany and Cotton, 1981; Kautz et al., 1982; Roseland and Selhang, 1984; Stenzel, Schrameyer and Safrany, 1985; Escourrou et al., 1987). In biliary pancreatis, selective cannulation of the common bile duct and EPT are often technically easy. In 160 patients in whom biliary pancreatitis was suspected on clinical grounds, common bile duct stones were identified in 141 and EPT was successful in 138. Complications included five bleeds requiring transfusion but none requiring surgery. At first contrast medium was injected into the common bile duct, avoiding the pancreatic duct, but later the pancreatic duct was occasionally filled and we learned that cautious filling does not have an adverse effect on the pancreas. We found additional pathological findings in the pancreas (such as necrotic cavities and pseudocyst) in 14 cases. Nineteen cases of pancreatitis of non-biliary aetiology were not harmed by ERCP and visualization of the pancreatic duct may even give useful information about the need for surgery, such as fistulization (Tonak, Lutz and Gebhardt, 1986).

The first prospective randomized study shows that ERCP/EPT in acute pancreatitis is of benefit and is safe (Neoptolemos *et al.*, 1986). Mortality from biliary pancreatitis was restricted entirely to patients predicted to have severe attacks but randomized to the group not treated by EPT.

REFERENCES

Acosta, J. M. and Ledesma, L. (1974) Gallstone migration as a cause of acute pancreatitis. *New Engl. J. Med.*, **290**, 484–7.

Acosta, J. M., Rossi, R., Galli, O. M. R. *et al.* (1978) Early surgery for acute gallstone pancreatitis: evaluation of a systemic approach. *Surgery*, **83**, 367–70.

Boey, J. H. and Way, L. W. (1980) Acute cholangitis. *Ann. Surg.*, **190**, 264–70.

Classen, M. and Demling, L. (1974) Endoskopische Sphinkterotomie der Papilla Vateri und Steinextraktion aus dem Ductus Choledochus. *Dtsch. Med. Wochenschr.* **99**, 496–7.

Cotton, P. B. (1984) Endoscopic management of bile duct stones (apples and oranges). *Gut*, **25**, 587–97.

Cotton, P. B., Burney, P. G. and Mason, R. R. (1979) Transnasal bile duct catheterization after endoscopic sphincterotomy: method for biliary drainage, perfusion and sequential cholangiography. *Gut*, **20**, 285–9.

Doyle, R. J., Ward-McQuaid, J. N. and McEwen-Smith, A. (1982) The value of routine preoperative cholangiography – a report of 4000 cholecystectomies. *Br. J. Surg.*, **69**, 617–9.

Escourrou, J., Cordova, J. A., Lazorthes, F. *et al.* (1984) Early and late complications after endoscopic sphincterotomy for biliary lithiasis with and without the gallbladder 'insitu'. *Gut*, **25**, 598–602.

Escourrou, J., Liquory, C., Boyer, J. and Sahu, J. (1987) Emergency endoscopic sphincterotomy in acute biliary pancreatitis: results of a multicenter study. *Gastrointest. Endosc.*, **33**, 187.

Gogel, H. K., Runyon, B. A., Volpicilli, N. A. and Palmer, R. C. (1987) Acute suppurative obstructive cholangitis due to stones: treatment by urgent endoscopic sphincterotomy. *Gastrointest. Endosc.*, **33**, 210–3.

Hawes, R., Vallon, A. G., Holton, J. M. and Cotton, P. B. (1987) Long term follow-up after duodenoscopic sphincterotomy (DS) for choledocholithiasis in patients with prior cholecystectomy. *Gastrointest. Endosc.*, **33**, 157.

Kautz, G., Kohaus, H., Keferstein, R. D. and Bunte, H. (1982) Zur Pathogenese und Endo-skopischen Therapie der akuten Biliaren Pankreatitis. *Klinikarzt*, **11**, 1202.

Kawai, K., Akasaka, Y., Murakami, K. *et al.* (1974) Endoscopic sphincterotomy of the ampulla of vater. *Gastrointest. Endosc.*, **20**, 148–51.

Kelly, T. R. (1980) Gallstone pancreatitis. The timing of surgery. *Surgery*, **88**, 345.

Laing, F. C. (1987) Ultrasound diagnosis of choledocholithiasis. *Semin. Ultrasound CT MR* **8**, 103–13.

Leese, T., Neoptolemos, J. P., Bakes, A. R. and Carr-Locke, D. L. (1980) Management of acute cholangitis and the impact of endoscopic sphincterotomy. *Br. J. Surg.*, **73**, 988–92.

Leung, J. W. C., Chung, S. C. S., and Li, A. K. C. (1987) Is there a role for urgent endoscopic drainage in acute suppurative cholangitis? *Gastrointest. Endosc.*, **33**, 157.

Lux, G., Riemann, J. F. and Demling, L. (1984) Biliare Pankreatitis – Diagnostische and Therapeutische Moglichkeiten durch ERCP and Endoskopische Papillotomie. *Z. Gastroenterol.*, **22**, 346–56.

McSherry, C. K. and Glenn, F. (1980) The incidence and causes of death following surgery for nonmalignant biliary tract disease. *Ann. Surg.*, **191**, 271–5.

Neoptolemos, J. P., Carr-Locke, D. L., Frazer, I. and Fossard, D. P. (1984) The management of common bile duct calculi by endoscopic sphincterotomy in patients with gallbladders in situ. *Br. J. Surg.*, **71**, 69–71.

Neoptolemos, J. P., Carr-Locke, D. L. and Fossard, D. P. (1987) Prospective randomized study of preoperative endoscopic sphincterotomy versus surgery alone for common bile duct stones. *Br. Med. J.*, **294**, 470–4.

Neoptolemos, J. P., London, N., Slater, N. D. *et al.* (1986) A prospective study of ERCP and endoscopic sphincterotomy in the diagnosis and treatment of gallstone acute pancreatitis. *Arch. Surg.*, **121**, 697–701.

Opie, E. L. (1901) The etiology of acute hemorrhagic pancreatitis, *Bull. Johns Hopkins Hosp.*, **12**, 182–8.

Palmer, K. R. and Hofman, A. F. (1986) Intraductal monooctanoin for the direct dissolution of bile duct stones: experience in 343 patients. *Gut*, **27**, 196–202.

Roseland, A. R. and Selhang, J. H. (1984) Early or delayed endoscopic papillotomy (EPT) in gallstone pancreatitis. *Ann. Surg.*, **199**, 165–7.

Safrany, L. (1978) Endoscopic treatment of biliary tract disease. *Lancet*, **ii**, 983–5.

Safrany, L., Neuhaus, B. S., Krause, S. *et al.* (1980) Endoskopische Papillotomie bei akuter, biliar bedingter Pankreatitis. *Dtsch. Med. Wochenschr.*, **105**, 115.

Safrany, L. and Cotton, P. B. (1981) A preliminary report: urgent duodenoscopic sphincterotomy for acute gallstone pancreatitis. *Surgery*, **89**, 424–8.

Safrany, L. and Cotton, P. B. (1982) Endoscopic management of choledocholithiasis. *Surg. Clin. North Am.*, **62**, 825–36.

Sauerbruch, T., Holl, J., Sackmann, M. *et al.* (1987) Treatment of bile duct stones by extracorporeal shock waves, *Semin. Ultrasound CT MR*, **8**, 155–61.

Sauerbruch, T., Stern, M. and the Study Group for Shock Wave Lithotripsy of Bile Duct Stones (1988) Fragmentation of bile duct stones by extracorporeal shock waves: a new approach to biliary calculi after failure of routine endoscopic measures, *Gastroenterology*, (submitted for publication).

Siegel, J. H., Safrany, L., Ben-Aoi, F. S. *et al.* (1988) Duodenoscopic sphincterotomy in patients with gallbladders in situ: report of a series of 1272 patients. *Am. J. Gastroenterol.*, **83**, 1255–8.

Siegel, J. H. and Yatto, R. P. (1984) Biliary endoprosthesis for the management of retained common bile duct stones. *Am. J. Gastroenterol.*, **79**, 50–4.

Spuy, van der, S. (1981) Endoscopic sphincterotomy in the management of gallstone pancreatitis. *Endoscopy*, **13**, 25.

Staritz, M., Poralla, T., Dormeyer, H. S. and Meyer zum Buschenfelde, K. H. (1985). Endoscopic removal of common bile duct stones through the intact papilla after medical sphincter dilation. *Gastroenterology*, **88**, 1807–11.

Stenzel, M., Schrameyer, B. and Safrany, L. (1985) Endoscopic therapy of acute biliary pancreatitis. *Am. J. Gastroenterol.*, **80**, 850.

Stone, H. H., Fabrian, T. C. and Dunlop, W. E. (1981) Gallstone pancreatitis: biliary pathology in relation to time of operation. *Ann. Surg.*, **194**, 305–10.

Thompson, J. E., Tompkins, R. K. and Longmire, W. P. (1982) Factors in management of acute cholangitis. *Ann. Surg.*, **195**, 137–45.

Tonak, J., Lux, G. and Gebhardt, C. (1986) A surgical approach to hemorrhagic necrotizing pancreatitis based on ERCP. *Gastrointest. Endosc.*, **32**, 104–6.

Vellacott, K. D. and Powell, P. H. (1975) Exploration of the common bile duct; a comparative study. *Br. J. Surg.*, **66**, 389–91.

CHAPTER TWENTY-THREE

Interventional biliary and pancreatic radiology

S. Somers

Developments in imaging, contrast media, catheters, needles, and embolization agents have made interventional procedures in the radiology department useful and safe. Cross-sectional imaging using computed tomography (CT) and ultrasound (US) provides easy localization of a mass. Instruments can then be used either to biopsy or drain the lesion. Biplane fluoroscopy also assists interventional procedures. The variety of available catheters and biopsy needles makes it easier to choose one that works best in any particular situation. Fine needle aspiration biopsies now have a sensitivity of 77% for pancreatic tumours and 60% for biliary tumours (Hall-Craggs and Lees, 1986). The non-ionic, intravenous contrast agents make procedures requiring opacification safer. This chapter will discuss the more commonly performed interventions that have been developed as a result of these improvements.

23.1 PERCUTANEOUS TRANSHEPATIC CHOLANGIOGRAM (PTC)

Percutaneous transhepatic cholangiography is performed to delineate both the intra- and extra-hepatic biliary trees. It is done most often in patients with obstructive jaundice to determine the anatomical location of the obstruction. If a complete or almost total obstruction is demonstrated it is best to proceed to

percutaneous drainage, a procedure often undertaken as a preliminary step in the insertion of a drainage catheter (Ferrucci, Mueller and Harbin, 1980).

The patients who need this procedure often have coagulation abnormalities, so clotting indices should be checked. If abnormal, vitamin K intramuscularly may correct them within 24 or 48 hours. However, if the clinical situation is urgent (e.g. an acute suppurative cholangitis) or coagulation is severely abnormal, the procedure may be possible after the administration of fresh frozen plasma.

The examination is performed after the patient has had nothing by mouth for at least 6 hours. For sedation pethidine (demerol) alone or in combination with Diazemuls may be used. As with all interventional procedures it is useful to have an intravenous line in place. Patients with an obstructed biliary system, should be given antibiotics prophylactically since they often develop a bacteraemia during the examination. Ampicillin and gentamicin in combination, or a broad-spectrum cephalosporin are appropriate. Our preference is to use amikacin 500 mg 8-hourly. The first dose is given before the procedure and subsequent doses for 48 hours, unless an infection develops when it is continued for up to 10 days. As this antibiotic is nephrotoxic as well as ototoxic, creatinine levels should be monitored.

The Chiba needle used for this study is

passed under local anaesthesia into the liver. The puncture site in the right midaxillary line is chosen after locating the position of the liver, lungs, and pleura by fluoroscopy. The puncture into the liver is made away from these structures during suspended respiration. Once the needle is in, the stilette is removed and contrast injected through the sheath under fluoroscopic control. The sheath is slowly withdrawn until a biliary radical is opacified. This is further filled until there is adequate visualization for diagnostic purposes. When the biliary radical is identified, the contrast is reduced from a concentration of 50% to about 25%. The patient may have to be tilted and the head elevated to fill the more distal ducts. Several punctures can be made until the intrahepatic biliary ducts are opacified, but it is wise not to exceed 10–15 attempts.

Complications of this procedure are uncommon, but are more likely if the biliary system is obstructed and not drained during the examination. They include biliary peritonitis, sepsis, bleeding and pneumothorax (Harbin, Mueller and Ferrucci, 1980). The patient should be closely monitored after the procedure for changes in temperature, pulse or blood pressure, increasing abdominal pain, or the onset of shoulder-tip pain. Local pain can be almost totally overcome by using bupivicaine for the local anaesthesia instead of lignocaine. Usually 10 ml 0.5% bupivicaine containing 1/200 000 adrenaline (epinephrine) infiltrated around the puncture site and adjacent liver capsule with a 25-gauge 3-cm needle is adequate (Lieberman and Sledor, 1986).

23.2 PERCUTANEOUS TRANSHEPATIC BILIARY DRAINAGE (PTBD)

The PTC examination can be converted to a drainage procedure if an obstructed biliary system is found. If obstruction is anticipated, the Accustick (Medi-Tech) or a Schwartz introduction system (Cook) should be used. These systems consist of a skinny needle, an 18-gauge guide-wire, and a dilator which allows the passage of a 38-gauge guide-wire.

The 18-gauge guide-wire can pass easily through the skinny needle. When a dilated biliary system is encountered during PTC no further contrast is injected (Figure 23.1(a)). The 18-gauge guide-wire is passed through the needle until it is well within the dilated biliary system, the skinny needle is removed, and the dilators passed over the guide-wire. When the dilator is within the dilated duct, a 38-gauge guide-wire is passed through it into the bile ducts. An attempt is then made to pass the guide-wire into the duodenum (Figure 23.1(b)). Once this has been accomplished a drainage catheter with end- and side-holes can be introduced over the guide-wire and advanced into the duodenum. If it is not possible to get the guide-wire into the duodenum, the drainage catheter is left in the most dilated part of the biliary system. Further attempts at passing the drainage catheter into the duodenum can be made subsequently when the system has been decompressed. Usually a second attempt, about 1–2 weeks after the initial procedure, is successful.

The drainage catheter should be soft and of the smallest size to maintain continuous drainage. Our preference is to use a 7- or 8-Fr Cope-loop biliary drainage catheter (Cook). This catheter has a reformable loop at one end with multiple side-holes along the loop as well as a portion of the straight part of the catheter. The loop is reformed by pulling a thread on the hub portion of the catheter. The loop limits movement of the catheter and prevents its being pulled out. This catheter can be changed for a larger size if prolonged drainage is required. A Ring–McLean biliary drainage catheter (Cook) may also be used for the same purpose (Figure 23.1 (c)). The disadvantage of this catheter is its stiffness which causes discomfort if drainage is prolonged. The catheter should, in any case, be changed every 3 months, and earlier if it obstructs. The indications of obstruction include leakage around the catheter, increasing jaundice and sepsis.

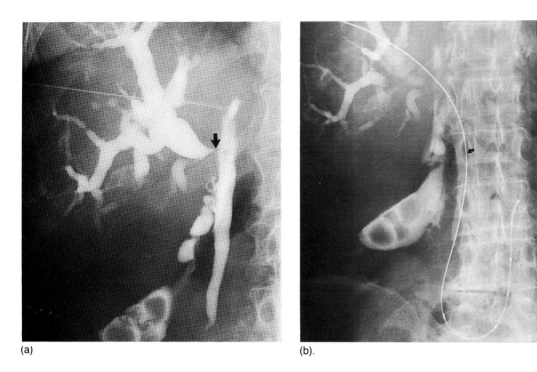

(a)

(b).

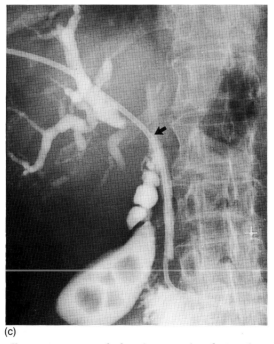

(c)

Figure 23.1 (a) Chiba needle percutaneous cholangiogram. An obstruction of the hepatic duct (arrow) with proximal dilatation of the intrahepatic ducts is demonstrated. The common bile duct is normal. Stones are present in the gallbladder. (b) A guide-wire (arrow) has been passed through the obstruction and into the duodenum. It is now ready for the drainage catheter to be passed over it. (c) A Ring–McLean biliary drainage catheter is shown in good position.

Following the drainage procedure the patient should be placed on broad-spectrum antibiotics for at least 5 days. Our choice is again amikacin, 500 mg three times a day.

The complications associated with this procedure are similar to those of PTC. However, biliary peritonitis and a pneumothorax are more likely if the catheter dislodges itself and some of the side-holes come to lie in the peritoneal cavity or pleural space: both these conditions can be fatal. Therefore, it is useful to check the position of the side-holes of the catheter with frequent plain radiographs of the right upper quadrant hepatic area.

23.3 COMBINED PERCUTANEOUS TRANSHEPATIC CHOLANGIOGRAM AND ENDOSCOPIC RETROGRADE PANCREATICOCHOLANGIOGRAM (ERCP)

Occasionally an ERCP may fail in a patient who needs to have a papillotomy or a stent placed in the common bile duct. In these patients the endoscopic procedure can be aided by passing a guide-wire and drainage catheter into the duodenum following PTC. The temporary dilatation of the ampulla by the drainage catheter facilitates the endoscopic papillotomy. Alternatively, a 400-cm guide-wire may be passed into the duodenum and withdrawn with the aid of an endoscope. A nasobiliary drain can then be introduced over the guide-wire as a temporary measure. Following this, endoscopic papillotomy and stent placement may be undertaken. Again the presence of the nasobiliary drain facilitates entry of the papillotome into the distal common bile duct.

23.4 PERCUTANEOUS PANCREATOGRAPHY

An ERCP may fail or inadequately opacify the pancreatic duct as a result of duct obstruction.

Percutaneous pancreatography then becomes an alternative, especially in suspected chronic pancreatitis with a pancreatic mass, when further delineation of the duct anatomy is necessary. This information is useful in the planning of appropriate pancreatic surgery (Wong, Schuman and Grodsinsky, 1980). Percutaneous fine needle biopsy is also aided by pancreatography as it more clearly defines the lesion, in particular the strictures (Lees and Heron, 1987). Percutaneous pancreatography is performed in the fasting patient after sedation with pethidine (demerol) and Diazemuls under ultrasound control using a 3.5- or 5-MHz transducer. The pancreatic duct is identified as a tubular structure within the gland and punctured with a 22-gauge needle in the midbody region where the main duct is usually less than 6 cm from the interior surface of the abdominal wall. The needle tip is manipulated until its echo is identified within the lumen. When the stilette is removed from the needle, pancreatic juice flows freely if it is under pressure, otherwise aspiration produces pancreatic juice. Contraindications to this procedure include acute pancreatitis, cholangitis, and abnormal coagulation indices.

23.5 HEPATIC BIOPSY

23.5.1 PERCUTANEOUS

In diffuse parenchymal liver disease a random biopsy is usually performed through a lower right intercostal space. This may be either a fine needle aspiration or a core biopsy. The core biopsy can be done manually with a Menghini needle or Tru-cut needle, or a Biopty gun (Radiplast Biopty, Henleys Medical Supplies Ltd, UK) which produces better and more consistent biopsies (Lindgren, 1982). The biopsy gun uses a special Tru-cut needle to obtain a core biopsy within a fraction of a second of releasing a trigger mechanism. Cook have developed a similar

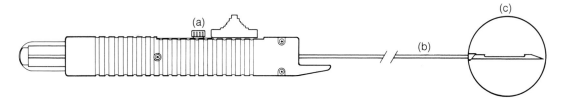

Figure 23.2   Roth biopsy device showing the trigger button (a), cutting cannula (b), and tissue stilette (c).

device called the Roth Biopsy device (Figure 23.2) which also uses a Tru-cut type of needle. It has the advantages of being cheaper than the Biopty gun, and its biopsy tip (tissue stilette) can be more accurately localized within the lesion. This is especially important for smaller nodules. Before the procedure the liver size and location should be accurately mapped using either ultrasound or fluoroscopy. The location of the liver is especially important if it is small and fibrotic as in chronic liver disease. In focal liver disease good biopsies of the area of interest can be obtained using either ultrasound or CT for guidance of the needle.

Accurate positioning of the needle can be accomplished with ultrasound. Often two people are necessary to do this. One radiologist locates the lesion and the needle tip as it is passed into the liver, and the other performs the biopsy. If a Roth biopsy device or a Biopty gun is used the procedure can be performed by one radiologist. As a general rule a biopsy under ultrasound control is quicker than with the aid of CT.

CT-controlled biopsies have the advantage of not only showing the location of the lesion but also permitting accurate measurement of its depth and size (Figure 23.3a, b). The easiest access avoiding pleura, lung and bowel is also easily demonstrated.

A cytotechnologist must be on hand to make a cytological smear immediately if a fine needle aspiration biopsy is performed. This ensures more consistent results on cytology. Core biopsies can be fixed in formalin by the radiologist.

23.5.2 TRANSJUGULAR

In any patient in whom there is a contraindication to a percutaneous biopsy the transjugular technique is an excellent alternative. It also has the advantage of being able to measure intrahepatic pressures and is the method of choice if this is desired.

The equipment for this procedure consists of a long Seldinger needle, a dilator with a sheath, the biopsy needle with a hollow stilette with side-holes near the tip, and a 9-Fr catheter. The biopsy is performed with the patient lying on a tilting fluoroscopic table. Sedation is not usually required, but if needed up to 50 mg of pethidine (demerol) or 5–10 mg of Diazemuls can be given intravenously. Before inserting the Seldinger needle into the internal jugular vein, the patient is tilted to 30° head down with the shoulders elevated about 15 cm with pads. Tilting engorges the internal jugular veins, and elevation of the shoulders stretches them, making the straight, relatively immobile veins easier to puncture. Once the right internal jugular vein has been punctured, a guide-wire is introduced and the 9-Fr catheter passed over it. The catheter is introduced into one of the veins of the right lobe of the liver (Figure 23.4 (a)). The right internal jugular vein is chosen as it forms the most direct line to the inferior vena cava into which the hepatic veins empty. The biopsies are usually taken from the right lobe as it is the largest part of the liver and perforation is unlikely.

When the catheter is in the right lobe hepatic vein pressures may be taken in both the

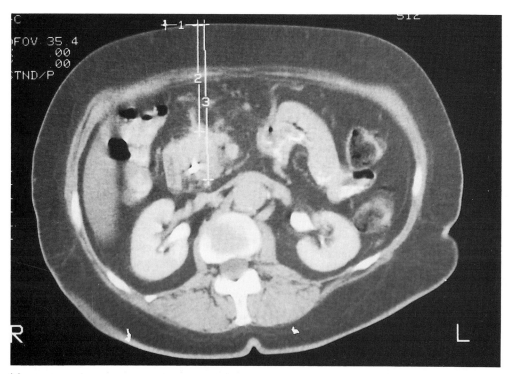

(a)

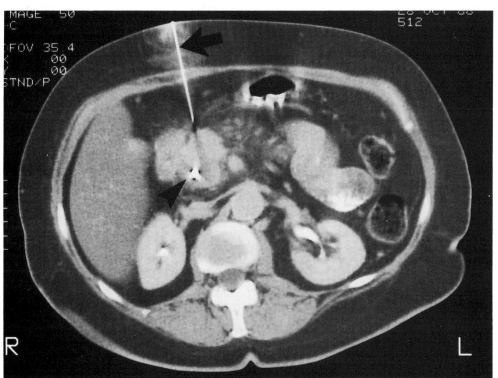

(b)

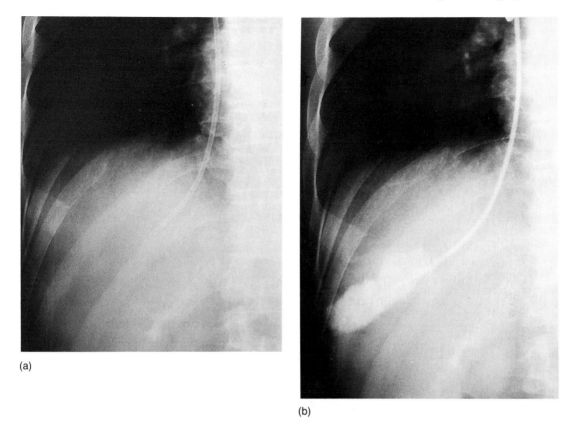

(a)

(b)

Figure 23.4   (a) A 9-Fr transjugular catheter in position in one of the right hepatic veins. (b) The wedged position of the catheter in the right lobe of the liver is demonstrated by the sinusoidogram.

free and wedged positions. The wedged position can be determined by the sinusoidogram that is seen when contrast is injected (Figure 23.4 (b)). The corrected sinusoidal pressure (CSP) may be calculated by subtracting the free hepatic vein pressure from the wedged pressure. The degree of portal hypertension, if present, can be assessed by the corrected sinusoidal pressure. The normal CSP is up to 5 mmHg. In mild portal hypertension the CSP ranges from 6 to 14 mmHg; moderate from 15 to 30 mmHg, and severe to above 30 mmHg (Viamonte, Warren and Famon, 1970). After pressures have been taken the biopsy needle

is introduced into the liver through the 9-Fr catheter with a syringe half filled with saline attached to it. A Menghini 'one second' technique (Menghini, 1958) is then used to obtain a biopsy while the patient maintains suspended respiration. The needle is withdrawn and the biopsy flushed out of the needle with saline. Several attempts to biopsy different areas of the liver can be made.

When adequate biopsies have been obtained it is important to inject contrast into the hepatic veins. If any extravasation is seen it indicates perforation of the liver capsule and the perforation can be embolised immediately

Figure 23.3   (a) A mass in the head of the pancreas has been localized and measurements taken showing its most proximal (2) and distal (3) surfaces from the anterior abdominal wall. These measurements are useful in planning the biopsy of the lesion. (b) The needle (arrow) has been localized within the lesion.

with Gelfoam (Riley *et al.*, 1984). Perforation does not occur more frequently than 3.5% (Colapinto, 1985).

The biopsy apparatus is removed at the end of the procedure and the patient is allowed to sit up. Little pressure is required over the puncture site as bleeding often stops spontaneously due to the low pressure in the venous system.

The success of the transjugular procedure often depends on the disease process in the liver. Good core biopsies are obtained from tissue that is relatively normal but when hepatic fibrosis is present specimens tend to fragment. This may explain the disparity in success rates reported by different authors using this technique. Bataille and Bercoff (1983) report 64%, whereas Gilmore, Bradley and Thompson (1977) claim a 100% success rate and in our own experience of 95 patients we have had no failures.

The complications of this procedure are minimal, but include bleeding at the puncture site with occasional haematoma formation; transient hoarseness, or Horner's syndrome, secondary to the infiltration of local anaesthetic; and transient cardiac arrhythmias as the catheter is passed through the right atrium. Rare but more serious complications are inadvertent puncture of the internal carotid artery and perforation of the liver capsule.

This technique can be performed by any skilled angiographer and has the added advantage of being able to obtain more representative tissue that lies deep in the liver (Sherlock, 1985). Another advantage of this technique is that biopsies can be done in a high-risk group of patients in whom conventional liver biopsy is contraindicated because of severe coagulation abnormalities and ascites.

23.6 ABSCESS DRAINAGE

Intra-abdominal abscesses used to have a mortality as high as 60% (Redfern, Close and Ellison, 1962) until the advent of percutaneous

drainage of the lesion which has dramatically improved the outcome (Altemeier *et al.*, 1973; Gerzof *et al.*, 1979; Haaga and Weinstein, 1980; Gerzof *et al.*, 1981; Gronvall *et al.*, 1982; Kuligowska, Connors and Shapiro, 1982; Martin *et al.*, 1982; van Sonnenberg *et al.*, 1982).

The advantages of percutaneous drainage include: performance under local anaesthesia, avoidance of prolonged postoperative hospitalization and, in seriously ill patients, immediate benefit which can reverse potentially fatal situations (Crass and Karl, 1982; Greenwood, Collins and Yrizarry, 1982).

Any abscess cavity identified, either by CT or ultrasound, can be drained (Figure 23.5 a, b). CT has the advantage of providing better localization not only of the abscess, but also of the surrounding structures. Therefore, if the abscess is deeply situated, CT guidance helps in avoiding passage of the drainage catheter through bowel or any other vital organ. Ultrasound guidance is just as useful as CT when the fluid collection is closer to the abdominal surface and interposing bowel can be excluded. Therefore, in the liver, CT has no particular advantage over ultrasound.

The drainage catheter is preceded by an introduction system such as the Accustick (Meditech). The system is used in the same manner as in biliary drainage except that for abscess drainage a sump drain is passed over the guide-wire into the abscess cavity. Before passing the sump catheter the track may need to be dilated. Our preference is to use a 12-Fr vanSonnenburg (Meditech) sump or a Ring–McLean (Cook) sump catheter. If the contents of the abscess are extremely viscous a 16-Fr sump catheter may be inserted. A CT or an ultrasound examination is done immediately after the drainage procedure. Multiloculated abscess cavities require multiple drains. The multiloculated nature may be apparent on the immediate postdrainage scan or when it is repeated a few days later. The catheter is left in place until the abscess resolves completely. Resolution can be monitored by regular sino-

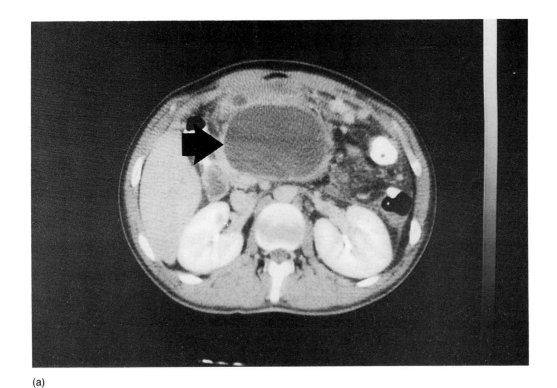

(a)

(b)

Figure 23.5 (a) A large pancreatic pseudocyst (arrow) seen on CT. (b) An immediate postdrainage CT scan shows the position of the drainage catheter and a partially empty abscess cavity with air in it.

grams, and the catheter position changed as required. Occasionally resolution may not occur, usually due to a tumour. If the abscess is a pancreatic pseudocyst it usually means that a main pancreatic duct is completely obstructed and surgery is then indicated.

Complications may be fatal if a mesenteric vessel is lacerated by the drain. Careful CT guidance avoids this complication. Sepsis and disseminated intravascular coagulation may also be encountered. Covering the procedure with broad-spectrum antibiotics, and continuing treatment for several days, usually avoids sepsis. The radiologist's task continues after the catheter has been secured, for the initial catheter may be too small or dislodge, requiring replacement. It may plug because of inadequate irrigation, so close surgical/radiological supervision is necessary.

23.7 FINE NEEDLE ASPIRATION BIOPSY – GENERAL COMMENTS

Biopsies of the pancreas and biliary system have a higher success rate if these areas can be visualized clearly, either by ultrasound or fluoroscopy. A biliary stent or a pancreatico-gram often points the way to a lesion. At least three passes should be made, and this is particularly important for the smaller lesions and reduces the sampling error. The presence of a cytotechnologist at the time of biopsy further improves the success rate by making a slide of the cells before the aspirate has had time to clot.

REFERENCES

Altemeier, W. A., Culbertson, W. R., Fullen, W. D. and Shook, C. D. (1973). Intra-abdominal abscesses. *Am. J. Surg.*, **125**, 70–9.

Bataille, C. and Bercoff, E. (1983) La Ponction bio-psie hepatique par voie transveineuse. Une experience portant sur 213 examens. *Acta Clin. Belg.*, **38**, 222–7.

Colapinto, R. F. (1985) Transjugular biopsy of the liver. *Clin. Gastroenterol.*, **14**, 451–67.

Crass, J. R. and Karl, R. (1982) Bedside drainage of

abscesses with sonographic guidance in the desperately ill. *A.J.R.*, **139**, 183–5.

Ferrucci, J. T., Mueller, P. R. and Harbin, W. P. (1980) Percutaneous transhepatic biliary drainage: technique, results and applications. *Radiology*, **135**, 1–13.

Gerzof, S. G., Robbins, A. H., Birkett, D. G. et al. (1979) Percutaneous catheter drainage of abdominal abscesses guided by ultrasound and computed tomography. *A.J.R.*, **133**, 1–18.

Gerzof, S. G., Robbins, A. H., Johnson, W. C. et al. (1981) Percutaneous catheter drainage of abdominal abscesses. *New Engl. J. Med.*, **305**, 653–7.

Gilmore, I. T., Bradley, R. D. and Thompson, R. P. (1977) Transjugular liver biopsy. *Br. Med. J.*, **2**, 100–1.

Greenwood, L. H., Collins, T. L. and Yrizarry, J. M. (1982) Percutaneous management of multiple liver abscesses. *A.J.R.*, **139**, 390–2.

Gronvall, S., Gammelgaard, J., Haubet, A. and Holm, H. H. (1982) Drainage of abdominal abscesses guided by sonography. *A.J.R.*, **138**, 527–9.

Hall-Craggs, M. A. and Lees, W. R. (1986) Fine needle aspiration biopsy: pancreatic and biliary tumours. *A.J.R.*, **147**, 399–403.

Harbin, W. P., Mueller, P. R. and Ferrucci, J. T. (1980) Transhepatic cholangiography: complications and use patterns of the fine-needle technique. *Radiology*, **135**, 15–22.

Haaga, J. R. and Weinstein, A. F. (1980) CT-guided percutaneous aspiration and drainage of absces-ses. *A.J.R.*, **135**, 1187–94.

Kuligowska, E., Connors, S. K. and Shapiro, J. H. (1982) Liver abscess: sonography in diagnosis and treatment. *A.J.R.*, **138**, 13–5.

Lees, W. R. and Heron, C. W. (1987) US guided percutaneous pancreatography: experience in 75 patients. *Radiology*, **165**, 809–13.

Lieberman, R. P. and Sledor, P. R. (1986) Pain control after percutaneous biliary drainage: local infiltration with bupivacaine and adrenalin. *A.J.R.*, **146**, 595–6.

Lindgren, P. G. (1982) Percutaneous needle biopsy. A new technique. *Acta Radiol. (Diagn.)*, **23**, 653–6.

Martin, E. C., Karlson, K. B., Fankuchen, E. I. et al. (1982) Percutaneous drainage of postoperative intrabdominal abscesses. *A.J.R.*, **138**, 13–15.

Menghini, G. (1958) One-second needle biopsy of the liver. *Gastroenterology*, **35**, 190–9.

Redfern, W. T., Close, A. S. and Ellison, E. H. (1962) Intra-abdominal abscess: a review of 100 consecutive patients. *Arch Surg.*, **85**, 278–84.

Riley, S. A., Ellis, W. R., Irving, H. C. et al. (1984) Percutaneous liver biopsy with plugging of needle track: a safe method for use in patients with impaired coagulation. *Lancet*, **ii**, 436.

Sherlock, S. (1985) *Diseases of the Liver and Biliary System*, 7th edn, Blackwell Scientific, Oxford, p. 33.

van Sonnenberg, E., Ferruci, J. T. Jr, Mueller, P. R. *et al*. (1982) Percutaneous drainage of abscesses and fluid collections: technique, results and applications. *Radiology*, **142**, 1–10.

Viamonte, M. Jr, Warren, W. D. and Fomon, J. J. (1970) Liver panangiography in the assessment of portal hypertension in liver cirrhosis. *Radiol. Clin. North Am.*, **VIII**, 147–67.

Wong, D. G., Schuman, B. M. and Grodsinsky, C. (1980) The value of endoscopic retrograde cholangiopancreatography in the surgical management of chronic pancreatitis. *Am. J. Gastroenterol.*, **73**, 353–6.

CHAPTER TWENTY-FOUR

Benign biliary obstruction: radiological intervention

H. J. Burhenne

The benign conditions leading to obstruction of the bile ducts are cholelithiasis, and stricture formation, or a combination thereof as in recurrent pyogenic cholangitis or oriental cholangitis. Biliary strictures are related, in order of frequency, to: cholangitis, bile duct anastomosis, injury (including iatrogenic) and sclerosing cholangitis. Stricturing of the common hepatic duct may also rarely be seen in the Mirizzi syndrome (Cruz *et al*, 1983).

24.1 DIAGNOSIS OF BENIGN BILIARY OBSTRUCTION

Bile duct obstruction can be deduced from clinical signs and symptoms as well as laboratory study. A definitive and specific diagnosis is then required using imaging techniques. The initial radiological technique for the identification of bile duct obstruction is ultrasonography which usually demonstrates the degree and extent of bile duct dilatation and often identifies the level of obstruction. Hepatolithiasis and choledocholithiasis can usually be diagnosed, although stone disease in the distal common duct may be obscured by overlying gas in the duodenum. Direct cholangiography follows ultrasonic imaging. Transhepatic cholangiography is used for lesions in and above the hepatic ducts, and endoscopic retrograde cholangiography for suspected obstructing lesions in the distal bile ducts. Computed tomography as an additional

procedure is rarely required, but is more sensitive in identifying calcified bile duct stones. Postoperatively retained stones in the bile duct are most easily demonstrated by T-tube cholangiography obtained 7–10 days after common duct exploration.

Contrast dilution to about 25% iodine content is utilized for cholangiography. This permits radiographic penetration, for stones may be hidden if dense contrast material is used (Figure 24.1). Particular attention must be directed to the distal common duct at the duodenal entrance where spasm of the intramural portion of the common duct and its muscular closing mechanism may obscure bile duct stones. A low-pressure hand injection is required for good filling of the distal end of the common duct, for overinjection will result in spasm. When spot filming of the distal common duct has been completed, filling of the intrahepatic radicals is required, and the cystic duct should also be filled if possible.

Other postoperative abnormalities diagnosed on cholangiograms include malposition of tubes, strictures, neoplasms and other retained material such as blood clot and bile sludge (Figures 24.2 and 24.3).

Intravenous cholangiography as an alternative to direct cholangiography is no longer used in North America because of a high incidence of reported complications. An improved contrast material for intravenous cholangiography, however, has given good

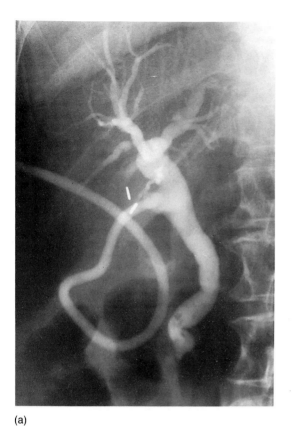

(a)

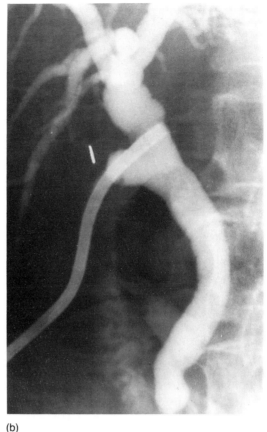

(b)

Figure 24.1   (a) Dilute contrast with radiographic penetration identifies multiple, very small, retained distal common duct stones. (b) Poor radiographic penetration in the same patient is inadequate to ensure that all retained stones were removed. Note that one of the two surgical clips was inadvertently removed with the wire basket during stone retrieval.

results in Europe (meglumine iotroxinate, Biliscopin, Germany). Of 286 patients, 1.3% developed transient skin rashes as the only recorded side-effect (Daly, Fitzgerald and Simpson, 1987).

24.2 RADIOLOGICAL STONE REMOVAL

Interventional radiological treatment for cholelithiasis is a recent but rapidly expanding field. A variety of new therapeutic techniques have been developed along two access routes, percutaneous or postoperative. The percutaneous approach developed from transhepa-

tic cholangiography. The postoperative interventional route utilizes postoperative sinus tracts or cholecystostomy openings.

The postoperative subhepatic approach through surgical drain tracts is less time consuming and less technically demanding than the direct percutaneous technique. It carries a lower complication rate when compared with the transhepatic approach. The subhepatic approach also has advantages in offering a larger access diameter for stenting catheters, for dilatation balloon catheters, and for retrieval instruments in the treatment of cholelithiasis.

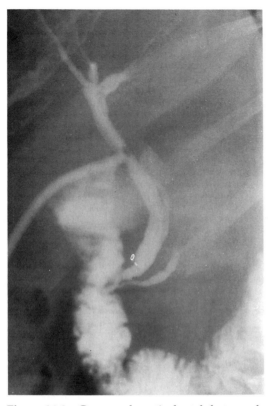

Figure 24.2 Common hepatic duct defect may be misinterpreted as a retained stone. It represents the cut-out in the T-tube at the junction of the long and short arms. Note that the T-tube was inserted into the common hepatic duct with a low insertion of a retained cystic duct stump. The operative report contains a statement that choledochotomy was performed.

Postoperative radiological techniques for stone extraction and stricture dilatation are usually done without anaesthesia and in the ambulatory patient. Complicated cases require short-term hospitalization and antibiotic cover, particularly if there is a previous history of postoperative pancreatitis. The transhepatic percutaneous approach, on the other hand, is usually painful and best performed under intravenous analgesia.

24.3 EQUIPMENT

A special catheter has been designed for easy instrumentation of sinus tracts and the biliary ducts (Burhenne, 1973). Wires in the wall of the catheter permit guidance of the catheter tip from the outside. Catheters are available in 8-, 10- and 13-Fr diameters (Medi-Tech Inc., USA). The lumen of only the largest 13-Fr steerable catheter allows passage of the Dormia stone extraction basket with its sheath. Smaller baskets from Cook and Medi-Tech are available for smaller catheters, but the difficulty of instrumentation increases as the size of the available sinus tract diminishes (Figure 24.4).

Dormia (V. Mueller, USA), Medi-Tech and Cook (Cook, Inc., USA) stone baskets are used (Figure 24.5). The first is available in only one size (13 Fr), the others come in three sizes. Larger baskets are required for large stones and large common ducts. Ideally, the wires of the open basket should touch the walls of the bile duct, resulting in easy stone engagement. Large baskets, therefore, are used even for retrieval of small stones if the bile duct system is dilated.

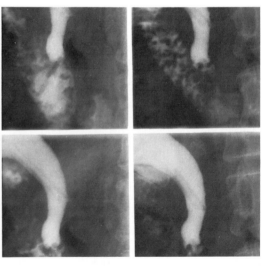

Figure 24.3 Good filling of the distal common duct with multiple spot films demonstrating that the duct inserts into a small duodenal diverticulum. This is not a retained stone.

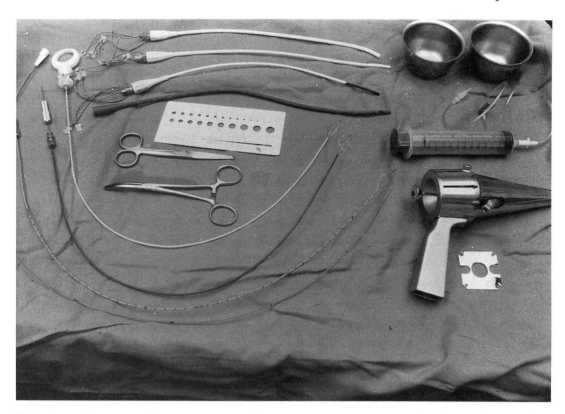

Figure 24.4   Equipment for non-operative stone retrieval. Left row top to bottom: steerable catheters in three sizes, straight catheter, catheter measuring template, scissors, artery-forceps, three different baskets, Fogarty balloon catheter. Right row top to bottom: 10-cm stainless steel bowls for mixing of contrast and saline, syringe for contrast injection with connecting tubing, pistol control handle and wobble plate for the steerable catheter.

24.4 TECHNIQUE (Figure 24.6)

Mondet (1962) pioneered the use of the post-operative T-tube tract for access to the bile ducts. He and Mazzariello (1970) used pliable forceps for stone extraction. The first use of the Dormia ureteral stone basket was described by LaGrave (LaGrave *et al.*, 1969). This basket is still the most commonly used instrument for biliary stone retrieval. The combination of the stone basket with the steerable catheter has made non-operative stone extraction more practicable and less time consuming. It also carries a lower complication rate.

The patient reports to the X-ray department about 5 weeks after operation. Almost all are treated as outpatients without premedication. Antibiotics are used only in patients with a history of previous pancreatitis, or if multiple intrahepatic stones require extraction.

The T-tube is extracted and the steerable catheter passed through the sinus tract. Turns in the tract are demonstrated under fluoroscopic control during contrast injection. The steerable catheter can be manoeuvred around 90° turns in the sinus tract. An angle of more than 90° between the sinus tract and the common duct can also be negotiated.

After manipulation of the steerable catheter into the bile duct, the position of the retained stone is identified by cholangiography. The tip of the catheter is then steered into that

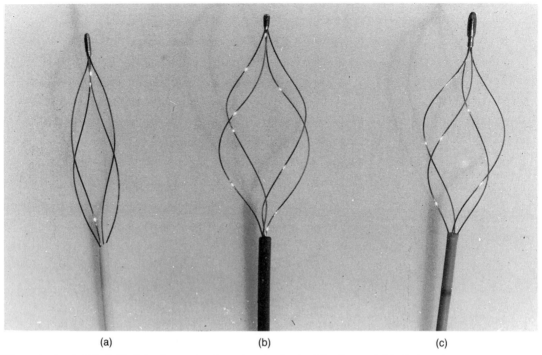

Figure 24.5   (a) Medi-Tech basket with white sheath. (b) Cook basket with black sheath. (c) Dormia basket with green sheath.

portion of the biliary tract containing the stone. It is positioned just beyond the stone if the duct diameter permits passage of the catheter alongside the stone. If the stone is blocking the duct, the steerable catheter is positioned with its tip just at the stone. The closed stone basket is then inserted through the steerable catheter and opened distal to the stone. Passage of the wire basket alongside the stone may be difficult, particularly if the duct is narrow and if the tip of the basket cannot be advanced parallel to the bile duct wall. Passage of the basket often requires making an obtuse angle between its tip and the duct wall. No perforations have occurred with this manoeuvre, but we do not advance the basket if it is at a right angle to the duct.

After opening the basket distal to the stone, it is slightly rotated during basket withdrawal. This usually results in stone engagement. We do not close the basket in the duct system after stone engagement. This used to be done, but it often resulted in stone fragmentation and the stone falling out of the basket. We now use a continuous extraction movement as soon as the stone is seen within the basket. Stones up to 6 mm diameter are usually extracted intact through the sinus tract of a No. 14 French T-tube. Larger stones require fragmentation.

Percutaneous transhepatic intervention for bile duct stone removal utilizes standard percutaneous transhepatic cholangiography technique to enter a right hepatic duct with a stylet and sheath as used in arteriography. After the sheath has been advanced into the hepatic duct, the transhepatic tract is enlarged with arterial dilators, followed by a guide-wire and stone extraction baskets. The basket is closed in position after stone engagement and the fragments are expelled or moved through the papilla into the duodenum (Clouse et al., 1986).

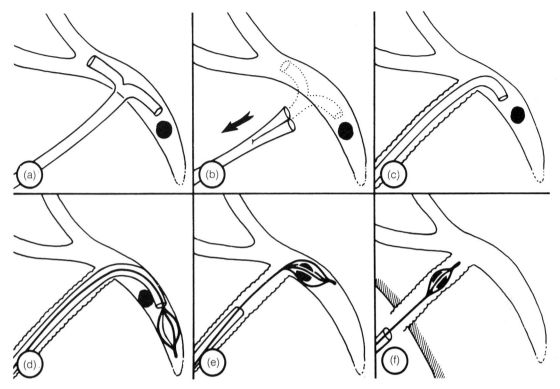

Figure 24.6   Technical steps of stone extraction. (a) Identification of retained stone on T-tube cholangiography. (b) Extraction of T-tube. (c) Insertion of steerable catheter through the sinus tract. (d) Open basket in position distally to the retained stone. (e) Stone engagement in the wire basket. (f) Extraction of the stone through the sinus tract. From Burhenne (1973), with permission.

Patients are only admitted as inpatients for extraction of difficult intrahepatic stones or if there is a history of previous postoperative pancreatitis. However, outpatients are asked to wait in the X-ray department for several hours after completion of the extraction procedure. This precaution was taken because some patients develop right upper quadrant pain following instrumentation of the distal common duct. This results from ampullary spasm and requires temporary external bile drainage.

24.5 RESULTS

Our personal experience consists of 2148 patients referred for retrieval of retained stones in the years 1972 and 1987. All patients underwent postoperative T-tube cholangiography for diagnosis.

Detailed analysis of 661 patients by Burhenne (1980) demonstrated that 80% of retained stones were in an extrahepatic location; 72.5% were solitary stones (Tables 24.1 and 24.2). An attempt is made to extract the stone and obtain a satisfactory closing cholangiogram in one sitting. This is often not possible.

Table 24.1   Incidence of multiple stones

Stones (no.)	Incidence (%)
Single	72.5
2–5	19.0
6–10	8.0
11–27	0.5

252 Benign biliary obstruction

Table 24.2 Location of stones

Location	No.	%
Extrahepatic	529	80
Intrahepatic	98	15
Combined	34	5
Total	661	

Blood clots or gas may accumulate in the duct system during stone removal. The patient is then asked to return several days later for a completion cholangiogram to ensure that all stones have been removed. A straight catheter is inserted through the sinus tract into the duct system during the interval (Figure 24.7).

24.6 MULTIPLE SESSIONS

The removal of several retained stones may require multiple extraction sessions. Indications for multiple sessions are:

1. Completion cholangiogram.
2. Fragmentation.
3. Multiple stones.

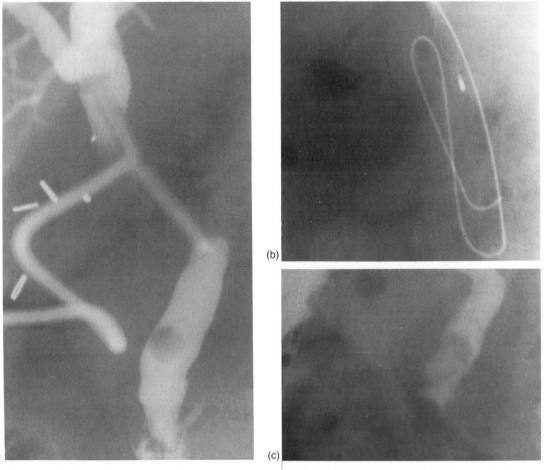

Figure 24.7 (a) A distal retained common duct stone. (b) Wire basket in place distal to the retained stone. Note that a guide-wire was placed through the sinus tract and common duct into the duodenum for easier recatheterization of the sinus tract after extraction. (c) The retained stone has been fragmented, some fragments and several blood clots are present, requiring conclusion cholangiography at a subsequent session.

4. Cystic duct stones.
5. Intrahepatic stones.
6. Tract manipulation.
7. Impacted stones.
8. Strictures.
9. Penrose drains.

If a stone larger than the diameter of the sinus tract is extracted, this can result in injury to the wall of the sinus tract, or bleeding. It is then best to insert a straight catheter and have the patient return a week later for further stone extraction. We have learned that multiple sessions in patients with multiple stones are more likely to succeed in the extraction of the final stone. If one stone remains behind, the procedure is considered a failure. About 40% of all patients undergoing stone retrieval now attend for multiple sessions.

If a Penrose drain is in place adjacent to the sinus tract, we prefer to extract the drain and have the patient return at a later date. We have found that cross-connections exist between Penrose drains and T-tube tracts. This makes tract catheterization more difficult, and extravasation from the sinus tract may occur during the procedure.

Stone extraction is not attempted on the first day if small stones are present proximal to the short arm of the intraductal T-tube. The T-tube is simply extracted and a straight catheter is placed. This gives small stones a chance to pass spontaneously into the gut in the interval before the second visit.

It may be impossible to extract intrahepatic stones in second or third division radicals because of poor access with the wire basket. We prefer these patients to be ambulant for several additional weeks to give the hepatic stone a chance to move distally. Waiting in this way has contributed significantly to our high success rate.

Retained stones in cystic duct remnants are usually not accessible to the stone basket. If a low junction of common hepatic and cystic duct is present, surgical exploration and T-tube insertion has usually been performed

into the common hepatic duct and the sharp angle from the common hepatic duct into the cystic duct remnant cannot be negotiated with the steerable catheter. Patients with stones retained in cystic duct remnants are positioned in a semierect or erect posture on the fluoroscopic table. This often results in downward movement of the retained stone so it can be extracted from the common duct. If this manoeuvre is unsuccessful, patients are asked to return several weeks later and the procedure is then started with the patient in a semierect position (Figure 24.8).

24.7 SMALL STONES

Small stones (up to 3 mm diameter) should pass from the common duct into the duodenum spontaneously if no ampullary narrowing is present. The T-tube can be clamped in almost all patients during the 4-week interval between T-tube cholangiography and stone extraction procedure. This increases the chance of passage of small stones or remaining fragments. Only rarely are distal common duct stones truly impacted, causing complete obstruction. We also clamp the indwelling straight tube between multiple sessions after fragmentation of large stones. This encourages the passage of stone fragments.

Small stones are sometimes difficult to demonstrate during fluoroscopy on the television screen. Multiple spot films are required for stone identification. Extraction with the open basket may then be a blind manoeuvre in the sense that the radiologist cannot see if the stone is being caught in the basket. Multiple passages with the basket may be required to engage and extract small stones. We select the basket size so that the wires of the open basket touch the duct wall during extraction as this facilitates the engagement of small stones. A rotating motion of the wire stem of the basket also helps (Figure 24.9).

24.8 LARGE STONES

Stones larger than the sinus tract and stones with a diameter of more than 7 mm usually

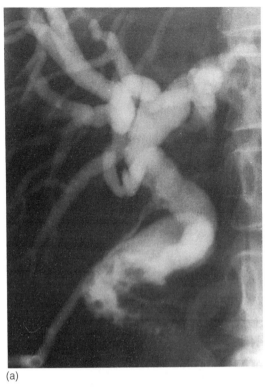
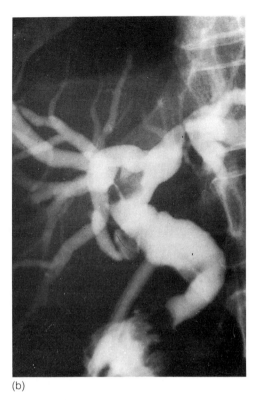

(a)   (b)

Figure 24.8   (a) Retained common hepatic duct stones and retained stone in cystic duct remnant. (b) Patient required two sessions for removal of all retained stones. The cystic duct stone was extracted with the patient in a semi-erect position on the fluoroscopic table.

require fragmentation. The stone is engaged in the basket and brought to the junction of bile duct and sinus tract. Resistance is felt at this point, and traction is applied. A steady, slow increasing pull on the basket always results in fragmentation because the wire baskets are sufficiently thin and sharp to cut large stones. None of our 661 patients had retained large stones which were calcified. Large stones are predominantly pigment and relatively soft, and can be crushed between the fingertips after extraction (Figure 24.10).

Extravasation of contrast from the sinus tract due to injury of its fibrous wall may be seen after stone fragmentation in this fashion. If so, we discontinue the procedure and place a straight catheter until the next extraction

session, about 1 week later. It is unnecessarily time consuming to remove all small pieces from the duct after fragmentation of a large stone. Major fragments are extracted, but small fragments are given a chance to pass spontaneously into the duodenum. As many as four sessions may be required if stone fragmentation involves several stones. Extracorporeal cholelithotripsy can now be employed for fragmentation of large stones.

24.9 IMPACTED STONES

Stones partially impacted (Figure 24.10(a)) in the distal common duct are more difficult to engage in the wire basket. We use a variety of manoeuvres to bring such a stone into a more proximal position in the duct before the basket can be opened distally to it. Suction through the steerable catheter may accomplish this change in stone location. A hand-held syringe is used for suction and the tip of the catheter is placed directly on the stone. Multiple attempts often succeed in moving the stone proximally. Other manoeuvres include rolling the stone proximally by bending the tip of the steerable catheter behind it, or injecting contrast forcefully behind the stone. As a final manoeuvre, we use a Fogarty balloon catheter (Figure 24.10(b)). The contrast-filled balloon is

positioned distal to the stone and gentle traction applied. The balloon is never inflated to a size greater than the bile duct diameter.

24.10 INTRAHEPATIC STONES

One or more stones may be retained in intrahepatic ducts after surgery. If a wire basket cannot be moved alongside the stone in the hepatic duct, or if the stone cannot be engaged by the basket, the stone has to be moved distally. This usually occurs after waiting for an interval longer than 5 weeks after surgery.

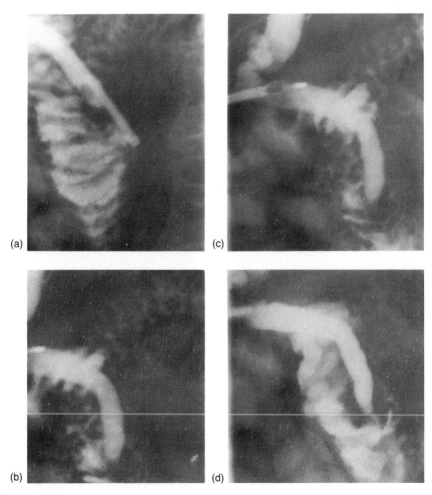

(a) (b) (c) (d)

Figure 24.9   Small distal retained common duct stone was engaged in the stone basket and extracted. The stone was difficult to visualize on the television monitor and multiple spot films throughout the procedure were required for visualization.

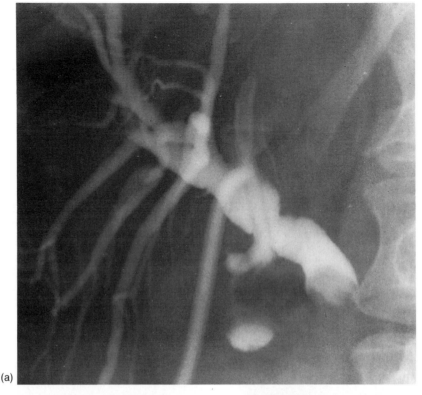

(a)

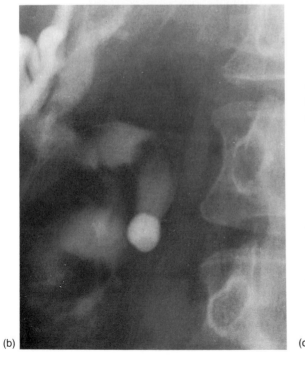

(b)

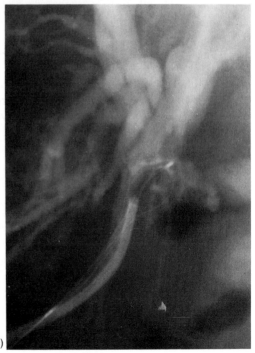

(c)

Multiple return visits may be required. As a final resort, the Fogarty balloon catheter is employed. It is opened distal to the stone and gently pulled. No attempt at strong traction is made if the stone is seen to be wedged against the hepatic duct wall. The Fogarty balloon is carefully inflated with contrast under fluoroscopic vision to ensure that its inflated diameter is less than the diameter of the duct (Figure 24.11).

We have removed as many as 27 intrahepatic stones in one patient in multiple sessions (Table 24.1).

The indwelling T-tube may be converted to a transhepatic U-tube if multiple and repeated non-operative stone extractions are required (Burhenne and Peters, 1978). This technique is particularly useful in patients suffering from oriental cholangitis (Park *et al.*, 1987). Percutaneous transhepatic stone removal can also be employed for treatment of intrahepatic stones (Clouse *et al.*, 1986).

24.11 COMPLICATIONS (Table 24.3)

A survey of 38 institutions was made to collect information on the complications of stone extraction (Burhenne, 1976). There was a 4.1% morbidity. This included postextraction fever, pancreatitis, sepsis and extraductal bile collection. Contrast extravasations from injury to the sinus tract were usually confined. Free extravasation into the peritoneal cavity was seen in two patients. All signs and symptoms in patients with complications subsided within 48 hours. Patients with pancreatitis and sepsis were placed on antibiotics.

Routine premedication with antibiotics is not used for our stone extraction procedures, but patients with a history of previous pan-

Table 24.3 Complications of stone extraction

Complication	No.
Sinus tract leak	7
Peritoneal spill	2
Bile collections	2
Fever	11
Sepsis	2
Pancreatitis	2
Vasovagal reaction	1
Total	27

creatitis and patients with multiple intrahepatic stones are placed on antibiotics before extraction is attempted.

No mortality occurred in our group of 2148 patients, although one death from acute pancreatitis following stone extraction has been reported in the literature (Polack, Fainsinger and Bonnano, 1977). (This group had experience of three extraction procedures before they attempted to remove a distal impacted common duct stone in a patient with a history of previous pancreatitis. The patient was transferred from one radiological room to another with instruments in place. Spot films were obtained in the second room where it was found that the stone had passed into the duodenum.)

24.12 SUCCESS AND FAILURE

All stones were removed in 97% of our 2148 patients, obviating reoperation. Our success rate has been duplicated by other investigators (Garrow, 1977). The procedure can readily be learned, but a radiologist usually requires experience of about 20 stone retrievals before his success rate rises above 80%.

Failure of stone extraction in a review of 661

Figure 24.10 (a) Partially impacted common duct stone. Note a leakage from the cystic duct stump. The proximal short arm of the T-tube is lying in the left hepatic radicle. (b) The large retained common duct stone was mobilized with use of a Fogarty balloon. The balloon was inflated with contrast. (c) Shows the stone in the wire basket. The deformity of the wire basket is due to traction required for stone fragmentation.

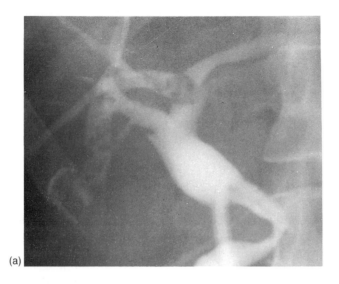

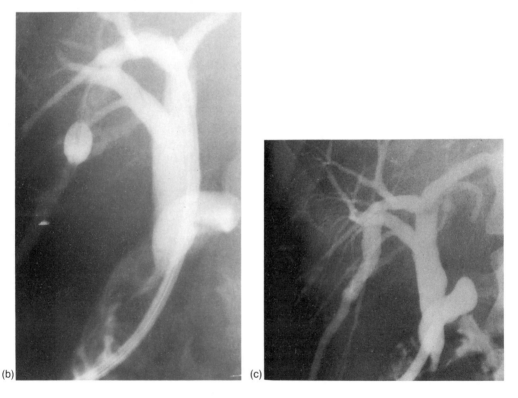

Figure 24.11 (a) Multiple retained stones in second division hepatic radical. (b) Fogarty balloon in place during mobilization of retained intrahepatic stones. (c) All stones have been retrieved from the dorsocaudal branch of the left hepatic radicle.

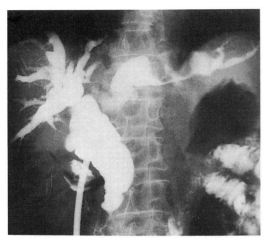

Figure 24.12   Large retained stone in enlarged left hepatic radicle with narrowing at the porta hepatis. We were unable to extract this retained stone.

patients showed that this occurred primarily in patients with intrahepatic stones (Figure 24.12, Tables 24.4 and 24.5). Other failures include distally impacted stones and stones retained in cystic duct stumps. It is sometimes impossible to enter the sinus tract of the T-tube, particularly in patients with T-tubes brought out through a midline incision. Failure may also result from injury to the sinus tract during removal of the first stone, and inability to re-enter the sinus tract for extraction of further stones. It is the extraction of the last remaining stone which determines success or failure.

Clouse *et al.* (1986) performed 38 procedures in 35 patients with obstructive jaundice, biliary colic and cholangitis for the removal of bile duct stones. The transhepatic technique for stone removal revealed a complication rate of 21% in this series.

24.13 SHOCKWAVE CHOLELITHOTRIPSY

The principle of electrohydraulic disintegration of stones in the urinary tract was tested in the nineteenth century (Riches, 1968), but the first successful fragmentation with shock-

Table 24.4   Failures of stone extraction

Extraction failure	No.
Inability to catheterize	5
Inability to recatheterize	7
Cystic duct remnant stones	4
Inability to engage hepatic stones	15
Impacted distal stones	2
Total	33

waves in cholelithiasis was reported *in vitro* and *in vivo* by Burhenne in 1975. Shockwaves applied extracorporeally are now employed successfully for cholelithotripsy (Sauerbruch *et al.*, 1986). Gallbladder stones are located by sonography, and common duct stones are targeted by endoscopic retrograde cholangiography. Endoscopic papillotomy may be added for fragment extraction, but fragments can also be extracted through an existing post-operative sinus tract. We have employed extracorporeal shockwave lithotripsy successfully for the removal of retained cystic duct stones (Becker *et al.*, 1987) (Figure 24.13).

Biliary lithotripsy is still in its infancy but its use is growing rapidly, although further investigation is required before the technique will find its proper place (Burhenne, 1987). Second-generation lithotriptor systems suitable for the biliary tract are available from six different manufacturers (Ferrucci, 1987). Most experience is available with the Dornier (Dornier Medical Systems, FR Germany) or Siemens (Siemens, FR Germany) lithotriptor system. The first uses a spark gap electrode and the second an electromagnetically produced shockwave.

Table 24.5   Failure of stone extraction by location

Location	No.	%
Extrahepatic	18	3.5
Intrahepatic and combined	15	11
Total	33	5

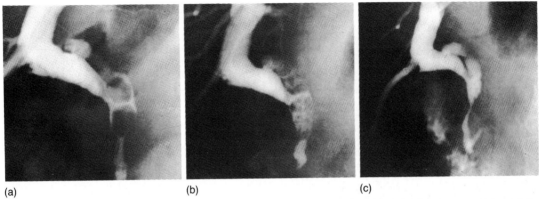

(a)   (b)   (c)

Figure 24.13   (a) Cholangiogram via T-tube tract demonstrates a large cystic duct remnant containing two impacted gallstones. The lower of the two stones is situated at the junction of the cystic duct remnant and common hepatic duct. (b) Shows fragmentation of the retained stones after 2350 shockwaves in two sessions. All fragments moved subsequently into the common bile duct, allowing basket extraction via the T-tube tract. (c) Conclusion cholangiogram showing that all fragments have been removed.

24.14 STRICTURE DILATATION

Radiological dilatation of biliary tract strictures causing obstruction was first reported with the use of radiological intervention by Burhenne in 1975 in seven patients. Several institutions have reported on this technique, giving their results by extension to a transhepatic approach (Molnar and Stockum, 1978) and via a choledochojejunostomy (Hutson *et al.*, 1984). Mueller *et al.* (1986) reported a multicentre review of clinical management in 73 patients with biliary stricture dilatation. This involved strictures at biliary-digestive anastomoses, cases with iatrogenic strictures, and strictures associated with sclerosing cholangitis. The patency rates 36 months after dilatation were 67%, 76% and 42%, respectively. Complications occurred in 7% of patients. However, no definite conclusion can be drawn about the utility of long-term stenting after radiological stricture dilatation. Percutaneous dilatation of biliary tract strictures is a promising technique with good long-term results and may be the best initial treatment in patients who have recurrent strictures after surgery (Moore *et al.*, 1987). Grüntzig-type angioplasty catheters are employed with 6- to 10-mm balloons. Balloons are inflated until the 'waisting' caused by the stricture can be eliminated. Multiple sessions may be required. Maintenance of radiologically dilated strictures is more successful in our experience if catheter stents are left in place through the dilated anastomosis for up to 2 months. Lasting patency following removal of biliary stents after stricture dilatation occurred in 73% of 49 patients reported from the Mayo Clinic (Williams, Bender and May, 1987). Stricture patency was more easily achieved in patients with primary ductal strictures than in those with biliary-enteric anastomotic strictures (Figure 24.14).

24.15 TRANSCHOLECYSTOSTOMY INTERVENTION

Percutaneous removal of gallstones can be employed as the definitive form of therapy in patients with acute cholecystitis by percutaneous cholecystolithotomy (Kerlan, LaBerge and Ring, 1985). The same percutaneous route is useful for gallstone dissolution and drainage of obstruction (vanSonnenberg *et al.*, 1986). The patient is prepared with a liquid diet and broad-spectrum

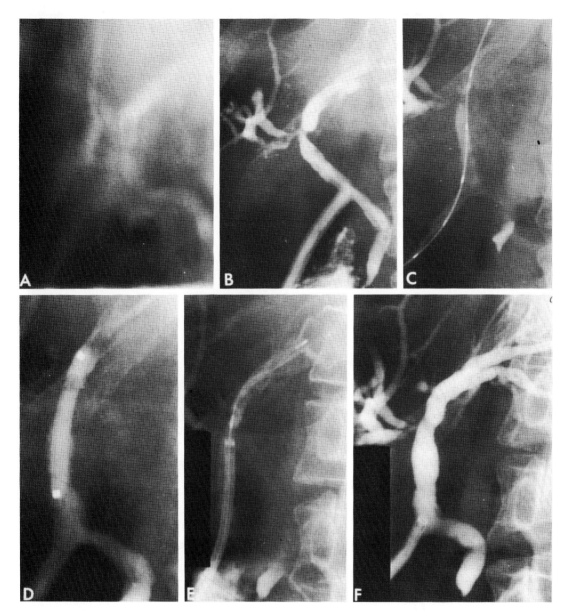

Figure 24.14 (a) Intravenous preoperative cholangiogram demonstrates a bile cast above an obstructing inflammatory stricture at the porta hepatis. (b) Postoperative T-tube cholangiogram shows the stricture at the porta hepatis clearly. (c) Using the T-tube tract for access, a guide-wire is passed through the stricture into the left hepatic radicle. (d) The stricture is dilated with a 4-mm angioplasty balloon catheter. (e) The hepatic duct stone is removed through the dilated stricture with a stone basket. (f) The stricture at the porta hepatis on the left side remains dilated whereas the right hepatic radicle stricture is unchanged.

antibiotics. Ultrasonic guidance is used to find the optimal position for percutaneous gall-bladder puncture, a point anterior to the liver edge. The needle should be passed through the hepatic parenchyma in order to avoid the possibility of peritoneal bile spillage.

We prefer a minicholecystostomy under local anaesthetic for placement of a cholecystostomy catheter and subsequent radiological stone extraction from the gallbladder and common duct in high-risk patients (Burhenne and Stoller, 1985). Patients with a high operative risk and diagnosis of gallstone disease underwent cholecystostomy under local infiltration anaesthesia. A small incision is made in the gallbladder fundus just large enough to accept a 24-Fr Foley catheter. It is important that the gallbladder wall be sutured into the abdominal wall. This prevents intraperitoneal bile leakage and permits early radiological stone removal (Figures 24.15 and 24.16). If common duct stones cannot be removed through cystic duct manipulation, endoscopic sphincterotomy is then added to relieve benign bile duct obstruction and permit stone removal.

Cholecystectomy for acute cholecystitis as a complication of cholelithiasis carries a 9.8% operative mortality in patients over 65 years of age (Glen, 1981). Our experience with 37 high-

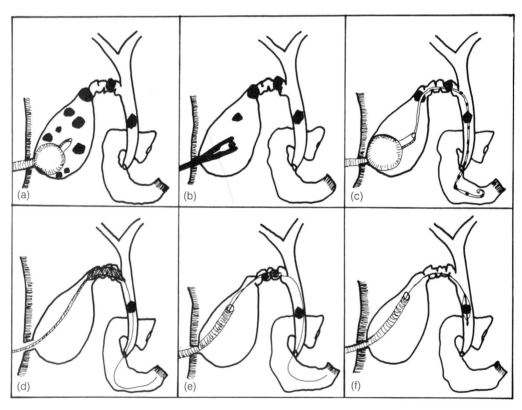

Figure 24.15   Representation of radiological stone removal from gallbladder, cystic duct and common duct via minicholecystostomy. (a) Cholecystostomy balloon in place. (b) One week after surgery, the gallbladder stones are removed. (c) The cystic duct is traversed with guide-wires and drainage catheters. (d) The cystic duct is dilated with an angioplasty balloon catheter. (e) Stones are removed from the cystic duct with the use of a contrast-inflated Fogarty balloon under fluoroscopic vision alongside an indwelling guide-wire. (f) Common duct stone is now removed via this transcholecystic approach.

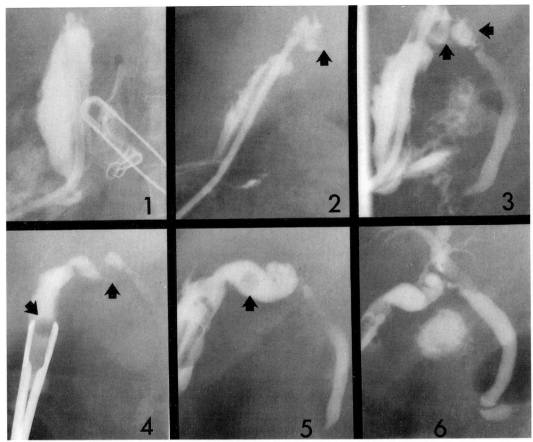

Figure 24.16   (1) Contrast injection into inflamed gallbladder 2 days after cholecystostomy under local anaesthetic. Note that the cystic duct is obstructed. (2), (3) Cystic duct stones now partially disimpacted with contrast flowing into the common duct. (4) Bile drainage through cholecystostomy into bile bag resulted in disimpaction of one cystic duct stone 10 days after cholecystostomy (stones are marked by arrows). (5) Further cystic duct stone disimpaction now permits access for retrieval. (6) The cystic duct is clear of gallstones and cholecystitis subsided under drainage and antibiotic therapy. The gallbladder is left in place.

risk patients undergoing minicholecystostomy and radiological stone removal had no mortality and no serious morbidity.

24.16 ANTEGRADE SPHINCTEROTOMY

Sphincterotomy with the endoscopic diathermy catheter is useful in patients with a history of previous gastric resection where an endoscopic retrograde approach is not feasible (Figure 24.17). This can be accomplished in an antegrade transcholecystic fashion as described by Burhenne and Scudamore (1986) or in an antegrade transhepatic approach (Günther, Klose and Störkel, 1984). Günther has also used electropapillotomy for transhepatic incision of stenoses after hepaticojejunostomy.

24.17 SURGICAL IMPLICATIONS

Successful non-operative retrieval of retained bile duct stones eliminates a problem for the surgeon, so his operative technique should

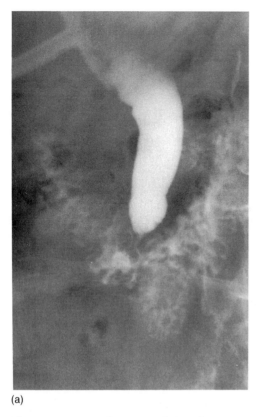
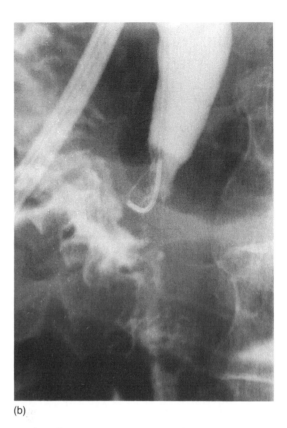

(a)   (b)

Figure 24.17   (a) Patient with intrahepatic stones 3 weeks after surgery with a T-tube in place. Note narrowing of the common duct entry due to fibrosis. (b) Endoscopic diathermy wire placed through a steerable catheter in the sinus tract is positioned at the sphincter in a 10 o'clock position for antegrade sphincterotomy.

be designed to facilitate postoperative stone removal.

A sufficiently large T-tube should be used routinely. The long arm of the T-tube should never be smaller than a No. 14 French. The short arms of the T-tube can usually be adjusted and bivalved to fit to a small bile duct. A T-tube with a large calibre long arm, originally described by Burhenne (1975), has now been made available by Moss, Whalen and Fry (1976) (Davol, USA).

The long end of the T-tube should be brought out through a lateral anterior stab wound in the abdominal wall. Placement through abdominal midline incisions often makes extraction procedures impossible.

Routine operative cholangiography and operative choledochoscopy are more reliable techniques for detection of common duct stones than reliance on probing with surgical instruments. The passage of probes, dilators or catheters through the distal end of the common duct into the duodenum is particularly unreliable for the demonstration of distal common duct stones. Our experience has shown that steerable catheters and baskets almost always pass easily alongside distal common duct stones into the duodenum.

24.18 OTHER INTERVENTIONS FOR TREATMENT OF CHOLELITHIASIS

The use of the T-tube tract for passage of an endoscope has been described, with basket instrumentation for stone retrieval. This method is more expensive, less successful and requires hospitalization because sinus tract dilatation is required in most patients (Yamakawa *et al.*, 1976). However, X-ray exposure is reduced because of direct vision and it is easy to distinguish between stones, air bubbles and blood.

Retained common duct stones after surgery may be extracted by endoscopic retrograde cannulation of the bile duct followed by sphincterotomy and basket extraction. This method is used in preference to radiologically retained stone intervention by many investigators in Europe. It is, however, more difficult to learn and shows a lower success rate for large and intrahepatic stones (Classen, Koch and Demling, 1975).

Non-operative percutaneous retrieval under fluoroscopic control carries the highest success rate and is associated with fewest complications. If a T-tube is in place, it is the therapeutic technique of choice for the retrieval of retained stones (Classen and Ossenberg, 1977).

Increasing experience in treating gallstones with dissolving agents is now available. Systematically administered compounds such as chenodeoxycholic acid and orthodeoxycholic acid are expensive and the cholelitholytic effect is only achieved in stones that are composed mainly of cholesterol and that do not have a significant admixture of calcium salts, pigments or mucus. A 10% recurrence rate has been reported within 1 year after discontinuation of bile acid medication (Fromm, 1986). Local application of dissolving agents via transhepatic or endoscopic catheter infusion involves the use of monoglyceride monooctanoin. This treatment is required in the hospitalized patient for several days and recent reports showed moderate to severe inflammation and ulceration.

REFERENCES

Becker, C. D., Fache, J. S., Gibney, R. G. *et al.* (1987) Treatment of retained cystic duct stones using extracorporeal shockwave lithotripsy. *Am. J. Roentgenol.*, **148**, 1121–2.

Burhenne, H. J. (1973) Nonoperative retained biliary tract stone extraction: a new roentgenologic technique. *Am. J. Roentgenol.*, **117**, 388–99.

Burhenne, H. J. (1975a) Dilatation of biliary tract strictures: a new roentgenologic technique. *Radiol. Clin.*, **44**, 153–9.

Burhenne, H. J. (1975b) Electrohydrolytic fragmentation of retained common duct stones. *Radiology*, **117**, 721–2.

Burhenne, H. J. (1975c) Nonoperative instrumentation of the postoperative biliary tract, in *Surgery of the Liver, Pancreas and Biliary Tracts* (eds J. S. Najarian and J. P. Delaney), Symposia Specialists, Miami, pp. 177–207.

Burhenne, H. J. (1976) Complications of nonoperative extraction of retained common duct stones. *Am. J. Surg.*, **131**, 260–2.

Burhenne, H. J. (1980) Percutaneous extraction of retained biliary tract stones: 661 patients. *Am. J. Roentgenol.*, **134**, 888–98.

Burhenne, H. J. (1987) Perspective. The promise of extracorporeal shockwave lithotripsy for the treatment of gallstones. *Am. J. Roentgenol.*, **149**, 233–5.

Burhenne, H. J. and Peters, H. E. (1978) Retained intrahepatic stones: use of the U tube during repeated nonoperative stone extractions. *Arch Surg.*, **113**, 837–41.

Burhenne, H. J. and Scudamore, C. H. (1986) Antegrade transcholecystic sphincterotomy: canine study of a new interventional technique. *Gastrointest. Radiol.*, **11**, 73–6.

Burhenne, H. J. and Stroller, J. L. (1985) Minicholecystostomy and radiologic stone extraction in high-risk cholelithiasis patients: preliminary experience. *Am. J. Surg.*, **149**, 632–5.

Classen, M., Koch, H. and Demling, L. (1975) Papillotomy and treatment of gallstones by means of endoscopy, in *Surgical Endoscopy* (ed. E. Seifert), Witzstrock, Baden-Baden, pp. 187–284.

Classen, M. and Ossenberg, F. W. (1977) Progress report: non-surgical removal of common bile duct stones. *Gut*, **18**, 760–9.

Clouse, M. E., Stokes, K. R., Lee, R. G. L. and Falchuk, K. R. (1986) Bile duct stones: percutaneous transhepatic removal. *Radiology*, **160**, 525–9.

Cruz, F. O., Barriga, P., Tocornal, J. and Burhenne, H. J. (1983) Radiology of the Mirizzi syndrome:

diagnostic importance of the transhepatic cholangiogram. *Gastrointest. Radiol.*, **8**, 249–53.

Daly, J., Fitzgerald, T. and Simpson, C. J. (1987) Pre-operative intravenous cholangiography as an alternative to routine operative cholangiography in elective cholecystectomy. *Clin. Radiol.*, **38**, 161–3.

Ferrucci, J. T. (1987) Perspective. Biliary lithotripsy: what will the issues be? *Am. J. Roentgenol.*, **149**, 227–31.

Fromm, H. (1986) Gallstone dissolution therapy. Current status and future prospects. *Gastroenterology*, **91**, 1560–7.

Garrow, D. G. (1977) The removal of retained biliary tract stones: report of 105 cases. *Br. J. Radiol.*, **50**, 777–82.

Glen, F. (1981) Surgical management of acute cholecystitis in patients 65 years of age and older. *Ann. Surg.*, **193**, 56–9.

Günther, R. W., Klose, K. J. and Störkel, S. (1984) Percutaneous antegrade electropapillotomy. Study in dogs. *Cardiovasc. Intervent. Radiol.*, **7**, 270–6.

Hutson, D. G., Russell, E., Schiff, E. *et al.* (1984) Balloon dilatation of biliary strictures through a choledochojejuno-cutaneous fistula. *Ann. Surg.*, **199**, 637–47.

Kerlan, R. K. Jr, LaBerge, J. M. and Ring, E. J. (1985) Percutaneous cholecystolithotomy: preliminary experience. *Radiology*, **157**, 653–6.

LaGrave, G. *et al.* (1969) Lithiase biliaire residuelle. Extraction à la sonde de Dormia par le drain de Kehr. *Mem. Acad. Chir.*, **95**, 430.

Mazzariello, R. (1970) Removal of residual biliary tract calculi without reoperation. *Surgery*, **67**, 566–73.

Molnar, W. and Stockum, A. (1978) Transhepatic dilatation of choledochoenterostomy strictures. *Radiology*, **129**, 59–64.

Mondet, A. (1962) Técnica de la extracción incuenta de los calculos en la litiasis residual del colédoco. *Bol. Trab. Soc. Circug. Buenos Aires*, **46**, 278–90.

Moore, A. V. Jr, Illescas, F. F., Mills, S. R. *et al.* (1987) Percutaneous dilation of benign biliary strictures. *Radiology*, **163**, 625–8.

Moss, J. P., Whalen, J. G. and Fry, D. E. (1976) Unsuccessful postoperative extraction of retained common duct stones. *Am. J. Surg.*, **135**, 785–9.

Mueller, P. R., vanSonnenberg, E., Ferrucci, J. T. Jr *et al.* (1986) Biliary stricture dilatation: multicenter review of clinical management in 73 patients. *Radiology*, **160**, 17–22.

Park, J. H., Choi, B. I., Han, M. C. *et al.* (1987) Percutaneous removal of residual intrahepatic stones. *Radiology*, **163**, 619–23.

Polack, E. P., Fainsinger, M. H. and Bonnano, S. V. (1977) A death following complications of roentgenologic nonoperative manipulation of common bile duct calculi. *Radiology*, **123**, 585–6.

Riches, E. (1968) The history of lithotomy and lithotrity. *Ann. R. Coll. Surg. Engl.*, **43**, 185–99.

Sauerbruch, T., Delius, M., Paumgartner, G. *et al.* (1986) Fragmentation of gallstones by extracorporeal shockwaves. *New Engl. J. Med.*, **314**, 818–22.

vanSonnenberg, E., Wittich, G. R., Casola, G. *et al.* (1986) Diagnostic and therapeutic percutaneous gallbladder procedures. *Radiology*, **160**, 23–6.

Williams, H. J. Jr, Bender, C. E. and May, G. R. (1987) Benign postoperative biliary strictures: dilation with fluoroscopic guidance. *Radiology*, **163**, 629–34.

Yamakawa, T. *et al.* (1976) An improved choledochofiberscope and non-surgical removal of retained biliary calculi under direct visual control. *Gastrointest. Endosc.*, **22**, 160–4.

CHAPTER TWENTY-FIVE

Papillary stenosis

M. V. Sivak

25.1 INTRODUCTION

The major duodenal papilla with the sphincter of Oddi is a complex structure that responds to humoral, and perhaps neural, stimulation. Because of its anatomical location and intricate structure, it has been implicated in a variety of disorders of the biliary tract and pancreas since the nineteenth century (Raskin, 1985).

The physiology and pathology of the sphincter of Oddi remain uncertain, despite great interest and considerable investigative work which has accrued greater importance with the development of ERCP, since endoscopic sphincterotomy affords a method of altering or eliminating function of the sphincter.

25.2 DEFINITION OF TERMS

Papillary stenosis is an imprecise term. Pathologically, papillary stenosis specifies inflammation and fibrosis of the major duodenal papilla (MDP), but the term is also used loosely to indicate a clinical syndrome characterized by recurrent abdominal pain after cholecystectomy. The terms sphincter of Oddi dysfunction, biliary dyskinesia and postcholecystectomy syndrome have also been applied to this disorder. This multiplicity of terms reflects a fundamental ignorance of the pathogenesis of papillary stenosis. In some cases actual stenosis, in the pathological sense, is absent. Whether papillary stenosis is a specific malady with diverse clinical manifestations, or a heterogeneous group of unrelated disorders is uncertain. It has been suggested that sphincter of Oddi disorders may range from purely functional to morphological alterations including inflammation and fibrosis, and that perhaps there are disorders with features of both.

Papillary stenosis has been suggested as a causative factor in pancreatitis and gallstones. However, evidence of pathological change in the major duodenal papilla or other indications of sphincter of Oddi dysfunction do not necessarily establish that these are the cause of a given biliary or pancreatic disorder. Choledocholithiasis is one of the possible clinical manifestations of papillary stenosis. However, the intimate relationship between bile duct stones and the sphincter of Oddi makes it difficult to establish cause and effect. Pathological changes at the sphincter of Oddi (or dysfunction without such changes) may lead to stone formation, or the passage of small stones might produce papillary stenosis. The problem of cause versus effect also applies to pancreatic diseases. For example, Toouli *et al.* (1985b) demonstrated the presence of manometric abnormalities of the sphincter of Oddi in 25 of 28 patients with idiopathic recurrent pancreatitis, but retrograde pancreatography was also abnormal in the majority. The relationship between papillary stenosis and recognized disorders of the biliary system and pancreas will not be considered in this review.

The term papillary stenosis will be used exclusively in the remainder of this discussion in its broad clinical sense, referring to a clinical syndrome including pain characteristic of biliary colic, or acute pancreatitis. The differential diagnosis of this symptom includes choledocholithiasis and recurrent acute pancreatitis, but patients with this syndrome have no evidence of bile duct stones or pancreatitis. Pathological changes may be present or absent in the major duodenal papilla, but none are evident in the liver, bile ducts or pancreas.

25.3 PAPILLARY STENOSIS

25.3.1 GENERAL DESCRIPTION

Papillary stenosis, as a clinical syndrome, denotes the intermittent occurrence of pain that suggests biliary colic or pancreatitis. The majority of patients are middle-aged women who have undergone cholecystectomy. The pain is usually episodic, and may be accompanied by transient abnormalities of liver function tests or serum amylase. There may be associated dilatation of the bile duct (Zimman, Ferrarg and Clement, 1978).

Histological abnormalities in the major duodenal papilla in patients with various biliary and pancreatic disorders, as well as those with pain alone, have been recognized for many years (Trommald and Seabrook, 1950; Cattell, Colcock and Pollack, 1957; Grage and Lober, 1960; Paulino and Cavalcanti, 1960; Nardi and Acosta, 1966). Moody, Becker and Potts (1983) reported on the results of surgical treatment of 92 patients with chronic, incapacitating upper abdominal pain and stenosis of the sphincter of Oddi, in 85 of whom an abnormality such as fibrosis and/or muscular hypertrophy of the major duodenal papilla was found. A functional stenosis without pathological findings occurred in only seven cases. Biopsies from the major duodenal papilla of patients with postcholecystectomy abdominal pain and a stenotic papilla were compared by Acosta et al. (1967) with biopsies from those of patients without biliary tract disease. The group with pain had a higher

frequency of inflammation and fibrosis than the control group. A classification of pathological findings with categories of ulcerous, granulomatous, adenomatous and sclerosing was recommended by Acosta and Nardi (1966).

Despite the occurrence of a spectrum of inflammatory and fibrotic changes in the MDP, there is poor correlation between these findings and clinical manifestations of disease. Although Nardi and Acosta (1966) did not find inflammation in a control group of 30 patients who underwent surgical biopsy of the major duodenal papilla, Grage et al. (1960) found fibrosis or inflammation in about 5% of biopsies from a control group of 31 patients without biliary tract disease. Grage et al. (1960) investigated 31 patients in whom it was impossible to pass a number 3 Bakes dilator and found that almost one-third had no histological changes. In surgical series in which biopsies were obtained from the major duodenal papilla pathological abnormalities were found in 50–75% of patients. Assuming that patients were carefully selected for operation, this frequency of pathological findings may be regarded as relatively low.

25.3.3 AETIOLOGY AND PATHOGENESIS

There is a close relation between papillary stenosis and choledocholithiasis. It is well established that acute inflammation of the major duodenal papilla may be associated with common bile duct stones, and Doubilet and Mulholland (1956) suggested that fibrosis of the distal common bile duct might be induced by stone impaction and/or transit. In animals, fibrosis of the major duodenal papilla can be produced by instrumentation (Branch, Bailey and Zollinger, 1939) and, experimentally, bile itself may induce acute inflammation and muscular hypertrophy (Das, 1965). These observations led to the theory that repetitive passage of small stones or lithogenic bile might cause papillary stenosis, but evidence of gallstone disease is absent in many patients with papillary stenosis (Allen and Wallace, 1940; Colcock, 1958; Prudhomme *et al.*, 1965).

Another theory suggests that the clinical manifestations of papillary stenosis may be explained by sphincter dysfunction leading to spasm and/or sphincter muscle hypertrophy. However, acute and/or chronic inflammation of the major duodenal papilla occur in many cases of papillary stenosis, and it is difficult to accept that functional spasm could induce pathological changes in the sphincter of Oddi.

25.3.4 DIAGNOSIS

(a) Surgical diagnosis

Resistance to passage of a probe of certain diameter (Bakes 3 mm dilator) through the major duodenal papilla at surgery has been accepted since the 1950s as indicative of papillary stenosis (Cattell and Colcock, 1953; Mahorner, 1959; Grage *et al.*, 1960; Autio and Parvinen, 1965; Acosta and Nardi, 1966). Although crude and invasive, this observation correlates roughly with the presence of papillary stenosis. Braasch and McCann (1967) measured the diameter of the normal choledochoduodenal junction in 201 subjects; in most cases a 6-mm dilator would pass without difficulty, while a 3-mm dilator could be passed in almost all subjects.

Various methods of measuring intrabiliary pressure and bile flow at surgery, with and without pharmacological manipulation of the Sphincter of Oddi, have been employed as tests for papillary stenosis (Madura *et al.*, 1981; Setakis *et al.*, 1984; Hastbacka *et al.*, 1986). However, there are many anaesthetic factors that can influence the major duodenal papilla and its sphincter so intraoperative tests of sphincter of Oddi (SO) function are remote from physiological conditions and their validity has been challenged (Dahl-Iversen, Sorenson and Westengaard, 1957; Grage and Lober, 1960).

(b) Provocative tests

Provocative tests of sphincter of Oddi dys-

function were first described in the late 1940s (Knight, Muether and Sommer, 1949; Myhre, Nesbitt and Hurley, 1949; Snape, Wirts and Friedman, 1949), but later investigations questioned their sensitivity and specificity (Burke, Plummer and Bradford, 1950; Wirts and Snape, 1951; Dreiling and Richman, 1954).

The morphine-neostigmine provocation test was described in 1965 (Sterkel and Knight, 1965). The objectives of this test are reproduction of the patient's pain and elevation of serum levels of pancreatic enzymes in response to the combined actions of morphine and neostigmine which respectively induce sphincter of Oddi spasm and stimulate pancreatic secretion, while a number of investigators have found it useful in the diagnosis of papillary stenosis (Nardi and Acosta, 1966; Gregg *et al.*, 1977; Raskin *et al.*, 1978; Broad, Gordon and Vernick, 1979; Madura *et al.*, 1981), others have challenged its validity (LoGiudice *et al.*, 1979; Steinberg, Salvato and Toskes, 1980; Warshaw *et al.*, 1985). Modifications of provocative testing include the use of other indices of abnormality, such as measurement of serum bile acids (Dolgin and Soloway, 1980), liver enzymes (Roberts-Thomson and Toouli, 1985), and pancreatic or bile duct diameter as measured by ultrasonography (Berezny *et al.*, 1985; Warshaw *et al.*, 1985).

Opinion varies as to what constitutes a positive morphine-neostigmine test. Nardi and Acosta (1966) accepted a four-fold increase in serum amylase or lipase plus reproduction of pain; Gregg *et al.* (1977) an increase in serum lipase to five times greater than basal; Raskin *et al.* (1978) and Madura *et al.* (1981) pain plus a four-fold increase in serum enzymes, or any pain identical to the patient's usual symptom. Broad, Gordon and Vernick (1979) accept a rise in serum enzyme levels of three times basal values plus reproduction of pain as positive. Using these various criteria, all of these authors found the morphine-neostigmine test to be of value in the diagnosis of papillary stenosis.

The efficacy of the morphine-neostigmine test was studied by Roberts-Thomson and Toouli (1985) in a complex investigation that included three patient groups: 40 post-cholecystectomy patients who had biliary dilatation and/or transient changes in liver enzymes after episodes of pain; 20 post-cholecystectomy patients with pain but no evidence of bile duct dilatation or spontaneous elevation of liver enzymes; and 20 patients with intact gallbladders and no evidence of biliary tract disease. A rise in serum enzyme levels to twice the upper normal limit was defined as a positive test result. Mild to severe pain occurred in 81% of patients when the three patient groups were compared collectively with controls. (Two control subjects experienced mild pain.) However, there was a significant difference in the frequency of severe pain when the first two patient groups were compared with the third. All patients who had an abnormal rise in the serum concentration of aspartate aminotransferase (AST) after morphine-neostigmine had either mild or severe pain, whereas a rise in amylase occurred in the absence of pain in two patients in the first patient group, five patients in the second group, and in two patients in one of the control groups (10 individuals without abdominal pain or prior biliary surgery). A positive result with respect to serum AST and amylase levels was significantly more frequent in the first patient group compared with controls.

The conclusions to be drawn are that determination of a liver enzyme (in this case AST) in response to morphine-neostigmine administration may have greater discriminatory value than serum amylase elevation. A positive morphine-neostigmine test (enzyme elevation plus pain) occurred more frequently in patients who were likely to have the post-cholecystectomy syndrome, but other investigators have questioned its discriminatory value (LoGiudice et al., 1979; Steinberg, Salvato and Toskes, 1980; Warshaw et al., 1985). Steinberg, Salvato and Toskes (1980) found a positive test in almost two-thirds of control patients; LoGiudice et al. (1979) noted a positive test in one-half of normal control subjects. None had pain, although some patients with irritable bowel syndrome had a positive test that included pain (Steinberg, Salvato and Toskes, 1980). No evidence of papillary stenosis was found at operation in a few of the patients reported by LoGiudice et al. (1979), whereas papillary stenosis was found at surgery in some patients who had a negative provocative test.

Warshaw et al. (1985) have described a provocative test based on ultrasonographic detection of changes in pancreatic and bile duct diameters in response to secretin stimulation or the administration of morphine and neostigmine. The effects of both pharmacological regimens on the diameter of the pancreatic duct were comparable, and there was a correlation between test results and the presence of papillary stenosis at surgery. However, the number of false-positive responses was greater with the morphine-neostigmine test than with secretin stimulation. After intravenous administration of secretin (1 unit/kg), dilatation of the pancreatic duct was demonstrated in 10 of 12 patients found at surgery to have a stenotic sphincter of Oddi (17 patients with pancreas divisum were also studied). A comparable degree of pancreatic duct dilatation was observed in 14% of control subjects in whom there was no suspicion of disease of the major duodenal papilla, and in none of 10 patients with surgically disproved stenosis. Concomitant elevation of serum amylase and reproduction of pain were found to have no discriminatory value. There was good correlation between test results and the response of patients to surgical sphincteroplasty.

Experience with provocative tests based on changes in pancreatic or bile duct diameter is limited, and some investigators (W. Lees, personal communication) have not found variations in duct diameter detected by ultrasonography useful.

(c) Cholescintigraphy

Radionuclide cholescintigraphy studies are being used as a method of defining functional obstruction of the bile duct (Lee *et al.*, 1985; Zeman *et al.*, 1985; Roberts-Thomson *et al.*, 1986; Shaffer *et al.*, 1986).

Roberts-Thomson *et al.* (1986) performed biliary scintigraphy using ^{99}Tc^m-di-isopropyl iminodiacetic acid (DIDA) in patients who had undergone cholecystectomy. There were 20 asymptomatic patients and 45 patients with biliary-type pain, some of whom also had bile duct dilatation and transient increases in liver enzymes. The results in asymptomatic individuals and those in patients with pain were compared with respect to the time at which counts in the common duct reached 50% of maximum activity (CBD T_{50}) and the time at which the isotope first entered the duodenum. Patients with bile duct dilatation and/or elevation of serum enzymes showed a significant prolongation of the CBD T_{50} and the time to first entry into the duodenum. The results in symptomatic patients without other features of sphincter dysfunction did not differ from control values.

Shaffer *et al.* (1986) found that the time required to reach maximal radioactivity in the biliary system was greater in nine patients with suspected sphincter of Oddi dysfunction compared with that in 35 postcholecystectomy subjects without symptoms. The percentage of radiotracer excreted at 45, 60 and 90 minutes was also less in the symptomatic patients, and the rate of emptying of the bile duct was prolonged.

(d) ERCP

ERCP affords an opportunity to observe and palpate the major duodenal papilla, to measure its function by means of sphincter of Oddi manometry, and to obtain radiographs of the ductal structures that might be affected by papillary stenosis.

The major duodenal papilla is normal by visual inspection in most patients with papillary stenosis.

Inability to cannulate the papilla has been considered as evidence of stenosis of the sphincter of Oddi (Gregg *et al.*, 1978; Zimmon, Falkenstein and Clemett, 1978; Gregg *et al.*, 1980). Gregg *et al.* (1978) reported that it was difficult to place the ERCP cannula in the orifice of the major duodenal papilla, and to obtain pancreatograms, except by wedge injection, in 74% of cases. Zimmon, Falkenstein and Clemett (1978) accepted unsuccessful cannulation as equivalent to a diagnosis of papillary stenosis, but in both these reports the correlation between endoscopic observations and findings at surgery was poor.

Other investigators have not detected any abnormalities of the major duodenal papilla at endoscopy by inspection, palpation with the ERCP cannula, or in relation to the ease of cannulation (Raskin *et al.*, 1978; LoGiudice *et al.*, 1979). The major duodenal papilla was described as normal to palpation in all surgically proved cases reported by Raskin *et al.* (1978). The inability to cannulate may result from any cause of obstruction, including tumour and common duct stone, or it may be due to technical failure. Furthermore, functional disorders of the sphincter of Oddi probably would not make cannulation appreciably more difficult.

Although papillary stenosis has no specific radiographic findings at ERCP (Gregg *et al.*, 1977; Raskin *et al.*, 1978; Zimmon, Falkenstein and Clemett, 1978; LoGiudice *et al.*, 1979), certain radiographic abnormalities including dilatation of the bile ducts and delayed drainage of contrast medium from the biliary system may suggest it. Abnormal pancreatograms may occur (Gregg *et al.*, 1978; Raskin *et al.*, 1978), the most frequent finding being stenosis of the main duct near the major duodenal papilla, but most reports do not mention these.

Delayed drainage of contrast medium from the biliary system is said to be present when the bile duct remains opacified for 45 minutes after retrograde injection in the absence of the gallbladder. However, the validity of this observation has not been tested extensively. In practice, it is unusual, even in the most obvious cases of papillary stenosis, for all the contrast injected to remain in the duct for three-quarters of an hour. Biliary retention of contrast is a matter of subjective judgement, and may, in any case, be influenced by other factors such as drugs used for sedation, duodenal atony, and patient position.

Compensatory dilatation of the extrahepatic bile ducts seems not to occur after cholecystectomy (Graham et al., 1980; Mueller et al., 1981), so if the diameter of the extrahepatic system is normal before removal of the gallbladder, it will remain so after surgery, even if surgical exploration of the bile duct is performed. If the bile ducts are dilated preoperatively, they will remain dilated, or in a few cases return to normal diameter after surgery. It has been suggested that this relates to the integrity of ductular elastic fibres which may be damaged as a result of longstanding obstruction. However, small undetected stones may account for persistent postoperative dilatation. If extrahepatic ducts increase in diameter after cholecystectomy, obstruction is probably present. If the patient is asymptomatic, the process may be low grade or intermittent and might be caused by a stone or perhaps dysfunction of the sphincter of Oddi.

Dilatation of the bile ducts should therefore be a reliable indicator of obstruction at the level of the major duodenal papilla, especially if a progressive increase in diameter can be demonstrated. Despite this there are patients with papillary stenosis in whom the bile duct is not dilated. Raskin et al. (1978), for example, found bile ducts of normal calibre in 83% of their patients.

(e) Sphincter of Oddi manometry

A typical normal manometric profile obtained by perfusion manometry includes a common bile duct pressure about 10 mm greater than intraduodenal pressure and a basal sphincter of Oddi pressure within the sphincter segment about 10–17 mm greater than intraduodenal pressure (Figure 25.1 and Table 25.1). Phasic pressure waves are superimposed on the basal sphincter of Oddi pressure. There is a wide range in reported normal values for phasic wave amplitude (Table 25.2), and their reported frequency ranges from 2.6 to 7.5 per minute (Csendes et al., 1979; Geenen et al., 1980; Carr-Locke and Gregg, 1981; Toouli et al., 1982; De Masi et al., 1984). A frequency of 8 per minute or greater is generally considered abnormal.

Other measurements that can be made include mean phasic wave height (mean difference between peak and trough values for pressure waves), mean duration of phasic waves, and mean phasic wave amplitude (peak pressure). If a triple lumen perfusion catheter is used, the direction of propagation of the sphincteric phasic waves can be determined.

Whether the sphincter of Oddi is functionally separate from the duodenal musculature is an important question that bears on the interpretation of endoscopic manometry. Embryologically the human sphincter of Oddi develops separately from the duodenal musculature, and the sphincter becomes incorporated into the duodenal wall during later development of the fetus (Boyden, 1937; Schwegler and Boyden, 1937). Several animal studies suggest that SO function is distinct from that of the duodenum (Hauge and Mark, 1965; Hedner and Rorsman, 1969; Ono, 1970;

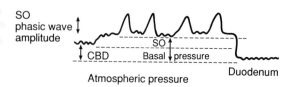

Figure 25.1 Schematic representation of a manometric recording (station pull through) from the sphincter of Oddi (SO) using the open tip perfusion method. A recording from a perfusion catheter with a single perfusion port is depicted. Modified from Geenen, Hogan and Dodds (1987).

Table 25.1 SO manometry values in normal subjects*

Reference	Subjects (no.)	Basal SO pressure (mmHg)		CBD/duodenum gradient (mmHg)	
Csendes *et al.* (1979)	12			11.4	(± 1.3)
Geenen *et al.* (1987)	26	4 > CBD		12.4	(± 1.5)
Carr-Locke and Gregg (1981)	25	15.2	(± 8.2)	3	(± 2.5)
Toouli *et al.* (1982)	20	17	(± 4)	8	(± 0.6)
Gregg and Carr-Locke (1984)	43	13.4	(± 6.2)	2.0	(± 1.7)
Meshkinpour *et al.* (1984)	9	14.9	(± 0.99)	8.6	(± 1.02)
Toouli *et al.* (1989a)	10	17	(10–35)		
Funch-Jensen *et al.* (1987)	9	10		5	

* Adapted from Lebovics, Heier and Rosenthal (1986) with permission.

La Morte *et al.*, 1980). For example, simultaneous electromyography of the SO and duodenum discloses that SO motor activity is not directly connected to that of the duodenum (Ishioka, 1959; Ono, 1970).

Animal (Persson, 1971) and human studies (Geenan *et al.*, 1980; Carr-Locke and Gregg, 1981) suggest an intrinsic automaticity for the SO which is not abolished by agents that block neural function. Experiments in rabbits indicate that the SO has a pacemaker separate from that which regulates duodenal motor activity (Sarles *et al.*, 1976).

After Vondrasek, Eberhardt and Classen (1974) reported endoscopic measurements of sphincter of Oddi pressure in 1974, Nebel (1975) demonstrated the high pressure zone within the duodenal papilla, the presence of which has been confirmed by other investigators (Csendes *et al.*, 1979; Carr-Locke and Gregg, 1981). Virtually all studies have demonstrated pressure gradients between the duodenum and the bile duct as well as the pancreatic duct (Rosch, Koch and Demling, 1976; Csendes *et al.*, 1979; Geenen *et al.*, 1980; Carr-Locke and Gregg, 1981). In addition, endoscopic manometric studies demonstrate phasic pressure waves when the recording catheter is within the sphincter zone (Bradley and Nebel, 1977; Funch-Jensen *et al.*, 1979; Geenen *et al.*, 1980; Carr-Locke and Gregg, 1981; Carr-Locke, Gregg and Aoki, 1983). Carr-Locke and Gregg (1981) described a pancreatic duct sphincter zone separate from the sphincter of Oddi and the distal choledochal sphincter, but this has not been confirmed (Okazaki, Yamamoto and Ito, 1986). In most studies the pancreatic-duodenal pressure

Table 25.2 SO phasic contractions in normal subjects*

Reference	Subjects (no.)	Amplitude (mmHg)		Frequency (per min)		Duration (s)	
Csendes *et al.* (1979)	12	110	(± 10.6)	7.5	(± 0.7)		
Geenen *et al.* (1987)	26	101	(± 50)	4.1	(± 0.9)	4.3	(± 1.5)
Carr-Locke and Gregg (1981)	25	52.7	(± 10.7)	5.6	(± 2.4)		
Toouli *et al.* (1982)	20	140	(± 13)	4	(± 0.5)	8	(± 0.6)
Gregg and Carr-Locke (1984)	43	51.2	(± 6.7)				
Meshkinpour *et al.* (1984)	9	113.0	(± 8.6)	6.89	(± 0.2)		
Toouli *et al.* (1989a)	10	188	(75–330)	4	(3–6)		
Funch-Jensen *et al.* (1987)	9	102.9		2.6	(1.3–4.6)	4.8	

* Adapted from Lebovics, Heier and Rosenthal (1986) with permission.

gradient is higher than that between bile duct and duodenum (Rosch, Koch and Demling, 1976; Bar-Meir *et al.*, 1979; Carr-Locke and Gregg, 1981; Tanaka, Ikeda and Nakayama, 1981).

Differences in the technique (e.g. different perfusion rates (Carr-Locke and Gregg, 1981)) explain some different results.

Methods of determining whether the catheter is within the bile duct include aspiration of bile (Staritz, Poralla and Ewe, 1985), injection of a small volume of contrast, or insertion of the catheter after retrograde injection with clearing of contrast medium (although the effects of contrast injection on the dynamics of the sphincter of Oddi are uncertain). In many studies the catheter was merely 'oriented' in the direction of the bile duct.

Many drugs, including some used routinely in endoscopy, but not diazepam (Webel, 1975), stimulate or inhibit the sphincter of Oddi, and are sometimes used to facilitate cannulation (Toouli *et al.*, 1985a).

Funch-Jensen, Kraglund and Djurhuus (1984) studied the effect of different catheter diameters on the results of sphincter of Oddi manometry in three anaesthetized dogs. No differences were seen in phasic wave amplitude, frequency, basal pressure or common duct pressure after cannulation with catheters of 1.0- and 1.3-mm diameter, but significant disturbances occurred with catheters of 1.6- and 1.9-mm diameter.

Whether these brief pressure measurements can be considered truly representative of sphincter of Oddi function is uncertain. For example, papillary stenosis appears clinically to be intermittent, so abnormalities of sphincter function might not be present during any given recording period.

A study of the frequency and cyclical pattern of human sphincter of Oddi motor activity (Torsoli *et al.*, 1986) sheds some light on this question.

Long recordings from bile-duct T-tubes showed that phasic activity varied in a cyclical fashion like the duodenal interdigestive motor complex. Phases of maximum sphincter of Oddi phasic activity (9–12 c/min) lasted for a mean of 168 seconds (2–4 minutes), and were followed by periods of absent phasic activity that lasted an average of 297 seconds (1–7 minutes). These quiescent periods were followed by periods of time during which there was an irregular and progressively increasing frequency of sphincter of Oddi phasic activity that lasted an average of 76.5 minutes (33–111 minutes). Maximum phasic activity coincided with phase III of the duodenal interdigestive migrating motor complex (MMC), while absent phasic activity coincided with phase I of the MMC. During phases I and II the sphincter of Oddi phasic activity appeared to be independent of the MMC, but during phase III sphincter activity and duodenal contractions were closely associated. A similar relationship between sphincter phasic activity and the MMC has been demonstrated in the opossum (Coelho, Moody and Senninger, 1985).

There is a difference of opinion regarding the effect of the phasic contractions of the sphincter of Oddi on bile flow. Some investigators hold that sphincter phasic activity is peristaltic and propels bile into the duodenum (Toouli and Watts, 1972), but others believe, on the contrary, that it retards emptying of the biliary and pancreatic ducts (Ono *et al.*, 1968).

Delicate (and expensive) microtransducers have also been used to record intraductal and sphincter of Oddi pressures at endoscopy (Tanaka, Ikeda and Nakayama, 1981); pressures were lower than those obtained with perfusion systems.

Simultaneous myoelectric and manometric recordings demonstrated that sphincter of Oddi myoelectric activity showed rhythmic bursts of action potentials that corresponded to the ascending phase of the sphincter phasic pressure waves (Bortolotti *et al.*, 1985).

It is important to know whether cholecystectomy alters the function of the sphincter of Oddi. Toouli *et al.* (1982) found no difference in sphincter pressures in patients with intact gallbladders compared with patients who had undergone cholecystectomy. However, Tanaka, Ikeda and Nakayama (1984) placed an indwelling microtransducer in the bile duct in seven patients before and after cholecystectomy and induced sphincter spasm by morphine. Before cholecystectomy, morphine produced no spasm, although the additional administration of caerulein (a decapeptide 20 times more potent than CCK in animal studies) caused a rise in bile duct pressure as a result of gallbladder contraction. After cholecystectomy, however, morphine administration produced a rise in bile duct pressure that was eliminated by administration of caerulein. Basal bile duct pressure was also significantly higher after cholecystectomy. The findings in this study were attributed to a pressure reservoir effect of the gallbladder.

(f) Sphincter of Oddi disorders

Manometry of the sphincter of Oddi has been useful in assessing the long-term results of endoscopic sphincterotomy and the effectiveness of sphincterotomy as a method of eliminating sphincter function (Rosch, Koch and Demling, 1976; Geenen et al., 1977; Funch-Jensen et al., 1979; Tanaka, Ikeda and Nakayama, 1981). Although a few investigations have found the effect of endoscopic sphincterotomy to be unpredictable (Staritz, Ewe and zum Buschenfelde, 1986), most studies demonstrate such consistent results that there is usually no need for manometry after sphincterotomy unless there is recurrent pain (Ponce et al., 1983; Geenen et al., 1984a). Although manometry has been used in various disorders of the bile duct and pancreas (including common duct stones) (Csendes et al., 1979; Tanaka, Ikeda and Nakayama, 1981; Toouli et al., 1982; Guelrud et al., 1983; De Masi et al., 1984; Gregg and Carr-Locke, 1984), acute (Johnson and Doppman, 1967; McCutcheon, 1968; Tuzhilin, Podolsky and Dreiling, 1981; Toouli et al., 1985) and chronic pancreatitis (Novis et al., 1985; Okazaki,

Yamamoto and Iko, 1986), and miscellaneous disorders (Guelrud et al., 1983; Viceconte, Viceconte and Bogliolo, 1984), the technique is of only secondary importance for clinical diagnosis in these circumstances. Manometry of the sphincter of Oddi may have a more fundamental role in the difficult diagnosis of papillary stenosis, although its value has not been proved conclusively.

Manometric abnormalities of the sphincter of Oddi have been categorized into four types (Toouli, 1984): spasm (Bar-Meir et al., 1979), excessive frequency of phasic contractions (Berci and Johnson, 1965), an abnormal direction of propagation of phasic waves (Toouli et al., 1982) and paradoxical response to CCK-OP (Hogan et al., 1982).

Meshkinpour et al. (1984) found manometry abnormalities of the sphincter of Oddi in 10 patients with recurrent right upper quadrant pain, mild intermittent transaminasaemia, and radiographically normal pancreatic and biliary ducts. The basal pressure of the sphincter of Oddi was significantly greater than in nine healthy control subjects, and the frequency of retrograde phasic waves was increased. The amplitude and frequency of the phasic contractions were not different.

The complete spectrum of manometric abnormalities of the sphincter of Oddi was found by Toouli et al. (1985a) in 38 post-cholecystectomy patients (35 women) with episodic pain and either a dilated bile duct, transient changes in biochemical tests of liver function (10 patients), or both (six patients). Satisfactory recordings were obtained in 32 patients, and 25 of these disclosed manometric abnormalities of the sphincter of Oddi (compared with 10 control patients), including excess retrograde contractions (12 patients), high frequency phasic contractions (11 patients), elevation of basal pressure (eight patients), and a paradoxical response to CCK-OP (10 patients).

A paradoxical rise in pressure of the sphincter of Oddi after intravenous cholecystokinin or ceruletide was demonstrated by Rolny et al.

(1986) in 10 to 62 patients with suspected biliary dyskinesia.

Tanaka *et al.* (1985) used a bile duct microtransducer to compare 17 patients with postcholecystectomy pain and nine control subjects. Morphine was given to induce spasm of the sphincter of Oddi, and 30 minutes later caerulein was administered to relax the sphincter. Thirteen patients developed pain in response to morphine, with a concomitant rise in biliary pressure. Three had pain but no increase in pressure, and one patient experienced no pain although there was an increase in bile duct pressure. Because some patients developed pain at low levels of bile duct pressure the authors postulated a difference in the pain threshold for given degrees of spasm of the sphincter of Oddi.

In the study of Funch-Jensen *et al.* (1982), patients with the postcholecystectomy syndrome were found to have higher sphincter of Oddi pressures than controls, although there was no significant difference in common bile duct pressure.

25.3.5 APPROACH TO DIAGNOSIS

The validity of every diagnostic criterion for papillary stenosis can be challenged. At present, no single test or observation is sufficiently reliable for diagnosis, which is therefore, based on combined clinical, biochemical, radiographic and manometric criteria. When there is an indication of papillary stenosis by two or more of these criteria, the diagnosis is thought to be more likely. However, the occurrence of all or most of these criteria in a single patient is decidedly unusual. Although this approach to the diagnosis appears reasonable, it may be difficult to match the symptoms and findings in a given patient with established diagnostic criteria. Pain is common after cholecystectomy, often different from characteristic biliary pain; transient biochemical abnormalities are non-specific; the diameter of the bile duct is not absolute, and 'normal' values vary according to the

method of measurement; delayed clearance of contrast medium from the bile duct is a subjective assessment at best.

Whether mild to moderate degrees of inflammation and fibrosis of the sphincter of Oddi in the absence of more severe obstruction can be appreciated endoscopically is uncertain. Even in biopsies inflammation may be overlooked or underestimated. There may be a spectrum of disorders of the sphincter of Oddi with organic stenosis, manifested by an inability to cannulate, at one extreme, and functional disturbances without microscopic changes at the other. In patients with recognizable abnormalities of the biliary or pancreatic ducts (e.g. choledocholithiasis), it is probably impossible to determine whether manometric abnormalities of the sphincter of Oddi are a cause or an effect of the disorder.

25.3.6 THE CLINICAL PROBLEM

The magnitude of the clinical problem of postcholecystectomy syndrome is unknown, but the true syndrome is not common.

Bar-Meir *et al.* (1984) contacted 774 patients who had undergone cholecystectomy consecutively during a 5-year period. Of 454 patients (58.7%) who responded, 29 (6.7%) were found to have typical abdominal pain, suggestive of papillary stenosis. Seventeen (10 had abnormal enzyme levels) accepted ERCP. Cannulation was successful in 16 (94%) cases, and manometry in 15 patients. An elevated basal pressure of the sphincter of Oddi was found in two patients, and elevated common duct pressure in one patient. The authors concluded that papillary stenosis (postcholecystectomy syndrome) occurs in less than 1% of patients who have undergone cholecystectomy.

25.3.7 TREATMENT

(a) Medical

Non-operative measures (diet and anticholinergics) are not very effective in the treatment of postcholecystectomy syndrome. It has been known for some time that nitrates have an effect on the sphincter of Oddi (Butsch, McGowan and Walters, 1936; Staritz *et al.*, 1985), and offer some prospect of improved medical treatment (Bar-Meir, Halpern and Bardan, 1983).

(b) Surgical

The reported results of surgical sphincterotomy with a variety of modifications are generally good (Gregg *et al.*, 1977; Moody, 1977; Raskin *et al.*, 1978; Madura *et al.*, 1981), although not in all series. In the report of Moody, Becker and Potts (1983) of 92 patients with pain due to stenosis of the sphincter of Oddi, surgery gave complete relief of pain in only 43% and 24% experienced no relief of pain at all.

(c) Endoscopic sphincterotomy

Tanaka *et al.* (1985) performed endoscopic sphincterotomy on 12 patients with papillary stenosis who had both pain and elevation of bile duct pressure in response to morphine. This resulted in complete relief in eight patients, a moderate decrease in symptoms in three, and slight relief of pain in one. Intrabiliary transducer manometry with morphine stimulation was repeated 1–2 weeks after endoscopic sphincterotomy. No elevation of biliary pressure was found in three patients, although slight elevations were recorded in the others. Mild, transient pain occurred with morphine administration in two patients, one of whom underwent a repeat endoscopic sphincterotomy. The average follow-up was 23 months (2–50 months), during which time a slight degree of pain recurred in one patient who initially had complete relief, and in one patient who had experienced only slight relief of pain immediately after endoscopic sphincterotomy.

Further data from the study by Geenen *et al.* (1984b) on the efficacy of endoscopic sphincterotomy in relieving postcholecystectomy pain has been reported recently (Geenen *et al.*, 1987). Forty-seven patients had been randomized to undergo endoscopic sphincterotomy or a sham procedure. At 1 year, endoscopic sphincterotomy was performed in 12 symptomatic patients from the group of 24 patients who were initially randomized to the sham procedure. The sphincter pressure was high in seven and normal in five of these patients. Forty patients were available for analysis at 4-year follow-up. Overall, 17 of 18 patients (96%) with manometric disorders of the sphincter of Oddi were benefited by endoscopic sphincterotomy. In patients with normal sphincter pressure, endoscopic sphincterotomy did not result in pain relief beyond the expected placebo effect of the sham procedure. However, almost one-third of patients with normal sphincter pressure (five sphincterotomy, two sham) were lost to follow-up at 4 years. Even if it were assumed that all lost patients responded to sphincterotomy, only 59% of the group with normal sphincter pressures would have benefited from sphincterotomy.

Roberts-Thomson (1984) reported on the results of endoscopic sphincterotomy in 300 patients. In the 15% with presumed dysfunction of the sphincter of Oddi sphincterotomy resulted in sustained relief of symptoms in only 51%. Four patients with a positive morphine-neostigmine test (Roberts-Thomson and Toouli, 1985) had a second provocative test 6–18 months after endoscopic sphincterotomy. Serum enzyme levels remained within the normal range in two patients, although serum amylase concentrations were mildly elevated in two patients. Two patients were pain free at the second provocative test, while the other two had pain of lesser severity than that experienced in response to morphine-neostigmine before sphincterotomy.

Roberts-Thomson *et al.* (1986) (see above) also reported the results of a study in which six patients with papillary stenosis underwent biliary cholescintigraphy before and after endoscopic sphincterotomy. The time at which radioactivity in the common duct reached

50% of the maximum activity (CBD T_{50}), and the time for initial appearance of the isotope in the duodenum, decreased in all patients after sphincterotomy.

In the biliary cholescintigraphy study of Shaffer et al. (1986) (see above), the time required to reach maximal radioactivity in the biliary system was significantly greater in nine patients with suspected papillary stenosis compared with 35 asymptomatic subjects who had undergone cholecystectomy. Sphincterotomy (eight endoscopic, one surgical) resulted in a significant decrease in the time to peak activity in the bile duct, as well as a significant increase in the amount of radiotracer excreted at 45 minutes. The basal emptying rate also increased, but this was not significant. Relief of pain occurred in eight of nine patients after sphincterotomy. Radiotracer uptake and emptying were normal before sphincterotomy in the one patient with persistent pain after sphincterotomy. Biliary cholescintigraphy demonstrated deterioration in uptake and emptying in one patient with recurrent symptoms after a period of pain relief following sphincterotomy.

In the study of Rolny et al. (1986) hydrostatic balloon dilatation of the sphincter of Oddi in one patient, and endoscopic sphincterotomy in eight patients, produced relief of pain at 11–16 months follow-up.

Thatcher et al. (1987) reviewed the records of 51 patients with presumed dysfunction of the sphincter of Oddi from three centres. Elimination of abdominal pain occurred in 31 of 46 patients available for follow-up. The presence of bile duct dilatation and/or delayed drainage of contrast medium were the best predictive factors for a favourable outcome of sphincterotomy. There was no correlation between the results of manometry and a favourable outcome for sphincterotomy, especially in patients with a dilated bile duct and/or delayed drainage of contrast medium.

There were complications of endoscopic sphincterotomy in seven patients (13.7%) with presumed papillary stenosis. A complication occurred in three of 34 patients (8.8%) with dilated bile ducts and/or delayed drainage of contrast, while four of 17 patients (23.5%) with normal bile ducts sustained a complication of sphincterotomy. The difference in complication rates for these two groups was statistically significant. These authors concluded that the complication rate of endoscopic sphincterotomy was significantly higher when the indication was papillary stenosis as compared to choledocholithiasis, especially when the bile duct is not dilated.

REFERENCES

Acosta, J. M., Civantos, F., Nardi, G. I. and Castleman, B. (1967) Fibrosis of the papilla of Vater. Surg. Gynecol. Obstet., 124, 787–94.

Acosta, J. M. and Nardi, G. L. (1966) Papillitis. Inflammatory disease of the ampulla of Vater. Arch. Surg., 92, 354–61.

Allen, A. W. and Wallace, R. H. (1940) The surgical management of stone in the common bile duct. Ann. Surg., 111, 838.

Autio, V. and Parvinen, T. (1965) Results of surgical treatment of stenosis of the sphincter of Oddi. J. Int. Coll. Surg., 44, 656–9.

Bar-Meir, S., Geenen, J. E., Hogan, W. J. et al. (1979) Biliary and pancreatic duct pressure measured by ERCP manometry in patients with suspected papillary stenosis. Dig. Dis. Sci., 24, 204–13.

Bar-Meir, S., Halpern, Z. and Bardan, E. (1983) Nitrate therapy in a patient with papillary dysfunction. Am. J. Gastroenterol., 78, 94–5.

Bar-Meir, S., Halpern, Z., Bardan, E. and Gilat, T. (1984) Frequency of papillary dysfunction among cholecystectomized patients. Hepatology, 4, 328–30.

Berci, G. and Johnson, N. (1965) Functional studies of the extrahepatic biliary system in the dog by use of a controlled biliary fistula. Ann. Surg., 161, 286–92.

Berezny, G. M., Beck, I. T., DaCosta, L. R. et al. (1985) Ultrasound in the diagnosis of sphincter of Oddi spasm. J. Clin. Gastroenterol., 7, 528–32.

Bortolotti, M., Caletti, G. C., Brocchi, E. et al. (1985) Endoscopic electromyography and manometry of the human sphincter of Oddi. Hepatogastroenterology, 32, 250–2.

Boyden, E. A. (1937) The sphincter of Oddi in man and certain representative mammals. Surgery, 1, 25–37.

Braasch, J. W. and McCann, J. C. (1967) Normal luminal size of choledochoduodenal junction as determined by probe at choledochostomy. *Surgery*, **62**, 258–9.

Bradley, V. D. and Nebel, O. T. (1977) Clinical evaluation of sphincter of Oddi manometry. *Gastrointest. Endosc.*, **24**, 27–9.

Branch, C. D., Bailey, O. T. and Zollinger, R. (1939) Consequences of instrumental dilation of the papilla of Vater; experimental study. *Arch. Surg.*, **38**, 358.

Broad, L. T., Gordon, S. J. and Vernick, J. J. (1979) Papillary stenosis: predictability of anatomic involvement by provocative testing. *Gastroenterology*, **76**, 1107.

Burke, J. O., Plummer, K. and Bradford, S. (1950) Serum amylase response to morphine, mecholyl and secretin as a test of pancreatic function. *Gastroenterology*, **15**, 699.

Butsch, W. L., McGowan, J. M. and Walters, W. (1936) Clinical studies on the influence of certain drugs in relation to biliary pain and to the variations in intrabiliary pressure. *Surg. Gynecol. Obstet.*, **63**, 451–6.

Carr-Locke, D. L. and Gregg, J. A. (1981) Endoscopic manometry of pancreatic and biliary sphincter zones in man. Basal results in healthy volunteers. *Dig. Dis. Sci.*, **26**, 7–15.

Carr-Locke, D. L., Gregg, J. A. and Aoki, T. T. (1983) Effects of exogenous glucagon on pancreatic and biliary ductal and sphincteric pressures in man demonstrated by endoscopic manometry and correlation with plasma glucagon. *Dig. Dis. Sci.*, **28**, 312–20.

Cattell, R. B. and Colcock, B. P. (1953) Fibrosis of the sphincter of Oddi. *Ann. Surg.*, **137**, 797–806.

Cattell, R. B., Colcock, B. P. and Pollack, J. L. (1957) Stenosis of the sphincter of Oddi. *N. Engl. J. Med.*, **246**, 429–35.

Coelho, J. C., Moody, F. G. and Senninger, N. (1985) A new method for correlating pancreatic and biliary duct pressures and sphincter of Oddi electromyography. *Surgery*, **97**, 342–9.

Colcock, B. P. (1958) Stenosis of the sphincter of Oddi. *Surg. Clin. North Am.*, **38**, 631.

Csendes, A., Kruse, A., Funch-Jensen, P. et al. (1979) Pressure measurements in the biliary and pancreatic duct systems in controls and in patients with gallstones, previous cholecystectomy, or common bile duct stones. *Gastroenterology*, **77**, 1203–10.

Dahl-Iversen, A., Sorenson, H. and Westengaard, E. (1957) Pressure measurement in the biliary tract in patients after cholecystolithotomy and in patients with dyskinesia. *Acta Chir. Scand.*, **11**, 181–90.

Das, P. N. (1965) An experimental study of disturbances of the sphincter of oddi. *J. Pathol. Bacteriol.*, **90**, 135–50.

De Masi, E., Corazziari, E., Habib, F. I. et al. (1984) Manometric study of the sphincter of Oddi in patients with and without common bile duct stones. *Gut*, **25**, 275–8.

Dolgin, S. M. and Soloway, R. D. (1980) Serum bile acid response to morphine-neostigmine in controls and in patients with biliary dyskinesia. *Gastroenterology*, **78**, 1158.

Doubilet, H. and Mulholland, J. H. (1956) Eight-year study of pancreatitis and sphincterotomy. *J.A.M.A.*, **160**, 521–8.

Dreiling, D. A. and Richman, A. (1954) Evaluation of provocative blood enzyme tests in diagnosis of pancreatic disease. *Arch. Intern. Med.*, **94**, 197.

Funch-Jensen, P., Csendes, A., Kruse, A. et al. (1979) Common bile duct and Oddi sphincter pressure before and after endoscopic papillotomy in patients with common bile duct stones. *Ann. Surg.*, **190**, 176–7.

Funch-Jensen, P., Kraglund, K. and Djurhuus, J. C. (1984) The influence of measuring catheter diameter on direct manometry in the canine sphincter of Oddi. *Scand. J. Gastroenterol.*, **19**, 926–30.

Funch-Jensen, P., Kruse, A., Csendes, A. et al. (1982) Biliary manometry in patients with postcholecystectomy syndrome. *Acta Chir. Scand.*, **148**, 267–8.

Funch-Jensen, P., Kruse, A. and Ravensbaek, J. (1987) Endoscopic sphincter of Oddi manometry in healthy volunteers. *Scand. J. Gastroenterol.*, **22**, 243–9.

Geenen, J. E., Hogan, W. J. and Dodds, W. J. (1987) Sphincter of Oddi, *Gatroenterologic Endoscopy* (ed. M. V. Sivak Jr), W. B. Saunders, Philadelphia, pp. 735–51.

Geenen, J. E., Hogan, W. J., Dodds, W. J. et al. (1980) Intraluminal pressure recording from the human sphincter of Oddi. *Gastroenterology*, **78**, 317–24.

Geenen, J. E., Hogan, W. J., Dodds, W. J. et al. (1987) Long-term results of endoscopic sphincterotomy (ES) for treating patients with sphincter-of-Oddi (SO) dysfunction. A prospective study. *Gastroenterology*, **92**, (abstr.), 1401.

Geenen, J. E., Hogan, W. J., Shaffer, R. D. et al. (1977) Endoscopic electrosurgical papillotomy and manometry in biliary tract disease. *JAMA*, **237**, 2075–8.

Geenen, J., Hogan, W., Toouli, J. et al. (1984a) A prospective randomized study of the efficacy of endoscopic sphincterotomy for patients with presumptive sphincter of oddi dysfunction. *Gastroenterology*, **86**, (abstr.), 1086.

Geenen, J. E., Toouli, J., Hogan, W. J. *et al.* (1984b) Endoscopic sphincterotomy: follow up evaluation of effects on the sphincter of Oddi. *Gastroenterology*, **87**, 754–8.

Grage, T. B., Lober, P. H., Imamoglu, K. and Wangensteen, D. H. (1960) Stenosis of the sphincter of Oddi. A clinicopathologic review of 50 cases. *Surgery*, **48**, 3–4–17.

Graham, M. F., Cooperberg, P. L., Cohen, M. M. and Burhenne, H. J. (1980) The size of the normal common hepatic duct following cholecystectomy: an ultrasonographic study. *Radiology*, **135**, 137–9.

Gregg, J. A. and Carr-Locke, D. L. (1984) Endoscopic pancreatic and biliary manometry in pancreatic, biliary, and papillary disease, and after endoscopic sphincterotomy and surgical sphincteroplasty. *Gut*, **25**, 1247–54.

Gregg, J. A., Clark, G., Barr, C. *et al.* (1978) The association of ampullary stenosis, pancreatitis and retained common duct stone with the postcholecystectomy syndrome. Diagnosis by ERCP and morphine-Prostigmine test (MPT). *Gastrointest. Endosc.*, **24**, 199.

Gregg, J. A., Clark, G., Barr, C. *et al.* (1980) Postcholecystectomy syndrome and its association with ampullary stenosis. *Am. J. Surg.*, **139**, 374–8.

Gregg, J. A., Taddeo, A. E., Milano, A. F. *et al.* (1977) Endoscopic pancreatography in patients with positive morphine Prostigmine tests. *Am. J. Surg.*, **134**, 318–21.

Guelrud, M., Bettarello, A., Cecconello, I. *et al.* (1983) Sphincter of Oddi pressure in chagasic patients with megaesophagus. *Gastroenterology*, **85**, 584–8.

Hastbacka, J., Jarvinen, H., Kivilaakso, E. and Turunen, M. T. (1986) Results of sphincteroplasty in patients with spastic sphincter of Oddi. Predictive value of operative biliary manometry and provocation tests. *Scand. J. Gastroenterol.*, **21**, 516–20.

Hauge, C. W. and Mark, J. B. D. (1965) Common bile duct motility and sphincter mechanism: I. Pressure measurements with multilumen catheter in dogs. *Ann. Surg.*, **162**, 1028–38.

Hedner, P. and Rorsman, G. (1969) On the mechanism of action for the effect of CCK on the choledochoduodenal function in the cat. *Acta Physiol. Scand.*, **76**, 248–54.

Hogan, W., Geenen, J. E., Dodds, W. J. *et al.* (1982) Paradoxical motor response to cholecystokinin (CCK-OP) in patients with suspected sphincter of Oddi dysfunction. *Gastroenterology*, **82**, 1085.

Ishioka, T. (1959) Electromyographic study of the choledochoduodenal junction and duodenal wall muscle. *Tohoku J. Exp. Med.*, **70**, 73–84.

Johnson, R. H. and Doppman, J. (1967) Duodenal reflux and the etiology of pancreatitis. *Surgery*, **62**, 462–7.

Knight, W. A. Jr, Muether, R. O. and Sommer, A. J. (1949) Chronic recurrent pancreatitis: serial serum diastase levels following Prostigmine stimulation. *Gastroenterology*, **12**, 24.

La Morte, W. W., Gaca, J. M., Wise, W. E. *et al.* (1980) Choledochal sphincter relaxation in response to histamine in the primate. *J. Surg. Res.*, **28**, 373–8.

Lebovics, E., Heier, S. K. and Rosenthal, W. S. (1986) Sphincter of Oddi motility: developments in physiology and clinical application. *Am. J. Gastroenterol.*, **81**, 736–43.

Lee, R. G., Gregg, J. A., Koroshetz, A. M. *et al.* (1985) Sphincter of Oddi stenosis: diagnosis using hepatobiliary scintigraphy and endoscopic manometry. *Radiology*, **156**, 793–6.

LoGiudice, J. A., Geenen, J. E., Hogan, W. J. and Dodds, W. J. (1979) Efficacy of the morphine-Prostigmin test for evaluating patients with suspected papillary stenosis. *Dig. Dis. Sci.*, **24**, 455–8.

McCutcheon, A. D. (1968) A fresh approach to the pathogenesis of pancreatitis. *Gut*, **9**, 296–310.

Madura, J. A., McCammon, R. L., Paris, J. M. and Jesseph, J. E. (1981) The Nardi test and biliary manometry in the diagnosis of pancreaticobiliary sphincter dysfunction. *Surgery*, **90**, 588–95.

Mahorner, H. (1959) Supra and transduodenal exploration of the common bile duct. *Am. J. Gastroenterol.*, **32**, 182–9.

Meshkinpour, H., Mollot, M., Eckerling, G. B. and Bookman, L. (1984) Bile duct dyskinesia. Clinical and manometric study. *Gastroenterology*, **87**, 759–62.

Moody, F. G. (1977) Surgical therapy for gallstones and their complications, in *Disease of the Gallbladder and Biliary System* (ed. L. J. Schoenfield), John Wiley, New York, pp. 268–9.

Moody, F. G., Becker, J. M. and Potts, J. R. (1983) Transduodenal sphincteroplasty and trans-ampullary septectomy for postcholecystectomy pain. *Ann. Surg.*, **197**, 627–36.

Mueller, P. R., Ferrucci, J. T. Jr, Simeone, J. F. *et al.* (1981) Postcholecystectomy bile duct dilatation: mytho or reality? *A. J. R.*, **136**, 355–8.

Myhre, J., Nesbitt, S. and Hurley, J. T. (1949) Response of serum amylase and lipase to pancreatic stimulation as a test of pancreatic function. *Gastroenterology*, **13**, 127.

Nardi, G. L. and Acosta, J. M. (1966) Papillitis as a

cause of pancreatitis and abdominal pain: role of evocative test, operative pancreatography and histologic evaluation. *Ann. Surg.*, **164**, 611–21.

Nebel, O. T. (1975) Manometric evaluation of the papilla of Vater. *Gastrointest. Endosc.*, **21**, 126–8.

Novis, B. H., Borman, P. C., Girdwood, A. W. and Marks, I. N. (1985) Endoscopic manometry of the pancreatic duct and sphincter zone in patients with chronic pancreatitis. *Dig. Dis. Sci.*, **30**, 225–8.

Okazaki, K., Yamamoto, Y. and Ito, K. (1986) Endoscopic measurement of papillary sphincter zone and pancreatic main ductal pressure in patients with chronic pancreatitis. *Gastroenterology*, **91**, 409–18.

Ono, K. (1970) The discharge of bile into the duodenum and electrical activities of the muscle of Oddi and duodenum. *Jpn. J. Smooth Muscle Res.*, **6**, 123–8.

Ono, K., Watanabe, K., Suzuki, H. *et al.* (1968) Bile flow mechanism in man. *Arch. Surg.*, **96**, 869–74.

Paulino, F. and Cavalcanti, A. (1960) Anatomy and pathology of the distal common duct. Special reference to stenosing odditis. *Am. J. Dig. Dis.*, **5**, 697–713.

Persson, C. G. A. (1971) Adrenoceptor functions in the cat choledochoduodenal junction *in vitro*. *Br. J. Pharmacol.*, **42**, 447–61.

Ponce, J., Sala, T., Pertejo, V. *et al.* (1983) Manometric evaluation of sphincter of Oddi after endoscopic sphincterotomy, and in patients with previous surgical sphincterotomy. *Endoscopy*, **15**, 249–51.

Prudhomme, P., Niloff, P., Skoryna, S. C. and Webster, D. R. (1965) Experimental studies on fibrosis of the sphincter of Oddi and on sphincterotomy. *Can. J. Surg.*, **8**, 201–7.

Raskin, J. B. (1985) Papillary stenosis in *Gastroenterology* (eds. J. E. Berk, W. S. Haubrich, M. H. Kalser *et al.*), W. B. Saunders, Philadelphia, pp. 3799–807.

Raskin, J. B., Kafka, E., Maladonado, A. and Levi, J. V. (1978) Endoscopic retrograde cholangiopancreatography (ERCP) findings in ampullary stenosis. *Gastrointest. Endosc.*, **24**, 208.

Roberts-Thomson, I. C. (1984) Endoscopic sphincterotomy of the papilla of Vater: an analysis of 300 cases. *Aust. N.Z. J. Med.*, **14**, 611–7.

Roberts-Thomson, I. C. and Toouli, J. (1985) Abnormal responses to morphine-neostigmine in patients with undefined biliary type pain. *Gut*, **26**, 1367–72.

Roberts-Thomson, I. C., Toouli, J., Blanchett, W. *et al.* (1986) Assessment of bile flow by radioscintigraphy in patients with biliary-type pain

after cholecystectomy. *Aust. N.Z. J. Med.*, **16**, 788–93.

Rolny, P., Arleback, A., Funch-Jensen, P. *et al.* (1986) Paradoxical response of sphincter of Oddi to intravenous injection of cholecystokinin or ceruletide. Manometric findings and results of treatment in biliary dyskinesia. *Gut*, **27**, 1507–11.

Rosch, W., Koch, H. and Demling, L. (1976) Manometric studies during ERCP and endoscopic papillotomy. *Endoscopy*, **8**, 30–3.

Sarles, J. C., Bidart, J. M., Devaux, M. A. *et al.* (1976) Actions of cholecystokinin and caerulein on the rabbit sphincter of Oddi. *Digestion*, **14**, 415–23.

Schwegler, R. A. and Boyden, E. A. (1937) The development of the pars intestinalis of the common bile duct in the human fetus with special reference to the origin of ampulla of Vater and the sphincter of Oddi. 2: The early development of the musculus proprius. *Anat. Rec.*, **68**, 17–40.

Setakis, N., Vennart, W., Gardner, A. M. and Nayak, P. (1984) A peroperative test of the function of the sphincter of Oddi. *Ann. R. Coll. Surg.*, **66**, 175–8.

Shaffer, E. A., Hershfield, N. B., Logan, K. and Kloiber, R. (1986) Cholescintigraphic detection of functional obstruction of the sphincter of Oddi. Effect of papillotomy. *Gastroenterology*, **90**, 728–33.

Snape, W. J., Wirts, C. W. and Friedman, M. H. (1949) Evaluation of pancreatic function by means of induced hyperamylasemia following morphine and secretin. *Am. J. Med.*, **7**, 417–8.

Staritz, M., Ewe, K. and zum Buschenfelde, K. H. (1986) Investigation of the sphincter of Oddi before, immediately after and six weeks after endoscopic papillotomy. *Endoscopy*, **18**, 14–6.

Staritz, M., Poralla, T., Ewe, K. and Meyer zum Buschenfelde, K. H. 1(985) Effect of glyceryl trinitrate on the sphincter of Oddi motility and baseline pressure. *Gut*, **26**, 194–7.

Steinberg, W. M., Salvato, R. F. and Toskes, P. P. (1980) The morphine-Prostigmine provocative test: is it useful for making clinical decisions? *Gastroenterology*, **78**, 728–31.

Sterkel, R. L. and Knight, W. A. (1965) The value of a provocative serum enzyme test in 'pancreatic dyspepsia'. *South. Med. J.*, **58**, 56–61.

Tanaka, M., Ikeda, S., Matsumoto, S. *et al.* (1985) Manometric diagnosis of sphincter of Oddi spasm as a cause of postcholecystectomy pain and the treatment by endoscopic sphincterotomy. *Ann. Surg.*, **202**, 712–9.

Tanaka, M., Ikeda, S. and Nakayama, F. (1981) Nonoperative measurement of pancreatic and common bile duct pressures with a microtransducer catheter and effects of duodenoscopic sphincterotomy. *Dig. Dis. Sci.*, **26**, 545–52.

Tanaka, M., Ikeda, S. and Nakayama, F. (1984) Change in bile duct pressure responses after cholecystectomy: loss of gallbladder as a pressure reservoir. *Gastroenterology*, **87**, 1154–9.

Thatcher, B. S., Sivak, M. V. Jr, Tedesco, F. J. *et al.* (1987) Endoscopic sphincterotomy for suspected dysfunction of the sphincter of Oddi. *Gastrointest. Endosc.*, **33**, 91–5.

Toouli, J. (1984) Sphincter of Oddi motility. *Br. J. Surg.*, **71**, 251–6.

Toouli, J., Geenen, J. E., Hogan, W. J. *et al.* (1982) Sphincter of Oddi motor activity: a comparison between patients with common bile duct stones and controls. *Gastroenterology*, **82**, 111–7.

Toouli, J., Roberts-Thomson, I. C., Dent, J. and Lee, J. (1985a) Manometric disorders in patients with suspected sphincter of Oddi dysfunction. *Gastroenterology*, **88**, 1243–50.

Toouli, J., Roberts-Thomson, I. C., Dent, J. and Lee, J. (1985b) Sphincter of Oddi motility disorders in patients with idiopathic recurrent pancreatitis. *Br. J. Surg.*, **72**, 859–63.

Toouli, B. and Watts, J. M. (1972) Actions of cholecystokinin-pancreozimin, secretin and gastrin on extra-hepatic biliary tract motility *in vitro*. *Ann. Surg.*, **175**, 439–47.

Torsoli, A., Corazziari, E., Habib, F. I. *et al.* (1986) Frequencies and cyclical pattern of the human sphincter of Oddi phasic activity. *Gut*, **27**, 363–9.

Trommald, J. P. and Seabrook, D. B. (1950) Benign fibrosis of the sphincter of Oddi. *West. J. Surg. Obstet. Gynecol.*, **58**, 89–94.

Tuzhilin, S., Podolsky, A. and Dreiling, D. A. (1981) The role of insufficiency of the sphincter of Oddi in the pathogenesis of pancreatitis. *Mt. Sinai J. Med.*, **48**, 133–6.

Viceconte, G., Viceconte, G. W. and Bogliolo, G. (1984) Endoscopic manometry of the sphincter of Oddi in patients with and without juxtapapillary duodenal diverticula. *Scand. J. Gastroenterol.*, **19**, 329–33.

Vondrasek, P., Eberhardt, G. and Classen, M. (1974) Endoscopic semiconductor manometry. *Int. J. Med.*, **3**, 188–92.

Warshaw, A. L., Simeone, J., Schapiro, R. H. *et al.* (1985) Objective evaluation of ampullary stenosis with ultrasonography and pancreatic stimulation. *Am. J. Surg.*, **149**, 65–72.

Wirts, C. W. and Snape, W. J. (1951) Evaluation of pancreatic function tests. *J.A.M.A.*, **145**, 876.

Zeman, R. K., Burrell, M. I., Dobbins, J. *et al.* (1985) Postcholecystectomy syndrome: evaluation using biliary scintigraphy and endoscopic retrograde cholangiopancreatography. *Radiology*, **156**, 787–92.

Zimmon, D. S., Falkenstein, D. B. and Clemett, A. R. (1978) Endoscopic diagnosis and management of papillary stenosis. *Gastrointest. Endosc.*, **24**, 214.

Zimmon, D. S., Ferrarg, T. P. and Clement, A. R. (1978) Radiology of papilla of Vater stenosis. *Gastrointest. Radiol.*, **3**, 343–8.

CHAPTER TWENTY-SIX

Management of biliary obstruction

G. W. Stevenson

The investigation and management of patients with biliary tract disease have undergone dramatic changes in the last 10–15 years. In the early 1970s the diagnosis of extrahepatic obstruction was made by serum chemistry, which was then followed by either percutaneous cholangiography with a large sheathed needle, by liver biopsy, or by laparotomy. The ability to measure the bile duct, and frequently to define the level and nature of pathology with ultrasound, CT scanning and needle aspiration or biopsy, has brought a satisfying degree of precision to the initial assessment of these patients. In borderline cases the ultrasound fat provocation test may add further support for invasive investigation (Darweesh *et al.*, 1988). At the same time there have been developments in interventional endoscopic and radiological percutaneous techniques that allow the treatment of many patients with 'surgical' jaundice without the need for formal surgery (Mueller, 1988; Summerfield, 1988).

The five biliary chapters in this book (Chapters 23–28) leave an overwhelming sense that endoscopy, radiology and surgery are so closely intertwined in the diagnosis and management of these disorders that only a team approach involving the three disciplines will permit selection of the most appropriate procedure, utilization of optimum technique during the procedure, and the avoidance of unnecessary complications.

The chapters on gallstone disease (Chapters 22 and 24) describe the radiological and endoscopic techniques for treating stones. The radiological paper describes the astonishing variety of approaches that can now be utilized by an innovative radiology group working closely with surgeons, and concentrates on the technical aspects of the various methods which they and others have developed, rather than discussing in detail the indications for radiology, surgery or endoscopy in these patients. Therefore it does not provide insight for the general reader wondering how the various methods discussed compare with surgical or endoscopic approaches. The endoscopic chapter illustrates some of the endoscopic possibilities and emphasizes the crucial importance of good radiological technique during ERCP, but does not address and evaluate the place for competing radiological techniques, or the ways in which interventional radiology can contribute to increased success in achieving sphincterotomy. Thus these chapters provide an exceptional review of what can be achieved by a highly developed part of the team. However, a broader perspective is also required to place these techniques in the context of a team of surgeons, radiologists and gastroenterologists, so that the reader can estimate how they may fit into clinical practice.

Chapters 27 and 28 on malignant biliary obstruction can be read as a pair, giving the endoscopic and radiological approaches to the problem. Both of these authors come from institutions and backgrounds where the team approach has been even stronger (and perhaps easier to implement than in the North American and German medical environments). Both discuss the place for radiological and endoscopic stenting, and each stresses the particular advantages of the competing technique, as well as emphasizing the benefits of their own subject matter.

The chapter on the controversial topic of papillary stenosis (Chapter 25) leads to the uncomfortable conclusion that it may not be possible to investigate and treat these patients safely without sphincter of Oddi manometry. Without manometry, and using current criteria to decide on the need for sphincterotomy, the clinical response rate to sphincterotomy was only 68% (with a 30% response from the placebo effect in a control group having a sham sphincterotomy), but the response rate in those with increased sphincter pressure at manometry was 91% (Geenan et al., 1984, 1987); although not all authors have found manometry to be so helpful (Krims and Cotton, 1988). That the accurate prediction of response to sphincterotomy is important is indicated by the complication rate of sphincterotomy being much higher in patients with papillary stenosis than in those with choledocholithiasis (Leese, Neoptolemos and Carr-Locke, 1985; Classen, 1986) – in one series, 14% versus 9%, and as high as 24% in patients with papillary stenosis and no duct dilatation (Thatcher et al., 1987). The condition is uncommon, although quite often suspected, but there does seem to be a case for referring to a centre that can do biliary manometry any patient suspected of having papillary stenosis before deciding upon sphincterotomy in the absence of stones. This suggests that more university centres providing therapeutic ERCP services will need to establish biliary manometry.

For the future, it is clear that the techniques discussed in these five chapters have great potential. There are few hospitals in which all these techniques are available, particularly the advances discussed by Burhenne and Sivak. Two problems persist in encouraging their widespread implementation.

26.1 DEVELOPMENT IN ISOLATION

These new procedures have tended to be developed in subspecialty isolation by enthusiasts. Endoscopic sphincterotomy and stenting have been introduced principally by gastroenterologists, and the percutaneous methods by radiologists (Cope, 1988). This has led to the extraordinary spectacle of papers appearing on the emergency management of acute cholangitis by percutaneous drainage, with excellent results, that do not even refer to the fact that the same result can be achieved endoscopically; and of papers by gastroenterologists reporting similarly good results with endoscopic sphincterotomy that do not refer to the possible role of the percutaneous approach. A similar phenomenon has occurred with percutaneous gastrostomy with radiologists and endoscopists ignoring each other's results. Eventually, from hospitals in which radiologists and endoscopists work together, came reports describing how the percutaneous technique can allow failed endoscopic sphincterotomy to be completed, so that by judicious application of the two approaches by a team including radiologists and endoscopists, sphincterotomy can be accomplished in virtually all patients (Passi and Rankin, 1986). A further advance from closer association has been the development of a safer method of placing large stents in high obstructions (McLean, 1989). The passage of large catheters transhepatically is associated with complications of bleeding and biliary leakage, but the combined approach suggested by Kerlan et al. (1984) and described by Chapman (Chapter 28) allows large percutaneous transhepatic stents, up to 14 Fr, to be placed across biliary obstructions with only a small 3- or 5-Fr access track through the liver. Several of the new techniques developed by Burhenne (Chapter 24) have arisen from close association with surgeons, such as the transcholecystostomy interventions for dealing with stones in gallbladder or even in the ducts in frail elderly patients.

26.2 ISOLATION OF SURGEONS FROM THESE DEVELOPMENTS

Although there are some surgeons who perform endoscopic sphincterotomy and percutaneous transhepatic interventional procedures, the majority of these treatments are administered by gastroenterologists and radiologists. Many of these procedures replace operations, and the wisdom of the decision is not always clear cut. For example, a few years ago we tended to stent endoscopically any patient with obstructive jaundice due to pancreatic carcinoma. Several patients returned with acute symptoms from blocked stents that needed changing, or from duodenal obstruction. Our enthusiasm has waned, and relatively fit patients with small carcinomas or duodenal narrowing are now more likely to be treated with surgical biliary bypass and duodenal bypass, with stenting being reserved for intolerable itching or malnutrition in the frail elderly patient with more advanced disease, or for high inoperable obstruction.

In the early stages of introduction of these techniques within a hospital two scenarios may develop. First, patients already under the care of surgeons may continue to have 'inappropriate' operations, as the surgeons are unconvinced of the safety or effectiveness of the new approach, to the frustration of the avant-garde endoscopist or radiologist. Patients may be referred with reluctance from surgeons who are not involved in the decision making and in the gradual evaluation, modification and development of confidence in the new approaches. Surgical clinical guidance has a great deal to offer radiologists as they learn to take a more active interventional role in acute abdominal problems, not only in the bile duct. Second, patients being cared for by gastroenterologists or other physicians tend to have the endoscopic or radiological procedure, sometimes without a surgical opinion (perhaps because it is assumed that the surgeon will attempt to take over the patient and operate). Gastroenterologists may on occasion be tempted to treat their surgical and radiological colleagues as their personal technicians, rather than to plan ahead with radiologist and surgeon. This individualistic approach will have some dramatic successes but inevitably eventually leads to a surgeon being called to perform an emergency operation on an unknown patient who is bleeding or has perforation of the duodenum or bile duct. Both scenarios tend to cause hardening of suspicion into confirmed belief in the recalcitrance or irresponsibility of the other specialist.

Various strategies may be used to hasten the integration of care of patients with biliary obstruction. Surgeons, gastroenterologists and radiologists may hold regular working rounds to discuss management of both diagnostic and therapeutic plans. Joint biliary outpatient clinics can be organized in which initial assessment and diagnostic sequences are planned; patients with sphincterotomy, stents or surgical bypass are followed up; and patients referred for a specific treatment (such as sphincterotomy in a patient with three attacks of pancreatitis and small stones in the gallbladder) are reviewed for joint decision on the appropriateness of the proposed treatment. This clinic and the weekly rounds will help to ensure that interdisciplinary communication is both frequent and regular so that all members of the team have the opportunity for input and remain comfortable with the evolution of changing patterns of care. This critical interchange has great potential for joint evaluation, or investigation of new modifications of technique. Radiologists who wish to be part of this exciting world have to be prepared to work at inconvenient hours and to take some responsibility on the wards, for example in the care of catheters. Surgeons and gastroenterologists may feel little responsibility for a catheter placed by the radiologist, who will have to continue to visit the ward to ensure its optimal function. For example, when should it be capped to convert external to internal drainage, should it be irrigated and how often, and have the nurse or patient pulled it out a little and converted the internal biliary drainage into a pleurobiliary communication? Surgeons also have an adjustment to make to be comfortable with fewer operations and more consultations, and to be willing to pick up the urgent complications from their gastroenterology and radiology colleagues. Surgeons will be pleased if gastroenterologists and radiologists do not embark on therapeutic biliary procedures without a surgical consultation, so that there can be joint approval of the appropriateness of the proposed manoeuvre.

Many of the techniques described in these biliary chapters are only available in a few hospitals, and as they gradually spread, the problems of development in isolation and absence of surgical involvement may tend to occur afresh if not anticipated in advance. Nevertheless, for those hospitals which are already developing a multidisciplinary team approach, the five biliary chapters in this book open an exhilarating vista of new opportunity in the care of patients with biliary obstruction (Chespak *et al.*, 1989).

REFERENCES

Chespak, L. W., Ring, E. J. and Shapiro, H. A. (1989) Multidisciplinary approach to complex endoscopic biliary intervention. *Radiol.*, **170**, 961–7.

Classen, M. (1986) Endoscopic papillotomy – new indications, short and long term results. *Clin. Gastroenterol.*, **15**, 457.

Cope Constantin (1988) Needle endoscopy in special procedures. *Radiol.*, **168**, 353–8.

Darweesh, R. M. A., Dodds, W. J., Hogan, W. J. *et al.* (1988) Fatty meal sonography for evaluating patients with suspected partial common duct obstruction. *A.J.R.*, **151**, 63–8.

Geenan, J., Hogan, W. J., Dodds, W. J. *et al.* (1987) Long term results of endoscopic sphincterotomy for treating patients with sphincter of Oddi dysfunction. *Gastroenterology*, **92**, (abstr.), 1401.

Geenan, J., Hogan, W. J. and Toouli, J. (1984) A prospective randomised study of the efficacy of endoscopic sphincterotomy for patients with presumptive sphincter of Oddi dysfunction. *Gastroenterology*, **86**, (abstr.), 1086.

Kerlan, R. K., Ring, E. J., Pogany, A. C. and Brooke Jeffrey, R. (1984) Biliary endoprostheses: insertion using a combined peroral-transhepatic method. *Radiology*, **150**, 828–30.

Krims, P. E. and Cotton, P. B. (1988) Papillotomy and functional disorders of the sphincter of Oddi. *Endoscopy*, **20**, 203–6.

Leese, T. J. P., Neoptolemos, P. C. and Carr-Locke, D. (1985) Successes, failures, early complications and their management following endoscopic sphincterotomy: results in 394 consecutive patients from a single centre. *Br. J. Surg.*, **72**, 215.

McLean, G. K., Burke, D. (1989) Role of endoprostheses in the management of Malignant Biliary obstruction. *Radiol.*, **170**, 961–7.

Mueller, P. R. (1988) Interventional radiology of the biliary tract: A decade of progress. *Radiol.*, **168**, 328–30.

Passi, R. B. and Rankin, R. N. (1986) The transhepatic approach to a failed endoscopic sphincterotomy *Gastrointest. Endosc.*, **32**, 221–5.

Summerfield, J. A. (1988) Biliary obstruction is best managed by endoscopists. *Gut*, **29**, 741–5.

Thatcher, B. S., Sivak, M. V., Jr, Tedesco, F. J. *et al.* (1987) *Gastrointest. Endosc.*, **33**, 91–5.

CHAPTER TWENTY-SEVEN

Endoscopic stenting in malignant biliary obstruction

B. H. Laurence

27.1 INTRODUCTION

Malignant biliary obstruction is rarely curable and treatment of the most common manifestations, jaundice and pain, is usually palliative. In the young and fit patient with a localized tumour, surgical resection can give excellent palliation of jaundice over a long period (Leung *et al.*, 1983). The majority of patients with pancreatic or cholangiocarcinoma are, however, elderly and frail and in this group conventional surgical management carries considerable risk – less than 20% of the tumours are resectable and palliative resection or biliary bypass have a mortality of 20–40% (Lerut *et al.*, 1984; Saar and Cameron, 1984). Non-surgical methods of biliary decompression with an endoprosthesis can provide relief of jaundice, with potentially fewer early complications. Percutaneous drainage or a transhepatic internal stent, although less invasive than surgery, still have a relatively high morbidity related to hepatic puncture. This can be avoided using the transpapillary approach, with the endoscopic, retrograde insertion of a stent. Since the early descriptions of this technique (Laurence and Cotton, 1980; Soehendra and Reynders-Frederix, 1980), developments have enabled the use of large stents leading to significant improvement in the clinical results, so that it is now an acceptable alternative to other methods of biliary drainage.

27.2 EQUIPMENT

Ideally two duodenoscopes, one with a 2.8- or 3.8-mm channel (Olympus JF1T10, Fujinon DUOI-XL2, DUO-XT, Pentax FD-34H) and one with a large 4.2-mm channel (Olympus TJF10) should be available, together with the appropriate light source and a diathermy unit. A high-resolution image intensifier, preferably with a tilt table is essential. Standard ERCP and sphincterotomy accessories, including a needle knife are required; a Y-connector (Cook PSFLL-PCF-MLL 30) for injecting contrast down the catheter without removal of the guide-wire is useful. Paediatric biopsy forceps and a sheathed cytology brush should be available; a Dormia basket and toothed biopsy forceps are needed for the removal of blocked stents. Cannulation and dilatation of the stricture and the introduction of a prosthesis require – straight and J, floppy-tipped safety, Teflon-coated guide-wires (0.035, 300 cm), a tapered Teflon guide catheter (6.5 Fr, 250 cm), tapered Teflon dilatation catheters (8, 10, 11.5 Fr, 200 cm), dilatation balloons (4, 6 mm), polyethylene pushing catheters (8, 10, 11.5 Fr, 200 cm) and a range of straight stents with flaps (8, 10, 11.5 Fr; 5 cm, 7.5 cm, 10 cm and 15 cm). Double pigtail stents (8, 10 Fr; 5 cm, 10 cm) may occasionally be needed.

27.2.1 ENDOPROSTHESES (Leung, Del Favero and Cotton, 1985; Rey, Maupetit and Greff, 1985)

Endoprostheses (stents) are available in polyethylene, polyvinylchloride, polyurethane and Teflon. All are suitable and the differences in their chemical and physical characteristics (such as surface smoothness) do not seem to affect their performance.

The internal diameter of the prosthesis is the critical factor determining bile flow and long-term patency. At physiological flow rates, the volume of bile passing through the prosthesis obeys Poiseulle's Law and increases by the 4th power of the radius. A small increase in the luminal diameter is followed by a substantial increase in the flow rate, e.g. the flow of bile through a 10-Fr tube (in. diam. 2.2 mm) is more than double that through an 8-Fr tube (int. diam. 1.75 mm).

To prevent displacement of the stent through the tumour, loops, pigtails or flaps are incorporated into either end. The number and size of side-holes varies with the design, but multiple side-holes increase the resistance to bile flow and are undesirable. Pigtails and C-loops reduce the flow of bile through the stent by up to 50%; they are more difficult to insert and with large stents, the pigtail often fails to form above the obstruction. Straight polyethylene stents with double flaps and a single side-hole at either end are probably the most satisfactory.

A variety of stents, of differing materials and design, are commercially available in a range of diameter and length (Wilson-Cook, USA; Microvasive, USA; Olympus, Japan; MIW, Fr. Germany; Surgimed, Denmark; Biotrol, France) (Figure 27.1). Stents can be made cheaply and easily with a cutting jig

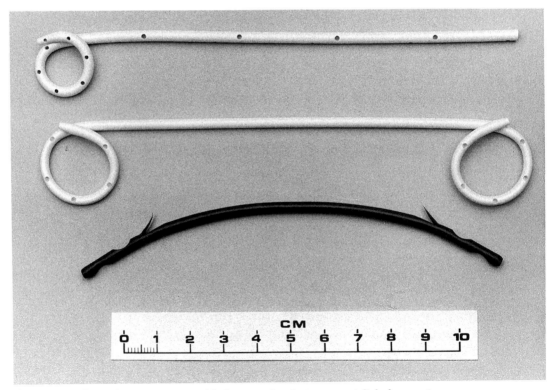

Figure 27.1 Stents in common use with flaps or pigtails to prevent dislodgement.

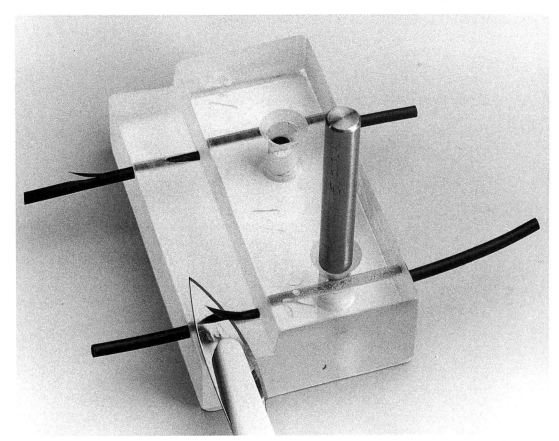

Figure 27.2   Stent jig for cutting flaps and side-holes.

which allows the precise positioning of side-holes and flaps (Figure 27.2).

27.3 EQUIPMENT PREPARATION

The duodenoscopes should be disinfected before the procedure to minimize the risk of introducing organisms, e.g. *Pseudomonas aeruginosa*, into the obstructed duct systems. The recommended practice is to thoroughly clean the instruments and then soak them in glutaraldehyde for 20 minutes; the water bottles should also be disinfected and filled with sterile water. All reuseable accessories are sterilized with either heat or gas (ethylene oxide). Disposable equipment such as guide-wires should not be reused; organisms can gain access to the core of the wire through a break in the Teflon coating and may remain viable even after heat sterilization.

Since the biopsy channel of the duodenoscope becomes contaminated by the bacterial flora of the mouth and upper gastrointestinal tract, it is not possible to maintain sterility of equipment which is passed through the instrument. Contamination of guide-wires and catheters during handling can be minimized by assistants working in sterile gloves from a sterile-draped Mayo table positioned above the patient's head.

27.4 STAFF REQUIREMENTS

In addition to the endoscopist, a radiologist or a skilled radiographer and two assistants are required. One of the assistants is responsible for the monitoring and care of the patient; the use of a self-retaining patient mouthguard (Endoguard, Microvasive) also enables this assistant to provide general help. The other assistant is retained for the special tasks involved in the insertion of the prosthesis; valuable experience in the skills needed can be gained by assisting with transhepatic and angiographic procedures.

27.5 PATIENT PREPARATION

The patients who are referred for this procedure form a high-risk group. The majority are elderly (70 years or more) and often have other serious medical problems such as ischaemic heart disease or respiratory insufficiency. Most are deeply jaundiced and many have lost a substantial amount of weight. Some have had recurrent cholangitis and 20% or more have abnormal renal function. Careful medical assessment prior to the procedure is essential, with special attention to evidence of infection – cholangitis, septicaemia or hepatic abscess – clotting abnormalities or renal failure. Significant sepsis is particularly likely if biliary drainage has been previously attempted. Upper abdominal ultrasound is of value in demonstrating the site and nature of the obstruction and defining the diameter of intrahepatic ducts for future comparison. Prophylactic antibiotics (mezlocillin, cephamandole or cephotaxime or gentamicin with amoxycillin and metronidazole) are administered before the procedure. Parenteral vitamin K is given as indicated by coagulation measurements. Because of the harmful effects of dehydration on renal function in obstructive jaundice, intravenous fluids are given to ensure an adequate urine output.

27.6 TECHNIQUE (Huibregtse and Tytgat, 1982)

Endoscopic retrograde cholangiography is carried out with the patient semiprone. Intravenous (i.v.) sedation is used routinely, usually pethidine (demerol) 50 mg, diazepam (Diazemuls) 10 mg or midazolam 5 mg, the dose being modified according to the response; in the elderly, frail and deeply jaundiced patient, a reduced dose of sedation is often adequate. Forceful dilatation of the malignant stricture can be painful and additional analgesia may be needed at that stage. General anaesthesia is rarely necessary. Duodenal relaxation is induced by giving hyoscine-N-butylbromide (Buscopan) 20–40 mg i.v. and this may need to be repeated. Buscopan is contraindicated in glaucoma or ischaemic heart disease and glucagon (0.5–1 i.u.) i.v. is a useful alternative. Naloxone hydrochloride (Narcan) 0.2–0.4 mg i.v. is given if the patient develops respiratory depression or is still heavily sedated at the end of the procedure.

The initial diagnostic phase is carried out with a small-channel (2.8- or 3.8-mm) duodenoscope and the larger instrument is used for insertion of the prosthesis. Depending upon the experience of the endoscopist, a large-channel duodenoscope tends to be more difficult to use for routine ERCP or sphincterotomy; the instrument is stiffer and standard cannulae have less directional stability over the wider elevator. This can be partially resolved by using a larger diameter cannula (8 Fr) or a standard cannula or sphincterotome passed through an oversleeve (10 Fr). The large-channel duodenoscope is the instrument of choice for the removal and replacement of a blocked prosthesis.

To avoid possible difficulties in recannulation with the bigger instrument, a technique has been used in which endoscopes are exchanged over a guide-wire (Martin, 1987; Carr-Locke, 1988). After diagnostic cholangiography with a 2.8-mm channel instrument (e.g. Olympus JFITIO) a 0.035 or 0.038 in Teflon-coated 400 mm guide-wire is passed through the ERCP catheter, and positioned above the obstruction. The ERCP catheter is removed and a 6-Fr pigtail catheter inserted over the guide-wire. The endoscope is then withdrawn under fluoroscopic control leaving the catheter and guide-wire in position. Endoscopic biopsy forceps are passed down the channel of the large-channel endoscope (e.g. Olympus TJFl0), grasp the guide-wire, and the wire and catheter are fed up the channel by withdrawing the forceps. The endoscope is then guided into place over the catheter. The stent can then be passed over the catheter.

As the duodenoscope is being introduced, the upper gastrointestinal tract is carefully examined. A large volume of fasting gastric contents may indicate malignant duodenal stenosis and the fluid should be removed to reduce the risk of pulmonary aspiration. Inflammation and erosions of the duodenal bulb are not uncommon with longstanding obstructive jaundice. A prominent, submucosal bile duct impression may indicate a low duct obstruction due to peri-ampullary malignancy. Stenosis of the duodenal lumen, thickened nodular mucosa or frank ulceration of the duodenal wall or the papilla may be due to malignant infiltration and should be biopsied. Malignant distortion or narrowing of the duodenal loop can make access to the papilla extremely difficult and is a major cause of failure of the procedure.

On cannulation of the papilla, duct stenosis or obstruction with typical malignant features can be demonstrated. The length of the biliary stricture and its relation to the bifurcation should be carefully outlined so that a stent of the appropriate length and shape is selected.

27.6.1 SPHINCTEROTOMY

Once the diagnosis has been established radiologically, a small sphincterotomy should be performed. This facilitates further manipulations in the bile duct and is essential if an endoprosthesis, 10 Fr in diameter or larger, is to be used; it is not usually necessary for 8-Fr stents. Dilatation of the papilla with a balloon catheter (4–6 mm) is possible but may cause acute pancreatitis, presumably due to local

trauma. Without a sphincterotomy, great force may be required to push the prosthesis through a tight papilla, or the leading edge of the prosthesis may impact on the papilla, making further progress impossible. A sphincterotomy also allows free drainage of bile or pancreatic juice around the prosthesis and may lessen the risk of pancreatitis due to obstruction of the pancreatic duct by the stent.

A sphincterotomy is performed with an Erlangen sphincterotome, using the standard technique. In pancreatic carcinoma where the obstruction is close to or involves the papilla, the distal segment of the bile duct may be too short or too distorted to permit adequate cannulation. This occurs in 20% or more of procedures and may necessitate sphincterotomy using a needle knife (Classen and Phillip, 1984). The needle is extended 2–3 mm beyond the insulating sheath and with the needle just lifting the roof of the papilla, diathermy is applied until short, 2–3-mm cuts are made in an 11 to 12 o'clock direction. As the roof of the papilla opens up, the direction and depth of the needle is adjusted until further incision allows a conventional cannula to be inserted into the bile duct. This technique should be used with caution; it is difficult to control and there is a risk of entering the submucosal plane or inducing perforation. If all attempts to cannulate the bile duct fail, retrograde insertion of a prosthesis may still be possible using a combined transhepatic and endoscopic technique.

Following the sphincterotomy, brush cytology or forceps biopsy of duct strictures should be possible (Figure 27.3). A positive cytological or histological diagnosis of malignancy may be established using these methods in about 30% of cases. They are more likely to succeed in the bile duct where obstruction is due to luminal tumour (e.g. cholangiocarcinoma) than to external compression (e.g. pancreatic carcinoma or hilar metastases); a negative result does not exclude malignancy. In the bile duct, cytological specimens can be obtained by passing the sheathed brush

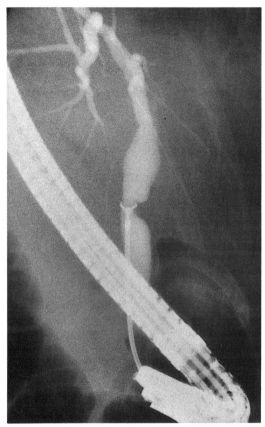

Figure 27.3   Forceps biopsy of common bile duct stricture.

beyond the obstruction and withdrawing the extended brush through the tumour. Paediatric biopsy forceps are sufficiently flexible to be introduced into the bile duct for biopsies to be taken under fluoroscopic control. The diagnostic yield from these techniques in pancreatic carcinoma is low and percutaneous fine needle cytology or biopsy – with ultrasound guidance or using the endoprosthesis as a target – are of more value (Lees, Hall-Craggs and Manhire, 1985).

The first part of the procedure takes about 15 minutes but may be substantially longer when cannulating the bile duct is difficult. When this phase is unduly prolonged and there is a need for repeated sedation, it may be in the interest of the patient to terminate

the procedure and complete it 24–48 hours later. If contrast has been introduced above the obstructed bile duct, however, there is a risk of cholangitis and biliary drainage, with a nasobiliary or transhepatic catheter or an endoprosthesis, must be established.

27.6.2 CANNULATION OF THE STRICTURE

To enable insertion of the largest diameter prosthesis possible (11.5 Fr) a large-channel duodenoscope must be used. Careful fluoroscopic control is required throughout this stage of the procedure, which usually takes about 15–20 minutes. The bile duct is cannulated with a tapered Teflon catheter (6.5 Fr, 250 cm) containing a straight, floppy-tipped Teflon guide-wire (0.035 diam., 300 cm); a metal marker incorporated into the tip of the catheter makes fluoroscopic recognition easier. The catheter is introduced into the lower end of the stricture and the guide-wire advanced into the dilated duct system beyond; this is often possible, even when contrast has failed to pass the stricture (Figure 27.4). Long and tortuous or acutely angulated strictures may be difficult to cannulate and multiple passes with the wire may be necessary before being successful. When the tip of the wire fails to progress, it should be withdrawn and redirected; if the wire becomes impacted in the tumour, its further advance may cause perforation. When a straight wire repeatedly impacts in an acutely angulated stricture, a J-tipped wire may be of value. The catheter is advanced to the limit of the straight wire and is replaced by a J-wire that can often be made to negotiate the lumen beyond. Torque-controlled guide-wires are available (Advanced Cardiovascular Systems, Wilson-Cook) but the long distance over which they operate endoscopically makes them little more responsive to torque than the standard guide-wires.

Once the wire has traversed the stricture, the catheter is advanced over the wire until it the catheter is withdrawn or advanced over the wire, because of frictional resistance, the wire will be pulled or pushed with it. This can lead to the wire being pulled out of the stricture or being pushed into the periphery of the liver; puncture of the bile duct or the liver capsule by the wire is uncommon because of the flexible tip. The endoscopist should advance or withdraw the catheter slowly and in small increments. This allows the assistant watching the fluoroscope monitor to pull or push the wire as required to keep the position of the tip constant. Care must be taken not to kink the wire since this will make it difficult to pass the catheter over it. If the catheter is being withdrawn through the endoscope, the wire should be gripped with the elevator to reduce the risk of dislodging it from the bile duct.

27.6.3 STRICTURE DILATATION

The stricture must be dilated to the same diameter as the proposed prosthesis. Omission of this step – except when replacing a blocked stent – may lead to the prosthesis becoming impacted in the stricture. Dilatation can usually be achieved by passing a stiff, tapered Teflon catheter of the appropriate diameter over the guide catheter and wire. While applying firm external pressure to the dilator, it is essential to keep the tip of the endoscope as close to the papilla as possible. If the tip is too far away from the papilla, the dilator will bow in the duodenal lumen, which may prevent its further passage through the stricture. Major resistance to dilatation may be encountered, particularly in hilar tumours. Considerable upward force can be applied to the dilator at the papilla by lifting the catheter with the elevator or flexing the tip of the endoscope; with these manoeuvres, the dilator can often be made to advance a few millimetres at a time through the stricture. Controlled withdrawal of the endoscope with its tip close to the papilla will also force the catheter upwards; this should be carried out with great care since

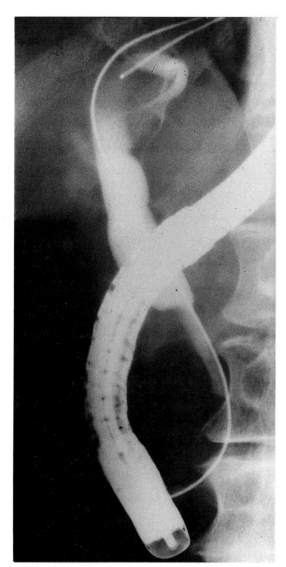

Figure 27.4 Guide-wire through stricture due to pancreatic carcinoma, preparatory to advancing guide catheter.

is well above the obstruction; this provides a stiffer guide than the wire alone. The guide catheter should ideally be of a different colour (e.g. white) than the dilatation catheter, prosthesis or pushing catheter, to allow easier recognition in the duodenum. This part of the procedure requires careful co-ordination between the endoscopist and the assistant. As it can easily result in dislodgement of the 'scope from the duodenal loop and withdrawal of the catheter from the bile duct.

Malignant hilar strictures may be extremely difficult to dilate with a catheter, because of their firmness and the distance over which the dilating force must be applied. If this method is unsuccessful, dilatation with graded balloon catheters (4–6 mm) should be attempted. The guide-catheter is removed and the balloon dilator is passed over the wire until the metal markers on either side of the balloon lie above and below the stricture (Figure 27.5). The balloon is dilated a number of times at the recommended pressure and is then replaced by the original guide-catheter.

27.6.4 INSERTION OF PROSTHESIS

The largest diameter endoprosthesis compatible with the diameter of the dilated lumen is selected. A 10- or 11.5-Fr prosthesis can usually be inserted in pancreatic tumours; in hilar obstruction, particularly if the bifurcation is involved, it may not be possible to use a stent larger than 8 Fr. The length of the prosthesis between the retaining flaps should be equivalent to the distance between the upper end of the obstruction and the papilla. This must be corrected for radiological magnification (about 30%) against the known diameter of the duodenoscope. Any major changes in the angle of the lumen, e.g. in a blockage of the main hepatic ducts, may need to be taken into account, to prevent impaction of the end of prosthesis against the duct wall. The appropriate shape can be incorporated after the prosthesis has been softened with hot air (e.g. from a hot air paint stripper). If the prosthesis is too short and its lower end lies within the bile duct, future retrieval can be difficult. The upper end of a prosthesis which is too long may impinge on the duct wall and compromise drainage; the lower end may impact on the opposite duodenal wall with the risk of traumatic ulceration or perforation.

The prosthesis is pushed over the guide

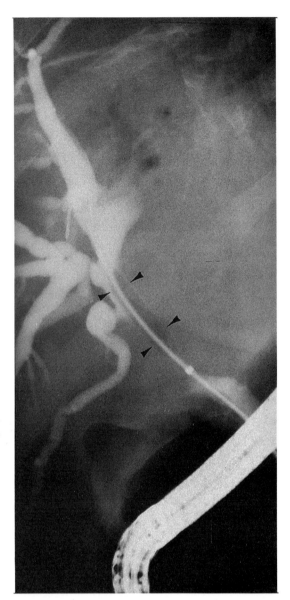

Figure 27.5 Balloon dilatation of hilar stricture; outline of distended balloon arrowed with metal market indicating lower end of balloon.

with a following catheter of the same diameter and advanced through the obstruction, until the lower flap is at the papilla; resistance to the passage of the prosthesis through the stricture is overcome with the methods described for dilatation. When the prosthesis has been

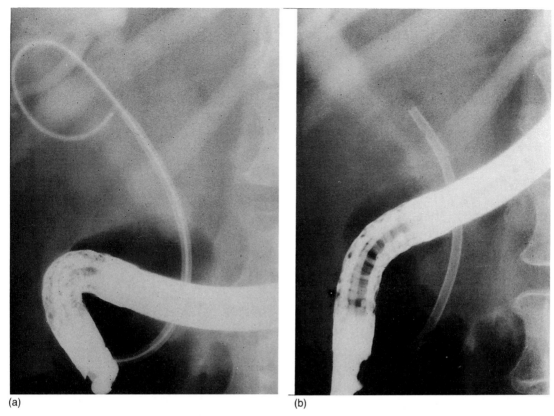

(a)   (b)

Figure 27.6   Stent passed over guide catheter wire (a) with removal of guides (b).

accurately positioned across the obstruction, the guide catheter with its wire and the pushing catheter are removed, leaving the lower 1 cm of the prosthesis protruding into the duodenum (Figure 27.6). If the position of the prosthesis is in doubt, dilute contrast (25–50%) can be injected down the guide catheter once the wire has been removed. Bile and contrast usually gush from the prosthesis, confirming its patency (Figure 27.7); bile should be aspirated through the duodenoscope and collected in a suction trap for bacteriological examination. A plain abdominal radiograph with the patient supine is taken as a reference for stent position (Figure 27.8).

When the bifurcation is obstructed, selective insertion of stents into both right and left hepatic ducts is indicated but is only possible

in about 10% of attempts. Drainage of only one lobe of the liver can provide adequate palliation of pruritus and jaundice but there is a risk of infection developing in the undrained lobe.

Endoscopic biliary drainage can be achieved after a Billroth II gastrectomy and is facilitated by use of a large 3.7-mm channel forward-viewing endoscope (Olympus GIF IT10, Fujinon UGI-CT2, Pentax FG-34JH). It is often easier in this situation to carry out a sphincterotomy with a needle knife.

27.7 COMBINED TRANSHEPATIC AND ENDOSCOPIC TECHNIQUE

When the endoscopic technique has failed or has been only partially successful, e.g. the inability to pass a guide-wire through the

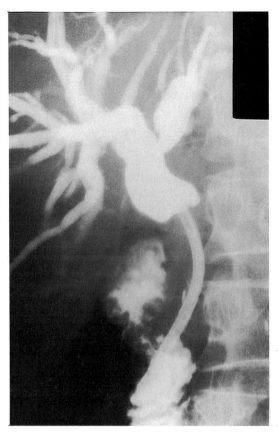

Figure 27.7 Drainage of contrast into duodenum through 10-Fr stent.

stricture or to drain both lobes of the liver, a combined transhepatic and endoscopic approach may be appropriate (Shorvon *et al.*, 1986). This method has the advantage of being able to insert a large diameter prosthesis, without the complications inherent in passing it through the liver substance. Depending upon the patient's general condition and the ability to pass a guide-wire and catheter through the stricture at the initial procedure, the combined technique can be carried out either in one or two stages, 48 hours apart.

A transhepatic cholangiogram is performed using a standard technique (Butch and Mueller, 1985). A long (0.035, 300-cm) straight Teflon-coated guide-wire is passed through the stricture into the duodenum. Ideally, the

hepatic duct should be punctured as high as possible (at least 4–5 cm) above the obstruction if at the hilum. This allows an adequate length of wire between the duct wall and the obstruction to accommodate the upper end of the dilatation catheter or prosthesis; without it, there is a risk that the prosthesis may pass over the wire, and into the hepatic parenchyma. A catheter (6.5 Fr) is passed over the wire to prevent the liver capsule, the duct wall and papilla from being cut when traction is applied to the wire. The duodenal end of the wire is grasped endoscopically with a Dormia basket and withdrawn through the biopsy channel (Figure 27.9); a sufficient length of wire is required outside the endoscope to allow the guide catheter to be passed over it without losing control of its upper end. With gentle traction on both ends of the wire, the guide can be passed through the stricture as

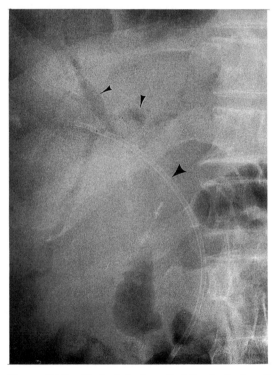

Figure 27.8 Air in intrahepatic bile ducts (small arrows) indicating patency of 8-Fr stent in hilar stricture.

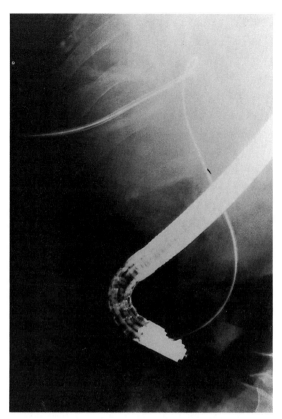

Figure 27.9 Combined percutaneous and endoscopic approach. The transhepatic guide-wire has been withdrawn up the instrument channel.

the transhepatic catheter is withdrawn. The stricture is then dilated and a prosthesis inserted endoscopically over the guide catheter and wire, taking advantage of the taut wire. On completion of the procedure, the wire is removed; the transhepatic catheter is usually left in the hepatic duct above the obstruction until patency of the prosthesis can be confirmed by injection of contrast on the following day. Each step of the procedure must be carried out carefully to prevent tearing of the liver capsule or duct wall.

27.8 PROSTHESIS REMOVAL

Blockage of the endoprosthesis occurs in up to 20–30% of patients in the long term. This can result in cholangitis and is an indication for immediate removal of the prosthesis and its replacement by a new one. Antibiotic therapy should be commenced before the procedure, after blood cultures have been taken. A large-diameter-channel duodenoscope is used. The end of the blocked prosthesis is captured in a Dormia basket, pulled firmly up to the endoscope and secured with pressure from the elevator; it is then slowly removed by withdrawing the endoscope. Too rapid removal can traumatize the tumour or the papilla and induce bleeding, making subsequent access to the papilla difficult. If the lower end of the prosthesis has impacted in the opposite wall of the duodenum, it may not be possible to remove it with a basket; in this situation, it can usually be grasped and removed with toothed forceps. A new prosthesis can be inserted immediately, often without dilatation of the stricture.

27.9 POSTPROCEDURE PATIENT CARE

The patient usually recovers from the procedure within a few hours and can commence a normal diet and full activity as tolerated. Prophylactic antibiotics are given for a further 48 hours, or for a full course should fever or other signs of cholangitis develop. Pruritus often resolves within 48 hours and its persistence suggests incomplete biliary drainage. Jaundice frequently disappears within 3 weeks, although the rate of resolution is variable; it depends not only on the adequacy of large duct drainage but also on the presence of significant cholangitis, hepatic metastases or hepatocellular failure. A plain abdominal radiograph to demonstrate air in the biliary tree and a repeat ultrasound to confirm duct decompression are taken before the patient is discharged. The patient is warned about the possibility of stent blockage and is advised to return as soon as possible should fever, rigors or cholestatic symptoms develop.

27.10 EARLY COMPLICATIONS (Safrany et al., 1982; Haber and Kortan, 1985; Tytgat et al., 1986)

Early complications usually develop within 48 hours and occur in up to 25% of procedures.

27.10.1 CHOLANGITIS

Cholangitis is the most common early complication (8–27%) with clinical manifestations ranging from low-grade fever to fulminant septicaemia and death. Most episodes resolve rapidly with antibiotic therapy alone, although pseudomonas cholangitis may be particularly slow to respond; occasionally improved drainage (by insertion of a larger stent or a transhepatic catheter) may be necessary before infection can be controlled.

The use of sterile equipment and prophylactic antibiotics reduce the risk of introducing infection or prevent it from becoming established. Adequate biliary drainage is probably the most important factor in avoiding serious cholangitis. Early cholangitis occurs significantly less frequently with 10-Fr stents (5%) than with 8-Fr stents (34%); it is also less common after stent drainage of low bile duct obstructions (8%) than of obstructions of the bifurcation (27%).

27.10.2 PROSTHESIS BLOCKAGE OR DISLODGEMENT

Early blockage of the prosthesis, e.g. from blood clot or impaction on the bile duct wall, or dislodgement, are uncommon. Significant dislodgement can be confirmed by an abdominal radiograph. Blockage is suggested by the absence of air in the biliary tree; the diameter of the intrahepatic ducts will be unchanged or increased on ultrasonography. Deterioration in liver function from an occluded stent may be difficult to distinguish from the effects of severe cholangitis with intrahepatic cholestasis or hepatic metastases. Although an isotope (HIDA) biliary scan may help to resolve this problem, blockage should be confirmed by cannulation at repeat ERCP before the prosthesis is removed.

27.10.3 TUMOUR PERFORATION

Perforation of the tumour or bile duct wall or penetration of the liver with a guide-wire or catheter does not usually cause serious problems but can result in a subphrenic abscess. If perforation occurs during the procedure, every attempt should be made to establish adequate biliary drainage and the patient should be given a full course of antibiotics.

27.10.4 SPHINCTEROTOMY COMPLICATIONS

Complications related directly to the sphincterotomy occur in 3–4% of procedures. Bleeding, pancreatitis or perforation are less frequent following sphincterotomy for stent insertion than for stone removal, probably because of the smaller incision.

27.11 LATE COMPLICATIONS

27.11.1 PROSTHESIS BLOCKAGE (Speer et al., 1985)

Occlusion of the prosthesis by biliary sludge is by far the most common long-term complication, occurring in 20–30% of cases. A prosthesis can function satisfactorily for 10 months or longer, but this is uncommon; the average duration of a stent's useful life is approximately 4 months and depends upon its internal diameter. The median survival of 10-Fr stents (32 weeks) is significantly longer than that for 8-Fr stents (12 weeks).

Progressive blockage of the stent causes deterioration in liver function and cholangitis and presents clinically with fever, rigors and cholestatic symptoms. When these occur, the stent should be removed as soon as possible and replaced; flushing or brushing the stent is not adequate and may precipitate a severe attack of cholangitis.

27.11.2 DUODENAL OBSTRUCTION

Obstruction of the duodenal lumen occurs in 4–7% of patients with pancreatic carcinoma. This incidence is lower than that reported in surgical series and reflects exclusion of patients with significant duodenal stenosis at the time of the initial endoscopy. Its occurrence is an indication for surgical bypass of both the stomach and biliary tree since the endoscopic replacement of a blocked stent is no longer possible.

27.11.3 PROSTHESIS DISLODGEMENT

Migration of the prosthesis either upwards or downwards is infrequent (1–2%). When the lower end of a blocked prosthesis lies above the papilla, retrieval is difficult but should be attempted with a Dormia basket or snare. If this is not successful, it is often possible to pass a new, but smaller diameter stent alongside the old.

27.11.4 PERFORATION

Silent perforation of the tumour or bile duct by the stent, diagnosed at autopsy or cholangiography, has been observed. Ulceration and perforation of the duodenal wall can also occur.

27.11.5 CHOLECYSTITIS

Acute cholecystitis, presumably due to malignant cystic duct obstruction, has been described, occurring up to 6 months after the insertion of the prosthesis.

27.12 RESULTS

Experience with endoscopic stenting in malignant biliary obstruction is now extensive (Riemann *et al.*, 1981; Cotton, 1982; Laurence,

1982; Siegel, Harding and Chateau, 1982; Clasen and Hagenmuller, 1984; Cotton, 1984; Hagenmuller, 1984; Zimmon and Clement, 1985; Huibregtse *et al.*, 1986; Speer and Cotton, 1986; Speer, Cotton and Dineen, 1986). Some of the early reports (Riemann *et al.*, 1981; Cotton, 1982; Laurence, 1982; Siegel, Harding and Chateau, 1982; Cotton, 1984; Hagenmuller, 1984; Zimmon and Clement, 1985) are either collected series or are difficult to compare because of insufficient patient data (e.g. risk factors, site of obstruction) or the use of small stents (5–8 Fr) of varying design (C-shaped, pigtails). The largest series of patients managed by this technique is that of Tytgat and colleagues (1986). They have treated 1250 patients, with the successful insertion of a 3.2-mm prosthesis (10 Fr) in 90% – a result similar to the 84–89% overall success rate with 8–10-Fr stents reported by others. Failure was due to duodenal stenosis, the inability to perform a sphincterotomy or to pass a guide-wire through the stricture. Jaundice resolved or diminished in 90% of patients and the overall 30-day mortality was 15%. The long-term incidence of stent blockage was 21%, which is similar to that described in other series.

The endoscopic insertion of a prosthesis in high bile duct obstruction is undoubtedly technically more difficult than in low strictures and the outcome is less satisfactory. Biliary drainage is not as adequate and therefore predisposes to early complications (such as cholangitis) and reduced early survival. For these reasons, the results of this procedure are better in pancreatic carcinoma than in malignant hilar obstruction and should be considered separately.

27.12.1 PANCREATIC CARCINOMA (Huibregtse *et al.*, 1986; Speer and Cotton, 1986) (Table 27.1)

In 221 consecutive patients with pancreatic carcinoma (median age 70 years), Tytgat's group were able to insert a 3.2-mm (10-Fr) prosthesis in 90%, with disappearance of

Table 27.1 Endoscopic stent drainage – pancreatic carcinoma

| | Stent insertion (%) | Successful drainage (%) | 30-day mortality (%) | Early cholangitis (%) | Late complications | | Survival (weeks) |
					Stent block (%)	Duodenal stenosis (%)	
Tytgat et al. (1986) n = 221	90	94	10	8	21	7.5	26
Speer et al. (1986) n = 102	89	88	9	9	29	6	21
Laurence (unpublished) n = 67	82	80	5	17	17	5	21

jaundice in 94%. Cholangitis occurred in only 8% and the 30-day mortality was 10%. The prosthesis became clogged in 219 and surgical bypass for late duodenal obstruction was required in 7.5%; the mean survival time was 26 weeks.

Speer and Cotton have reported their results in 102 patients with unresectable pancreatic cancer. This was a high-risk group with a median age of 76 years; most were deeply jaundiced and 25% had renal impairment. Previous attempts to relieve biliary obstruction by other means had failed in 17. Stents were successfully inserted in 89% of patients with the relief of jaundice in 88%. Early complications, mainly cholangitis, occurred in 9% and eight patients (9%) died within 30 days of the procedure – three from direct complications, three from disseminated malignancy and two following upper gastrointestinal bleeding. Blockage of the stent necessitating endoscopic replacement developed in 29%; 6% underwent surgical bypass for duodenal obstruction. The median duration of survival was 21 weeks.

At the Sir Charles Gairdner Hospital we have treated 67 elderly patients with pancreatic carcinoma by endoscopic drainage. Their median age was 69 years and 42% had other serious, medical problems; all were deeply jaundiced and 18% had renal insufficiency. A stent (8, 10, 11.5 Fr) was successfully inserted in 82% with either complete (80%) or

partial resolution of jaundice (18%). The procedure was complicated by cholangitis in 17%; one developed duodenal perforation after the sphincterotomy. The median duration of hospitalization after the uncomplicated insertion of a stent was 7 days, increasing to 15 days in those patients with cholangitis. The 30-day mortality was 5%. Late stent blockage occurred in 17% and duodenal obstruction in 5%; the mean survival time was 21 weeks.

27.12.2 MALIGNANT HILAR OBSTRUCTION (Speer, Cotton and Dineen, 1986; Tytgat et al., 1986) (Table 27.2)

Tytgat has treated over 500 patients with malignant hilar obstruction – 46% with strictures of the mid common bile duct and 54% with strictures of the bifurcation. Stents were successfully inserted in 70–75% with disappearance of jaundice in 71–72%. Early cholangitis occurred in 27% of the patients with obstruction of the bifurcation and the 30-day mortality was 20%. The median survival for patients with mid common duct strictures was 5 months and for those with strictures of the bifurcation, 6 months.

The Middlesex Hospital group have attempted endoscopic stenting in 64 patients with malignant hilar obstruction – 42 with cholangiocarcinoma, 10 with carcinoma of the gallbladder and 12 with hilar metastases. The

Table 27.2 Endoscopic stent drainage – malignant hilar obstruction

	Stent insertion (%)	Successful drainage (%)	30-day mortality (%)	Early complications (%)	Survival (weeks)
Tytgat *et al.* (1986) n = 512					
Mid CBD	70–75	71	20	14	20
Bifurctn		72	20	17	24
Speer *et al.* (1986) n = 64					
CHD	100	93	7	14	16
Bifurctn	76	62	16	14	
Laurence (unpublished) n = 48					
CHD	95	86	14	22	12
Bifurctn	65	54	17	19	

stricture involved the common hepatic duct alone (type 1) in 14, the bifurcation alone (type 2) in nine and both the right and left hepatic and intrahepatic ducts (type 3) in 41; previous attempts to bypass the obstruction surgically had failed in 17%.

The overall success rate for stent insertion was 81% and was higher in type 1 (100%) than type 3 strictures (73%); biliary drainage was also significantly more successful, in 93% and 56% respectively. Early complications, mainly cholangitis, occurred in 16% and the 30-day mortality was 13%; neither were influenced by the site of the stricture. Removal of a blocked prosthesis was necessary in 25%; two developed cholangitis in undrained segments of the liver which was managed by percutaneous drainage. The median survival for the whole group was 16 weeks.

At the Sir Charles Gairdner Hospital we have used this technique in 48 patients with hilar obstruction – 21 with cholangiocarcinoma, 19 with hilar metastases, and eight with carcinoma of the gallbladder. The bifurcation was obstructed in 55% and surgical bypass had been attempted without success in 25%. The overall success rate for endoscopic stent insertion (8–10 Fr) was 79%; 95% in strictures below the bifurcation but only 65% when the bifurcation was involved. Jaundice resolved in 86% with common hepatic duct strictures but only in 55% when the right and left ducts were obstructed. Cholangitis occurred in six (13%) and two developed pancreatitis; blocked stents were replaced in 16%. The 30-day mortality was 16% – 14% in type 1 and 25% in type 3 strictures; the median survival was only 12 weeks.

27.13 ENDOSCOPIC OR PERCUTANEOUS STENT DRAINAGE?

The percutaneous insertion of an internal draining biliary catheter can provide effective palliation in malignant obstructive jaundice (Nakayama, Ikeda and Okuda, 1978; Hoevels and Lunderquist, 1984; May *et al.*, 1985) (Chapter 28). Some of the long-term disadvantages of this technique, in particular bile leakage and catheter dislodgement, can be overcome by the insertion of an endoprosthesis by the same route (Burcharth, 1978). The percutaneous approach is, however, associated with a significant incidence of immediate complications (6–38%) (Wittich, Van Sonnenberg and Simeone, 1985), the most frequent of which, haemorrhage (13.8%) (Monden *et al.*, 1980) and bile leakage (16%) (Carrasco, Zornoza and Bechtel, 1984), are directly related to hepatic puncture. The endoscopic technique seems to have fewer early complications but because of technical variations (e.g. size of stent) and differences in

Table 27.3 Endoscopic versus percutaneous drainage

Stent	Stent insertion (%)	Clinical improvement (%)	30-day mortality (%)	Early complications (%)
Endoscopic n = 39	89	81	15	18
Percutaneous n = 36	76	61	33*	61**

*P = 0.016.
**P = 0.0037.
From Speer et al. (1987) with permission.

patient selection, comparison of the two methods is difficult.

A randomized trial of the two techniques in poor-risk elderly patients has been reported (Speer et al., 1987) (Table 27.3). Thirty-nine were treated endoscopically and 36 percutaneously with 10-Fr and 12-Fr stents respectively; there was a higher proportion of patients with hilar strictures in the endoscopic group but otherwise they were well matched. Stents were inserted by both techniques with equal success but drainage was more successful after the endoscopic procedure (81% versus 61%). There was a significant increase in the incidence of early complication, particularly bile leakage and haemorrhage, in the percutaneous stent group (33% versus 6%), with a significant increase in the 30-day mortality (34% versus 15%). There was no significant difference in the median survival of the two groups (endoscopic 119 days, percutaneous 88 days). Although this study suggests that the endoscopic procedure is the method of first choice in the poor-risk patient with malignant jaundice, because of the very high incidence of early complications in the percutaneous stent group, this conclusion requires confirmation. Where endoscope placement is not possible, the combined endoscopic-percutaneous technique can be used successfully (Robertson et al., 1987).

27.14 ENDOSCOPIC STENT OR SURGICAL BILIARY BYPASS?

Malignant biliary obstruction is essentially a disease of the elderly (Fraumeni, 1975; Maruchi et al., 1979) and in most patients, confirmation of the diagnosis or suitability for attempted curative resection can be decided without a laparotomy. Pancreatic carcinoma is not often resectable (20% or less)) Edis, Kiernan and Taylor, 1980; Morrow, Hilaris and Brennan, 1984) and even when it is, in the elderly, poor-risk patient, the operative mortality is high (40–58%) (Andren-Sandberg and Ihse, 1983; Lerut et al., 1984). Palliative surgery involving biliary bypass without re-

Table 27.4 Endoscopic stent versus surgical bypass

	Hospital stay (days)	Clinical improvement %	30-day mortality %	Complications %	Survival (days)
Endoscopic stent n = 18	6	78	5	22	176
Surgical bypass n = 19	11.5*	73.6	21	36	128

*P<0.05
From Shepherd et al. (1986) with permission.

section also has a high morbidity and mortality (12–19%) (Saar and Cameron, 1984), although this may be lower in the younger, good-risk patient (Leung *et al.*, 1983). Less than 20% of patients with cholangiocarcinoma are suitable for attempted curative surgery and palliative procedures to bypass the obstruction have an operative mortality between 11% and 35% (Evander *et al.*, 1980; Blungart *et al.*, 1984).

Surgical biliary bypass has been compared with endoscopic stenting in a randomized trial involving 46 patients with malignant obstruction of the distal bile duct (Shephard *et al.*, 1986) (Table 27.4). The median duration of initial hospitalization was significantly less in the group treated by endoscopy (6 versus 11.5 days). Endoscopic stenting or surgical bypass were equally successful, involving jaundice – in 78.9% and 73.6% respectively. There was no significant difference in results of the endoscopic and surgical approach in the complication rate (22% versus 36%), total hospital stay (225 days versus 286 days), the 30-day mortality (5% versus 21%) or the overall median survival time (176 days versus 128 days).

Radvan, Hewson and Denham (1986), in a non-randomized trial of the two techniques in 41 patients also demonstrated a significantly shorter period of hospitalization after the endoscopic insertion of a stent (3.7 versus 21 days); the incidence of procedure-related complications was higher after surgical biliary bypass (37.5% versus 8.0%). It was estimated that the mean cost of surgical treatment was five times that of endoscopic stenting.

These studies suggest that in elderly frail patients with unresectable disease, the endoscopic insertion of a stent should be attempted before the other drainage procedures; it seems to provide as effective palliation as percutaneous drainage or surgical bypass but with a lower initial morbidity. Further trials assessing the results in pancreatic cancer and malignant hilar obstruction separately are required to support this conclusion.

27.15 FUTURE DEVELOPMENTS

Although the basic technique for inserting a stent endoscopically is now established, the high incidence of cholangitis and stent blockage and the short survival time remain major challenges. Developments which allow the insertion of larger stents, an understanding of the mechanisms of stent blockage and the use of intraluminal irradiation may help to resolve these problems.

27.15.1 STENT SIZE

The risk of early cholangitis and of stent blockage are largely determined by the stent diameter, which in turn is limited by the diameter of the instrument channel. Developments in duodenoscope design have resulted in a progressive increase in channel size and have made possible the routine use of large-channel stents with an improvement in the clinical results. Standard duodenoscopes with a 2.8-mm channel initially limited stent size of 7–8 Fr; the subsequent introduction of 3.7- and 4.2-mm channel instruments which accommodate 10- and 11.5-Fr stents, has led to a reduced incidence of cholangitis and significantly longer stent life. A method has been described for the insertion of 15-Fr stents over a self-retaining guide-wire, positioned above the stricture with a conventional duodenoscope (Kautz, 1983). Experience with this technique is limited; it is likely to be superseded by the use of duodenoscopes with even larger, 5.5-mm channels, prototypes of which are under evaluation.

27.15.2 STENT BLOCKAGE

Chemical analysis of biliary sludge from blocked stents shows it to be composed mainly of calcium bilirubinate with some calcium palmitate and cholesterol crystals, embedded in a fibrous, protein matrix (Wosiewitz, Schrameyer and Safrany, 1985). Protein makes up about 25% of the dried

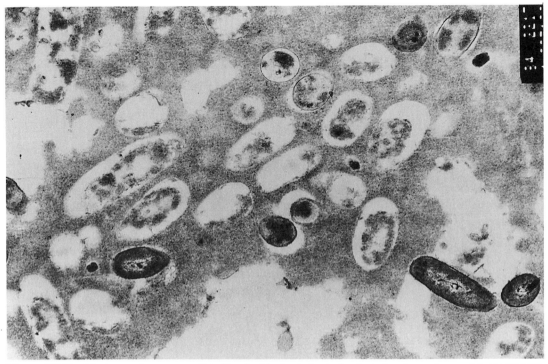

Figure 27.10   Electron microscopy of biofilm for blocked stent – bacteria in glycocalyx matrix (× 21 000).

sludge and some protein adheres firmly to the wall of the stent; the sludge contains up to 20% of plant fibre which has refluxed up from the duodenum and could contribute to rapid stent blockage (Groen *et al.*, 1987).

Examination of the occluding material by transmission electron microscopy reveals features typical of a bacterial biofilm; with bacteria adhering to each other within a matrix of polysaccharide, glycocalyx, Gram-positive and Gram-negative organisms, both cocci and bacilli, can be identified (Speer *et al.*, 1986) (Figure 27.10). Scanning electron microscopy shows that both surfaces of the stent are covered with this biofilm (Leung, 1986). These findings strongly suggest that colonization of the stent with a mixed bacterial population leads to the adherence and progressive build up of a biofilm. Bacterial enzymes such as glucuronidase and phospholipase are subsequently responsible for the formation and deposition of insoluble calcium bilirubinate and

palmitate within the stent, causing its eventual blockage.

The biofilm protects the bacteria from luminal antibiotics and the long-term use of a broad-spectrum antibiotic, even in high dosage, does not prevent stent blockage. The development of safe bactericidal agents, incorporated into the stent surface and released slowly, may inhibit the growth of bacterial biofilm (Kingston, Seal and Hill, 1986). Furthermore, stent patency may be prolonged by aspirin or doxycycline (Smit *et al.*, 1989).

27.15.3 INTRALUMINAL IRIDIUM-192 IRRADIATION

In spite of adequate biliary decompression with a stent, patients with pancreatic and bile duct cancer often develop intractable pain and their survival time remains short. External radiotherapy can prolong survival in cholangiocarcinoma (Hanna and Rider, 1978) and give good palliation of pain in pancreatic cancer (Dobelbower and Milligan, 1984). Intracavitary irradiation delivers a high radiation dose to a small volume of tissue in a short period of time, usually with significantly less morbidity than with conventional external radiotherapy. Intraluminal irradiation has been used to treat malignant bile duct obstruction, with iridium-192 or radium being inserted transhepatically (Herskovic *et al.*, 1981; Conroy *et al.*, 1982; Laurence *et al.*, 1984; Mornex *et al.*, 1984; Molt *et al.*, 1986); in hilar cholangiocarcinoma, this may double the survival time (Karani *et al.*, 1985). To avoid the morbidity of the transhepatic approach, we have used iridium-192 wire inserted down a nasobiliary tube.

(a) Technique

A large-diameter 11.5-Fr stent is inserted as described, except that a guiding catheter with a distal pigtail is used. When the stent is in position across the obstruction, the pushing catheter and guide-wire are removed, allowing the pigtail on the guiding catheter to form above the stent. The duodenoscope is removed over the catheter, and the catheter re-routed through the nose; bile drains both externally and through the stent, around the catheter.

The radiation source is prepared by removing the central stilette from a straight 0.035 guide-wire and inserting a length of iridium-192 wire (Amersham, UK) into the distal end of the outer sheath. The length of iridium wire used is equal to one and a half times the length of the malignant obstruction and gives a 25% overlap of wire at either end.

The upper end of the obstruction is outlined with a nasobiliary cholangiogram and the active end of the loaded guide-wire then advanced down the catheter under fluoroscopic control until the iridium wire is positioned across the stricture; this is facilitated by iridium having a higher radiodensity than the guide-wire (Figure 27.11).

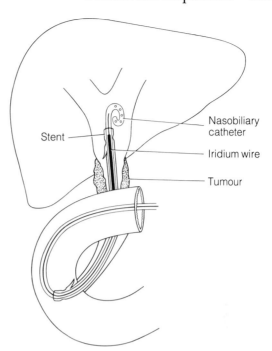

Figure 27.11 Intraluminal irradiation – diagram of combined stent and nasobiliary catheter with iridium-192 wire across the stricture.

A total of 6000 cGy is administered, with 100% of the dose delivered 0.5 cm from the wire; this necessitates 3–4 days of treatment, the duration depending upon the activity of the wire. On completion of therapy, the pigtail was straightened with the wire and the catheter removed, leaving the stent to drain into the duodenum.

(b) Results

Experience with this technique is limited. Phillip and colleagues have treated three patients – two with cholangiocarcinoma, one with hilar metastases – with intraluminal iridium-192 (6000 cGg) followed by an endoscopic stent; all were alive 4–5 months after treatment and there were no complications (Philip *et al.*, 1984). A patient with cholangiocarcinoma has also been treated by combined external beam (4500 cGy) and intraluminal irradiation (2100 cGy), with a 50% increase in the internal diameter of the stricture and normal liver function tests 1 year after therapy (Venu *et al.*, 1987).

We have treated 25 patients with this method – 12 with pancreatic carcinoma, seven with cholangiocarcinoma, three with hilar metastases, two with carcinoma of the gallbladder and one with carcinoma of the papilla. Two patients with cholangiocarcinoma were given a second course of intraluminal irradiation for local extension of the disease, 15 and 35 months after the initial treatment; five patients with pancreatic carcinoma received additional external radiotherapy (3000 cGy) 1–4 weeks after intraluminal irradiation.

There were no immediate (e.g. nausea, leucopenia) or long-term (e.g. fistula) complications directly attributable to radiotherapy. Early cholangitis developed in 29% but all responded to antibiotics. Blockage of the prosthesis was the most common late complication; the overall median survival of the first prosthesis was 4.4 months and in 60%, bile drainage was still adequate at the time of death. In two patients, blocked stents were removed but not replaced with liver function remaining normal, 2 and 4 months later. Duodenal obstruction requiring surgical bypass developed in two patients with pancreatic carcinoma, 16 and 34 weeks after radiotherapy.

Twenty patients have died of their malignancy from between 60 and 532 days after treatment; five are still alive after 150, 240, 285, 317 and 1340 days. The overall median survival for patients with pancreatic carcinoma was 250 days (approximately 8.3 months) and for cholangiocarcinoma 300 days (10 months). The significance of these survival figures is difficult to assess in the absence of a control group of patients treated by endoscopic stenting alone. Intraluminal irradiation of biliary malignancy by the transduodenal route is certainly technically feasible and safe; a controlled trial is required to determine its real value in improving palliation and survival.

27.16 CONCLUSION

The endoscopic method for inserting large-bore endoprostheses is a significant advance in the management of malignant biliary obstruction. In the elderly, poor-risk patient, it promises rapid relief of jaundice with low morbidity and short hospitalization. Endoscopic stenting in unresectable pancreatic carcinoma is at least as effective as surgical bypass or percutaneous drainage and is probably the drainage method of first choice. The results in strictures of the bifurcation are not as good but are likely to improve with the increased use of a combined percutaneous and endoscopic approach. Early infection and late stent blockage are continuing problems which hopefully will be partially resolved by the use of larger diameter stents and new stent materials.

In the search for increasing refinement in methods to relieve jaundice, it must be remembered that this is only one aspect of the palliation of malignant biliary obstruction. The control of pain, provision of nutritional support and the psychosocial aspects of malignancy and terminal care are at least of equal importance and are worthy of the same careful attention.

REFERENCES

Andren-Sandberg, A. and Ihre, I. (1983) Factors influencing survival after total pancreatectomy in patients with pancreatic cancer. *Ann. Surg.*, **198**, 605–10.

Blumgart, L. H., Hadjis, N. S., Benjamin, I. S. and Beazley, R. (1984) Surgical approaches to cholangiocarcinoma at confluence of hepatic ducts. *Lancet*, **i**, 66–70.

Burcharth, F. (1978) A new endoprosthesis for non-operative intubation of the biliary tract in malignant obstructive jaundice. *Surg. Gynecol. Obstet.*, **146**, 76–8.

Butch, R. J. and Mueller, P. R. (1985) Fine-needle transhepatic cholangiography: State of the Art. *Semin. Intervent. Radiol.*, **2**, 1–20.

Carr-Locke, D. L. (1988) Endoscope exchange in biliary prosthesis procedures. *Lancet*, **ii**, 903.

Carrasco, C. H., Zornoza, J. and Bechtel, W. J. (1984) Malignant biliary obstruction: complications of percutaneous biliary drainage. *Radiology*, **152**, 343–6.

Classen, M. and Hagenmuller, F. (1984) Endoscopic bililary drainage. *Scand. J. Gastroenterol.*, **19,** suppl. 2, 76–83.

Classen, M. and Phillip, J. (1984) Endoscopic retrograde pancreatography (ERCP) and endoscopic therapy in pancreatic disease. *Clin. Gastroenterol.*, **33,** 3819–42.

Conroy, R. M., Shahbazian, A. A., Edwards, K. C. *et al.* (1982) A new method for treating carcinomatous biliary obstruction with intracatheter radium. *Cancer*, **49,** 1321–7.

Cotton, P. B. (1982) Duodenoscopic placement of a biliary prostheses to relieve malignant obstructive jaundice. *Br. J. Surg.*, **69,** 501–3.

Cotton, P. B. (1984) Endoscopic methods for relief of malignant obstructive jaundice. *World J. Surg.*, **8:** 854–61.

Dobelbower, R. R. and Milligan, A. J. (1984) Treatment of pancreatic cancer by radiation therapy. *World J. Surg.*, **8,** 919–28.

Edis, A. J., Kiernan, P. and Taylor, W. F. (1980) Attempted curative resection of ductal carcinoma of the pancreas. Review of Mayo Clinical Experience, 1951–1975. *Mayo Clin. Proc.*, **55,** 531–40.

Evander, A., Fredlund, P., Hoevels, J. *et al.* (1980) Evaluation of aggressive surgery for carcinoma of the extrahepatic bile ducts. *Ann. Surg.*, **191,** 23–9.

Fraumeni, J. F. (1975) Cancers of the pancreas and biliary tract. Epidemiological considerations. *Cancer Res.*, **35,** 3437–46.

Groen, A. K., Out, T., Huibregtse, K. *et al.* (1987) Characterization of the content of occluded biliary prosthesis. *Endoscopy*, **19,** 57–9.

Haber, G. B. and Kortan, P. P. (1985) Complications of endobiliary prosthesis. *Gastrointest. Endosc.*, **31,** 168.

Hagenmuller, F. (1984) Results of endoscopic bilioduodenal drainage in malignant bile duct stenoses, in *Non Surgical Biliary Drainage* (eds M. Classen, J. Geenen and K. Kawai), Springer, Berlin, pp. 93–104.

Hanna, S. S. and Rider, W. D. (1978) Carcinoma of the gallbladder or extrahepatic bile ducts: the role of radiotherapy. *Can. Med. Assoc. J.*, **118,** 59–61.

Herskovic, A., Heaston, D., Engler, M. J. *et al.* (1981) Irradiation of biliary carcinoma. *Radiology*, **139,** 219–22.

Hoevels, J. and Lunderquist, A. (1984) Results of percutaneous internal-external drainage, in *Non Surgical Biliary Drainage* (eds M. Classen, J. Geenen and K. Kawai), Springer, Berlin, pp. 43–6.

Huibregtse, K., Katon, R. M., Coene, P. P. and Tytgat, G. N. J. (1986) Endoscopic palliative treatment in pancreatic cancer. *Gastrointest. Endosc.*, **32,** 334–8.

Huibregtse, K. and Tytgat, G. N. (1982) Palliative treatment of obstructive jaundice by transpapillary introduction of large bore bile duct endoprosthesis. Experience in 45 patients. *Gut*, **23,** 371–5.

Karani, J., Fletcher, M., Brinkley, D. *et al.* (1985) Internal biliary drainage and local radiotherapy with Iridium 192 wire in the treatment of hilar cholangiocarcinoma. *Clin. Radiol.*, **36,** 603–6.

Kautz, G. (1983) Transpapillary bile duct drainage with a large calibre endoprosthesis. *Endoscopy*, **15,** 312–5.

Kingston, D., Seal, D. V. and Hill, I. D. (1986) Self-disinfecting plastics for intravenous catheters and prosthetic inserts. *J. Hyg. Camb.*, **96,** 185–98.

Laurence, B. H. (1982) Endoscopic transpapillary drainage in malignant bile duct obstruction. *Aust. N.Z. J. Med.*, **12,** 103.

Laurence, B. H. and Cotton, P. B. (1980) Decompression of malignant biliary obstruction by duodenoscopic intubation of the bile duct. *Br. Med. J.*, **1,** 522–3.

Laurence, B. H., Kilburn, M., Cameron, F. and Collins, D. (1984) The treatment of malignant bile duct obstruction with transpapillary Iridium 192 wire. *Aust. N.Z. J. Med.*, **14,** 917.

Lees, W. R., Hall-Craggs, M. A. and Manhire, A. (1985) Five years experience of fine-needle aspiration biopsy: 454 consecutive cases. *Clin. Radiol.*, **36,** 517–20.

Lerut, J. P., Gianello, P. R., Otte, J. B. and Kestens, P. J. (1984) Pancreaticoduodenal resection. Surgical experience and evaluation of risk factors in 103 patients. *Ann. Surg.*, **199,** 432–7.

Leung, J. W. C. (1986) Mechanism of biliary prosthesis blockage: scanning electron microscopy evidence. *Gut*, **27,** A602.

Leung, J. W. C., Del Favero, G. and Cotton, P. B. (1985) Endoscopic biliary prosthesis: a comparison of materials. *Gastrointest. Endosc.* **31,** 93–5.

Leung, J. W. C., Emery, R., Cotton, P. B. *et al.* (1983) Management of malignant obstructive jaundice at The Middlesex Hospital. *Br. J. Surg.*, **70,** 584–6.

Martin, D. F. (1988) Catheter and wire guided endoscope exchange for biliary stents. *Lancet*, **ii,** 542–4.

Maruchi, W., Brian, D., Ludwig, J. *et al.* (1979) Cancer of the pancreas in Olmsted County, Minnesota, 1935–1974. *Mayo Clin. Proc.*, **54,** 245–9.

May, G. R., Bender, C. E., Williams, H. J. and Maccarty R. L. (1985) Percutaneous biliary decompression. *Semin. Intervent. Radiol.*, **2,** 21–30.

Molt, P., Hopfan, S., Watson, R. C. *et al.* (1986)

Intraluminal radiation therapy in the management of malignant biliary obstruction. *Cancer*, **57**, 536–44.

Monden, M., Okamura, J., Kobayashi, N. *et al.* (1980) Haemobilia after percutaneous transhepatic biliary drainage. *Arch. Surg.*, **115**, 161–4.

Mornex, F., Ardiet, J. M., Bret, P. and Gerard, J. P. (1984) Radiotherapy of high bile duct carcinoma using intracatheter Iridium 192 wire. *Cancer*, **54**, 2069–73.

Morrow, M., Hilaris, B. and Brennan, M. F. (1984) Comparison of conventional surgical resection, radioactive implantation and bypass procedures for exocrine carcinoma of the pancreas, 1975–1980. *Ann. Surg.*, **199**, 1–5.

Nakayama, T., Ikeda, A. and Okuda, K. (1978) Percutaneous transhepatic drainage of the biliary tract: techniques and results in 104 cases. *Gastroenterology*, **73**, 554–9.

Philip, J., Hagenmuller, F., Manegold, J. *et al.* (1984) Endoscopic intraductal radiotherapy of high bile duct carcinoma. *Dtsch. Med. Wochenschr.*, **109**, 422–6.

Radvan, G. H., Hewson, E. G. and Denham, J. M. (1986) Palliative biliary drainage in obstructing carcinoma: endoscopy versus surgery. *Aust. N.Z. J. Med.*, **16**, 613.

Rey, J. F., Maupetit, P. and Greff, M. (1985) Experimental study of biliary endoprosthesis efficiency. *Endoscopy*, **17**, 145–8.

Riemann, J. F. Lux, G., Rosch, W. and Beickert-Sterba, A. (1981) Non-surgical biliary drainage – technique, indications and results. *Endoscopy*, **13**, 157–61.

Robertson, D. A. F., Hocking, C. N., Birch, S. *et al.* (1987) Experience with a combined percutaneous and endoscope approach to stent insertion in malignant obstructive jaundice. *Lancet*, **ii**, 1449–52.

Safrany, L., Schott, B., Krause, S. *et al.* (1982) Endoskopische transpapillare Gallengangs drainage bei tumorbedingten Verschlussikterus. *Dtsch. Med. Wochenschr.*, **107**, 1867–71.

Sarr, M. G. and Cameron, J. L. (1984) Surgical palliation of unresectable carcinoma of the pancreas. *World J. Surg.*, **8**, 906–18.

Shepherd, H. A. D., Diba, A., Ross, A. P. *et al.* (1986) Endoscopic biliary prosthesis in the palliation of malignant biliary obstruction – a randomized trial. *Gut*, **27**, A1284.

Shorvon, P. J., Cotton, P. B., Mason, R. R. *et al.* (1986) Percutaneous transhepatic assistance for duodenoscopic sphincterotomy. *Gut*, **26**, 1373–6.

Siegel, J. H., Harding, G. T. and Chateau, F. (1982) Endoscopic decompression and drainage of benign and malignant biliary obstruction. *Gastrointest. Endosc.*, **28**, 79–82.

Smit, J. M. Out, M. J., Goen, A. K. *et al.* (1989) A placebo-controlled study on the efficiency of aspirin and doxycycline in preventing clogging of biliary endoprosthesis. *Gastrointest. Endosc.*, **35**, 485–9.

Soehendra, N. and Reynders-Frederix, V. (1980) Palliative bile duct drainage. A new endoscopic method of introducing a transpapillary drain. *Endoscopy*, **12**, 8–11.

Speer, A. G. and Cotton, P. B. (1986) Endoscopic biliary prosthesis in 102 poor risk patients with carcinoma of the pancreas. *Gut*, **27**, A1278.

Speer, A. G., Cotton, P. B. and Dineen, L. P. (1986) Endoscopic palliation of malignant hilar strictures. *Gut*, **27**, A601.

Speer, A. G., Cotton, P. B., Russell, R. C. *et al.* (1987) Randomized trial of endoscopic versus percutaneous stent insertion in malignant obstructive jaundice. *Lancet*, **ii**, 57–62.

Speer, A. G., Farrington, H., Costerton, J. W. and Cotton, P. B. (1986) Bacteria, biofilms and biliary sludge. *Gut*, **27**, A601.

Speer, A. G., Leung, J. W. C., Yin, T. P. and Cotton, P. B. (1985) 10 French gauge straight biliary stents perform significantly better than 8 French gauge pigtail stents. *Gastrointest. Endosc.*, **31**, 140.

Tytgat, G. W., Bartelsman, J. F., Den Hartog-Jager, F. C. *et al.* (1986). Upper intestinal and biliary tract endoprosthesis. *Dig. Dis. Sci.*, **31**, suppl. 57S–76S.

Venu, R. P., Geenen, J. E., Hogan, W. J. *et al.* (1987) Intraluminal radiation therapy for biliary tract malignancy – an endoscopic approach. *Gastrointest. Endosc.*, **33**, 236–8.

Wittich, G. R., Van Sonnenberg, E. and Simeone, J. F. (1985) Results and complications of percutaneous biliary drainage. *Semin. Intervent. Radiol.*, **2**, 39–49.

Wosiewitz, U., Schrameyer, B. and Safrany, L. (1985) Biliary sludge: its role during bile duct drainage with an endoprosthesis. *Gastroenterology*, **88**, 1706.

Zimmon, D. S. and Clemett, A. R. (1985) Experience with 5 French biliary and pancreatic endoscopic stents. *Gastrointest. Endosc.*, **30**, 168.

CHAPTER TWENTY-EIGHT

Radiological stenting of malignant biliary obstruction

A. H. Chapman

Malignant disease obstructing the biliary tree usually presents late when curative surgery is no longer possible. Age and unrelated medical conditions may also preclude surgery but even when they do not, palliative by-pass surgery for pancreatic and bile duct carcinoma has been shown to carry a mortality of 18–33% (Blumgart *et al.*, 1984; Sarr and Cameron, 1984) and be associated with prolonged hospitalization (Feduska, Dent and Lindenauer, 1971). This has encouraged the use of endoprostheses placed by a percutaneous, endoscopic or combined techniques. Re-establishing bile drainage to the duodenum using one or more endoprostheses (Figure 28.1) results in clearing of jaundice and the troublesome pruritus that accompanies it. The patient will no longer experience malabsorption and appetite improves.

The endoscopic method of placing an endoprosthesis using a wide 4.2-mm channel side-viewing duodenoscope had largely replaced the percutaneous method, as by avoiding trauma to the liver parenchyma, it results in fewer complications, requires a shorter hospital stay and has a lower 30-day mortality (Table 28.1). When using this endoscopic method difficulty may be encountered in crossing tumours at the porta hepatis and even then the duct entered may be of insufficient size to provide worthwhile drainage. The endoscopic method may also fail in the presence of a peri-ampullary diverticulum,

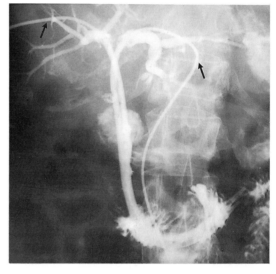

Figure 28.1 Bile duct carcinoma involving the porta hepatis. One endoprosthesis drains a left hepatic duct and one drains a right hepatic duct. Contrast medium has been injected through the two external drainage catheters (arrows) and is seen passing through the endoprostheses to the duodenum.

previous gastric or biliary-enteric surgery or tumour encasement of the duodenum. An endoscopic-radiological technique has been devised for such situations which only involves traversing the liver with a 5-Fr catheter and so causes less trauma than the percutaneous method of pushing a 12-Fr stent through the liver. This combined technique

Table 28.1 Method of stent placement

	Percutaneous*	Endoscopic†
Relief of jaundice (%)	61	81
Early complications (%)	67	19
Minimum hospital stay (days)	5	1
Median survival (days)	88	119
30-day mortality (%)	33	15
Stent replacement	Difficult	Easy
	Painful	Uncomfortable

Adapted from Spear *et al.* (1987) with permission.
*$n = 36$.
†$n = 39$.

requires the radiologist, after performing a percutaneous transhepatic cholangiogram, to catheterize a suitable intrahepatic duct. A guide-wire is passed through the tumour to the duodenum for the endoscopist to catch and pull back through the channel of endoscope, and then over this wire an endoprosthesis is pushed into position. The essence of this technique is for the wire to be held taut by the radiologist as it enters the percutaneous catheter and by the endoscopist's assistant as it exits from the channel of the endoscope, as this allows the stent to be pushed through the hardest of tumours. One unit was able to improve their success rate for stent placement from 67% to 97% by introducing this combined technique (Robertson *et al.*, 1987). When a tumour at the porta hepatis involves multiple ducts then two of the largest obstructed segments may be chosen for drainage and with this method two endoprostheses can easily be placed side by side. Draining a single segment can provide worthwhile palliation but leaving segments without drainage risks cholangitis. Lindström *et al.* (1988) failed to show an improvement with multiple stents but in another recent study by Deviere *et al.* (1988) it was found that treating malignant hilar strictures involving both left and right hepatic ducts (type II or III) with two stents instead of one, reduced the incidence of early cholangitis by over a half and reduced the 30-day mortality from 29% to 8%. In the presence of previous gastric

surgery and a long afferent loop, the endoscopist may not be able to reach the ampulla but the technique can still be performed provided the radiologist can advance the guide-wire to the end of the duodenoscope so it can be caught with a wire basket by the endoscopist. Effective biliary drainage depends on the internal diameter of the stent, and although 10–12 Fr is the size most frequently used, the endoscopic placement of a 15-Fr stent has been advocated (Ayela *et al.*, 1988). This usually requires a papillotomy, and stents of this size will not pass through the channel of the endoscope which must withdraw so that the stent can be pushed into position over the wire. When an endoscopist experienced in stent placement is available, percutaneous radiological stenting is rarely called for and in the last 2 years in my department it has only been used for patients with previous biliary-enteric surgery and a long roux loop.

Bile salts encrust and eventually block the endoprosthesis which has a half-life of about 7 months (Speer *et al.*, 1985), but in the presence of pancreatic or gallbladder carcinoma or obstruction by periductal lymph node metastases the patient will invariably die from tumour spread before the endoprosthesis stops functioning. The exception is the slowly growing bile duct or ampullary carcinoma, when replacement of the endoprosthesis may become necessary. This is easily achieved by the endoscopic method and even when a combined technique has been required to insert the stent because of the presence of a hilar tumour, subsequent replacement can often be achieved by the endoscopic method alone. The percutaneously introduced internal/external drainage catheter (Mendez *et al.*, 1979) can be passed through a tumour to the duodenum and with suitably placed side-holes will allow drainage of bile (Ring *et al.*, 1979) (Figure 28.2). In most centres today, these catheters are reserved for temporary drainage as, although easily changed, they need to be of at least 10-Fr size to provide adequate long-term drainage (Kerlan *et al.*, 1984) and so are difficult for the patient to tolerate.

Percutaneous transhepatic stenting carries a significant morbidity and mortality (Table 28.2) which is comparable to that of surgery (Table 28.3) (Bornman *et al.*, 1986), but it can often be performed when palliative surgery would be difficult or impossible. Endoscopic stenting has a lower morbidity and mortality than radiological stenting (Table 28.1) (Speer *et al.*, 1987) and recovery time is shorter making this the preferred technique. The combined endoscopic-radiological technique is likely to have a morbidity and mortality somewhere between the two.

New metallic percutaneous stents which are introduced over a 7-Fr delivery catheter and expanded within the tumour hold promise as their insertion results in less liver trauma and they are thought to have a longer half life than plastic stents. Such stents may find a place in the management of hilar tumours as an alternative to combined endoscopic-radiological stenting (Adam *et al.*, 1989).

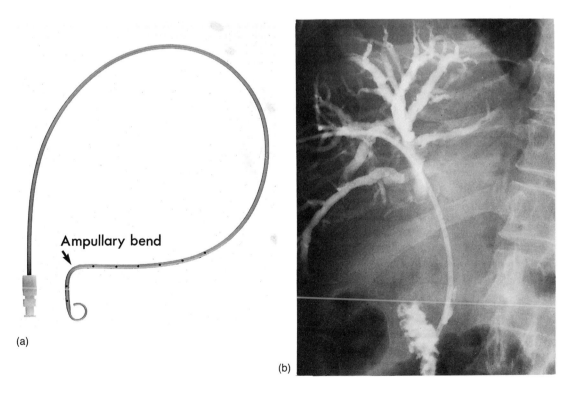

(a)

Ampullary bend

(b)

Figure 28.2   (a) Ring internal/external drainage catheter. (b) Ring catheter drains obstructed right hepatic ducts, in case of bile duct carcinoma involving porta hepatis.

Table 28.2 Transhepatic endoprosthesis placement for biliary obstruction secondary to pancreatic, bile duct and gallbladder carcinomas and lymph node metastases: results from three studies

	Reference		
	Dick et al. (1987)*	Mueller et al. (1982)†	Lammer and Neumayer (1986)‡
30-day mortality	10 (11.5%)	11 (9.7%)	25 (15.4%)
30-day mortality (excluding deaths caused by tumour spread)	3 (3.5%)	1 (0.9%)	6 (3.7%)
Mean survival (weeks)	22	—	20

*n = 87.
†n = 113.
‡n = 162.

28.1 PROCEDURE AND TECHNIQUE

28.1.1 PATIENT PREPARATION

Consented patients should have coagulation factors checked. The prothrombin time should not be prolonged by more than 3 seconds and the platelet count should be above 50 000. A prolonged prothrombin time should be corrected by a course of vitamin K (10 mg i.v. for 3–5 days), but if despite this the prothrombin time is prolonged by more than 5 seconds an infusion of fresh frozen plasma is required prior to the procedure. A low platelet count can be corrected with a platelet infusion. Half an hour before the procedure an antibiotic which has good bile penetration (such as mezlocillin 2–5 g by i.v. injection

should be given (Dooley et al., 1984). The patient should be kept well hydrated.

28.1.2 THE PERCUTANEOUS TRANSHEPATIC CHOLANGIOGRAM

The importance of an adequate cholangiogram cannot be overemphasized. This should not only demonstrate the extent and confirm the nature of the obstruction but should also demonstrate the best site for the catheter to enter the biliary tree. On the basis of this cholangiogram a skin puncture site is chosen which will enable the catheter to follow a smooth path from the punctured intrahepatic bile duct to the porta hepatis and to the common duct, avoiding awkward sharp angles

Table 28.3 Results of controlled trial comparing transhepatic endoprosthesis placement with surgical bypass in patients with incurable carcinoma of head of the pancreas

	Transhepatic endoprosthesis*	Surgical bypass*
Technical success (no.)	21 (84%)	19 (76%)
Median postprocedure hospital stay (days)	7	10.5
Median postprocedure hospital stay including readmissions (days)	9	11
30-day mortality (no.)	2 (8%)	5 (20%)
Median survival (weeks)	19	15
Late duodenal obstruction (no.)	3 (12%)	—

From Bornman et al. (1986) with permission.
*n = 25.

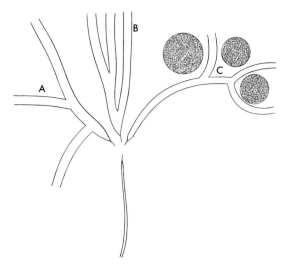

Figure 28.3 Segment A should be chosen for drainage. Segment B shows crowding of dilated ducts indicating parenchymal atrophy. Segment C contains metastases.

which might be difficult to negotiate with catheters and guide-wires. A tumour at the porta hepatis may obstruct multiple intrahepatic ducts, in which case the major duct systems can be chosen which will effectively drain the liver. When assessing the suitability of an obstructed segment for drainage, consideration should be given to the presence of parenchymal atrophy or metastases, as the drainage of such segments results in a poor return of function (Figure 28.3). After sedating the patient a cholangiogram is obtained with a 23-gauge Chiba needle. A puncture site is chosen by fluoroscopy approximately midway between the right inferolateral margin of the liver and the right costophrenic recess, just anterior to the midaxillary line, and the inferior part of the intercostal space is injected with local anaesthetic. When choosing the puncture site it is important to realize that the lateral costophrenic recess as it is traced from the front to the back of the patient moves caudally (Figure 28.4), otherwise the pleural space may be traversed. With the patient lying supine and breathing quietly the Chiba needle is advanced horizontally towards the right

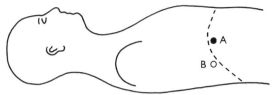

Figure 28.4 Pleural reflection (dotted line). Too posterior a puncture (point B rather than point A) will traverse the pleural space.

cardiophrenic angle so as to avoid hitting a distended gallbladder or extrahepatic duct. The needle should not be advanced beyond the midline as it may pass out of the posterior aspect of the left lobe or come close to the capsule where contrast injection will lift the capsule from the liver parenchyma causing pain. Contrast is injected as the needle is slowly withdrawn, but if no bile duct has been entered the needle is not removed from the liver but re-angled and advanced once again. This procedure is repeated so that each needle pass comes closer to the porta hepatis. Contrast oozes into a bile duct and persists once the injection is stopped, whereas it rapidly clears from the portal and hepatic veins. Hepatic veins if entered are seen running towards the right atrium, whereas contrast

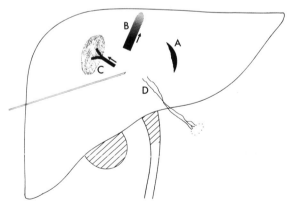

Figure 28.5 Subcapsular injection (A) hepatic vein (B), a portal vein producing a parenchymal blush (C), lymphatics and lymph node (D). Puncture should avoid the gallbladder and extrahepatic ducts (shaded).

injected into a portal vein produces a parenchymal blush (Figure 28.5). Lymphatics are also occasionally demonstrated and these run to glands at the porta hepatis which in turn drain to the cisterna chyli. The left duct system, if separately obstructed, can also be filled from a right-sided puncture but here the needle will have to be directed anteriorly to avoid passing posteriorly out of the back of the left lobe. It is often easier to perform an anterior subcostal puncture to demonstrate an obstructed left duct system. The puncture is made just inferior and to the left of the xiphoid process while the patient holds his breath in inspiration to bring the left lobe as far below the costal margin as possible.

Overdistension of the bile ducts with contrast should be avoided, and the amount of contrast injected can often be reduced if table elevation or rotation of the patient are used to move the denser contrast within the bile-distended ducts. Overdistension of ducts carries the risk of forcing endotoxins or bacteria from the bile ducts into the systemic circulation.

Sedation may not be required for a percutaneous cholangiogram but a combination of fentanyl (a short acting synthetic narcotic) and midazolam (a short acting benzodiazepine) are suitable for the following procedures (Vogelzang, 1989).

28.1.3 CANNULATION OF THE BILIARY TREE

A point is chosen for puncture of the biliary tree and the puncture is made with a needle-cannula consisting of an 18-gauge needle and a 5-Fr cannula. To achieve the smooth downwards curve desired for easy catheterization, it may be necessary to choose a different skin puncture site to that of the percutaneous cholangiogram. Alternatively an 0.046 mm guide-wire can be passed through a Chiba needle to facilitate the subsequent introduction of a larger cannula into the biliary tree (One-Stick 2 Introducer System, Cat. No. 05–

2) (Vogelzang, 1986). This may be the only way to cannulate the narrow bile ducts involved by sclerosing cholangitis but most operators find such fine guide-wires awkward to use. Although the use of the larger sheathed needle is more traumatic if multiple passes have to be made before the desired duct is entered, this is rarely necessary when the ducts are distended, especially if lateral screening is available. As the needle approaches the duct it will distort and finally puncture it so that removal of the needle results in the flow of bile from the cannula (Figure 28.6(a)). Blood-stained bile can be differentiated from pure blood as it oozes from the end of the cannula whereas blood drips. The distal 2 cm of a Lunderquist wire (Lunderquist Wire Guide, SFW, 23, 125, LQT; William Cook Europe) is curved between finger and thumb to produce a right-angle bend and the wire is then run down the cannula into the bile duct and towards the porta hepatis (Figure 28.6(b)). The cannula is then advanced over the wire to the porta hepatis, the guide-wire is removed, and the bile duct decompressed. The bile is sent for culture.

28.1.4 NEGOTIATING THE TUMOUR

The same guide-wire can now be used again to find a way through the tumour by gently advancing and rotating it. This may be facilitated by varying the shape of the bend on the end of the wire. A heavy hand at this stage may produce a false passage which often hinders further attempts at negotiating the tumour. Should this occur, or should it not be possible to pass through the tumour, the patient should be left for 48 hours on external drainage by which time catheterization is usually possible. On occasions we have had to wait as long as a week before being able to cannulate a tumour.

28.1.5 EXTERNAL DRAINAGE

External drainage will result in resolution of the patients's itching and jaundice but the

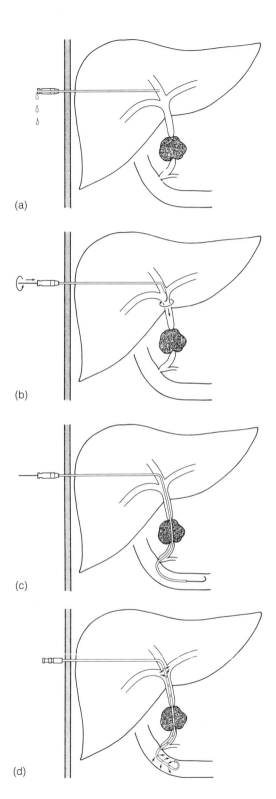

(a)

(b)

(c)

(d)

patient remains anoretic and experiences continued malabsorption as bile fails to reach the bowel. Problems are often encountered in maintaining an adequate fluid and electrolyte balance due to bile loss which can be particularly serious in the first 24 hours following the establishment of external drainage when the patient may have a 'biliuresis' and lose several litres of bile. In the presence of cholangitis it is important to establish external drainage, yet to minimize trauma to the biliary tree and the risk of inducing septicaemia, so attempts are not made to transverse the tumour until the infection has cleared.

28.1.6 INTERNAL-EXTERNAL DRAINAGE

An 8.3-Fr Ring catheter (P8.3, 38, 50, P, 32S, Ring; William Cook Europe) can be inserted when for technical or logistical reasons it is not possible to proceed straight to endoprosthesis placement. When a Lunderquist wire has reached the far side of the tumour the catheter is advanced, the wire removed and contrast injected to define the anatomy. The wire can be used again to advance the catheter as far as the third part of the duodenum (Figure 28.6(c)). The stent may now be placed by a combined endoscopic-radiological technique but if it is to be placed solely by the percutaneous route it is usual to insert a Ring catheter to provide internal-external drainage for 48 hours, as this allows a tract to develop through the liver and the tumour, which makes endoprosthesis placement easier and it is therefore better tolerated by the patient. Before insertion of the Ring catheter, the wire and catheter are advanced to the third part of the duodenum. Should the wire become trapped in duodenal folds, the duodenum can be distended by injecting fluid down the catheter; this makes passage of the wire to the third part of the duodenum easier. The

Figure 28.6   (a)–(d) Stages in placement of a Ring catheter.

Lunderquist wire is now withdrawn inside the catheter until its tip lies at the ampulla and the wire is bent at the point at which it leaves the hub of the catheter. It is then withdrawn further until its tip lies at the site at which the catheter enters the bile duct and the wire is bent again. The distance between the two bends marks the length from the ampullary bend on the Ring catheter (Figure 28.2(a)) over which side-holes need to be made with a punch. The radiologist is now ready to insert the 8.3 Fr Ring catheter to establish internal/external drainage (Figure 26.6(d)). A Lunderquist exchange 'coat-hanger' wire (Lunderquist Exchange Guide, CF, 35, 125, 10; William Cook Europe) is gently passed down the catheter, ensuring that it does not kink above the tumour or as it turns from the second to the third part of the duodenum. A gentle bend made immediately proximal to the solder point will help to prevent this stiff wire kinking the catheter. The catheter is removed over the wire and replaced by the Ring catheter so that the ampullary bend on the Ring catheter lies at the ampulla. The wire is removed and contrast injected to ensure that the catheter side-holes are suitably placed.

28.1.7 CATHETER FIXATION

Should the catheter inadvertently be pulled out before a tract has formed between the liver capsule and the chest wall the patient will almost certainly develop biliary peritonitis, so careful attention should be paid to securing the catheter. A strip of Elastoplast along a length of the catheter as it exits from the patient provides a purchase for a 0 silk suture which can be applied as a pursestring (Figure 28.7). It is a simple and effective technique but other equally effective means of securing the catheter have been devised (Athanasouis *et al.*, 1982; Coons and Carey, 1983). The catheter is allowed to drain into a bile bag. The Ring catheter was originally designed for its end to be capped for internal drainage but this may lead to cholangitis and others have found

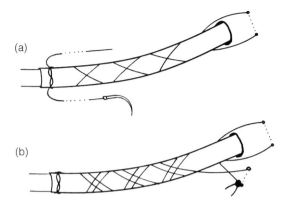

Figure 28.7 (a) A skin stitch is twisted around the Elastoplast-covered catheter and tied. (b) The suture is again twisted around the Elastoplast, back down the length of the catheter and secured with a further stitch.

that prolonged internal drainage requires catheters of at least 10-Fr calibre (Mueller *et al.*, 1982). Should prolonged drainage of this type be contemplated then, if possible, the catheter should be placed by the anterior subcostal route to avoid the discomfort that accompanies intercostal catheters.

28.2 ENDOPROSTHESIS PLACEMENT

Percutaneous endoprostheses are also introduced over a Lunderquist exchange wire. The liver is usually drained for 48 hours with a Ring catheter which is then removed over an exchange wire and replaced by a 12-Fr Teflon tear-away sheath (Multipurpose Peel-away Introducing Sheath, PLVW, 13.0, 38, 30 VAD 5; William Cook Europe) and dilator which makes a larger tract through the tumour. The inner dilator is then removed leaving the Teflon sheath through the tumour with its end in the duodenum. A Carey–Coons endoprosthesis (Carey-Coons Soft Stent, CSS, 12F, 15 cm length; Medi-tech, Incorporated) (Coons and Carey, 1983) is assembled behind its pushing catheter and over its introducing catheter (Figure 28.8). This is inserted over the exchange wire, down the middle of the 'tear-

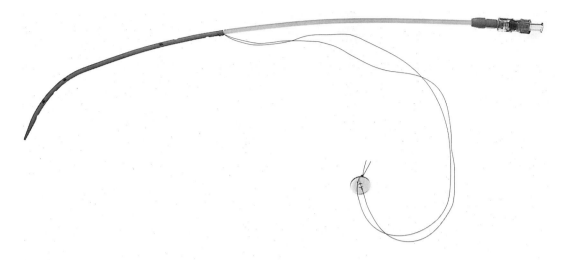

Figure 28.8   The Carey–Coons endoprosthesis and its pushing catheter are mounted on an introducing catheter.

away' sheath (Figure 28.9(a)). When satisfactorily positioned the sheath is slowly withdrawn and torn apart at skin level (Figure 28.9(b)). The introducing catheter is now unlocked from the pushing catheter and slowly withdrawn, followed by the withdrawal of the pushing catheter. A 5-Fr external drainage catheter with a number of side-holes along the distal end of its shaft is inserted so that its tip lies within the end of the endoprosthesis and only then is the exchange guide-wire removed (Figure 28.10). This catheter is stitched in position as previously described. The endoprosthesis has a fine thread attached to its upper end which is connected to a silastic button (Figure 28.11). The silastic button, which has a hole in the middle through which the external drainage catheter can pass, is designed to be implanted subcutaneously to prevent distal migration of the prosthesis. It is important not to have the mersilk thread taut between the prosthesis and the button as movement of the liver with respiration might result in the liver capsule being torn. We only rarely find it necessary to use the button, as the lengthy

endoprosthesis makes proximal migration unlikely; it is only used if it is felt that the endoprosthesis is unstable as is sometimes the case with soft tumours or when there has been a previous endoscopic papillotomy. A check cholangiogram is performed at 48 hours and if the endoprosthesis is stable in position the external drainage catheter is removed.

A technique has been devised for cutting down on silastic buttons and running a catheter along the thread to gain entry to the prosthesis (Brown *et al.*, 1986). This facilitates replacement of a blocked endoprosthesis as the old endoprosthesis can be pushed into the duodenum and replaced by a new one or even withdrawn through the skin after dilating the tract. In patients with a cholangiocarcinoma, where the patient might outlive the life-span of the endoprosthesis, the use of the silastic button may be an advantage. When placing two endoprostheses percutaneously for tumours of the porta hepatis, it may be necessary to run both 'tear-away' sheath dilator systems through the tumour simultaneously with the help of a second operator.

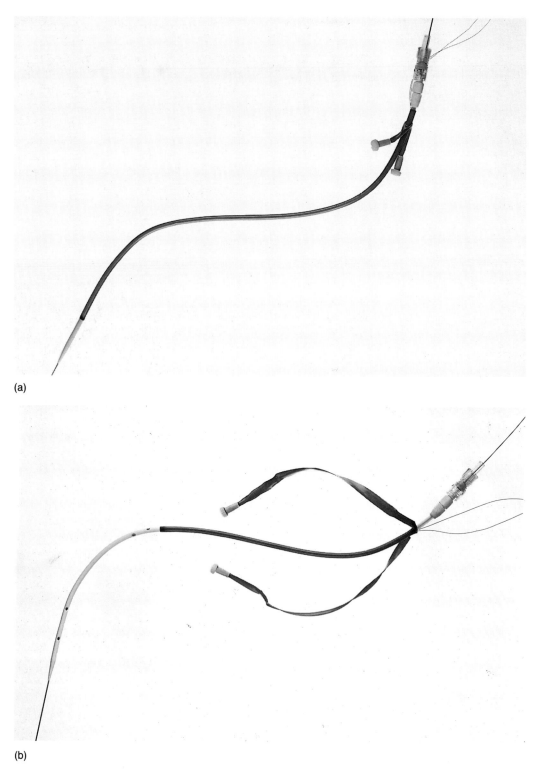

(a)

(b)

Figure 28.9 (a) The Carey–Coons endoprosthesis introduced through a tear-away sheath. (b) This can be torn apart at skin level leaving the endoprosthesis in place.

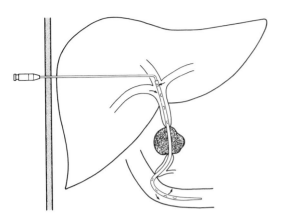

Figure 28.10 Endoprosthesis and external drainage catheter in place.

28.3 COMBINED PERCUTANEOUS–ENDOSCOPIC ENDOPROSTHESIS PLACEMENT

In the presence of a tumour at the porta hepatis, the segment of liver which will provide the most satisfactory biliary drainage is cannulated by an intercostal approach or an anterior subcostal approach to the left lobe. It may be necessary to drain a segment from both the left and the right lobe. As previously described a 5-Fr catheter is introduced percutaneously into the selected bile duct and the catheter is advanced over a guide-wire through the tumour to the duodenum. Bends are placed on the guide-wire, to determine the length of the endoprosthesis required, allowing an extra centimetre for protrusion of the endoprosthesis from the ampulla. A 400-cm guide-wire (400 cm Guide Wire Cat. No. 832200; Meadox Surgimed A/S) is inserted through the catheter to the duodenum and the patient is turned into a semiprone right posterior oblique position. Endoscopy is then performed and, with a wide-channel side-viewing duodenoscope, the wire is grasped using a wire basket and pulled out through the channel of the endoscope (Figures 28.12(a) and (b)). A 6-Fr Teflon catheter (6F guiding Cathet Cat. No. 832161; Meadox Surgimed A/S) is advanced through the endoscope over the wire and run up the bile duct

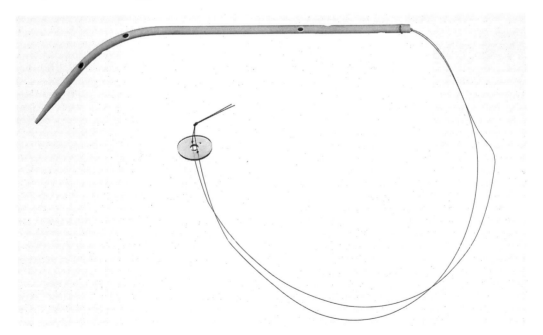

Figure 28.11 The Carey–Coons endoprosthesis has a silastic button attached by a thread to its proximal end.

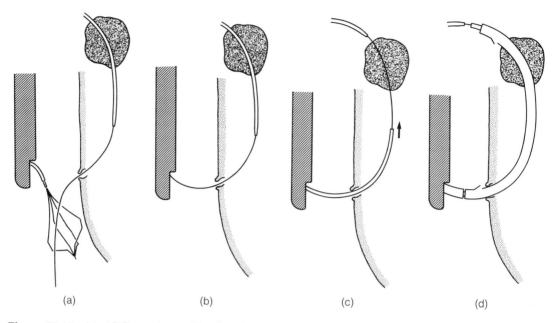

Figure 28.12   (a)–(d) Stages in combined endoscopic-radiological stent placement.

with the guide-wire held taut at both ends (Figure 28.12 (c)). A 10-Fr catheter (10.2F Pusher Catheter, Cat. No. 832162; Meadox Surgimed A/S) is advanced over the taut wire and catheter, to make a tract through the tumour and by fluoroscopy the radiologist checks that its end is not pushed into the liver parenchyma. The endoprosthesis is cut from a length of 10-Fr Teflon catheter tubing and a short tangential cut is made close to both ends so a spur can be pulled out. These spurs, located above the tumour and below the ampulla, will prevent the stent falling out. The 10-Fr catheter is removed and the endoprosthesis is inserted over the wire and 6-Fr catheter using the 10-Fr catheter to push it into position (Figure 28.12(d)). The 6- and 10-Fr catheters and the guide-wire can be removed through the endoscope. Contrast medium is injected through the external drainage catheter before it is removed to ensure the endoprosthesis is correctly positioned. An endoscopic papillotomy may be necessary if two 10-Fr endoprostheses are to be placed side by side or when a larger endoprosthesis is used.

28.3.1 ASPIRATION CYTOLOGY

A 22 gauge spinal needle is inserted percutaneously into the tumour using an anterior subcostal approach and aspirates obtained (Hall-Craggs and Lees, 1986). This is often best performed immediately after stent placement while the patient is still well sedated and before the external drainage catheter is removed. It is always important to ensure that the diagnosis has been confirmed by cytology or histology as otherwise there is a risk that an inflammatory or lymphomatous stricture will be misdiagnosed as a carcinoma.

28.4 COMPLICATIONS (Table 28.4)

Cholangitis and septicaemia are the most frequently encountered complications of percutaneous biliary drainage procedures. In two-thirds of cases with malignant biliary obstruction the bile is sterile at the time of initial drainage. A Ring catheter allows transient increases in duodenal pressure to force bacteria into the biliary tree, or bacteria enter

Table 28.4 Transhepatic endoprosthesis placement: incidence of significant complications taken from two studies

	Reference	
Complication	Dick et al. (1987)*	Lammer and Neumayer (1986)†
Cholangitis	12 (13.8%)	33 (20.4%)
Prosthesis migration	3 (3.4%)	5 (3.1%)
Prosthesis occlusion	12 (13.8%)	10 (6.2%)
Marked haemobilia	3 (3.4%)	5 (3.1%)
Biliary peritonitis	2 (2.3%)	4 (2.5%)
Bowel wall perforation	2 (2.3%)	1 (0.6%)
Tumour deposits at skin puncture site	2 (2.3%)	—
Biliary – cutaneous fistula	3 (3.4%)	—

*n = 87.
†n = 162.

via the external limb of the catheter. Should prolonged internal-external drainage be required, perhaps to see if the patient's general condition will improve sufficiently to allow definitive surgery, then the 8.3-Fr Ring catheter is often found to be of insufficient diameter to allow satisfactory internal drainage of viscous bile so cholangitis develops when the external end of the catheter is capped. Prolonged external drainage allows the bile to become less viscous and internal drainage may then be achieved; alternatively larger catheters can be used but these are uncomfortable, particularly when introduced through an intercostal space. External contamination may be reduced by adding povidone-iodine to the 'bile bag' (Blenkharn, McPherson and Blumgar, 1980). In the presence of tumours of the porta hepatis it is often impossible to satisfactorily drain all segments of the biliary tree, and segments that remain obstructed are at risk of becoming infected. In such situations it is usually possible to manage the infection with antibiotics. Cholangitis following placement of an endoprosthesis generally indicates failure of the endoprosthesis because of silting by biliary sludge, blockage by further tumour growth, or movement of the endoprosthesis out of position (Figure 28.13). It is important to remember that, in the elderly in particular, the clinical features of cholangitis can be subtle with the patient afebrile and just feeling unwell or becoming confused. Placement of the endoprosthesis at the first sitting does carry the theoretical advantage that the bile is likely to be sterile and therefore the procedure is less likely to cause septicaemia or septic shock.

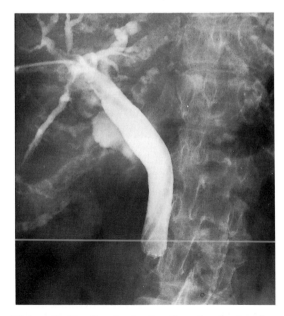

Figure 28.13 Proximal migration of a short endoprosthesis into a common duct obstructed by a pancreatic carcinoma.

Bile and blood may leak into the subphrenic space during a percutaneous drainage with the subsequent risk of a subphrenic abscess. The aetiology of acute renal failure is usually multifactoral Bacterial endotoxins cause renal cortical vasoconstriction and intravascular coagulation. Jaundiced patients have increased circulating endotoxin levels through increased absorption of gastrointestinal endotoxins due to the absence of bile salts in the small bowel, reduced endotoxin clearing capacity of the Kupfer cells of the liver and endotoxin release from bile into the bloodstream during the course of the procedure. Other factors predisposing to renal failure include hypovolaemia and hypotension, pre-existing renal disease, and the use of antibiotics (particularly tetracyclines and aminoglycosides). It may be possible to reduce the risk of endotoxaemia by careful technique, minimizing trauma and by avoiding overdistention of the biliary tree. The patient must be kept well hydrated during the procedure and mannitol (0.5 – 1 g/kg body weight) may be infused during and after the procedure to maintain a diuresis. It is important that an adequate saline infusion is given with mannitol to avoid hyponatraemia. (Allison *et al.*, 1979).

When a patient is on external biliary drainage a watch should be kept for dehydration and electrolyte imbalance. A 'biliuresis' may occur after the relief of obstruction, resulting in fluid and electrolyte depletion (particularly sodium and bicarbonate). A 'bile bag' that has been lowered to the level of the floor may syphon not only bile but large volumes of duodenal juice which can result in the patient rapidly becoming dehydrated.

Leakage of bile into the peritoneal cavity classically causes severe abdominal pain, peritonitis and shock but in some patients the bile is well tolerated (bile ascites) producing abdominal distension and only mild discomfort. Puncture of the obstructed distended gallbladder or the extrahepatic ducts at the time of the percutaneous transhepatic cholangiogram

(PTC) may be responsible. Should it be recognized that such a puncture has been made it is best not to withdraw the needle but to leave it in position draining bile and only remove it when the biliary tree has been decompressed by establishing external drainage by another route. Should an external drainage catheter or a Ring catheter inadvertently be pulled out or displaced before a tract has had time to develop between the liver capsule and the chest wall, it is likely that bile will leak into the peritoneal cavity. External drainage catheters are particularly at risk of becoming displaced if the patient makes a large diaphragmatic movement (Figure 28.14). The use of a pigtail catheter is therefore advocated with as much of the catheter as possible placed in the biliary tree. It normally takes at least 2 days for a tract to develop between the liver capsule and the chest wall, so displacement of an external drainage catheter during this time constitutes an emergency; drainage needs to be re-established as quickly as possible. It may be possible to renegotiate the sinus tract with a

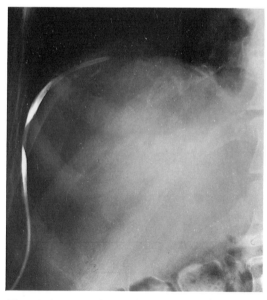

Figure 28.14 A bout of coughing dislodged this external drainage catheter which lies in the subphrenic space.

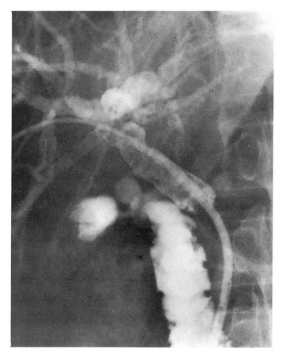

Figure 28.15 'Ghosting' of the biliary tree caused by blood clot.

catheter and guide-wire but a fresh puncture of the biliary tree often has to be made. Should an internal/external drainage catheter be capped to allow internal drainage and the duodenal end of the catheter subsequently block, then bile may leak back along the catheter to the skin. Should biliary peritonitis develop then this requires urgent laparotomy for peritoneal drainage. Bile ascites on the other hand can be managed by percutaneous drainage if the underlying cause can be identified and corrected.

Trauma at the time of the initial biliary drainage procedure may result in the biliary tree filling with blood clot (Figure 28.15). In such cases the catheter should be flushed with 10 ml of normal saline every 2 hours until the biliary tree is clear of blood which normally takes about 12 hours. Slight displacement of the catheter or decompression of a very distended biliary tree may result in a proximal side-hole slipping back into the liver paren-

chyma. This may allow blood from hepatic blood vessels to enter the catheter via a proximal side-hole and so fill the biliary tree. This problem can be identified if contrast medium is injected through the catheter as blood vessel filling will be seen and in such cases the catheter may need to be replaced or repositioned. Percutaneous biliary drainage is known to cause intrahepatic arterial aneurysms, arterioportal and arteriohepatic venous fistula in about 25% of cases (Hoevels and Nilsson, 1980). Should haemobilia result from these lesions they can be successfully managed by hepatic artery embolization. A portobiliary fistula is a rare cause of haemobilia and has been successfully managed by inflating a separately introduced balloon catheter beside the drainage catheter, at the site of the fistula, and leaving it inflated for 5 days to allow time for the fistula to close (Sniderman et al., 1985).

Misplaced side-holes in the catheter may allow air, blood or bile to enter the pleural space, if this has been traversed, resulting in a pneumothorax, haemothorax or biliary-pleural effusion. It is likely that the tip of the pleural space is commonly traversed but in practice this rarely causes problems.

We have encountered perforation of the duodenum at two sites. The lateral wall of the second part of the duodenum can be perforated as the guide-wire and catheter leave the ampulla, especially if a tumour at this site is pressing into the duodenum (Figure 28.16). Perforation is then usually extraperitoneal and rarely causes problems. The exchange guide-wire is sometimes difficult to negotiate from the second to the third part of the duodenum and we have had one incident where this part of the duodenum, which was infiltrated by tumour, was perforated by the wire causing peritonitis (Figure 28.17).

Pain can be a problem at the catheter entry point. When prolonged percutaneous catheterization is considered necessary an anterior subcostal approach to the left hepatic ducts is better tolerated than intercostal

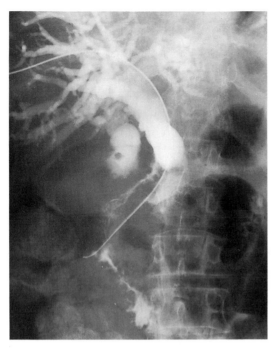

Figure 28.16 This guide-wire has perforated the lateral wall of the second part of the duodenum.

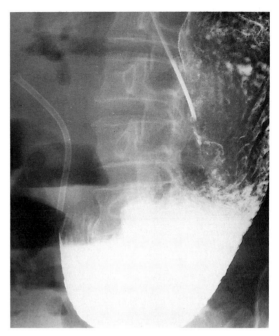

Figure 28.18 Carcinoma of the pancreas palliated by an endoprosthesis. The tumour has progressed to obstruct the third part of the duodenum. A gastro-enterostomy was performed.

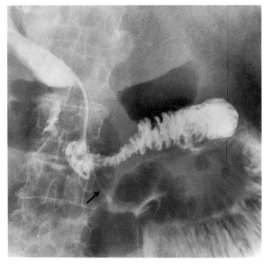

Figure 28.17 Perforation of the third part of the duodenum causing peritonitis. Contrast medium can be seen leaking from the duodenum into the peritoneal cavity (arrow).

catheterization. Severe pain from intercostal catheters may require an intercostal nerve block. A subcapsular haematoma often follows biliary drainage procedures, but usually resolves spontaneously, although it can become infected. Pancreatitis is a surprisingly rare complication even when multiple catheters pass through the ampulla. An endoprosthesis may satisfactorily drain the biliary tree but the tumour may obstruct the duodenum, in which case a gastroenterostomy will be required (Figure 24.18). Prolonged percutaneous catheterization can also result in the production of skin granulomas at the catheter entry point. These can be cauterized with a silver nitrate stick. Tumour seeding is a rare complication of biliary catheterization but may lead to the development of subcutaneous metastases at the catheter entry point or peritoneal metastases.

REFERENCES

Adam, A., Yeung, E., Chetty, N., El Din, A., Wallsten, H., Benjamin, I. S. and Allison, D. J. (1989) Wallstent Self-expanding biliary endoprosthesis for the treatment of malignant hilar strictures. *Clin. Radiol.*, **40**, 6, 645.

Allison, M. E. M., Prentice, C. R. M., Kennedy, A. L. and Blumgart, L. H. (1979) Renal function and other factors in obstructive jaundice. *Br. J. Surg.*, **66**, 392–7.

Athanasoulis, C. A., Pfister, R. C., Green, R. E. and Robertson, G. H. (1982) *Interventional Radiology*, W. B. Saunders, Philadelphia, p. 542.

Ayela, P., Ponchon, T., Valette, P. J. *et al.* (1988) A combined endoscopic and radiological method of biliary drainage. *Gastrointest. Endosc.*, **34**, 42–4.

Blenkharn, J. I., McPherson, G. A. D. and Blumgart, L. H. (1980) An improved system for external biliary drainage. *Lancet*, **ii**, 781–2.

Blumgart, L. H., Hadjis, N. S., Benjamin, I. S. and Beasley, R. (1984) Surgical approaches to cholangiocarcinoma at confluence of hepatic ducts. *Lancet*, **i**, 66–70.

Bornman, P. C., Harries-Jones, E. P., Tobias, R. *et al.* (1986) Prospective controlled trial of transhepatic biliary endoprosthesis verses bypass surgery for incurable carcinoma of the pancreas. *Lancet*, **i**, 69–71.

Brown, A. S., Mueller, P. R. and Ferrucci, J. T. (1986) Transhepatic removal of obstructed Carey–Coons biliary endoprosthesis. *Radiology*, **159**, 555–6.

Coons, H. G. and Carey, P. H. (1983) Large-bore, long biliary endoprostheses (biliary stents) for improved drainage. *Radiology*, **148**, 89–94.

Deviere, J., Baize, M., de Toeuf, J. and Cramer, J. (1988) Long-term follow-up of patients with hilar malignant stricture treated by endoscopic biliary drainage. *Gastrointest. Endosc.*, **34**, 95–101.

Dick, R., Platts, A., Gilford, J. *et al.* (1987) The Carey–Coons percutaneous biliary endoprosthesis: three-centre experience in 87 patients. *Clin. Radiol.*, **38**, 175–8.

Dooley, J. S., Hamilton-Miller, J. M. T., Brumfitt, W. and Sherlock, S. (1984) Antibiotics in the treatment of biliary infection. *Gut*, **25**, 988–98.

Feduska, N. J., Dent, T. L. and Lindenauer, S. M. (1971) Results of palliative operations for carcinoma of the pancreas. *Arch. Surg.*, **103**, 330–3.

Hall-Craggs, M. A. and Lees, W. R. (1986) Fine-needle aspiration biopsy: pancreatic and biliary tumors. *Am. J. Radiol.*, **147**, 399–403.

Hoevels, J. and Nilsson, U. (1980) Intrahepatic vascular lesions following non-surgical percutaneous transhepatic bile duct intubation. *Gastrointest. Radiol.*, **5**, 127–35.

Kerlan, R. K., Stimac, G., Pogany, A. C. and Ring, E. J. (1984) Bile flow through drainage catheters: an *in vitro* study *A.J.R.*, **143**, 1058–87.

Lammer, J. and Neumayer, K. (1986) Biliary drainage endoprostheses: experience with 201 placements. *Radiology*, **159**, 625–9.

Lindström, E., Anderberg, B., Olaison, G. and Ihse, I. (1988) Endoscopic biliary drainage in malignant bile duct obstruction. *Acta Chir. Scand.*, **154**, 277–82.

Mendez, G., Russell, E., Lepage, J. R. *et al.* (1984) Abandonment of endoprosthetic drainage technique in malignant biliary obstruction. *A.J.R.*, **143**, 617–22.

Mueller, P. R., vanSonnenberg, E. and Ferrucci, J. T. (1982) Percutaneous biliary drainage: technical and catheter related problems in 200 procedures. *A.J.R.*, **141**, 17–23.

Ringer, E. J., Husted, J. W., Oleaga, J. A. and Freiman, D. B. (1979) A multihole catheter for maintaining long-term percutaneous antegrade biliary drainage. *Radiology*, **132**, 752–4.

Robertson, D. A. F., Ayres, R., Hacking, C. N. *et al.* (1987) Experience with a combined percutaneous and endoscopic approach to stent insertion in malignant obstructive jaundice. *Lancet*, **ii**, 1449–52.

Sarr, M. G. and Cameron, J. L. (1984) Surgical palliation of unresectable carcinoma of the pancreas. *World J. Surg.*, **8**, 906–18.

Sniderman, K. W., Morse, S. S., Rapoport, S. and Ross, G. R. (1985) Haemobilia following transhepatic biliary drainage: occlusion of an hepatoportal fistula by balloon tamponade. *Radiology*, **154**, 827.

Speer, A. G., Cotton, P. B., Russel, R. C. G., Mason, R. R. Hatfield *et al.* (1987) Results of a prospective trial of rejected surgical patients with carcinoma of the pancreas and bile ducts. *Lancet*, **ii**, 57–62.

Speer, A. G., Leung, J. W. C., Yin, T. P. and Cotton, P. B. (1985) 10 French gauge straight biliary stents perform significantly better than 8 French pigtail stents. *Gastrointest. Endosc.*, **31**, A140.

Speer, A. G., Cotton, P. B., Russel, R. C. G. *et al.* (1987) Randomised trial of endoscopic versus percutaneous stent insertion in malignant obstructive jaundice. *Lancet*, **ii**, 57–62.

Vogelzang, R. L. (1986) A modified Cope introducing dilator to allow straight guide wire introduction. *A.J.R.*, **46**, 381–2.

Vogelzang, R. L. (1989) Pain control for percutaneous biliary procedures. *Seminars in Interventional Radiology*, **5**, 3, 207–12.

EQUIPMENT

Lunderquist Wire Guide
  (SFW, 35, 125, LQT)
  William Cook Europe
Lunderquist Exchange Guide
  (CF, 35, 125, 10)
  William Cook Europe
Ring catheter
  (P8.3, 38, 50, P, 32S, Ring)
  William Cook Europe
Multipurpose Peel-away Introducing sheath
  (PLVW, 13.0, 38, 30, VAD5)
  William Cook Europe
Carey-Coons Soft Stent
  (CSS, 12, 15 (12F, 15 cm length))
  Medi-tech, Incorporated.

One-Stick 2 Introducer System
  Cat. No. OS-2
  Medi-Tech, Incorporated.
400 cm Guide Wire
  Cat. No. 832200
  Meadox Surgimed A/S
6F guiding Catheter
  Cat. No. 832161
  Meadox Surgimed A/S
10.2F Pusher Catheter
  Cat. No. 832162
  Meadox Surgimed A/S

CHAPTER TWENTY-NINE

Jejunal biopsy

D. G. Colin-Jones

Small intestinal biopsy and aspiration is a vital part of the investigation and management of patients with malabsorption and suspected small intestinal disease. It used to be necessary to take biopsies using one of several commercially available capsules but these are not always easy to use and may cause complications, so in recent years gastroenterologists have tried to improve on the techniques for jejunal biopsy using the endoscope. Fortunately, because most small intestinal disease is diffuse, affecting much of the proximal small intestine, biopsies obtained from the distal duodenal or proximal jejunum are usually representative of more distal small intestine.

29.1 INDICATIONS

The most common indication for small intestinal biopsy is malabsorption. Malabsorption can be usefully divided into maldigestion, where there is a deficiency of an intraluminal or brush border enzyme, and true malabsorption where there is a defect in the absorptive process at the mucosal level. It is in this latter group that small intestinal biopsy is particularly valuable. Table 29.1 sets out the indications with the most frequent indication in the developed world being coeliac disease/dermatitis herpetiformis. People who have lived or travelled in tropical climates are at risk from parasitic infestation and tropical sprue where again biopsy is of great value. Samples may be analysed histologically using specific

Table 29.1 Indications for small intestinal biopsy

Common suspected diagnoses
Brush border membrane diseases
   disaccharidase deficiency
Small intestinal disorders
   coeliac disease
   dermatitis herpetiformis
   tropical sprue
   parasite infestation

Less common suspected diagnoses
Whipple's disease
Lymphangiectasia
Radiation enteritis
Intestinal lymphoma
Hypogammaglobulinaemia
Eosinophilic gastroenteritis
Amyloidosis
Proximal Crohn's disease

Complex disorders
Bacterial overgrowth in the small bowel
Postgastrectomy
Diabetes mellitus
Scleroderma
Endocrinopathies
Drugs such as neomycin, mefenamic acid

stains (such as PAS for amyloid) but also using the samples for enzyme assays such as in brush border disorders, where disaccharidase deficiencies may be readily detected.

29.2 CONTRAINDICATIONS

The most important contraindications to jejunal biopsy are lack of cooperation on the part of the patient and an uncorrectable coagulation disorder. Occasionally the procedure may be technically difficult where there is pyloric stenosis. Care should be taken if there are multiple proximal duodenal diverticula, for fear of biopsying within a diverticulum which has a thin wall and might be perforated. Special care is also needed for biopsy in small babies as perforation is more common unless a capsule with a small port is used.

29.3 CAPSULE BIOPSY

The traditional method of obtaining tissue for analysis is employing a capsule with a port into which a knuckle of small intestinal mucosa is sucked by aspiration with a syringe connected to the oral end of the capsule tubing. A spring-loaded knife then slices this thin layer of mucosa off for retrieval and analysis.

29.3.1 CROSBY–KUGLER CAPSULE

The Crosby capsule is a metal cylinder with a single 3-mm port attached to fine plastic tubing. This plastic tubing is of crucial importance. It is usually supplied as radiopaque tubing which is of soft consistency so that passage of the capsule through the pylorus is dependent on gravity and intestinal motility. This may well take several hours, so the majority of gastroenterologists change the soft tubing to angiographic tubing, the stiffness of which makes it possible to direct the capsule through the pylorus. The capsule passes to the duodenojejunal flexure where a sample is taken by suction which, by creating a vacuum, sucks the mucosa into the port and depresses a rubber diaphragm above a rotating knife blade (Figure 29.1). The pressure of this diaphragm disengages a spring hook within the capsule, causing the knife to rotate and a sample is taken. This mechanism can be fragile, with premature firing or failure to fire if the connecting tubing occludes with mucus. However, the major problem is getting the capsule into the distal duodenum/jejunum, which may take several hours (indeed some-

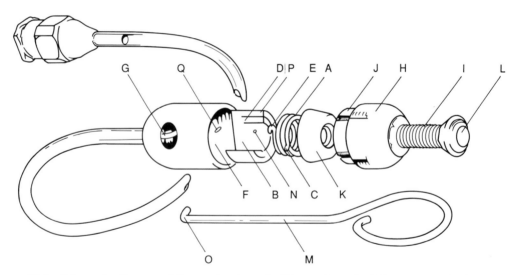

Figure 29.1 Schematic diagram of the mechanism of a Watson intestinal biopsy capsule. A, spring; B, central boss; C, spring hook; D, slot; E, spring loop; F, open end of body; G, stake; H, cap; I, allen screw; J, skirt, K, collar; L, port in screw; M, loading rod; N, hole in knife; O, prong; P, groove; Q, stake. A rubber diaphragm is inserted between the spring (A) and the tightening collar (K). Suction simultaneously pulls the intestinal mucosa into the port of the capsule and depresses the rubber diaphragm, which then presses on the blade and disengages the spring from the stake (Q). The spring then rotates the blade across the port in the capsule. Reproduced from Ravenscroft and Swan with permission.

times it is passed overnight) if dependent on natural gut movements. Various methods to reduce this time and improve reliability have been developed.

Shortening the time for passage of the capsule

By replacing the soft tubing with stiffer angiographic tubing the capsule can frequently be more accurately directed towards and sometimes through the pylorus, hastening its movement and so shortening the time required for the procedure. This is probably better achieved using an outer sheath, for example, a Scott–Harden outer tube (Figure 29.2) which, once advanced into the stomach, allows free movement of the inner angiographic semi-stiff tube without irritating the pharynx, thus minimizing patient discomfort. This method usually permits a sample to be obtained within half an hour.

An alternative method uses an internal stiffening wire for the same purpose, and in one report 20 such cases had their biopsies taken within 14 minutes (Law, 1984). A modification of the same technique has been used for children (Maki, 1984).

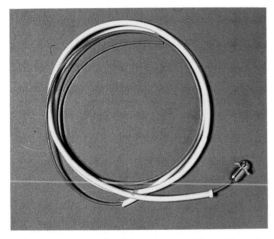

Figure 29.2 Standard biopsy capsule with outer stiffening sheath. The capsule is mounted on a semistiff angiographic catheter which is inserted through an outer sheath (radiopaque Scott–Harden).

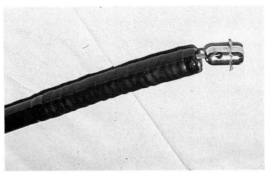

Figure 29.3 Muzzle loading of the capsule onto an endoscope which can then be used to guide the capsule into the small intestine.

29.3.2 ENDOSCOPIC GUIDANCE OF CAPSULE METHOD

The capsule is muzzle loaded onto a forward-viewing panendoscope by retrograde threading of the arteriographic catheter (semistiff, as mentioned before) so that the catheter protrudes from the biopsy channel at the top of the instrument. The capsule is positioned just ahead of the tip of the endoscope (Figure 29.3), and the procedure then follows the usual pattern for upper gastrointestinal endoscopy. Thus, usually under light sedation, the capsule is carried just ahead of the endoscope over the back of the throat and into the oesophagus. This has to be done relatively blind as the capsule obscures the view, but once in the oesophagus the capsule can be pushed 2–3 cm ahead of the instrument, to give clear views. The capsule and endoscope are then passed through the stomach and the pylorus into the second part of the duodenum from where the capsule may then be pushed onwards beyond view of the endoscope into the third part of the duodenum and the jejunum. The capsule may be screened to check on its position if that is required, but is not normally necessary. After firing the capsule as previously described, the endoscope is withdrawn, trailing the capsule. The advantage of this technique is the rapidity with which the biopsy may be taken, and the avoidance of radiation.

29.4 ALTERNATIVE CAPSULES

A number of modifications have been made to the basic Crosby–Kugler capsule. The Watson capsule is similar; both capsules having a spring-loaded blade which is fired by external aspiration. The Birmingham or Cooke capsule contains no moving blade but one edge of the biopsy port is sharpened so that on aspiration a knuckle of mucosa is pulled into the orifice and then as the capsule is withdrawn, so the sharp edge of the port severs the mucosa. It is important to keep the edge sharp for fear of tearing the mucosa. For this reason it is not widely used. The Carey capsule is used most in paediatrics, and requires constant suction to keep the port closed during withdrawal after biopsy.

29.5 MULTIPLE BIOPSY CAPSULE

A major drawback of the capsules mentioned above is that they are only capable of taking a single biopsy, and then not with 100% reliability. The sophisticated Quinton–Rubin hydraulic capsule tries to overcome this. It is a larger tube which has two or four holes distally and uses a hydraulically operated blade which may be reloaded while still inside the patient. The sample is delivered without removal of the tube, so that reassurance is obtained that some tissue has been acquired. This capsule is most commonly used in research procedures because of the multiple pieces of tissue that can be removed. This has been reviewed by Lembcke, Schneider and Lankisch (1986), who undertook 1007 hydraulic small bowel biopsies on 342 occasions over an 11-year period. The major complication was haemorrhage with an incidence of 1.5%, transfusion being required in one case. There was one perforation. It is a bulky tube for the patient to swallow, and the

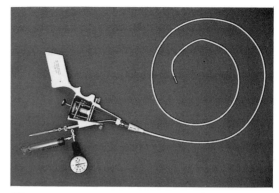

Figure 29.4 Steerable biopsy capsule. Capsule at the tip has two small ports with a blade that is operated from a wire running centrally through the catheter. The tip can be manoeuvred using the control handle proximally.

mechanism is not completely reliable so that it is not widely used nowadays.

29.6 STEERABLE CATHETER (Medi-Tech) (Figure 29.4)

This steerable catheter is made of Teflon and carries four very fine wires in its sheath. There is a central lumen down which suction can be applied and a wire travels. The wire operates a blade in the capsule. The catheter fits to a standard handle which is used for other Medi-Tech steerable catheters. Using this catheter a considerable degree of movement of the tip can be achieved. It is 5 mm in diameter and is well tolerated. It can be steered through into the duodenum with minimum screening and considerable saving of time. The tip has two ports, so that two modest-sized biopsies can be achieved. Its advantages are speed – in our experience, we obtained a biopsy within 15 minutes in every one of our 100 cases (Shepherd and Colin-Jones, 1982). The disadvantage is that vigorous movement of the tip causes the very fine wires to cut through the Teflon coat, so that the life expectancy is limited to between 20 and 40 uses.

29.7 ENDOSCOPY

There has been a growing literature on biopsies taken in the conventional way with biopsy forceps at endoscopy (Gillberg *et al.*, 1982; Mee *et al.*, 1985; Achkar *et al.*, 1986; Dandalides *et al.*, 1989). Small intestinal biopsy through the endoscope requires standard preparation, and a forward-viewing pan-endoscope is passed into the duodenum with biopsies being taken from the distal second part of the duodenum. These samplers are, however, difficult to orientate and may be small, and so it is normal practice to take four samples from different sites as far distally as possible. A better result can be achieved using a large channel instrument, through which large biopsy forceps which open to 10 mm across can be passed to obtain good sized samples (Figure 29.5).

29.8 ENTEROSCOPY

The shaft of the routine upper gastrointestinal endoscope is relatively stiff to facilitate its

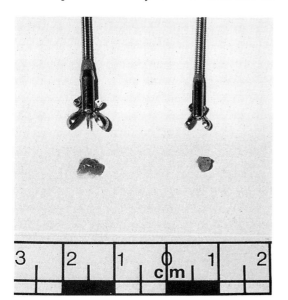

Figure 29.5 Endoscopic biopsy specimens. The smaller specimen has been taken with standard biopsy forceps whilst the larger specimen has been taken using the large channel instrument.

passage and manoeuvrability within the stomach. This means that it is difficult to pass beyond the third part of the duodenum. To get round this an enteroscope, which is longer and more supple, has been designed, which can be manoeuvred down the small intestine. This is a difficult technique and time consuming. It enables biopsies to be taken under direct vision, but the forceps used are small. However, this procedure has been undertaken by Barkin *et al.* (1985) who felt that it was indicated in patients where visualization was an important aid to making a firm diagnosis, and in order to take target biopsies. Any situation which inhibits the passage of the capsule or where radiology is contraindicated, might be considered for this technique. Alternatively a paediatric colonoscope can be passed to the duodenojejunal flexure and good-sized biopsies obtained.

29.9 PAEDIATRIC BIOPSY

Accurate diagnosis of small intestinal disease is nowhere more important than in infancy because a gluten-free or cow's milk-free diet is so successful in the appropriate case. However, such a diet is restrictive: it is important that a firm diagnosis should be made. Endoscopy is not usually carried out in these patients; either a small Crosby capsule with a port not greater than 2 mm, or a Carey capsule, is normally used under sedation. Again a number of techniques have been employed to minimize the problems associated with this procedure in young children. The largest series is that by Townley and Barnes (1973), who reported on 1172 children who had biopsies carried out over a 4-year period. They used a Watson paediatric capsule and relied upon motility for its passage through the stomach into the intestine. They used, however, a semistiff tube to enable some pushing effect to be applied. An alternative is to use an over-tube, as described by Collins *et al.* (1985). The advantage of the over-tube is that pushing and pulling on the inner catheter attached to the capsule does not cause gagging or disturb the child, who will often carry on sleeping once the over-tube is in place. Using this technique Collins *et al.* were able to minimize fluoroscopic time to less than 10 seconds in 75% of cases – a highly desirable feature in young children.

29.10 CARRYING OUT THE PROCEDURE

29.10.1 CAPSULE BIOPSY

A most important feature in passing a capsule is to ensure that it is firing reliably. It is essential, therefore, to load it, to check that it is firing with an appropriate degree of suction by placing a piece of rubber (not the investigator's finger!) over the port, and aspirating. Capsules that are not properly cared for may fire prematurely, may not fire at all or the spring may be fatigued so that the blade does not rotate with sufficient speed to make a clean cut and the mucosa is torn. The knife must be kept sharp. All these things need to be anticipated with very careful maintenance (Drossman, 1982; Ravenscroft and Swan, 1984). The procedure should be explained to the patient and written consent obtained. The throat should be sprayed with a local anaesthetic and the capsule, with either an outer stiffening tube or an inner guide, passed over the back of the tongue and the patient asked to swallow. A glass of water with a straw might help at this point but is not usually necessary. Once the capsule is past the cricopharyngeus it should be inserted relatively swiftly, until well down in the oesophagus; when the tube should be pushed to the side of the mouth so that it lies outside the teeth and inside the cheek. The patient should then close the teeth, avoiding any pressure on the tube, clench the jaw tightly and take slow, deep breaths, to diminish the gag reflex. Once the patient is comfortable the lubricated tube should be inserted further so that the capsule passes into the body of the stomach. Because the natural curvature of the lesser curve of the stomach tends to coil the capsule into the fundus it is preferable to do this with the patient sitting upright so that the capsule's tendency is to pass distally. The whole tube, including the stiffening sheath, is then passed round the greater curve and its position checked briefly by fluoroscopy. With the stiffening outer-tube the capsule can be placed in the gastric antrum and then, leaving the stiffening device static the capsule can be advanced. It usually passes through the pylorus quickly, and then tends to move swiftly into the distal duodenum where the biopsy can be taken. The tubing is cleared of any debris by inserting a small amount of water very gently through the connecting radiopaque tubing, followed by air, and vigorous suction is then applied using a 20-ml syringe. The sample is retrieved by withdrawing the capsule, which may occasionally catch at the cardia, when the patient should be asked to swallow whilst gentle traction is applied. On retrieving the sample it should be orientated on the upturned aspect of the index finger, so that the villi are down on the surface of the finger, and then the base of the biopsy is applied to a ground-glass slide or a flat plastic container (Colley *et al.*, 1982).

29.10.2 STEERABLE CATHETER

The catheter needs to be checked carefully as the direction control wires can fracture the Teflon coating, especially near the bending section of the distal tip. Enthusiastic newcomers to the technique should be dissuaded from vigorous movement of the tip as this shortens the life of the catheter assembly. The catheter should be mounted on the handle and the suction tested with the vacuum gauge. The knife should be checked. The tube is passed in the same way as for the capsule but the steerable tip makes positioning at and then passage through the pylorus very easy. It does, however, require some initial skill in interpreting a two-dimensional picture on the fluoroscopic screen into a three-dimensional movement of the tip of the catheter. It is helpful in training to practise outside the patient by lining up the Medi-Tech catheter on the X-ray table, the tube being held by an assistant, while the operator stands in his usual position were the patient present. The bends that the instrument acquires in the patient should be reproduced so that distortion in the movement of the tip can be observed on the couch, prior to its use in a patient. The posterior direction of the second part of the duodenum is often forgotten. Once in the distal third of the duodenum the biopsy can be taken by suction and pulling on the wire controlling the blade. The steerable catheter can be used in both adults and children (Ferry and Bendig, 1981).

29.11 UPPER GASTROINTESTINAL ENDOSCOPY

Preparation is by the standard method employed for oesophagogastroduodenoscopy with the patient starved and usually with topical pharyngeal anaesthesia and intravenous sedation with diazepam or midazolam. It is best to use a large-channel instrument such as the Olympus GIF 1T, Pentax FD-34H 3.8 mm, Fuji UGI-CT2 3.7 mm. After insertion of the endoscope a formal examination of the upper gastrointestinal tract to the proximal second part of the duodenum is carried out. Modification of the standard endoscopic technique will often allow the tip of the instrument to advance beyond the junction between the second and third parts of the duodenum. This is achieved by passing the instrument in the usual way so that the tip lies in the second part of the duodenum, inevitably with a large loop around the greater curve of the stomach. The endoscope is then withdrawn, at the same time turning it in a clockwise direction. This tends to straighten the loop which was in the greater curve of the stomach and so to advance the tip, although paradoxically the instrument shaft is being withdrawn. Then continue to turn the instru-

ment slowly through 180° whilst gently advancing the endoscope. The tip will usually advance to the distal second part, where, using the lateral control the tip can then be manoeuvred round the fold that marks the right-angle bend into the third part of the duodenum (Figure 29.6). The advantages of this technique are the speed with which the procedure can be performed (usually less than 15 minutes), the certainty with which multiple biopsies can be obtained from a precise location and the ability to inspect the gastrointestinal tract at the same time, which is often important where the individual is being investigated for iron-deficiency anaemia. When multiple (not less than four) biopsies are taken the tissue obtained is sufficient, although the larger forceps are preferable (Dandalides *et al.*, 1987). It is the author's practice to take four biopsies from different sites in the distal third part of the duodenum, one of which is examined under the dissecting microscope for macroscopic villous morphology. Duodenal aspiration can also be undertaken using a sterile tube, passing the catheter down the intestinal lumen as far as possible and then aspirating while it is withdrawn. Alternatively if duodenal juice is insufficient saline can be infused through the endoscope biopsy channel and duodenal aspiration subsequently made by regular suction with a sputum trap placed at the suction port on the endoscope umbilical to collect the aspirate for laboratory examination.

29.12 COMPLICATIONS

Lembcke, Schneider and Lankisch (1986) have reviewed the complication rate from small bowel biopsy and, from a detailed review of the literature, concluded that haemorrhage was the major complication. This was reported in up to 5.9% with only a minority of those patients requiring transfusion – the overall incidence is probably of the order of 1.5%. Fever has been reported rarely as has submucosal haematoma (Arthurs and

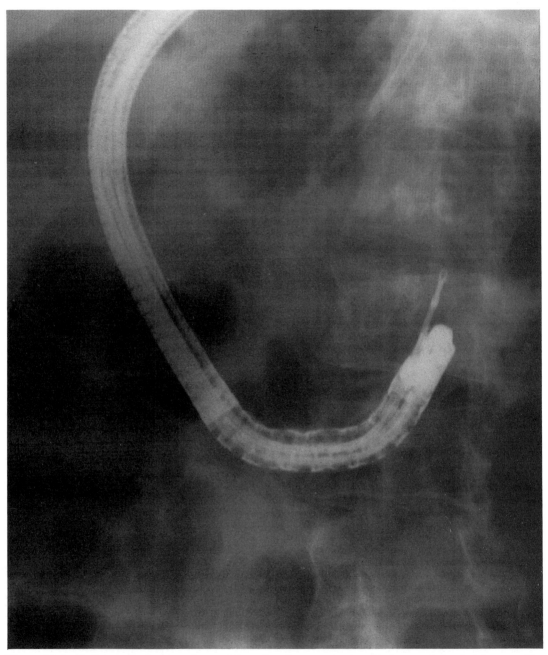

Figure 29.6 Radiograph showing the position of endoscope in the third part of the duodenum. The forceps can be advanced further up the duodenal lumen under direct vision. The endoscope used here is an Olympus GIF-K10 fore-oblique, which has the advantage of controllable direction of the forceps, with the disadvantage of just standard sized forceps.

Fielding, 1980). Perforation, too, has been an occasional experience being 0.3%, in Lembcke's review, particularly in young children, in whom the smaller capsule with a smaller biopsy port should be used. Failure to obtain a biopsy is one of the most irksome 'complications' – this occurs in about 12% (Ferry and Bendig, 1981), with a range of 2–22%; hence the trend towards endoscopically taken samples, where the complications of endoscopy are low.

29.13 INTERPRETATION OF THE BIOPSY

It is important to examine the biopsy sample under the dissecting microscope before fixation to look at the visual characteristics of the villous pattern. This can then be assessed with the histological appearance. Correct orientation of the biopsy is of great value when determining the length of the villi and the villous crypt ratio. This is most easily done using a capsule biopsy or a large endoscopic biopsy. It is difficult to achieve with the smaller endoscopy biopsies.

29.14 WHICH METHOD?

Each unit will have developed its own preferred method for taking biopsies of the small intestine and one method should be followed because that leads to improved skills, and therefore to the speed and success of the procedure. The Medi-Tech steerable capsule has many advantages in terms of speed, multiple biopsies and patient acceptability. Its drawback is its fragility (and hence cost), with regular replacement of the capsule being required. The multiple biopsy apparatus of Quinton–Rubin should probably only now be used for research purposes, where multiple moderate-sized specimens are needed. The passage of a Crosby capsule using a soft catheter, with progress being dependent upon natural motility, is no longer necessary. There can be no justification for exposing a patient to many hours of unnecessary waiting and probably many minutes of unnecessary radiation when several superior techniques are available. The combination of a capsule with an outer sheath to assist its passage through the plylorus is an improvement, or even better is muzzle-loading of the capsule onto an endoscope which can then be guided under direct vision into the distal duodenum. However, in the author's experience capsules are not completely reliable, with a failure rate of up to 20% owing to failure to fire or premature firing. This means that the whole procedure has to be repeated, much to the patient's discomfort. The use of the large-channel endoscope with large biopsy forceps is quick (less than 15 minutes), is safe, with virtually no complications other than those of routine oesophagogastroduodenoscopy, and as many biopsies as needed can be obtained at one session. An endoscope is expensive but may be used for routine work in addition.

To speed passage and minimize radiation, a modified (stiffened/sheathed) capsule for jejunal biopsies in children is the preferred method. In adults a large-channel endoscope is the method of choice. When a large-channel endoscope is not available the steerable catheter should be considered, or alternatively, standard endoscopic biopsies will suffice for most cases (Mee et al., 1985; Dandalides et al., 1987).

REFERENCES

Achkar, E., Carey, W. D., Petras, R. et al. (1986) Comparison of suction capsule and endoscopic biopsy of small bowel mucosa. Gastrointest. Endosc., 32, 278–81.

Arthurs, Y. and Fielding, J. F. (1980) Intramural hematoma of the duodenum complicating peroral jejunal biopsy with a Watson capsule. J. Clin. Gastroenterol., 2, 369–70.

Barkin, J. S., Schonfield, W., Thomsen, S. et al. (1985) Enteroscopy and small bowel biopsy – an improved technique for the diagnosis of small bowel disease. Gastrointest. Endosc., 31, 215–7.

Colley, S. J., Gledhill, T., Bone, R. et al. (1982) Porous containers for small biopsy specimens. Lancet, i, 773–4.

Collins, A. L., Brookfield, D. S. K., Hyde, I. and Rolles, C. J. (1985) Small bowel biopsy. *Arch. Dis. Child.*, **60**, 1082–5.

Dandalides, S. M., Carey, W. D., Achkar, E. and Petras, R. (1987) Endoscopic small bowel biopsy (EB): importance of forceps size and biopsy location. *Gastroenterology*, **92**, A-211.

Dandalides, S. M., Carey, W. D., Petras, R. and Achkar, E. (1989) Endoscopic small bowel mucosal biopsy: a controlled trial evaluating forceps size and biopsy location in the diagnosis of normal and abnormal mucosal architecture. *Gastrointest. Endosc.*, **35**, 197–200.

Drossman, D. A. (ed.) (1982) *Manual of Gastroenterologic Procedures*, Raven, New York.

Ferry, G. D. and Bendig, D. W. (1981) Peroral small-bowel biopsies in infants and children using a directable biopsy instrument. *Dig. Dis. Sci.*, **26**, 142–5.

Gillberg, R., Kastrup, W., Mobacken, H. *et al.* (1982) Endoscopic duodenal biopsy compared with biopsy with the Watson capsule from the upper jejunum in patients with dermatitis herpetiformis. *Scand. J. Gastroenterol.*, **17**, 305–8.

Law, R. L. (1984) Guide wire manipulation of Crosby jejunal biopsy capsule under fluoroscopic control. *Br. Med. J.*, **288**, 286–7.

Lembcke, B., Schneider, H. and Lankisch, P. G. (1986) How safe is small bowel biopsy? *Endoscopy*, **18**, 80–3.

Maki, M. (1984) Guide wire manipulation of Crosby jejunal biopsy capsule. *Br. Med. J.*, **288**, 862–3.

Mee, A. S., Burke, M., Vallon, A. G., Newman, J. and Cotton, P. B. (1985) Small bowel biopsy malabsorption: comparison of the diagnostic adequacy of endoscopic forceps and capsule biopsy specimens. *Brit. Med. J.*, **291**, 769–72.

Ravenscroft, M. M. and Swan, C. H. J. (1984) *Gastrointestinal Endoscopy and Related Procedures*, Chapman and Hall, London.

Shepherd, H. A. and Colin-Jones, D. G. (1982) Steerable catheter. *Dig. Dis. Sci.*, **27**, 474–5.

Townley, R. R. W. and Barnes, G. L. (1973) Intestinal biopsy in childhood. *Arch. Dis. Child.*, **48**, 480–2.

CHAPTER THIRTY

Tube placement under radiological guidance

M. K. Bilbao

This chapter describes the principles of ante-grade intestinal intubation, with radiological guidance, for diagnosis, feeding and intestinal decompression, and some methods of prevention and treatment of tube complications. The use of radiology enables the operator to see both tube and route during insertion. Special methods of catheter guidance, adapted from angiography, and the ability to exchange one catheter for another, make it possible to design a tube for its ease of placement or for its functional efficiency without attempting to combine these attributes in a single tube.

The blind passage of a tube is the simplest method even if not the most effective, and suffices in many instances. Where more sophisticated methods are needed, the advantages of fluoroscopically controlled gastro-intestinal intubation are that it is faster, safer, and surer than passing a tube blindly, and usually less traumatic and expensive than passing it endoscopically. Additionally, contrast material used during placement may allow a concomitant diagnostic study in cases of obstruction, and the demonstration of effectiveness when feeding tubes have been inserted.

The disadvantages are the added time, expense, and trouble in transporting the patient to the X-ray department and using the radiological resources. Additionally there is radiation exposure, although this is nearly all fluoroscopic, with few radiographs, and therefore less than that of a standard gastro-intestinal series.

30.1 INDICATIONS

Since most nasogastric tubes, feeding and intestinal decompression tubes are successfully placed by the ward personnel and only confirming radiographs are needed, a trial with blind placement makes sense and saves money. How long to try before seeking the radiologist's help depends on the referring physician's expectations and on the availability and skill of the radiologist. A trial of 8–12 hours for an intestinal decompression tube and 24 hours for a feeding tube are usual, but emergency placement is sometimes indicated, especially in infants and severely burned patients. Radiological guidance gives clear evidence of safe, appropriate positioning of feeding or decompression tubes. Fluoroscopically aided placement is indicated when blind passage has failed or is likely to be difficult, or dangerous; for example in patients with strictures, tumours, fistulae, injuries or surgical anastomoses, and in patients with swallowing difficulty, depressed gag reflexes or abnormal peristalsis. Radiologically guided intubation is faster. Duodenal intubation in 5 minutes and jejunal intubation in 10–30 minutes is usually possible with radiological aid (Edlich *et al.*, 1968; Bilbao and Dotter, 1975; Shipps *et al.*, 1979).

Relative contraindications to fluoroscopically controlled intubation are related to radiation exposure (especially in pregnant or young patients) and to the choice of contrast agent. Air is simplest but least effective.

Barium is the safest, most effective agent except in instances of suspected perforation or large bowel obstruction, or in positioning a tube for small intestinal biopsy where it may interfere with histological examination. Iodinated contrast agents, because of their high osmolarity (six times that of saline), are less safe. In infants they may cause hypovolaemic shock, as well as diarrhoea and vomiting (Harris, Newhauser and Gerth, 1964). Furthermore, because of dilution, they are less effective diagnostically (Nelson, 1965). Non-ionic iodinated contrast agents are so expensive that their use in the gastrointestinal tract, except for the occasional infant, is seldom considered.

There are circumstances where any method of intubation may be hazardous because of the risk of haemorrhage (bleeding diathesis, varices, anomalous mediastinal vessels), or perforation (recent surgical anastomoses, ulceration, tumours). If intubation is done at all in these instances fluoroscopic methods are safer than blind passage.

30.2 PRINCIPLES

Fluoroscopically aided tube passage is easy: the fluoroscopist 'sees' the route and controls the tube, moving the tube past obstacles, and shaping the tube and route into conformity. Afterwards he may exchange the tube for another which is more functional, comfortable, sturdier or cheaper. The tube is advanced partly by peristalsis and by gravity, but mainly by pushing, which requires that it be at least temporarily stiff enough. Stiffening is accomplished either coaxially by inner guide-wires or outer tubes, or by outrigged coupling to a pilot tube. These same techniques are used for tube exchanges. Coaxial layers are made movable and removable by straightening bends, and by lubrication. Passing obstacles can involve decongesting, lubricating (and anaesthetizing), smoothing and distending corrugated mucosal surfaces, and then 'dancing' the tube across them by revolving it and shaking it (or shaking the surface).

The tube is bent by gravity, by palpation, or by the use of steerable tube-tips or preshaped or steerable guide-wires. The shape of the route may be altered, using gravity to shift the viscera by positioning the patient and tilting the table, by palpation with either the fluoroscopist's or patient's hands, and by the patient's posturing – breathing, arching, stretching, flexing, leaning, 'undulating and fluttering' (like panting), and so forth. The patient may help more if he watches himself on the fluoroscopic monitor. Each sequential bend in the tract can be straightened in front of the advancing tube.

Nearly all feeding and decompression tubes are designed for blind intestinal passage and are 'gravity driven' by a weighted tip. Doing the simplest, cheapest thing first, the radiologist usually tries to advance the tip-weighted tube already in place in the patient by using fluoroscopy, contrast agent and guide-wires. If that fails, he tries (not necessarily at the same session) a non-weighted, more directable tube designed for radiological placement but which still fulfils the patient's original need for intubation. If that fails, he or she then tries placing a still more radiologically directable, but otherwise functionless, tube and exchanges it afterwards over a guide-wire for a tube that will serve the required function. These steps should be done in an orderly, expeditious, cost-effective sequence. The radiologist's understanding of the principles of advancing gravity-driven tubes and of the causes for failure can minimize delays, ineffective trials and patient discomfort.

The weighted tip of a gravity-driven tube must be induced to follow the stomach and duodenum as they drape back and forth over the central hump of the spine. The radiologist successfully intubates most patients, even after blind placement fails, by visualizing the anatomy with contrast agent, adjusting the patient's position in space in order to shape the route and put it sequentially dependent

under the weighted tip, and then stiffening the tube and pushing the tip in the **same direction** as gravity pulls.

30.3 TUBES

There is no perfect tube. Features which make it comfortable – small size, limpness, elasticity – also make it uncontrollable; features which make it easy to place, like stiffness and large size, also make it uncomfortable and more traumatic. Three general types of intestinal tubes are of interest to radiologists. **Diagnostic tubes**, used for rapid short-term nasoenteric intubation, are simple, versatile, easily placed, large-bore and inexpensive. **Feeding tubes** for long-term comfort and safety are soft, rubbery, and as small as possible while still allowing a liquid feed to be forced through them. **Decompression tubes** are to be propelled by the gastrointestinal tract, large bored enough for aspiration of intestinal content, yet soft enough for the patient to tolerate without undue discomfort and without ulcerating his mucosa.

30.3.1 CONSTITUTION

Materials used in gastrointestinal tubes include **natural rubber**, which is soft, flexible, and not irritating, but too elastic for use with a guide-wire and prone to get coated with and clogged by detritus. Also, it hardens and weakens when exposed to gut contents. **Polyvinylchloride** is soft, flexible, can be made radiopaque, and can be used with a guide-wire. Polyvinylchloride is excellent for short-term applications and for small feeding tubes, even though the plasticizer, which makes it soft, leaches out, irritates mucosal surfaces, and causes the tube to harden gradually after the first 2 weeks (Cowper, 1968; Duke and Vane, 1968; Editorial, 1975). **Polyurethane** is soft, flexible, inert, good for feeding tubes and can be used to a limited extent with guide-wires. **Silicone rubber** is extremely soft, durable, inert, comfortable, does not collect

detritus nor tend to plug, and does not harden. It is difficult to use with a guide-wire, but is excellent for a long-term feeding tube if it can be placed.

30.3.2 DESIGN

The length of the tube and guide is crucial, since every inch increases the friction. The lumen size affects performance, since flow through tubes varies with the fourth power of the diameter; thus reducing tube diameter to a half reduces the tube flow to a sixteenth. Flow through a hole varies with the square of the diameter (MacIntosh, Muskin and Epstein, 1963). Hole position is important. An end-hole is needed for coaxial exchange over a guide-wire and should be fabricated as needed.

For some purposes, like investigating strictures, side-holes in tubes for diagnostic studies are disadvantageous because they deliver contrast agent too far from the site to be examined, thereby obscuring the route. Feeding tubes should have holes located near the end to avoid delivery proximal to the target. Decompression tubes should have holes over a considerable length to decompress more than one segment of the gastrointestinal tract at a time.

30.3.3 FRICTION

Friction is the major impediment to gastrointestinal intubation. There is friction between tube and guide, tube and gastrointestinal tract, tube and coaxial tube, and tube and the fluid it carries. Friction increases directly with tube length, with every additional curve and with sharpness of curvature. Therefore, it is important to shorten the tube and make the curves fewer and gentler, especially while trying to move coaxial elements. One way is to move both guide and tube together around bends and advance the guide within the tube only when it is straight. Another way is to straighten the tube by external palpatation on the abdomen while the guide is advanced. Kinks or surface irregularities in either tube or guide increase friction. A guide considerably smaller than the tube reduces contact. Friction is greatest with the most elastic materials such as rubber, polyurethane and silicone rubber, less, but still considerable, with polyvinylchloride. Tubes and guides should be thoroughly lubricated to create surfaces which float instead of bind. Dobbhoff feeding tubes are already coated with a substance which becomes slippery when wet. For other tubes mineral oil is frequently used as a lubricant but if aspirated damages the lungs. Silicone fluid (medical grade) in a spray can with propellant is particularly useful (Figure 30.1). It can be sprayed directly on the tube and guide, and also into the tube; it can be sprayed on gauze and wiped on the guides. It may be put into a syringe and injected down the tube. Residual dissolved propellant boils out and carries the silicone forcefully to the tube's end. Using a 'Y' adaptor, this can be done while the tube is in the patient, even with a spring guide in

place. Silicone is inert, widely used in the food industry, and harmless in the gut. Silicone on the outside of the tube makes it less traumatic during passage, less irritating and less likely to get crusted with adherent blood and mucous. To emphasize: 'dripping wet' lubrication of tubes and guides is a crucial element in successful intubation.

30.3.4 SELECTION OF TUBE AND GUIDANCE METHOD

Usually the radiologist is asked to help after simpler methods have failed. Before trying to pass a tube, preliminary preparation saves time, trouble and money in the long run and is often essential to success. It is best to consult the referring clinician, see the patient and review the patient's anatomy as depicted on prior radiographs, looking for anything that might cause difficulty (such as Zenker's diverticulum, hiatal hernia, cascade stomach, duodenal malrotation, or previous gastro-

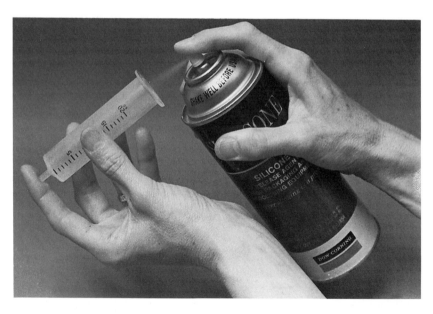

Figure 30.1 Silicone lubricant can be sprayed into a syringe and injected into a nasoduodenal tube to reduce friction between tube and guide. The residual dissolved propellant carries the silicone forcefully down the tube even with a guide-wire in the tube.

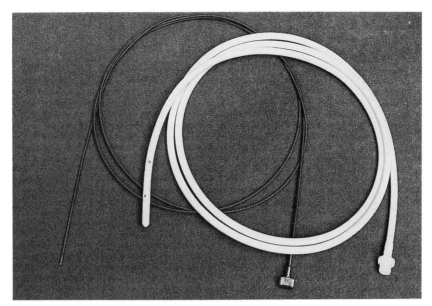

Figure 30.2 The original Bilbao–Dotter tube and guide, which have now been developed by gastro-intestinal radiologists into a family of radiologically guidable tubes and guides for the gastrointestinal tract.

intestinal surgery), or might otherwise influence the choice of tube and guide, such as an unusually tall patient. Answering these questions helps: What job is the tube to do? What has been tried so far? What can be deduced about the reasons for failure? What tube is already in the patient? (if the same tube is wanted, have a new one on hand). Will the physician allow a different tube to be used if you are unable to pass the one the patient has? Where possible, tube systems which separate placement features from functional features have advantages in versatility and cost.

It is useful to have on hand a supply of tubing, guides and fittings, as well as tools for their *ad hoc* fabrication (see Appendix).

Having decided what jobs the tube must do, how fast, for how long, in what order of priority, and what difficulties in placement are likely, the equipment and method is selected with regard to material, internal and external diameters, and position and size of holes, and length (to estimate nasojejunal length

measure nose to ear plus ear to xiphoid plus 25 cm). Manufacturers change and improve their tubes and also give instructions that are not only helpful but sometimes crucial. It is important to read the tube's instructions, and to practise with the tube and guide *in vitro*. How many bends can be put in the tube and still move the guide in it? What guides will it accept? Is it possible to overcome the tip's weight with a guide? What other tube characteristics will affect fluoroscopic placement, such as kinking at side-holes, ambiguous or absent radiopaque markings, inability to reinsert a guide once it is retracted and so on? To emphasize: preliminary bench trials – marking lengths, lubricating and testing the frictional resistance to tube and guide movement – are invaluable.

(a) Nasoduodenal diagnostic tubes

For radiological placement the Bilbao–Dotter intestinal tube and guide (Figure 30.2) have been useful. The original tube, intended for hypotonic duodenography, was made of

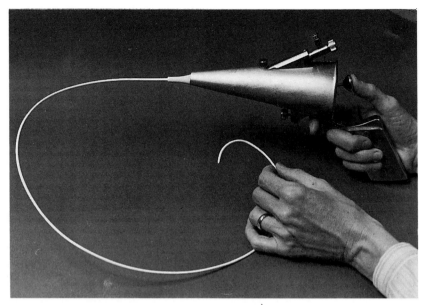

Figure 30.3   Medi-tech steerable catheter and control handle. 'Y' adaptor on the handle allows the apparatus to be used with a guide-wire and contrast injection simultaneously. The single end-hole allows cathether exchange over a guide-wire and helps with negotiating a narrowed lumen.

radiopaque polyvinyl chloride, 14-Fr size, 125-cm long, with a closed end- and side-holes near the tip. A Teflon-coated torque control guide-wire allowed directional control. Modifications have extended the tube's usefulness: There are now 8-Fr versions for enteral feeding (Frederick–Miller): longer 14-Fr and 12-Fr tubes for enteroclysis (Sellink, Nolan, Herlinger); balloon versions (Maglinte, Bilbao and Dotter); intestinal decompression tubes (Shipps); and coaxially placed intestinal biopsy apparatuses (Bilbao and Dotter). Guide-wires have been modified by designing bends and/or tapers into the tips (Shipps and Herlinger). Gianturco designed a much thicker yet still soft and very effective guide and Sargent an extra long guide-wire for intestinal decompression and catheter exchange.

A versatile, but more fragile and expensive, family of tubes is the Medi-tech system (Figure 30.3). A control handle attached to four wires in the tube wall makes the tip easy to control. Medi-tech controllable catheters are made of radiopaque polyvinylchloride in 5- to 13-Fr size and 30–270 cm long. Different varieties are used in the vascular system, biliary, bronchial, genitourinary and gastrointestinal tracts, along with accessory baskets, biopsy instruments, forceps and brushes. The gastrointestinal catheters include an adaptation for intestinal biopsy (Linscheer and Abele, 1976) and another for intestinal decompression. Gastrointestinal tubes accept guide-wires 0.6–1.3 mm (0.025–0.052 in) diameter. The Medi-tech system has a 'Y' adaptor in the handle allowing contrast agent injection while a guide is in place. The catheter has a single end-hole, useful for exchanging tubes over guide-wires, and helpful in threading strictured or difficult routes (Wendth *et al.*, 1973; Dodds *et al.*, 1976; Ho and Lipinski, 1978) by demonstrating the lumen with injected contrast material.

Medi-tech gastrointestinal catheters are sometimes not stiff enough to be effective but can be stiffened coaxially with a larger outer tube. At times it is difficult to manage the control handle and catheter simultaneously; these are minor disadvantages compared with its versatility and usefulness.

(b) Intestinal decompression tubes

Radiological placement methods can reduce the time required to pass a decompression tube from days to minutes. There are several types of decompression tubes. The **Shipps tube** (Figure 30.4(a)) is a long intestinal tube similar to the Bilbao–Dotter tube. It is made of radiopaque polyvinylchloride 14 Fr, 225 cm long, with a slit 150 cm from the tip for insert-ing a guide-wire. There are three Teflon-coated guide-wires, double wound for torque control, each designed specifically for nego-tiating a troublesome part of the gastro-intestinal route. Using this intubation system and 10 minutes fluoroscopic time, Shipps and his associates succeeded in reaching the jejunum in 39% and the duodenum in 76% of 400 cases (Shipps *et al.*, 1979).

Single-lumen tubes like the 16-Fr **Cantor** (Figure 30.4(b)), **Harris** or **Kaslow tubes** are made of radiopaque polyvinylchloride. They have a closed balloon for a mercury bolus and a lumen large enough for a curved-tip torque

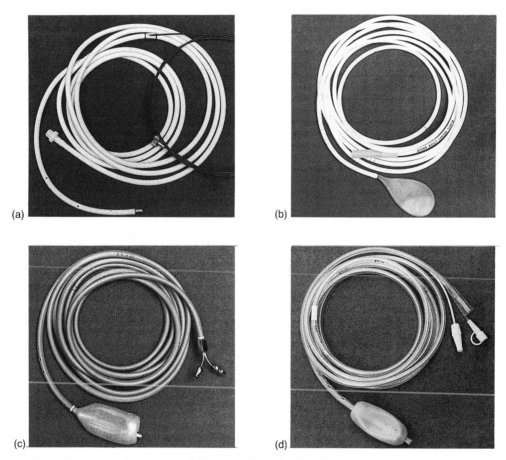

Figure 30.4 Decompression tubes. (a) Shipps 14-Fr polyvinylchloride single-lumen tube and guide. (b) Cantor 16-Fr polyvinylchloride single-lumen mercury-weighted balloon tube. (c) Miller–Abbott 16-Fr double-lumen natural rubber mercury-weighted inflatable balloon tube. (d) Medi-tech triple-lumen mercury-weighted inflatable balloon with sump conduit.

control guide-wire introduced through a side slit (Gianturco, 1967; Gelfand, 1978) or through the entire tube (Sargent and Meyers, 1969). A new tube should be used and the mercury bolus should be limited to 1.5 ml lest its weight interfere with guided placement. With these long tubes friction is a main difficulty. The well-lubricated tube must be forcibly 'milked' off the guide-wire into the duodenum lest the guide be trapped in the tube by additional friction from bending around the duodenal flexures. Using guided placement of a Cantor tube in 25 patients, Sargent succeeded in intubating the duodenum in all 25 and the jejunum in 11 (44%).

Double-lumen tubes like the **Miller–Abbott tube** (Figure 30.4(c)) have the advantage of a balloon which can pass through the pylorus with a mercury bolus and then be inflated with air for rapid propulsion through the small intestine. However, it is not possible to stiffen them with a guide-wire. The balloon is placed against the pylorus until peristalsis takes it through, a process taking hours or days but which is eventually successful in most patients (Smith, 1945; Deitel, 1967).

The **Medi-tech decompression tube** (Figure 30.4(d)) is an elegant version of one reported by Edlich in 1967. It is made of 16-Fr polyvinylchloride and has both end- and side-holes. It has a fine coiled spring throughout the forward end to reduce friction, a sump conduit for decompression and (optional) a doughnut-shaped terminal balloon with a conduit for inflation. It is guided by a Medi-tech 7-Fr steerable catheter which is inserted through a slit in the rear. Using his earlier tube Edlich succeeded in intubating the jejunum in less than 30 minutes in 96% of 30 cases with intestinal obstruction (Edlich et al., 1968).

Which tube is best? All these decompression tubes are large, uncomfortable and begin to stiffen after about a week as the toxic plasticizer leaches out. In a normal dog's jejunum Murata et al. (1967) found that the Cantor polyvinylchloride tube with mercury bolus progressed faster than others tested. In my experience, any tube that can be persuaded to pass the pylorus is acceptable; any tube that can be placed promptly in the jejunum is a fast tube; all tubes, once in the jejunum, proceed promptly to an obstruction.

Decompression tubes also have diagnostic value. Barium or iodinated contrast agent injected though the tube may show the site and often the nature of small intestinal obstruction; it can differentiate unequivocally between mechanical obstruction and paralytic ileus. Immediately afterwards the contrast agent can be removed by suction (Nelson and Christoferidis, 1968; Sargent and Meyers, 1969).

(c) Feeding tubes

Feeding tubes are made of polyurethane, silicone rubber or polyvinylchloride. The first two usually have a mercury bolus for passage by gravity. They have so much inherent friction that guide-wires are difficult to use, being hard to retrieve once the tube is passed. There are a number of methods for stiffening sticky tubes, all intended to overcome friction. Since frictional resistance increases with length, one way to make a stiffener retrievable is to insert it only a short distance inside the tube. A slit part way along the tube for guide insertion is one way (Figure 30.5(a)). Using the rearmost side-hole to insert it is another (Figure 30.5(b)). Once the tube is in position, the guide-wire is removed. One commercially available silicone rubber feeding tube is stiffened with an outer polyvinyl sheath (Figure 30.5(c)); once in place the feeding tube is extruded from the outer tube by a jet of water (flow-guided principle) (Griggs and Hoppe, 1979). There are several other ways to deliver feeding tubes (Figure 30.6). Silicone rubber and polyurethane tubes can be tip-connected using a gelatin capsule to a pilot tube. By cutting the ends off the capsules one can make a temporary ring-like coupler. The end-hole of the pilot tube, being free, can be passed over a guide or used for lumen seeking as described above. The capsule melts in a few minutes

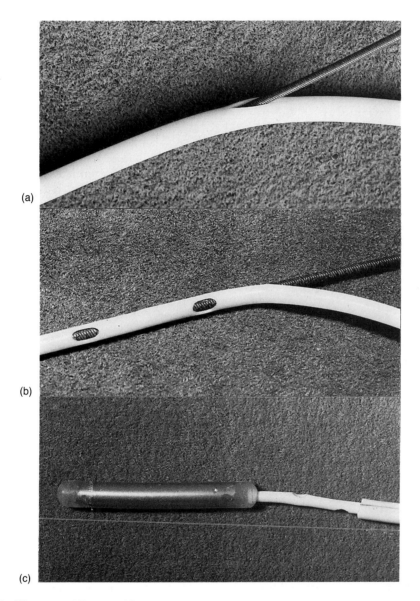

(a)

(b)

(c)

Figure 30.5 Ways to stiffen a rubbery tube (frictional resistance increases directly with length). (a) Teflon-coated guide-wire inserted through a slit 90 cm from the end of a Cantor polyvinyl tube. (b) Teflon-coated guide-wire inserted in the rearmost side-hole and advanced about 8 cm to the tip of a polyurethane feeding tube. (c) Polyvinyl 10-Fr outer sheath stiffens this mercury-weighted 5-Fr silicone rubber feeding tube. Once in place the inner catheter is extruded from the outer sheath by a jet of water (flow-guided principle).

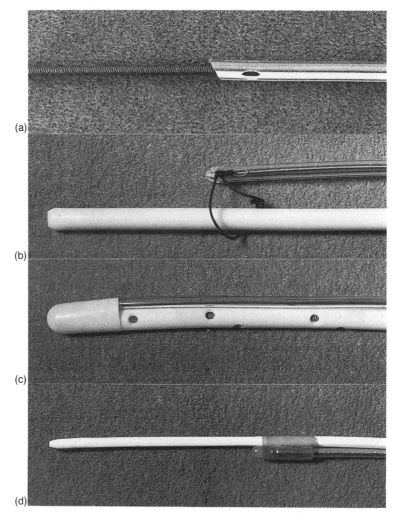

Figure 30.6   Ways to deliver a limp tube. (a) Coaxially, over a preplaced guide-wire. The tip has been cut off a polyvinychloride feeding tube. (b) Outrigged 'piggyback' style, tethered with a suture to a preplaced Bilbao–Dotter tube. The vinyl feeding tube has been stiffened with a guide-wire. (c) A polyvinylchloride feeding tube has been outrigged, jammed in half a gelatine capsule with a guide-wire stiffened Bilbao–Dotter pilot tube. (d) Silicone rubber feeding tube collared by an amputated gelatine capsule to the pilot, a steerable Medi-tech catheter. The front of the steerable catheter has been left free to move.

allowing removal of the pilot tube. Once placed, the tube should be tested for patency by injecting barium.

Some tubes designed for blind passage have been modified in recent years to be passed more easily fluoroscopically, if necessary. The **Dobbhoff** feeding tube is an excellent example. The tube is radiopaque polyurethane, which does not stiffen over time as does poly-

vinyl. It is prelubricated with a substance activated by water, and the stylet hub seats forcefully into the tube hub, thereby stretching and stiffening the tube. Contrast agent can be injected with the stylet in place. The tip is streamlined, short and scarcely larger than the tube, and flexibly weighted by a row of tungsten beads. Weights of 3 g and 7 g are available. The side-holes are situated just proximally and constructed in such a way that they cause no tendency for the tube to kink. The stylet seats smoothly and cannot exit through the side-holes. For fluoroscopic placement the biggest drawback is that the tube and stylet are sometimes not stiff enough and directable. This problem is easily corrected by substituting for the Dobbhoff stylet the much stiffer and also directable **Bilbao–Dotter guide-wire**. It fits easily and can be held in place by the tube's rear fitting. With a bend in the Bilbao–Dotter guide, the 3-g Dobbhoff tube is both directable and stiff, promptly solving many intubation problems (Bilbao and Mann, 1986).

A directable feeding tube equally or more functional than the Dobbhoff, since it is easier to clear when clogged, is the **Frederick–Miller tube**. Designed to be passed fluoroscopically, it has no weighted tip and is essentially independent of gravity. It is radiopaque polyvinyl, thin-walled and has side-holes near a smooth, closed end. It has a torque-control Teflon-coated guide-wire that is stiffer at the rear than at the front. Depending on the problem one can bend the tip of the guide to direct the tube or reverse the guide and use its stiffer rear end. In passing the tube it does not matter whether a loop or the tip leads as long as it is going in the right direction. The loop can be straightened later over the guide-wire (Miller and Sellink, 1986). Because it is polyvinyl, this tube stiffens over time and in some patients must be replaced every few weeks.

Argyle feeding tubes come in 5-Fr, 8-Fr and 10-Fr sizes. They are polyvinyl and radiopaque. They can be stiffened with a well-lubricated guide-wire but have more frictional resistance than the other tubes just mentioned.

30.4 METHODS

Premedication may make the stomach hypotonic and is best omitted except in infants where chloral hydrate is helpful. The patient normally lies supine. If the tube has a mercury weight, a 45° head-up tilt allows gravity to aid advancement.

The nasal fossa passes straight posteriorly from the nostril towards the ear. The passage is opened and gently intubated by using a nasal decongestant spray if needed and then filling it completely with a local anaesthetic agent in water-soluble lubricating jelly. Enough should be used to anaesthetize the pharynx also. While the patient widely opens his eyes (and thereby the inside of his nose), the tip of his nose is elevated and the tube passed backwards along the nasal floor with a gentle oscillating or rotational movement of the tube. During all ensuing tube advancements one should always push gently backwards and downwards, not up into the turbinates (Figure 30.7(a)).

The nasopharynx is straightened by extending the head. Although there is usually no problem intubating while the patient swallows a few sips of water, difficulties passing the pharynx may be resolved by fluoroscoping the patient in lateral view. It is then easy to advance the tube tip posteriorly past the epiglottis, even in a patient who cannot swallow. In frontal view the tube will be seen to curve laterally around the larynx. Any tube directly in the midline should be suspected of being misplaced in the trachea.

The oesophagus is more or less straight and a good place to hold the tube during insertion of a guide-wire. The tendency for the guide to exit through a hole is thus minimized (Gelfand, 1978). Before the wire is inserted, a little barium is injected into the stomach.

The gastroesophageal junction passes obliquely posterolaterally; it directs the tube into the fundus lying in the left paravertebral gutter where the tube often coils. This is avoided by first turning the patient right side down, or right prone oblique, allowing the stomach to fall toward the right, straightening the oesophagogastric junction, and directing the tube and guide towards the greater curvature (Figure 30.7(b)). Manoeuvring the tube through the pars media which passes

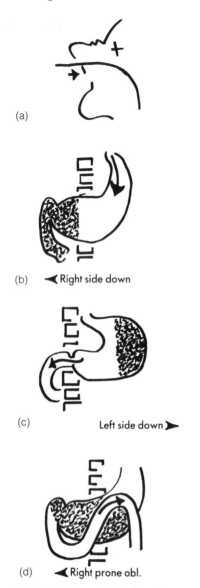

(a)

(b) ◄ Right side down

(c)

Left side down ➤

(d) ◄ Right prone obl.

Figure 30.7 Prototype intubation. Flexures in the gastrointestinal tract can be sequentially straightened in front of the advancing tube. (a) In the nose, push the tube straight back and down along the nasal floor, not up into the turbinates. (b) To pass the fundus, turn the patient to the far right lateral position. (c) To straighten the pylorus, turn the patient to the left lateral position ('lateral' means hips and shoulders). (d) To pass the duodeno-jejunal flexure at the ligament of Treitz, turn the patient to right prone oblique or right lateral position. Reproduced from Bilbao and Mann (1986) with permission.

ventrally over the spine is also aided by placing the patient right side down, injecting some barium and air to separate the walls and show the route, and inserting the stiffening wire. Rotating the tube, pushing cephalad on the greater curvature, turning the patient prone, even knee-chest or semi-upright, all help to allow the stiffened tube to fall ventrally and to the right across the spine into the antrum lying in the right paravertebral gutter. The tube now must pass cephalad and posteriorly to the pylorus. This can be aided by putting the patient supine, head down, and pushing cephalad along the greater curvature, and then turning the patient to the left supine oblique position (Figure 30.7(c)). By now barium should be showing in the pylorus which can be seen and straightened as the stomach slumps to the left. The tube is now lined up with the pylorus and pushed up and to the right of the greater curvature, shaking the stomach gently with the gloved hand as the tube advances.

Difficulties at the pylorus are usually related to poor radiological demonstration, malalignment, or the tube being impacted on a mucosal fold. The pylorus is most easily passed if it can be seen with contrast agent (a single 'end-hole' jet of contrast agent is ideal for this). Even when closed, it is not an impassable barrier. Emptying the stomach helps (Gianturco, 1967; Shipps et al., 1979), as does lining up the thrust of the tube with the presumed orifice. Often the tube tends to push adjacent to rather than against the pylorus. The patient's efforts at breathing, shaking and manoeuvring his own stomach can help here.

The superior duodenal flexure is straightened in the left supine oblique position. It is helpful to push on the patient's back behind his duodenal bulb while he alternately protrudes and retracts ('undulates') his abdomen as the tube is advanced. The inferior duodenal flexure is straightened in the left lateral position. The tube must then cross the spine again, passing anterior, left and cephalad to the duodenojejunal flexure. At the duode-nojejunal flexure the route is a hairpin-shaped bend passing anteriorly and caudally. The weight of an obese abdomen, abdominal mus-cles, pressure of the table top in the prone position and pressure from adjacent viscera all tend to keep the flexure acute. It is helpful to show the route with contrast agent, keep a little forward pressure on the tube, and try a number of manoeuvres to straighten the flex-ure long enough to allow the tube to pass. Right prone oblique position helps (Figure 30.7(d)). One can also have the patient 'belly roll' ('suck up, push forward, bear down'), or adopt the knee-chest position or its equivalent with pillows, palpate and shake his abdomen, and so on. Having him watch the fluoroscope helps. He has a strong vested interest in the success of the procedure!

30.5 SOME PARTICULAR PROBLEMS AND SOLUTIONS

Tip-weighted tubes cause difficulty when visi-bility, route and direction of tube advance-ment cannot be aligned with gravity (Figure 30.8), as in the following situations:

1. Inability to see the route except in a gravi-tationally disadvantageous position. For example, if the pylorus can be seen only with the patient on his left side, gravity will pull the tip leftward while one is try-ing to push it rightward under fluroscopic vision.
2. Inability to move the patient to align gravity optimally, as occurs, for instance, with burned or trauma patients in traction or from not having enough help present during the procedure to move and hold a helpless patient.
3. Inability to exert enough force with gravity and guide-wire combined.
4. Sometimes the optimal gravitational pos-ition causes other organs to press on the route and hold it shut. (The pylorus is seldom stenotic, and usually yields to suf-ficient force.)

5. Failure to align the pull of gravity and the direction of tube advancement so that the force vectors oppose each other.
6. Non-gravitational causes for failure in-clude atonic and/or distended stomachs, such as occur in diabetics or patients with ileus.

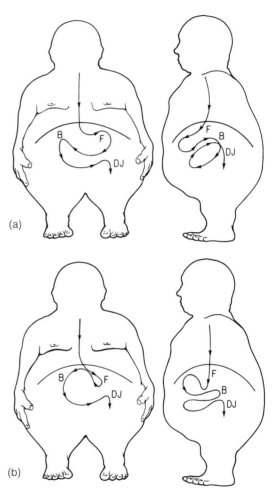

Figure 30.8 The route of a gravity-driven tip-weighted tube shown in a patient lying supine in frontal and in lateral views: (a) in the usual patient; (b) in a patient with a cascade stomach. It is necess-ary to rotate the patient and tilt the table (farther than one thinks) to make the tube tip dependent as it traverses the route. F, fundus; B, bulb: DJ, duo-denojejunal flexure. Reproduced from Bilbao and Mann (1986) with permission.

In these difficult situations it may help to vary the amount of weight at the tube tip.

Intestinal decompression tubes such as Cantor, Miller–Abbott or Dennis have multiple side-holes and on the tip a floppy balloon, which is weighted with mercury. In some tubes one can add or subtract mercury as needed; in others the balloon is sealed. Read the instructions and puncture such balloons **exactly as directed**. Otherwise, there is a risk of causing intestinal obstruction as the balloon swells with absorbed gas.

The use of a guide-wire may also help. When thoroughly lubricated, many intestinal decompression tubes will accept a guide-wire. A long guide-wire is available, or a shorter guide can be inserted through a small longitudinal slit made in the side of the tube. Again, practise *in vitro*.

30.5.1 GASTROJEJUNOSTOMY

Most Billroth II gastrojejunostomy anastomoses are antecolic, and the stoma is directly ventral to the stomach. Gravity is a liability here. It may help to turn the patient laterally (hips and shoulders), visualize the route, and use a Frederick–Miller tube and guide. Lead with a loop first, as previously mentioned. If that fails, try the Cobra method described below.

30.5.2 NARROW LUMEN

Threading a narrowed obstructed lumen is best done with a single end-hole angiography catheter with a small slightly curved tip, a 3-mm wire guide, and a Y adaptor to enable injection of contrast agent with the guide in place. To avoid perforating, **advance only where the lumen is already visibly outlined with contrast agent**. Exchange the tube afterwards for a more functional tube, either over a guide or by 'piggy-back' method.

30.5.3 BLOCKED TUBE

The piggy-back replacement method offers a simple solution for a plugged or a closed-end tube (Bilbao, 1983). Lubricate and then stiffen the new tube with an appropriate guide-wire. If possible, stiffen the old tube with a guide-wire, too. Tie securely onto the new tube's tip two or three loops of silk thread, each loop 2 cm in diameter. Tie them 2–4 cm apart. Pass these loops over the rear of the old tube, and, under fluoroscopic guidance, pass the new tube tethered by the silk loops alongside the old tube. If repeated, difficult replacements are expected, cut off the closed end of the new tube first so that the next replacement can be over a guide-wire.

30.5.4 CHILDREN

When intubating very young children, use chloral hydrate (40 mg/kg orally) to sedate the child but not his stomach. With his arms extended beside his ears, swaddle him with 12-cm wide elastic bandages to a 'brat' board, and use a Frederick–Miller tube and guide.

30.5.5 ATONIC STOMACH

In cases of atonic stomach, use metoclopramide 10–20 mg orally 30 minutes before attempting tube passage. Metoclopramide is not recommended in patients with intestinal obstruction.

30.5.6 IMMOBILE PATIENTS

In burned or orthopaedic patients who cannot be moved, gravity will be a liability. Use a Frederick–Miller tube plus water-soluble contrast agent and metoclopramide to stimulate peristalsis.

Use the Cobra catheter method for patients with atonic stomachs or for those who cannot be moved (Rosenkrantz and Healy, 1982). First, pass a soft, straight, single end-hole catheter to the fundus and exchange it over a 3-mmJ guide for a 9-Fr torcon directable Cobra catheter or a 7-Fr C2 or HIH catheter. After the catheter and guide have negotiated the duodenum, the catheter can be exchanged (over the guide) for a Frederick–Miller catheter with its end cut off.

When attempting a jejunal placement through a gastrostomy (McLean *et al.*, 1982), take out the mushroom catheter unless it has been too recently placed. Use a Cobra catheter and 3-mmJ guide. A Cook deflector and variable stiffness guide are helpful. If needed, use coaxially a stiff Teflon dilater to deflect the cant of the gastrostomy away from the fundus toward the pylorus.

30.6 COMPLICATIONS; RADIOLOGICAL MONITORING, DETECTION AND TREATMENT

Some tube complications can be prevented by radiological guidance; among them the misplaced feeding tube or the blindly advanced, knotted decompression tube. No 'blind' way to ascertain correct stomach tube placement is fool-proof. Listening over the stomach for injected air did not detect a misplaced small feeding tube in the right main bronchus of an asymptomatic patient (J. L. Rombeau, 1979, personal communication). Aspirating 'stomach' contents and listening for injected air did not detect decompression tubes passed inadvertently through basal skull fractures into the brain (Fremstad and Martin, 1976; Bouzarth, 1978; Gustavson *et al.*, 1978; Gregory *et al.*, 1978). Less spectacular, but more common, is the slightly misplaced tube with some of the side-holes above the cardia (making aspiration and reflux potential hazards). Because of the fallibility of these tests, nasogastric tube position should be checked radiographically before use in the following situations:

1. A basal skull fracture or gastrointestinal abnormality.
2. In any patient who has reduced consciousness or who is very young or very old.
3. In anyone in whom the ward tests were uncertain or whose intubation was difficult.

4. With the use of all feeding tubes, because even apparently alert patients have been unaware of feeding tubes in their lungs, mediastinum, or pleura.

Whenever chest and abdomen films are subsequently obtained during the course of the patient's care, radiologists should routinely report evidence of continued correct tube position and function. The report should include the position of the tube tip and the most rearward side-hole. A tip pointing down and on the right side of the spine in a supine film is assumed to be in the duodenum. Evidence of dysfunction, such as a stomach full of fluid or air in a patient with an enteric feeding tube or an intestinal decompression tube, should also be noted. The radiologist should routinely look for evidence of potential or actual complications, such as:

1. A tube midline behind the larynx producing cricoid ulceration. It should be repositioned laterally.
2. A tube pressing against anomalous great vessels, which may lead to fatal haemorrhage from vascular-oesophageal fistula.
3. Tube side-holes in the oesophagus or stomach, which may lead to reflux oesophagitis and aspiration pneumonia.
4. Tube loops in the fundus, which may lead to knot formation.
5. A tube tip protruding against the gut wall, which may lead to ulceration and perforation, especially in infants.
6. A kinked or knotted tube.
7. Perforated gastrointestinal tract producing an anatomically inconsistent tube pathway, perhaps pleural effusions, mediastinal widening, or air in tissue planes.
8. An enlarging balloon of an intestinal decompression tube, which may lead to obstruction.

Some tube complications can be treated with radiological guidance. Obstructed feeding tubes can sometimes be cleared with guide-wires. If this fails, they can be replaced using the 'piggyback' catheter exchange system already described. Long tubes tied into knots in the stomach can sometimes be untied by judicious manoeuvring under fluoroscopy. The manoeuvres used depend on individual circumstances, but useful principles include making the tube radiopaque enough to be clearly visible fluoroscopically, reducing friction with silicone, and using guide-wires or piggyback stiffeners to aid control of the tube. Catheter fragments in the jejunum can be snared via a guideable long intestinal tube (Bilbao, Krippachne and Dotter, 1971). Since 1971 improved equipment has become available, such as the Medi-tech catheter, stone retrieval baskets and snares developed for vascular catheters. A tube complication readily treated under radiological guidance is gaseous distention of the balloon of a single-lumen long intestinal tube (Rozanski and Klenfeld, 1975; Fricke and Niewodowski, 1976). This complication may occur after prolonged intubation of 10 days days or more and may cause intestinal obstruction. The balloon can be easily and safely decompressed percutaneously using a Chiba 22 gauge 'skinny' needle (Coleman et al., 1977).

In summary, because of fluoroscopic, anatomical and technical skills, the radiologist is uniquely able to place tubes safely and gently where they are most needed and to shorten intubation time and hospital stays. A knowledge of fluoroscopic anatomy and having skills with a range of tube methods are the keys to success.

REFERENCES

Bilbao, M. K. (1983) Interventional radiology of the GI tract, in I: Alimentary Tract Radiology (eds A. R. Margulis and H. J. Burhenne), C. V. Mosby, St Louis, pp. 2283–99.

Bilbao, M. K. and Dotter, C. T. (1975) Reflux cholangiography in sphincteroplasty or enterobiliary anastomosis. Radiology, 115, 585–8.

Bilbao, M. K. et al. (1975) Small bowel biopsy by coaxial catheter. Radiology, 116, 199–201.

Bilbao, M. K. et al. (1967) Hypotomic duodenography. Radiology, 89, 438–43.

Bilbao, M. K., Krippaehne, W. W. and Dotter, C. T. (1971) Catheter retrieval of a foreign body from the gastrointestinal tract. Am. J. Roentg. Radiat. Ther. Nucl. Med., 111, 473–5.

Bilbao, M. K. et al. (1968) Hypotonic duodenography in the diagnosis of pancreatic disease. Semin. Roentgenol., 3, 280–7.

Bilbao, M. K. and Mann, F. A. (1986) Gastrointestinal intubation, in Radiology, vol. 4 (eds J. M. Taveras and J. T. Ferucci), J. B. Lippincott, Philadelphia, ch. 7, pp. 1–10.

Bouzarth, W. F. (1978) Intracranial nasogastric tube insertion. (Editorial.) J. Trauma, 18, 818–9.

Coleman, S. L. et al. (1977) Nonoperative retrieval of an impacted long intestinal tube. Am. J. Dig. Dis., 22, 462–4.

Cowper, S. G. (1968) What's in PVC? (letter to editor). Lancet, ii, 221.

Deitel, M. (1967) Successful use of the Miller–Abbott tube. Can. J. Surg., 10, 245–57.

Dodds, W. J. et al. (1976) Use of steerable catheter for intubating patients with Zencker's diverticulum. Am. J. Dig. Dis., 21, 47–8.

Duke, H. N. and Vane, J. R. (1968) An adverse effect of polyvinylchloride tubing used in extracorporeal circulation. Lancet, ii, 21–3.

Editorial (1975) PVC, plasticizers and the pediatrician. Lancet, ii, 1172.

Edlich, R. F. et al. (1968). New long intestinal tube for rapid nonoperative intubation. Arch. Surg., 95, 443–50.

Fremstad, J. D. and Martin, S. H. (1976) Lethal complication from insertion of nasogastric tube after severe basilar skull fracture. J. Trauma, 18, 820–2.

Fricke, F. J. and Niewodowski, M. A. (1976) Hazardous gaseous distension of intestinal balloons. JAMA, 235, 2611–3.

Gelfand, D. W. (1978) An easy method for passing an intestinal intubation tube under fluoroscopic guidance. Radiology, 129, 532.

Gianturco, C. (1967) Rapid fluoroscopic duodenal intubation. Radiology, 88, 1165–6.

Gregory, J. A., Turner, P. T. and Reynolds, A. F. (1978) A complication of nasogastric intubation: intracranial penetration. J. Trauma, 18, 823–4.

Griggs, B. A. and Hoppe, M. C. (1979) Nasogastric tube feeding. Am. J. Nurs., 3, 481–5.

Gustavson, S. et al. (1978) The accidental introduction of a nasogastric tube into the brain. Acta Chir. Scand., 144, 55–6.

Harris, P. D., Newhauser, E. B. D. and Gerth, R. (1964) The osmotic effect of water soluble contrast media on circulating plasma volume. Am. J. Roentgenol. Radiat. Ther. Nucl. Med., 91, 694.

Ho, C. S. and Lipinski, J. K. (1978) Selective intubation of the afferent loop. *Am. J. Roentgenol. Radiat. Ther. Nucl. Med.*, **130**, 481–4.

Linscheer, W. G. and Abele, J. E. (1976) A new directable small bowel biopsy device. *Gastroenterology*, **71**, 575–6.

MacIntosh, R., Muskin, W. W. and Epstein, H. G. (1963) *Physics for the Anesthesiologist*, 3rd edn, F. A. Davis, Philadelphia, pp. 157–237.

McLean, G., Rombeau, J. and Caldwell, M. *et al.* (1982) Transgastrostomy jejunal intubation for enteric alimentation. *Am. J. Roentgenol. Radiat. Ther. Nucl. Med.*, **139**, 1129–33.

Miller, R. and Sellink, J. (1979) Enteroclysis, the small bowel enema. *Gastrointest. Radiol.*, **4**, 269–83.

Murata, A. *et al.* (1967) The rate of progression of long intestinal tubes in a dog with jejunal fistula. *Am. J. Dig. Dis.*, **12**, 1091–4.

Nelson, S. W. (1965) Facts versus folklore. *Am. J. Surg.*, **109**, 543.

Nelson, S. W. and Christoferidis, A. J. (1968) The use of barium sulfate suspensions in the diagnosis of acute disease of the small intestine. *Am. J. Roentgenol. Radiat. Ther. Nucl. Med.*, **104**, 505–21.

Rosenkrantz, H. and Healy, J. (1982) Rapid placement of small bowel tubes using modified angiographic techniques and equipment. *Radiology*, **143**, 564.

Rozanski, J. and Kleinfeld, M. (1975) A complication of prolonged intestinal intubation: gaseous distention of the terminal balloon. *Dig. Dis.*, **20**, 1067–70.

Sargent, E. N. and Meyers, H. I. (1969) Wire guide and technique for Cantor tube insertion: rapid small bowel intubation. *Am. J. Roentgenol. Radiat. Ther. Nucl. Med.*, **107**, 150–5.

Sellink, J. L. (1971) *Examination of the Small Intestine by Means of Duodenal Intubation*, H. E. Stenfert Kroese, Leiden.

Shipps, F. C. *et al.* (1979) Fluoroscopic placement of intestinal tubes. *Radiology*, **132**, 226–7.

Smith, B. C. (1945) Experiences with the Miller-Abbott tube. *Ann. Surg.*, **122**, 253–9.

Wendth, A. J. *et al.* (1973) Hypotonic duodenography; a modified technique using the selector catheter system. *Radiology*, **108**, 274.

Intubation equipment and suppliers

Medications

Item	Purpose, remarks	Suppliers
1.4% Adrenaline	Shrink nasal mucosa	Winthrop Laboratories, USA
2% Viscous lignocaine (lidocaine)	Topical anaesthetic agent, anaesthetizes and lubricates nasal mucosa	Astra Pharmaceutical, USA
Cetacaine spray	Pharyngeal anaesthetic agent	Cetylite Industries, USA
Silicone spray	Tube and guide lubricant spray. Can also be injected into and outside the tube	Dow Corning, USA
Elemental mercury	Decompression tube balloon. Follow instructions packaged with tube!!	Hospital pharmacy
Barium	GI visualization	
Renografin-60, gastrografin	GI visualization, stimulates peristalsis	ER Squibb & Sons, USA
Metoclopramide hydrochloride	GI visualization, stimulates peristalsis. Give 10 mg p.o. 30 min before or 10 mg i.v. immediately before intubation	As Reglan, A. H. Robins, USA
Alcohol	Clean tubing and patient before taping	
Tincture of benzoin	Apply to tube and patient before taping	
Chloral hydrate syrup 100 mg/ml	Sedate small children. Give 40 mg/kg p.o.	McKesson Laboratories, USA
Empty gelatin capsules	Temporary tube attachment	Pharmacy

Tubes and tubing

Item	Material*	Size (Fr)	Length (cm)	Side ports (no.)	Tip	Purpose	Supplier
Nasal topical anaesthesia tube	PV	14	15	0	metal end hole	Nasopharyngeal anaesthesia	Homemade
Bilbao–Dotter	PV	14	125	6	Closed end	Hyptonic duodenography	Cook, USA
Bilbao–Dotter	PV	14	125	6	Open end		Cook
Oregon Intestinal biopsy set	PV	14	125	12	Open end	Suction biopsy	Cook
Bilbao–Dotter	PV	14	125	0	Open end	Ad hoc fabrication	Cook
Bilbao–Dotter Nolan modification	PV	12	135	6	Closed end	Enteroclysis	Cook
Bilbao–Dotter: Herlinger modification	PV	14	135	0	Open end	Enteroclysis	Cook
Bilbao–Dotter	PV	12	135	0	Open end	Enteroclysis, ad hoc fabrication	Cook
Frederick–Miller	PV	8	110	3	Closed end	Feeding tube	Cook
Dobbhoff no. 14-7160	PU	8	43	2	7-g tungsten	Feeding tube	Biosearch Med Products, USA
Dobbhoff no. 14-7230	PU	8	43	2	3-g tungsten	Feeding tube directable with bent Bilbao–Dotter guide	Biosearch Med Products
Keofeed feeding tube	SR	6–18	92		Mercury bolus		Hedeco, USA
Medpro feeding tube	SR	10, 7	92		Closed end		Medpro, USA
Argyle feeding tube	PV	5, 8, 10	92		Closed end		Sherwood Medical, USA
Cantor decompression tube	PV	16, 12	247, 183		Balloon	Decompression	Clay Adams of Beckton, USA

Tubes and tubing

Item	Material*	Size (Fr)	Length (cm)	Side ports (no.)	Tip	Purpose	Supplier
Shipps decompression tube	PV	14	228		Closed end	Decompression	Cook, USA
Medi-tech intestinal decompression tube	PV	18	247		Balloon	Steerable catheter placement	Medi-tech Cooper Scientific, USA
Medi-tech steerable catheters	PV	13, 10, 8, 7	30–170		Directable	Multipurpose	Medi-tech
Medi-tech biopsy set		10	150		Biopsy capsule		Medi-tech
Assorted silicone rubber tubing							
Polyethylene angiography		9F	150		Cobra-shaped open end	To be exchanged over wire guide after placement	Cook
Polyethylene		7F	125		C2 or HIH		
		8.2F	125		Cobra-shaped open end	To be exchanged over wire guide after placement	Cook

*PV, polyvinylchloride; PU, polyurethane; SR, silicone rubber.

Wire guides

Item	Size (in)	Length (cm)	Purpose, remarks	Supplier
Angiography wire guides, fixed core	0.052 3 mmJ	400 3 mmJ	Fits 9-Fr cobra catheter for exchange or wire guide	Cook, USA
Frederick–Miller wire guide	0.045	145	Teflon-coated torque control hubless	Cook
	0.065	125	Teflon-coated torque control with hub	
Gianturco	0.095	125		
Bilbao–Dotter Nolan modification	0.065	135	For 12-Fr enteroclysis tube	Cook
Sargent	0.065	345	Use with intestinal decompression tubes	Cook
Gianturco wire guide	0.095	345	Use with intestinal decompression tubes	Cook
	0.065	345	Hubless for catheter exchange	Cook
	0.095	345	Hubless for catheter exchange	Cook

Connectors, accessories, miscellaneous items

Item	Purpose, remarks	Supplier
Side-arm fitting	Closes flow around wire guide during contrast injections	Cook, USA
Assorted suture silk and suture set	Piggyback loop method	
Hole punch, flaring tool 1.14 mm, 0.45	Ad hoc fabrication	
Iris scissors	Ad hoc fabrication	
Gauze 4 × 4 s, no cotton filling	Traction on slippery tubes	
Elastic bandage, 15 cm wide	Immobilizing infants	
Brat boart	Immobilizing infants	
Fluoroscope		
Tilting table		
Shoulder braces		
Foot board		
Lead gloves		
Lead shield on table top	Protects operator's hands during pharyngeal intubation under fluoroscopy	

CHAPTER THIRTY-ONE

Endoscopic tube insertion

C. J. Mitchell

31.1 INTRODUCTION

It is usually not difficult to intubate the stomach or rectum without endoscopic or radiological guidance. Nursing staff regularly pass nasogastric or flatus tubes without supervision and only rare mishaps occur. Similarly, trained nursing staff encounter little difficulty in accurately positioning tubes for gastric function tests or enteral feeding unaided except for confirmation of the position. The time required for adequate training is amply rewarded by savings in medical time and endoscopic or radiological resources. Endoscopists and radiologists have perhaps become overzealous in their use of the techniques available for tube placement and should first stop to consider whether their involvement is necessary.

Some advocate guided tube placement because it is faster and less unpleasant for the patient. However, many patients find the operator's manipulations which cause movement of the tube in the oropharynx a most unpleasant sensation, and prefer to swallow the tube themselves with a little encouragement. They may then rest quietly in an appropriate position until the tube reaches its destination. The position of the tube can be quickly checked radiologically and often reaches the duodenum in 60 minutes or so. Any initial retching rapidly settles when the tube is not being externally manipulated. This 'passive' method of intubation is a better start to a function test and obviates the need for administration of drugs which may themselves affect the test results. Personal experience of a considerable number of function tests performed in this way is that the tube is better tolerated and less likely to move during the test period, which is a prerequisite for a valid test result. Incorrect tube positioning or displacement is the major cause of test failures and occurs in up to 10% of cases with even experienced operators performing a pancreatic function test (Mitchell, 1981).

The principle is to keep intubation simple wherever possible and to avoid the temptation to overelaborate.

31.2 INDICATIONS FOR GUIDED TUBE PLACEMENT

Whilst a substantial proportion of intubations do not require guidance, there is a variety of situations in which unguided intubation is inappropriate. Some specialized units in which guided tube placement is the rule rather than the exception have often developed more specialized techniques (Mathus-Vliegen and Tytgat, 1983).

The main indications for guided tube placement include:

1. **Failure of 'blind' intubation.** The reasons for this include those discussed below. Many others come under the loose category of the 'uncooperative' patient. The patient may be too ill to help or is semi-comatose, but more often is apprehensive or frightened, in which case explanation and reassurance are of more

use than 10 mg of diazepam. In other instances the tube may have been passed but confirmation of its correction position is required.

2. An **obstructing lesion**, such as stenosis or neoplasm, where the risk of perforation contraindicates a blind intubation.
3. **Previous surgery.** Correct placing of a tube beyond the stomach in patients with, for example, a gastroenterostomy is often difficult and some form of guidance will be required. It is also unwise to contemplate unguided tube placement in patients who have recently had surgery involving the route of the tube.
4. **Variant anatomy** – such as a diverticulum, incarcerated hiatus hernia or a prominent prepyloric fold.
5. If a **coexistent procedure** is indicated, such as diagnostic endoscopy or radiology, it is a pity not to take the opportunity to place a tube. The opportunity to place aspiration or feeding tubes at operation should not be missed.
6. Where **precise siting** of a tube is needed then endoscopic and radiological confirmation of its position is required. This particularly applies to double-lumen tubes for a secretin-pancreozymin test or an enteral feeding tube. Frequently a check plain radiograph or screening will suffice but the tube may need to be screened or watched into position.
7. Where there is a **danger of aspiration**, particularly when the swallowing or gag reflexes are impaired or vocal cord paresis is present.
8. The intubation of **more remote sites**. To pass tubes through the sigmoid flexure is most safely carried out under guidance because of the risk of perforation.
9. In some situations, **speed of intubation** is paramount. This category includes the critically ill and those at immediate risk of aspiration or perforation.

31.3 ENDOSCOPIC OR RADIOLOGICAL GUIDANCE

There is no inherent superiority for either method, although the performance of a simultaneous endoscopic or radiological procedure may determine the choice. In terms of safety there is little to choose between endoscopy and radiological guidance except in a few circumstances. The unavailability of a small calibre ('paediatric') endoscope to negotiate a stenosed segment would tilt the balance towards a radiological procedure using narrow calibre instrumentation. Conversely, if a patient required frequent reintubation consideration would be given to the cumulative radiation exposure – although this can be reduced by using an image intensifier – remembering particularly that such patients might already have undergone a considerable number of other radiological investigations. This applies to patients requiring long-term enteral feeding, since up to 50% of feeding tubes become misplaced (Keohane, Attrill and Silk, 1983). Although guided procedures are difficult to cost, there is probably little to choose between endoscopy or radiology since the equipment required will be available to either department. The choice will usually depend upon more mundane considerations, including the geographical location of the patient and the respective departments, staff or equipment availability and the relative expertise and enthusiasm of the endoscopist or radiologist. In complicated situations the two techniques are complementary. If the patient cannot be easily transported from the ward (e.g. those on a ventilator or traction), endoscopic guidance is preferable since it is easier to bring the endoscopic trolley to the bedside (Pleatman and Nannheim, 1987). Review of the author's personal experience shows no advantage in either endoscopic or radiological tube guidance (Table 31.1). The choice of technique is normally governed by practical considerations.

Table 31.1 Results of tube placement

	'Blind'			Endoscopic			Radiological		
	Total	Failed	Comps.	Total	Failed	Comps.	Total	Failed	Comps.
Nasogastric tubes	78	4	1	14	0	0	3	1	0
Gastric function tests	36	6	0	9	1	0	—	—	—
Pancreatic function tests	126	8	1	17	2	0	4	2	0
Jejunal biopsy and aspiration	29	5	0	69	1	0	8	0	0
Enteral feeding tubes	43	2	5	14	0	0	7	2	0

Failures of 'blind' intubation are included in other columns.
Comps. = complications.

31.4 INSTRUMENTS AND EQUIPMENT

Endoscopes are expensive, so that most of us have to adapt our methods to the equipment available. Nevertheless, most units have a large-channel (3.7/4.2 mm) instrument, a paediatric and an oblique viewing endoscope. The former are best for insertion of fine-bore feeding tubes via the biopsy channel. A paediatric endoscope is preferred to pass a large calibre (e.g. aspiration) tube alongside the endoscope because there is less friction between them; it can also be used initially to negotiate a stenosing lesion, perhaps with a balloon dilator in front to ease the passage. An oblique viewing endoscope has two advantages; first the angled field of view makes visualization of the tip of the tube easier so that it does not have to be so far in advance of the endoscope, and secondly the bridge enables more precise manoeuvring of the tube in difficult situations. A side-viewing instrument is rarely used (except for pancreatic juice collection) but may help intubate an awkwardly placed or very scarred pylorus and duodenal bulb or the loops of a retrogastric anastomosis.

For all endoscopic intubation procedures, adequate lubrication of the tube to be inserted is most important – whilst it helps during introduction, it is even more important during endoscopic withdrawal which is the time at which most tubes will become displaced. Both water-miscible lubricating jellies and silicone (as fluid and aerosol) should be available for application to tubes, endoscope casings and biopsy channels.

There is a considerable variety of tubes available for each procedure. Most operators have their own favourites and many of these will be homemade or modifications of commercially available equipment. The use of stiffeners (well lubricated) even for quite inflexible tubes is a great aid to manoeuvrability, although the increased potential for perforation should be borne in mind. The simplest stiffener is a pair of biopsy forceps whose jaws can be held open during intubation to maintain the position within the tube (thus allowing smaller calibre forceps to be used). Some tubes have their own introducer or a flexible-tipped guide-wire can be employed. Finally we are indebted to the radiologists, especially angiographers, who now have a large variety of tubes, introducers and guide-wires available of which most endoscopists are unaware. Consultation and advice from a radiologist before tackling a difficult intubation can be invaluable.

31.5 PATIENT PREPARATION

Preparation of the patient is as described for a routine endoscopy (Chapter 1). The major hazard is aspiration in an inadequately fasted patient. A clear explanation of the procedure to the patient is not only good medical practice but also renders the patient less apprehensive and more cooperative – it also obviates or reduces the need for medication. Intravenous sedation without premedication or local anaesthetic spray is preferable, since a common request after the procedure is for fluid (where appropriate). If sedation is contraindicated then a lignocaine spray may be used. Intravenous buscopan, or occasionally glucagon is helpful in negotiating a spastic pylorus and duodenum but the experienced endoscopist rarely requires it. For function test intubations no parenteral drug should be administered, but pharyngeal anaesthesia may be used.

31.6 TUBE PLACEMENT TECHNIQUES

There are two basic options.

31.6.1 THROUGH THE BIOPSY CHANNEL OF THE ENDOSCOPE

The tube may be passed through the biopsy channel of the endoscope. Limitations of this technique are the biopsy channel diameter and, in the presence of a stenotic lesion, the size of endoscope which can be passed. Most units will now possess a large channel (3.7-mm) endoscope, if not a therapeutic (4.2-mm channel) instrument, either of which comfortably accommodates a fine-bore feeding tube. It is desirable that there is some tolerance between the diameter of the biopsy channel and the tube to be inserted in order to minimize the chance of tube displacement during endoscope withdrawal. The technique is simple and increasingly familiar to endoscopists as it is analogous to that used for guide-wire insertion prior to oesophageal dilatation. The endoscope is manoeuvred to the desired position and the tube to be placed (well lubricated and over twice the length of the endoscope) is passed down the biopsy channel and the tip positioned under direct vision. After

careful measurement of the protruding tube with reference to a fixed point, the endoscope is withdrawn over the tube left in its correct position. The tube's tendency to be pulled out of position by the endoscope can be diminished in two ways; a thin, lubricated wire can be left inside the tube until the endoscope has been withdrawn, or suction can be applied to the proximal end of the tube so that it adheres tightly to the mucosa. Alternatively, if the tube to be passed is too large for the biopsy channel, a guide-wire alone can be passed and the tube passed over this after the endoscope has been withdrawn (Kautz, Kohaus and Langhans, 1981; Mathus-Vliegen and Tytgat, 1983). If the tube to be inserted cannot be longer than the endoscope, it can be 'back loaded' up the biopsy channel and maintained in position by extruding it with a pair of forceps pushed antegradely down the biopsy channel during endoscope withdrawal (Stiegmann and Pearlman, 1986).

'Through-the-scope' tubes inserted by a colonoscope have been used for radiological retrograde studies of the terminal ileum (Frimberger, 1987; Whorwell, Maxton and Martin, 1988).

31.6.2 ALONGSIDE AN ENDOSCOPE

The tube may be passed alongside an endoscope, either together or in succession, when the tube is of larger calibre. The major problem to be overcome is the friction between the two tubes, particularly during endoscope withdrawal, which is lessened by the use of an introducer or stiffener. A variety of techniques have been described but commonly the tube is carried down alongside the endoscope using a pair of biopsy grasping forceps or a snare protruding from the biopsy channel to hold the end of the tube to be positioned; the forceps can either be used to grasp the tube itself or be inserted into an aspiration hole and held open during insertion. 'Alligator' or 'rat tooth' forceps may be better than standard biopsy forceps. This may damage the tube during placement and other techniques are described.

The method described 15 years ago by Keller (1973) using a nylon line passed through the biopsy channel and attached externally to the tube to draw it down alongside the endoscope into position had several problems. Atkinson, Walford and Allison (1979) inserted fine-bore feeding tubes by grasping the distal end with forceps and withdrawing the tip into the biopsy channel prior to introduction of the whole assembly. Suture material can be tied to the tube tip and the loose ends grasped by forceps to carry the tube down or to manoeuvre it into position (Tympner and Rosch, 1974; Meissner and Weissenhofer, 1978). Others have used a slip knot to tie the tube and endoscope together distally, enabling release of the tube after successful delivery (Siu, Lee and Wong, 1984).

31.7 NOTES ON INDIVIDUAL TECHNIQUES

31.7.1 INSERTION OF SENGSTAKEN–BLAKEMORE OR LINTON TUBES

These tubes can usually be passed blindly, but if bleeding varices are discovered at endoscopy, it is as easy to pass the tube at that time and check the position visually after inflation. Furthermore, if active bleeding is occurring during sclerotherapy the use of a Linton tube with manual traction by an assistant can facilitate the procedure. These tubes have been traditionally kept in a refrigerator prior to use to render them stiffer, but it is just as easy to stiffen them with narrow calibre forceps.

31.7.2 INSERTION OF NASOGASTRIC ASPIRATION TUBES

The requirement for guidance is unusual except as previously indicated (section 31.2). The tube must aspirate properly so that the largest calibre consistent with comfort should be used; the side-holes may be enlarged for function testing. The position for routine gastric aspiration is checked by auscultation during injection of air. For function testing, the water recovery test (Findlay, Prescott and Sircus, 1972) is preferable and whilst the exact position of the tube is claimed to be unimportant (Hassan and Hobsley, 1971), the test is usually less troublesome when the tube is in the gastric fundus, the patient lying on the left side and slightly head down.

31.7.3 INSERTION OF TUBES FOR PANCREATIC FUNCTION TESTS

The type of tube used depends upon the test being performed. The double-lumen Dreiling tube is the best available commercially for direct stimulation (secretin ± pancreozymin) tests, although specialist centres often employ homemade versions; complete separation of gastric from duodenal contents is vital for accurate results, so the tube must be positioned correctly. Guidance is routinely used and usually performed radiologically, but endoscopic positioning is equally effective employing the general techniques previously described (Tympner and Rosch, 1974). Intubation for the Lundh test requires a single-lumen weighted tube; many tubes can be introduced passively with a radiological check of position.

31.7.4 INSERTION OF FEEDING TUBES

The use of large-bore feeding tubes is associated with an unacceptable incidence of complications (Jones, 1986). Fine-bore tubes are the best choice but, although perforation is rare, these tubes are more likely to be misplaced (Bastow, 1986) or become displaced (Keohane, Attrill and Silk, 1983) and their calibre prevents aspiration being used to check position. Guidance is needed when blind intubation fails or is contraindicated. Endoscopic methods of guidance have been described previously and recently reviewed (Rives et al., 1989). The details are available elsewhere, including introduction of tubes alongside the endoscope (Pleatman and Nannheim, 1987) using forceps or retrograde insertion (Atkinson, Walford and Allison, 1979; Keohane, Attrill and Silk, 1983) or a suture (Meissner and Weissenhoffer, 1976), directly down the biopsy channel (Mann *et al.*, 1984; Gallo *et al.*, 1985) and over an endoscopically inserted guide-wire (Kautz, Kohaus and Langhans, 1981; Mathus-Vliegen and Tytgat, 1983), or using a biopsy brush to push the tube out of the endoscope (Stiegmann and Pearlman, 1985). Inserting the feeding tube with a stiffener or guide-wire down the biopsy channel minimizes the possibility of tube displacement during withdrawal.

31.7.5 INSERTION OF DECOMPRESSION TUBE

These are large-calibre tubes so must be passed alongside the endoscope. For the small bowel the main limitation in placement is that of endoscope length, but endoscopists who practise ERCP can usually progress further after 'shortening' the endoscope and peristalsis often takes the tube further. Alternatively, a paediatric colonoscope may be used because of its greater length. A balloon catheter may be successfully passed with the decompression tube and then inflated to enable peristalsis to propel the tube further down the small bowel; after the correct position is shown fluoroscopically the balloon catheter may be deflated and withdrawn. For colonic decompression the tube is passed under direct colonoscopic vision to the desired site. The colon in such circumstances is usually fragile and friable so that great care is required.

31.7.6 TUBE INSERTION IN THE PRESENCE OF A STRICTURE

Most strictures will have been dilated prior to tube insertion so that at least a paediatric endoscope can be passed. If this is not the case, the dilatation can be combined with passage of a feeding tube using a coaxial endoscopic balloon dilator preceding the tube. This technique has been used to pass a feeding tube through a stenotic segment of duodenal Crohn's disease.

REFERENCES

Atkinson, M., Walford S. and Allison (1979) Endoscopic insertion of fine-bore feeding tubes. *Lancet*, **ii**, 829.

Bastow, M. D. (1986) Complications of enteral nutrition. *Gut*, **27**, (S1), 51–5.

Findlay, J. M., Prescott, R. J. and Sircus, W. (1972) Comparative evaluation of water recovery test and fluoroscopic screening in positioning a nasogastric tube during gastric secretory studies. *Br. Med. J.*, **4**, 458.

Frimberger, E. (1987) Balloon probe for the colonoscopic small intestinal enema. *Endoscopy*, **19**, 169–70.

Gallo, S., Ramirez, A., Elizondo, J. *et al.* (1985) Endoscopic placement of enteral feeding tubes. *J. Parent. Enter. Nutr.*, **9**, 747–9.

Hassan, M. A. and Hobsley, M. (1971) The accurate assessment of maximal acid secretion in control subjects and in patients with duodenal ulcer. *Br. J. Surg.* **58**, 171–6.

Jones, B. J. M. (1986) Enteral feeding: techniques of administration. *Gut*, **27**, (S1), 47–50.

Kautz, G., Kohaus, H. and Langhans (1981) Endoscopic insertion of feeding tubes: a new method for the management of upper digestive tract stenosis. *Endoscopy*, **13**, 121–3.

Keller, R. T. (1973) A technique of intestinal intubation with the fibreoptic endoscope. *Gut*, **14**, 143.

Keohane, P. P., Attrill, H. and Silk, D. B. A. (1983) Endoscopic placement of fine bore nasogastric and nasoenteric feeding tubes. *Clin. Nutr.*, **1**, 245–6.

Mann, N. S., Nair, P. K., Mann, S. K. *et al.* (1984) Nasoenteral feeding tube insertion via fibreoptic endoscope for enteral hyperalimentation. *J. Am. Coll. Nutr.*, **3**, 333–9.

Mathus-Vliegen, E. M. H. and Tytgat, G. N. J. (1983) The role of endoscopy in the correct and rapid positioning of feeding tubes. *Endoscopy*, **15**, 78–84.

Meissner, K. and Weissenhofer, W. (1978) The effective placement of Miller–Abbott tubes under endoscopic guidance. *Endoscopy*, **10**, 13–6.

Mitchell, C. J. (1981) *Pancreatic Disease in Clinical Practice*, Pitman Medical, London.

Pleatman, M. A. and Nannheim, K. S. (1987) Endoscopic placement of feeding tubes in the critically ill patient. *Surg. Gynecol. Obstet.*, **165**, 69–70.

Rives, D. A., LeRoy, J. L., Hawkins, M. L. and Bowden, T. A. (1989) Endoscopically assisted nasojejunal feeding tube placement. *Am. Surg.*, **55**, 88–91.

Siu, K. F., Lee, N. W. and Wong, J. (1984) A simple method of endoscopy – guided insertion of naso-gastric tubes. *Endoscopy*, **16**, 24–5.

Stiegmann, G. V. and Pearlman, N. W. (1986) Simplified endoscopic placement of nasoenteral feeding tubes. *Gastrointest. Endosc.*, **32**, 349–50.

Tympner, F. and Rösch, W. (1974) Pancreatic function test in patients with Bilroth II resection with the end of an endoscope. *Endoscopy*, **6**, 245–8.

Whorwell, P. J., Maxton, D. G. and Martin, D. F. (1988) Post-colonoscopic retrograde ileography. *Lancet*, **i**, 738–9.

CHAPTER THIRTY-TWO

Colonoscopic polypectomy

J. D. Waye

32.1 THE RATIONALE OF COLONOSCOPIC POLYPECTOMY

'Polyp' is a term used to describe any protuberance on the surface of a mucous membrane. Polyps may be inflammatory, neoplastic or non-neoplastic, but the final determination of the nature of a polyp rests on its proper histopathological identification. A classification scheme for colonic and rectal tumours is presented in Figure 32.1. The majority of colonic polyps are adenomas, or non-malignant neoplasms, and only approximately 5% of colonoscopically removed adenomas are found to have invasive malignancy (Muto, Bussey and Morson, 1975; Gillespie *et al.*, 1979; Shinya and Wolff, 1979).

Polypectomy interrupts the well-established 'adenoma–carcinoma sequence' (Konishi and Morson, 1982). Current opinion holds that in the absence of polyps, carcinoma does not occur in the non-colitic colon (Fung and Goldman, 1970; Fenoglio and Lane, 1974; Kurzon, Ortega and Rywlin, 1974; Muto, Bussey and Morson, 1975; Morson, 1976; Spjut and Estrada, 1977). Although it is not necessary to remove non-neoplastic polyps, the true histopathology will not be correctly determined until the entire specimen has been examined in the pathology laboratory. Biopsy of polyps is not considered worthwhile since the small pieces of tissue may not accurately represent the histopathology from the entire polyp (Livestone, Troncale and Sheahan, 1977). Any polyp encountered during colonoscopic examination should be removed, since the endoscopist cannot reliably assess a polyp's histology on visual impression alone (Ameri-

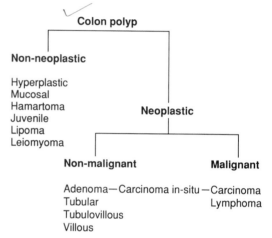

Figure 32.1 Classification scheme for colonic and rectal tumours.

can Society for Gastrointestinal Endoscopy, 1980). Once a polyp is encountered, it is unfair to the patient, placing them at additional risk (not to mention the increased discomfort), to require another colon preparation and endoscopic examination to remove colon polyps. So it is the responsibility of the colonoscopist to have the capability and equipment available to remove polyps as they are encountered during 'diagnostic' colonoscopy. Cost-benefit considerations preclude performing colonoscopy in a setting where the capability for polypectomy is not available.

Inspection of the entire colon must be performed whenever an adenoma is discovered, since 50% of patients with one adenoma will have another (Fox *et al.*, 1981; Fruhmorgen, Laudage and Matek, 1981). The most efficient method for discovering the synchronous polyp is to perform a total colonoscopic examination on each patient, but if this is not technically feasible, a barium enema can usually demonstrate the non-visualized portion of the colon (Williams, Macrae and Bartram, 1982).

32.2 PREPARATION AND SAFEGUARDS

Good patient care requires that the patient be informed of the major risks of colonoscopy. These are:

- Medication reaction.
- Bleeding.
- Perforation.

Infection occurs so rarely following polypectomy that this is not a topic which need be discussed. However, the major and common complications should be detailed for the patient. Alternative therapies should be discussed, and a record should be made that these discussions were held. Advances in endoscopic instrumentation and techniques have rendered obsolete the use of barium studies to monitor polyps and our knowledge of the adenoma–carcinoma sequence makes it unwise to ignore the potential risk of carcinoma developing within a colonic adenoma. Risk disclosures need not be made in a manner threatening to the patient, but should be presented fairly and factually. The likelihood of the patient requiring surgery after colonoscopic polypectomy is, of course, considerably less than the risk of having surgery if the patient were to have an exploratory laparotomy. Death following colonoscopic polyp removal is extremely unusual, whereas the mortality from surgical colon resection ranges from 0.5% to 2%. The alternatives to endoscopic polypectomy are to do nothing, to have surgical polypectomy or to follow polyps radiographically.

To reduce the incidence of complications during polypectomy, the colon should be prepared in such a manner that explosive levels of gases are not present (Nagy, 1981), by avoiding the use of fermentable sugars such as mannitol and cleansing the colon of bacteria and faecal matter. Carbon dioxide colonic insufflation, once thought necessary for avoidance of spark-induced explosion, is now considered optional with most endoscopists not using it (Fruhmorgen and Demling, 1979; Fruhmorgen, 1981).

Testing for bleeding disorders prior to colonoscopic polypectomy is not necessary as a routine. A history of bleeding disorders should be enquired about from the patient, including a tendency to bleed excessively from lacerations, after surgical procedures, or after tooth extraction. Laboratory testing is necessary when a positive answer to these questions is obtained. Aspirin should be avoided for 1 week before the endoscopic examination, since the antiplatelet properties may promote bleeding. Patients on anticoagulants may be safely colonoscoped, but polypectomy should not be performed because of the risk of bleeding. If polyps are discovered in an anticoagulated patient, hospitalization is required with heparin substitution until prothrombin levels have normalized, and heparin itself discontinued two hours before polypectomy. If good haemostasis is achieved at polypectomy, heparin may be re-started 4 hours later, and oral anticoagulation that night. The patient should remain on heparin in the hospital until prothrombin times return to therapeutic levels.

32.3 THE SNARE

Colon polyps are removed with either a wire snare-cautery device or with a specially insulated biopsy forceps providing electrocautery desiccation of the polyp base while a biopsy is simultaneously obtained (Cohen and Waye, 1986). This latter procedure is called a 'hot biopsy forceps' technique, and is useful for removal of polyps less than 8 mm in diameter (approximately 40% of all polyps). Larger polyps are removed by encircling the lesion with a wire loop, and applying electrocautery current to prevent bleeding as the snare is closed around the polyp. Most electrosurgical cautery units are not precisely calibrated as to their energy output, and a specific dial-control setting on one may not provide the same power output as on a similar unit even by the same manufacturer. The endoscopist must therefore become familiar with each unit available in the endoscopy suite. In most instances the power output, once set in the optimal range, need not be re-adjusted when switching between a hot biopsy forceps or a snare for polypectomy, nor for the size of the lesion encountered. Some endoscopists use a blended current of both coagulation and cutting, but the most experienced endoscopists rely on coagulation current solely during polypectomy as guillotine pressure of the wire snare severs the polyp stalk (Fruhmorgen, 1981). Any polyp can be severed with either cutting or coagulation current, or a blend of the two, but transecting a polyp too rapidly, with cutting current, for instance, may result in subsequent bleeding from the polypectomy site because of inadequate haemostasis. Since polyp transection is achieved by guillotine pressure as the wire snare is withdrawn into its plastic sheath, it is important that the wire snare retracts deeply enough into the sheath to permit transection. If the wire does not retract at least 1.5 cm into the plastic catheter *ex vivo*, then adequate guillotine transection may not be achieved during polypectomy, as the plastic sheath may 'accordian pleat' and shorten as the snare handle is closed (Waye and Bishop, 1984). Before the procedure begins the endoscopy assistant should test carefully that the snare conforms to these requirements. This pleating results in a shorter sheath, so that the snare wire, which appeared to retract properly inside the tip of the plastic catheter *ex vivo*, may protrude from the compressed catheter during polypectomy, even when the slide bar has been completely closed. The snare wire may then become stuck

around the polyp without transection, resulting in an incarcerated snare. If a wire does become incarcerated, switching to pure cutting current may result in transection; if it does not, the polyp may be severed by forcefully pulling on the sheath, shearing the wire through the polyp as the tissue is impacted onto the 'scope tip. Too much electrical current may result in perforation. An alternative to using more current or excessive force is to attempt removal of the snare wire and let the partially electrocoagulated polyp slough spontaneously. This may be difficult because the wire tends to become trapped in the desiccated polyp matrix if closure and electrocautery have been attempted.

32.4 TYPES OF POLYP

Approximately 40% of colon polyps are classified as 'diminutive', being less than 6 mm in diameter. It is frequently impossible for the endoscopist visually to estimate whether a diminutive colon polyp is hyperplastic, an excrescence of normal mucosa, or an adenoma. In the rectum and distal sigmoid colon, the majority of diminutive colon polyps are non-neoplastic, but throughout the remainder of the colon approximately 60–70% of small polyps are true adenomas, and therefore should be removed (Waye and Lewis, 1988). These small polyps should be removed by the hot biopsy forceps when seen on instrument introduction, since they may be missed during 'scope withdrawal. Pedunculated polyps are the easiest to remove, providing that the head of the polyp can be completely encircled within the snare loop. Pedicle length may vary up to several centimetres and transection should be directed to midstem or closer to the head than the colon wall. Sessile polyps may have various configurations. The majority are 'marble-type' adenomas, with a small attachment to the colon wall, and a base smaller than the widest diameter of the polyp (Cohen and Waye, 1986). These are relatively easy to transect and can almost always be removed by a single snare application. Other sessile polyps have the appearance of a 'mountain', where the base is the widest part of the polyp, with a diameter from 5 mm to 5 cm. Sometimes the base of a 'mountain-type' polyp may be clearly defined and the line of endoscopic polypectomy easily identified, but the removal may be difficult when the junction between the polyp base and the colon wall is diffuse and poorly delineated. Occasionally a polyp is seen wrapped around an interhaustral fold, extending on both sides like a 'clam-shell'. These may be difficult to remove, and the upper portion may be hidden from view. A flat sessile polyp may resemble a 'carpet' without much elevation, making these the most difficult polyps to remove because of the lack of a defined mass of tissue to grasp within the snare. Frequently, a combination of polyp types is encountered, some portions having the appearance of a 'mountain', with a surrounding 'carpet-like' configuration; the larger portions that protrude from the wall are easily ensnared, but the surrounding flat adenoma may be difficult to remove.

32.5 TECHNIQUE OF POLYPECTOMY (Waye, Geenen and Fleischer, 1987)

Removal of colon polyps is not painful. Patients are unaware that polypectomy is occurring, or that electrocoagulation current is being used. Other than the standard medications pethidine (meperidine) and diazepam (Diazemuls) or midazolam used for colonoscopy, no specific drugs need be administered when polypectomy is performed during colonoscopy. There is no role for antispasmodics. The colon contracts irregularly and infrequently, only rarely interfering with polypectomy. It is wise to have a solution of epinephrine (diluted 1:10 – final dilution 1:10,000) to spray on or inject into the polypectomy site should post-transection bleeding occur.

The hot biopsy forceps is the easiest tool used for removal of colon polyps, not only providing tissue sufficient for histology, but simultaneously ablating diminutive polyps by desiccation. Removal of diminutive polyps by multiple biopsy forceps application rarely results in total removal of the lesion since small fragments of viable adenoma may remain. The method for polypectomy of diminutive polyps with the hot biopsy forceps (Williams, 1973) is to grasp the polyp head and lift the closed forceps away from the wall by angling the tip of the colonoscope which results in 'tenting' the wall. An electrocautery current is applied, producing a surrounding zone of blanched thermal damage on the tented normal mucosa surrounding the polyp base. As the visible thermal injury enlarges to approximately 1–2 mm around the polyp base electrocautery current is stopped. Withdrawal of the biopsy forceps provides the specimen. Because the electrical pathway tends to flow around the tissue within the cups of the forceps, an adequate sample for histopathological investigation is almost always obtained.

It may be as quick and easy to remove diminutive polyps with a wire snare. Two main snare types are available: the 'standard' size loop which is 1.0 cm wide and 2.0 cm in length and the 'mini' snare, approximately 0.5 cm × 1.0 cm in length. The small snare is easy to manipulate around the head of a diminutive polyp. Occasionally the entire diminutive polyp may be desiccated during current application, resulting in no retrievable specimen. In order to avoid guillotining small polyps during snare closure before current application, it is useful for the endoscopic assistant to mark the snare handle at the point where withdrawal of the slide-bar coincides with snare loop retraction into the plastic snare catheter sheath (Waye and Bishop, 1984). Marking this point before polypectomy will allow the endoscopic assistant to close the snare rapidly to that point but stop before 'cold' transection of the small polyp. Although the large snare may be used for removal of diminutive polyps, it may be cumbersome since the loop does not open widely until a long segment of wire snare has passed outside the polyethylene sheath. Diminutive polyps on the edge of an interhaustral septum are more easily approached with the snare than hot biopsy forceps, since the wire loop can be positioned to encircle the polyp, whereas attempts at closure of biopsy forceps will result in an action similar to 'bobbing for apples', the small polyp bouncing out of the way when the forceps are closed.

Pedunculated polyps are usually easy to remove, providing that the head of the polyp can be completely encircled by the snare. Most commercial snares are large enough to encircle the largest pedunculated polyp by insinuating the loop over the polyp head using a combination of torque and control-wheel movement. It is important to maintain full direct vision of both snare and polyp as the capture and transection are occurring. Spatial relationships for successful polypectomy are optimal when the polyp is in the right lower portion of the visual field, since the snare enters the field at the 5 o'clock position from the biopsy channel of most colonoscopes.

The single most important factor in polypectomy is to advance the polyethylene catheter to the precise site on the pedicle where transection is desired (Cohen and Waye, 1986). Closure of the loop will result in seating the wire snare on the other side of the stalk opposite the polyethylene catheter. This principle holds even if the wire snare cannot be manipulated to surround a pedunculated polyp completely. If a pedunculated polyp is lying flat on the bowel wall, with the stalk in the foreground and the head remote, the opened snare may be placed over the head of the polyp, and the polyethylene catheter advanced to the desired closure site on the pedicle. With the catheter tip in this position, retraction of the slide-bar on the handle usually results in the wire's tip dragging along the colon wall, sliding under the polyp and retracting to the polyethylene sheath on the wall opposite the catheter tip. Pedunculated polyps with a head too large to encircle may be shaved down to ensnareable size by piecemeal resection as described in the section on sessile polyps (see below).

When removing pedunculated polyps, the endoscopist should seek a visible blanching of the stalk at the site of the wire loop when current is applied. If this is not observed, then a burn of approximately 10–15 seconds may be given prior to snare loop closure. Once whitening is seen, slow and steady snare closure should be performed until transection occurs. There is no need for 'on-and-off' current application during polypectomy by repeatedly depressing the foot switch, since that merely results in intermittent heating and cooling cycles, an inefficient method of polypectomy. This cycling of current during polypectomy has no scientific basis. Nor is it necessary to start current application with the electrosurgical unit at a low dial setting and increase it sequentially during polypectomy. One setting should be chosen and used for the entire polypectomy. The practice of sequential current increase may result in inadequate tissue heating for haemostasis during low current and, when high current is used, blood vessels may be disrupted with the explosive force of tissue vaporization. Utilization of a proper setting will permit heat to seal the coapted blood vessels within the polyp base ensnared by the wire loop. Tissue will be severed by both mechanical and thermal forces using guillotine pressure and cellular disruption by the heated wire which provides haemostasis.

Sessile polyps may be removed by a variety of techniques, and transection of the 'problem polyp' is best left to the more experienced endoscopist (Waye, 1987). The 'marble' type can be easily ensnared and the base usually transected with a single cautery current application. The 'mountain' type may require piecemeal resection, with one edge of the snare placed along a margin of the base, and the opposite wire positioned over a portion of the protruding portion. Snare closure will result in capture of a portion of the polyp which may then be transected. Several applications may be required, removing segments until satisfactory polypectomy is achieved. The technique for piecemeal polypectomy is similar to that for pedunculated polyps, with advancement of the polyethylene catheter tip to the point of desired separation prior to snare closure. An alternative technique is to centre the widely open snare over the polyp, and advance the polyethylene catheter as the assistant is closing the loop. This manoeuvre serves to keep the polyp in the centre of the loop during closure and is useful for polyps situated around folds, or where the angulated configuration of the colon does not permit full extension of a loop beyond the polyp. The decision as to whether any given broad-based polyp should be removed piecemeal or with one transection is not necessarily related to its size, but to the diameter of the 'bunched-up' base which forms a false pedicle after tight snare closure around the polyp. If the diameter of the false pedicle is less than 1.5 cm, transection with one application of the wire snare will frequently be successful (Waye, Geenen and Fleischer, 1987). Occasionally, after piecemeal transection of a wide-based sessile polyp, some visible fragments of ragged tissue may remain at the base; these should be left, without further attempt at polypectomy. Repeat examination after 6–12 weeks may show that the polyp has disappeared, heating during initial polypectomy having sloughed the residual tissue. If some viable tissue is present, it can be removed by further snare applications.

The 'clam-shell' polyp is best dealt with by shaving off the portion on the fold nearest the endoscope. The angulation of the endoscope tip, in conjunction with rotational torque, should manoeuvre the tip at right angles to the long axis of the colon to facilitate capture of the polyp on the far wall. If that is not possible, the residual polyp may be captured by placing the open snare over the fold, and

deflecting the endoscope tip onto the fold to flatten it, permitting snare closure under direct vision. In the right colon, further portions may be removed by performing a 'U-turn' manoeuvre in the ascending colon; a similar view can be achieved in the rectum and lower sigmoid using a gastroscope which has a greater tip deflection. Although it is desirable to remove all segments of every polyp, there are occasions when this is not technically feasible, especially in the case of some 'clam-shell' polyps. At reinspection of the site in 8–12 weeks, cicatrization of the base may have everted the proximal portion, providing an excellent position for subsequent removal.

The 'carpet-type' polyp may be approached by using the large snare in an attempt to create a false pedicle to the polyp, but if this cannot be done the surface may be extensively fulgurated with the shank of a hot biopsy forceps by applying electrocautery current while moving the side of the forceps across the polyp's surface. This 'paint-brush' technique can deliver sufficient thermal energy to necrose the adenomatous tissue, and biopsies may be taken as desired.

Laser vapourization of polyps may be possible, but this does not seem to be a suitable alternative in most instances because tissue is not obtained for histopathology.

32.6 POLYP RECOVERY

Histological examination of the resected specimen is necessary for categorization of the lesion. Five per cent of resected colon polyps contain invasive carcinoma, and the accurate histological grade and extent of invasion, and assessment of whether lymphatics or venules are involved needs to be ascertained. Follow-up plans after polypectomy depend on whether the polyp was hyperplastic or an adenoma. Specimens removed and fulgurated with the hot biopsy forceps are all recovered immediately. Because of the current pathway through the tip of the biopsy forceps, only 0.2% of specimens obtained by this method suffer thermal damage and are coagulated beyond histopathological recognition (Waye *et al.*, 1988). Small polyps removed with the wire snare may be rapidly recovered by sucking them through the accessory channel into a specimen trap placed on the suction port of the instrument's umbilical. This recovery technique permits colonoscopy to continue after small polyps have been transected. Larger polyps, over 8 mm in diameter, are best retrieved by re-lassooing the severed polyp head with the wire snare, and removal of the instrument and snare together. Once the transected polyp is ensnared, the snare tip should be extended several centimetres beyond the end of the endoscope during withdrawal to permit visualization of the lumen and colon wall. An alternative method is to suck the transected polyp onto the endoscope tip, and remove them both together. This method results in obliteration of the visual field by the polyp as the instrument is withdrawn, making a repeat colonoscopy up to the polypectomy site necessary for full colon inspection.

It is not acceptable accidentally to lose a transected polyp. All polyps may be located by a methodical search, even though hidden within haustral folds. The water-gravity method will aid in locating almost every 'lost' polyp following transection. A bolus of water is injected through the accessory channel while watching the lumen. If a stream of water is seen falling away from the instrument tip, the scope must be advanced with attention directed towards the site of water accumulation. If water injection results in a blurring of vision, this indicates a flow over the lens, and back along the shaft of the instrument. The blurred image means that the tip is pointed upward, and indicates that withdrawal of the colonoscope is necessary to locate the polyp submerged in the first pool of fluid. The endoscopist may choose to leave some resected polyps, or portions of a resected polyp, in the colon without total recovery, but this option should be chosen infrequently, only when

intubation has been difficult, or when several polyps of varying size have been removed. After resection of multiple polyps from the right colon, especially with a tortuous and fixed left colon, the smaller, obviously benign lesions may be left, but the largest or most irregular polyps should be ensnared and removed. If a large polyp is removed in piecemeal fashion, the portion nearest the base should be identified and removed. During most piecemeal polypectomies, several small fragments are usually present together with larger portions. Most of the small fragments may be sucked into a trap, and then the largest, most irregular, or basal portion can be snared and removed. It may be possible to ensnare several large portions of a resected polyp within a standard snare loop. Wire baskets are of little benefit for polyp retrieval

32.7 COMPLICATIONS OF POLYPECTOMY

The widespread use of colonoscopic polypectomy is related to the safety of the procedure and the low incidence of complications when compared to laparotomy and surgical polypectomy. The incidence of complications has been investigated, with perforation (the most serious problem) occurring in 0.1% (Macrae, Tan and Williams, 1983; Gilbert *et al.*, 1984). Perforation at the polypectomy site is usually related to entrapment of the puckered serosal surface caught within the wire loop as electrocautery current is being applied. This occurs when a deep portion of the wall is caught within the snare. Even if the serosal surface is not directly trapped by the snare, electrical current may be transmitted from the wire snare through the submucosa of a sessile polyp to the serosal surface resulting in full-thickness coagulation and subsequent necrosis of the wall. Lesser degrees of thermal bowel wall injury may result in a full thickness burn without perforation (Waye, 1981); the patient may develop symptoms of localized peritonitis with abdominal pain, rebound tenderness, fever, leucocytosis, and abdominal distension. If free air is not present on the X-ray, the patient should be treated conservatively since most of these 'colon electrocoagulation syndromes' will subside spontaneously without progressing to free perforation.

Bleeding occurs more frequently than perforation and is seen in 2% of polypectomies. Bleeding from a transected pedicle is treated by resnaring the pedicle and applying pressure for successive 5-minute intervals until haemostasis occurs. There should be no further attempt to retransect the pedicle since it may become too short, preventing the possibility of resnaring if bleeding persists. Haemostasis may be achieved by injecting adrenaline (epinephrine) or absolute alcohol into the base of a bleeding sessile polyp, or by impacting a catheter passed through the accessory channel onto the bleeding site and slowly infusing epinephrine.

The hot biopsy forceps may cause either perforation or bleeding (Wadas and Sanowski, 1988). The risk of perforation may be minimized by tenting the entrapped polyp into the lumen and away from the serosal surface, stretching the loose areolar tissue and increasing the distance through which current must pass to reach the serosal surface. Under no circumstances should current activation occur when the forcep's tip is pushed toward the mucosal surface, resulting in apposition of the mucosal and serosal surfaces.

32.8 POSTPOLYPECTOMY CARE

After polypectomy patients should avoid aspirin for at least 1 week to diminish the possibility of bleeding. If a single polyp is cleanly transected, the patient may return to normal activities immediately, but after removal of a large sessile polyp with a piecemeal technique the patient should continue on a liquid diet for the next 24 hours, in case a deep burn of the colon wall has occurred. The majority of patients undergoing colonoscopic polypectomy can return to normal activity the day after polypectomy.

Most patients have polyps successfully removed as outpatients, and it is rarely necessary for them to be admitted, unless they have difficulty with ambulation, are extremely elderly, require preparation in the hospital, have a bleeding diathesis, or will require multiple doses of intravenous antibiotics. If no complications of the procedure are evident at the time of polypectomy, and the patient feels well, having recovered from the effects of medication, the patient may return to their home within a short period in the company of a companion.

32.9 FOLLOW-UP AFTER POLYPECTOMY

A polyp grows slowly, and it takes several years to progress to a 1.0-cm lesion, at which size the incidence of invasive carcinoma may be approximately 1% (Waye and Braunfeld, 1982). So once a single benign adenoma has been removed from a patient with no other risk factors the next follow-up examination may be scheduled in 3 years, providing that the entire colon was well seen. A shorter follow-up period is indicated when the patient has a strong family history of colon polyps or carcinoma, has multiple polyps, or if there was any question that the endoscopist did not perform a full investigation of the large bowel (Holtzmann *et al.*, 1987, Kronberg and Fenger, 1987, Nava *et al.*, 1987). Following piecemeal resection of a benign large sessile adenoma, examination of the site may take place between 3 and 6 months, realizing that residual portions of the adenoma are likely to require resection. If multiple colon polyps have been removed the patient should be seen in 1 year for follow-up examination since there is a strong possibility of there being either metachronous growths or missed synchronous polyps.

REFERENCES

American Society for Gastrointestinal Endoscopy (1980) *The Role of Colonoscopy in the Management of Patients with Colonic Polyps* (ASGE Guidelines for Clinical Applications), ASGE,

Cohen, L. B. and Waye, J. D. (1986) Treatment of colonic polyps – practical considerations. *Clin. Gastroenterol.*, **15**, 359–76.

Fenoglio, C. M. and Lane, M. (1974) The anatomical precursor of colorectal carcinoma. *Cancer*, 34, 819–23.

Fox, J., Andrews, M., Guthrie, M. *et al.* (1981) Significance of the small polyp detected on proctoscopy: a preliminary report. *Gastrointest. Endosc.*, **27**, 140.

Fruhmorgen, P. (1981) Therapeutic colonoscopy, in *Colonoscopy* (eds R. H. Hunt and J. D. Waye), Chapman and Hall, London.

Fruhmorgen, P. and Demling, L. (1979) Complications of diagnostic and therapeutic colonoscopy in the Federal Republic of Germany (results of an inquiry). *Endoscopy*, **11**, 146–50.

Fruhmorgen, P., Laudage, G. and Matek, W. (1981) Ten years of colonoscopy. *Endoscopy*, **13**, 162–6.

Fung, C. H. K. and Goldman, H. (1970) The incidence and significance of villous change in adenomatous polyps. *Am. J. Clin. Pathol.*, **53**, 21–5.

Gilbert, D. A., Hallstrom, J. P., Shaneyfelt, S. L. *et al.* (1984) The national ASGE colonoscopy survey – complications of colonoscopy. *Gastrointest. Endosc.*, **30** (abstr.), 156.

Gillespie, P. E., Chambers, T. J., Chan, K. W. *et al.* (1979) Colonic adenomas – a colonoscopic survey. *Gut*, **20**, 240–5.

Holtzmann, R., Poulard, J. B., Bank, S. *et al.* (1987) Repeat colonoscopy after endoscopic polypectomy. *Dis. Colon Rectum*, **30**, 1815–88.

Konishi, F. and Morson, B. C. (1982) Pathology of colorectal adenomas: a colonoscopic survey. *J. Clin. Pathol.*, **35**, 830–41.

Kronborg, O. and Fenger, C. (1987) Prognostic evaluation of planned follow-up in patients with colorectal adenomas. *Int. J. Colorect. Dis.*, **2**, 203–7.

Kurzon, R. M., Ortega, R. and Rywlin, A. M. (1974) The significance of papillary features in polyps of the large intestine. *Am. J. Clin. Pathol.*, **62**, 447–53.

Livestone, E. M., Troncale, F. J. and Sheahan, D. G. (1977) Value of a single forcep biopsy of colonic polyps. *Gastroenterology*, **73**, 1296–8.

Macrae, F. A., Tan, K. G. and Williams, C. B. (1983) Towards safer colonoscopy: a report on the complications of 5000 diagnostic or therapeutic colonoscopies. *Gut*, **24**, 376–83.

Morson, B. C. (1976) Genesis of colorectal cancer. *Clin. Gastroenterol.*, 505–25, **5**.

Muto, T., Bussey, H. J. B. and Morson, B. C. (1975) The evolution of cancer of the colon and rectum. *Cancer*, **36**, 2251–70.

Nagy, G. S. (1981) Preparing the patient, in *Colonoscopy* (eds R. H. Hunt and J. D. Waye), Chapman and Hall, London.

Nava, H., Carlsson, G., Petrelli, N. J. *et al.* (1987) Follow-up colonoscopy in patients with colorectal adenomatous polyps. *Dis. Colon Rectum*, **30**, 465–8.

Shinya, H. and Wolff, W. I. (1979) Morphology, anatomic distribution, and cancer potential of colonic polyps. *Ann. Surg.*, **190**, 679–83.

Spjut, H. J. and Estrada, R. G. (1977) The significance of epithelial polyps of the large bowel. *Pathol. Annu.*, (Part I), 147–68.

Wadas, D. D. and Sanowski, R. A. (1988) Complications of the hot biosy forceps technique. *Gastrointest. Endosc.*, **34**, 3237.

Waye, J. D. (1981) The postpolypectomy coagulation syndrome. *Gastrointest. Endosc.*, **27**, 184.

Waye, J. D. (1987) Techniques of polypectomy: hot biopsy forceps and snare polypectomy. *Am. J. Gastroenterol.*, **82**, 615–8.

Waye, J. D. and Bishop, D. (1984) Endoscopic polypectomy snares: a comparative clinical evaluation. *Endosc. Rev.*, **1**, 6–12.

Waye, J. D. and Braunfeld, S. (1982) Surveillance intervals after colonoscopic polypectomy. *Endoscopy*, **14**, 79–81.

Waye, J. D., Geenen, J. and Fleischer, D. (Co-Eds) (1987) *Techniques in Therapeutic Endoscopy*. W. B. Saunders Co and Gower Medical Publishing. Philadelphia and New York.

Waye, J. D., Lewis, B. S., Frankel, A., Geller, S. A. (1988) Small colon polyps. *Amer. J. Gastroenterol.*, **83**, 120–2.

Williams, C. B. (1973) Diathermy-biopsy – a technique for the endoscopic management of small polyps. *Endoscopy*, **5**, 215.

Williams, C. B., Macrae, F. A. and Bartram, C. I. (1982) A prospective study of diagnostic methods in adenoma follow-up. *Endoscopy*, **14**, 74–8.

Index

Page numbers in *italic* refer to illustrations; those in **bold** to tables